Communication

CORE INTERPERSONAL SKILLS FOR HEALTHCARE PROFESSIONALS

5th edition

Communication

CORE INTERPERSONAL SKILLS FOR HEALTHCARE PROFESSIONALS

5th edition

Gjyn O'Toole

DipTEFL, DipOccThy, BA, MEdStud
Senior Lecturer Occupational Therapy (retired)
The University of Newcastle, Newcastle, New South Wales, Australia

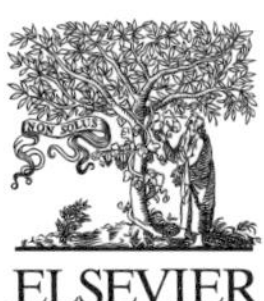

ELSEVIER

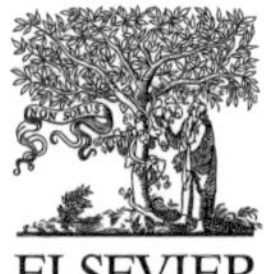

Elsevier Australia. ACN 001 002 357
(a division of Reed International Books Australia Pty Ltd)
475 Victoria Avenue, Chatswood, NSW 2067

Publisher's note: *Elsevier* takes a neutral position with respect to territorial disputes or jurisdictional claims in its published content, including in maps and institutional affiliations.

ISBN: 978-0-7295-4469-6

Notice

This publication has been carefully reviewed and checked to ensure that the content is as accurate and current as possible at time of publication. We would recommend, however, that the reader verify any procedures, treatments, drug dosages or legal content described in this book. Neither the author, the contributors, nor the publisher assume any liability for injury and/or damage to persons or property arising from any error in or omission from this publication.

National Library of Australia Cataloguing-in-Publication Data

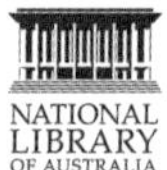

A catalogue record for this book is available from the National Library of Australia

Content Strategist: Melinda McEvoy
Content Project Manager: Fariha Nadeem
Edited by Margaret Trudgeon
Proofread by Sarah Newton-John
Copyrights Coordinator: Rupa Rai
Cover Designer: Gopalakrishnan Venkatraman
Index by Innodata
Typeset by GW Tech
Printed in China by 1010 Printing International Ltd

Last digit is the print number: 9 8 7 6 5 4 3 2 1

Contents

Section 3 Managing realities of communication as a healthcare professional 183

How to use this book

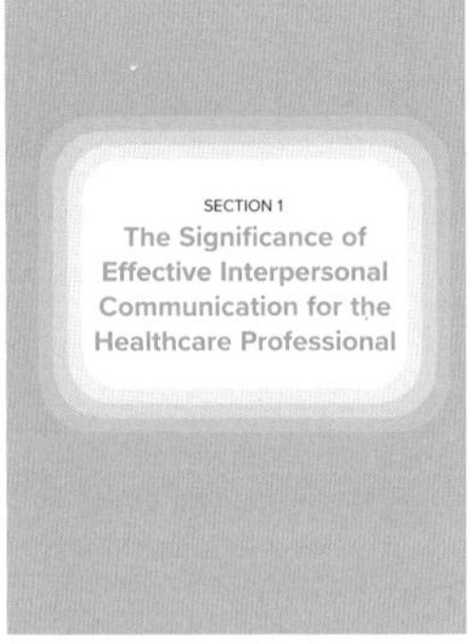	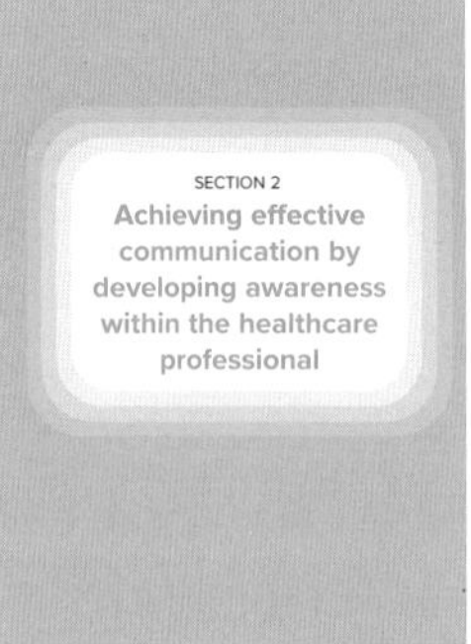	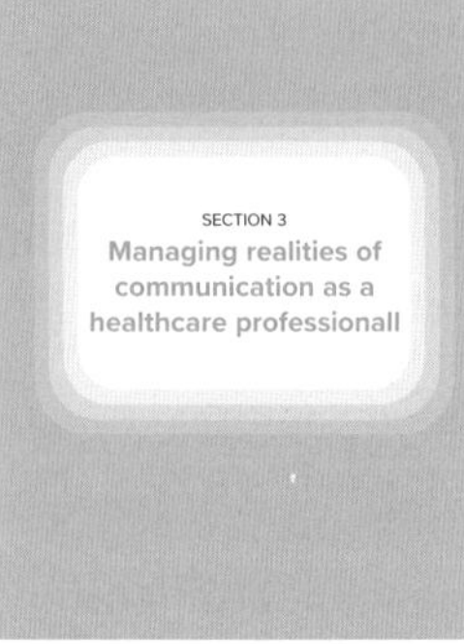	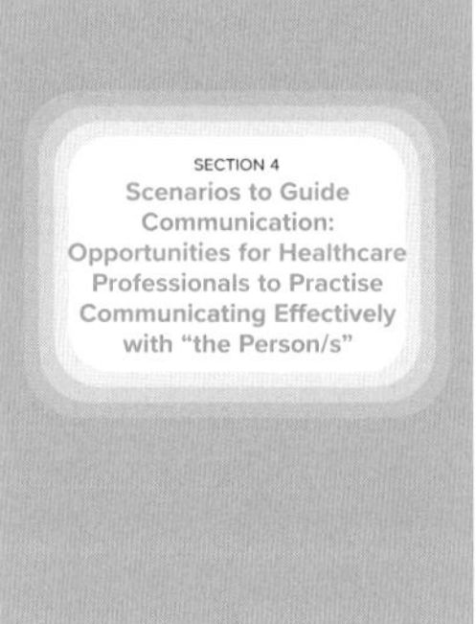
Section 1 explores the importance of studying communication when preparing to be an effective healthcare professional. It presents overall and specific goals typical of communication in healthcare.	**Section 2** highlights the importance of reflection and the resultant awareness of self and underlying personal biases and assumptions; of the individuals around the healthcare professional; of non-verbal elements of interactions; of the importance of listening and awareness of various environments affecting healthcare.	**Section 3** emphasises the realities of specific aspects of communication relevant to practice for the healthcare professional. These realities include holistic care, multidisciplinary teams, conflict; cultural variations; misunderstandings; ethical issues; communicating over distances; written documentation and electronic forms of communication, including social networking sites.	**Section 4** has 66 scenarios to encourage in-depth exploration of needs typical of encounters in healthcare. It provides opportunities using role-plays to both consider and practise communicating with such individuals. Potentially this will develop both confidence and competence when communicating as a healthcare professional.

Each section includes opportunities to explore elements of communication as individuals, in groups and from the perspective of a particular scenario. Various types of activities encourage reflection to promote deeper understanding of the requirements of communication. They also encourage increased awareness of personal tendencies during communicative events and skills development in preparation for communicating as a healthcare professional.

The following icons indicate the type of activity:

Group work or activity for a group

Individual activity or opportunity for individual reflection

Scenario or case study

Reviewers

Kay Fielden BSc(Hons), GradDipSocEcology, MSc, PhD
Lecturer, New Zealand School of Acupuncture and Traditional Chinese Medicine (Auckland)
Auckland, New Zealand

Narinder Verma, BSc(OccTher)(Hons), GradDip(TertEd), MProfPrac, NZROT, FHEA
Principal Lecturer/Fieldwork Team Lead, School of Occupational Therapy, Otago Polytechnic, Dunedin, New Zealand

Preface

Development of skills in communication is an ongoing journey for each person. It requires awareness of the needs of the "Person/s", awareness of personal biases and prejudice, awareness of the power of non-verbal aspects of communication, awareness of the effects of environments and background, as well as reflection about communicative practice. Even the best communicators have times when they experience unsatisfactory communication, regretting the effects of an interaction. The journey for a healthcare professional in developing communication skills is often eventful and sometimes difficult. However, commitment to perseverance in overcoming the barriers to effective communication is a beneficial and rewarding process for any individual, but essential for any healthcare professional.

This book contains four sections focusing on particular elements of communication. Section 1 examines the significance and goals of communication in the health professions. Section 2 highlights the importance of reflection and increased awareness of various factors when communicating as a healthcare professional. It indicates this awareness must be of "self", as well as the "Person" and the environment. Section 3 emphasises specific contexts, characteristics of and skills required for effective communication in the health professions.

Section 4 presents 66 scenarios, representing typical situations and people that a healthcare professional might encounter during their working week. This section challenges readers through role-plays to consider in-depth the circumstances and needs of the Person/s in the scenarios. Section 4 encourages readers to understand and validate the information found in the first three sections of the book, thus promoting application of the information learnt and consolidation of the skills developed in these sections.

All sections include presentation of information and opportunity for reflection, practice and discussion. They provide opportunities to communicate with both "self" and "others" in an attempt to promote awareness of the major factors contributing to effective communication.

Acknowledgements

I especially thank and acknowledge five people: Mitch, a wonderful model of a communicator in many forms; Esther, author, trainer, communicator and editor extraordinaire; Jasen, an interested and invaluable communicator, designer and trainer; ever-developing Zeke, who communicates in several languages with honesty, love and empathy; and Eden Joan, who continually communicates with acceptance and confidence. Your encouragement, understanding, acceptance and support empower and enable me, despite the challenges.

Thanks to the talented cartoonist Roger Harvey, who has used his talent to expertly capture particular points from each chapter.

Thanks to the people who assisted with the compilation of Section 4. These include all the many Person/s I have had the privilege to assist in practice and Esther Brooks (exceptional teacher), Matt Peters (talented healthcare professional) and Nell Harrison (creative and reliable healthcare professional) – all phenomenal people. To say thanks is not enough.

I also have students, colleagues, friends and other family members to thank for their commitment to both challenging and encouraging me in my journey towards becoming an effective communicator.

I am, however, most in debt and thankful to the Creator and Sustainer of the Universe, Yahweh.

SECTION 1

The significance of effective interpersonal communication for the healthcare professional

CHAPTER 1

Effective communication for healthcare professionals:
A model to guide communication

Chapter objectives

Upon completing this chapter, readers should be able to:

- explain the importance of effective communication for healthcare professionals
- describe a model of interpersonal communication relevant to healthcare professionals
- define effective communication
- demonstrate understanding of the importance of effective communication
- identify factors contributing to effective communication
- demonstrate understanding of the importance of considering relevant aspects of the "audience" to achieve effective communication.

Why learn how to communicate? Everyone can communicate!

Communication occurs constantly throughout the world. Indeed, most individuals from a young age participate daily in acts of communication regardless of their nationality, age, personality or interests. Communicative interactions are unavoidable and usually essential for satisfactory daily life, with even those unable to produce speech striving to effectively communicate. Well then, if everyone communicates so effectively in daily life, why is it necessary to learn how to communicate specifically in healthcare settings?

Ineffective communication in healthcare settings may not only result in complaints (Coad et al 2018; Hill 2015); adverse events (Shahid & Thomas 2018); delayed diagnosis (Rood & Elkin 2014); negative health outcomes (Vanderhooft 2021); it can also cause fatalities (Rucker & Windemuth 2019). Ineffective communication also has legal implications. These implications may affect the perceived competence of the **healthcare professional**. It can therefore affect the reputation of the particular healthcare professional. Interestingly, employers consider skills in **effective**

communication (spoken, non-verbal and written) to be the most important attribute when considering prospective employees (Graduate Careers Australia 2016). Effective communication is also connected to change (Lucas et al 2021). These realities indicate the relevance of exploring effective communication in healthcare.

In reality, when providing healthcare, many situations challenge the communication skills of communicating individuals. Effective communication in a healthcare setting is complex, requiring particular understanding of oneself and others (Moss 2020; Tamparo & Lindh 2017), along with developed skills in face-to-face and non-face-to-face communication. Individuals do not typically acquire such understanding or skill in everyday life. Thus, it is beneficial if preparing to be a successful healthcare professional, to learn how to achieve effective communication in healthcare settings (Henderson 2019).

Effective communication is an essential core skill for any healthcare professional, producing positive outcomes for all. It optimises development of the therapeutic relationship and provision of effective healthcare (Boggs 2023; Conroy et al 2017; Gilligan et al 2018). In contrast, ineffective communication produces **emotions** and thoughts potentially able to negatively affect **health** outcomes (Hill 2011a, 2011b; Rosen 2014). Certainly, evidence suggests the positive impact of effective communication when experiencing a health condition. These include increased recovery rates and decreased incidence of complications or further conditions (co-morbidities), along with increased motivation and satisfactory outcomes (Camerini & Schulz 2015; Henderson 2019; Pennebaker & Evans 2014; Rosen 2014; Stein-Parbury 2021). Generally, effective communication reduces the cost of healthcare (Duman 2015; Rosen 2014), ensuring positive outcomes (Prasad et al 2013; Vanderhooft 2021), thereby increasing satisfaction for all people relating to healthcare professionals (Chung et al 2018; Hall et al 2014; Hassan et al 2007; Koponen et al 2010; Levett-Jones et al 2020; Levinson et al 2010; Rosen 2014; Vanderhooft 2021). Therefore, with skills in effective communication being vital for positive outcomes in healthcare, it is crucial to understand both communication and the components of effective communication.

NOTE: In this book the word "**Person/s**" typically means those individuals and their families/carers and/or communities seeking the services of a healthcare professional. On some occasions it may refer to those individuals or colleagues working within or related to a healthcare service.

A guiding principle

Before defining communication, it is important to establish an underlying principle to guide communication for healthcare professionals. Critical **self-awareness** and self-knowledge (see Chapters 6–8) are necessary requirements for successful adherence to this principle. This guiding principle simply states:

Do not say or do anything to another person that you would not want said or done to you.

Adapted from Hillel around 15BC

Consistent consideration of and adherence to this principle is not always easy. However, consideration of the "audience" (the receiver of the message in health – usually the Person receiving care) and their response, generally produces effective communication and satisfying outcomes in both healthcare and life (Duman 2015). Cooper and colleagues (2015) suggest that effective communication should become a required component of guidelines for best practice in quality healthcare improvement recommendations. However, Lucas and colleagues (2021) highlight their obvious omission from quality improvement guidelines in healthcare. This indicates the need to consider effective communication as an essential component of effective healthcare.

Factors to consider when defining effective communication

Increasingly in the world today communication is one-way or linear. Text messages, emails, blogs and **social media** generally require a sender to "send" a message, with no immediate response and only some expectation of a response, and not necessarily from a specific individual (see Chapter 23). However, many dictionaries and communication theorists indicate that communication involves several interacting individuals simultaneously sending and receiving messages during an interaction. This understanding of communication appears to resemble aspects of a game of tennis. In the same way that tennis players hit a ball to each other, communicators send and receive messages in various forms. Initially this analogy seems appropriate; however, tennis players generally focus on the ball and the rules governing the game, typically avoiding personal interactions with each other. In addition, the tennis ball remains constant throughout the process, unlike messages, which tend to change and develop because of responses during interactions. These realities suggest that effective communication involves more than exchanging messages between communicators. Indeed, effective communication typically requires processing and understanding the messages, not merely sending and receiving them. Communication occurs in many forms or channels: auditory, verbal, **visual** and **non-verbal**. It includes vocalising without words (e.g. laughing or crying); non-verbal cues (e.g. **eye contact**, **facial expressions**, **gestures** and signing) and material forms (e.g. pictures, photographs, picture symbols, logos and written words) (Crystal 2008). Thus, it requires consideration of various forms and multiple factors from the perspective of all communicating individuals.

A communication model to guide interactions in healthcare: negotiating mutual understanding

Various communication models identify factors relevant to effective communication. Some models suggest a linear or one-way process (Shannon & Weaver 1949), some a circular process (Schramm 1954), and others a transactional process requiring ongoing processing of messages throughout an interaction, along with a relationship (Berlo 1960). Thus, transactional models require a connection between individuals and message-processing to achieve **mutual understanding**. This involves simultaneously sending and receiving messages, with the messages affecting the responses of every interacting individual. One exception to this is the context of communicating with an unresponsive Person. This limits the possibility of achieving mutual understanding. In these situations, it may be important to seek and supply information from and to a Carer.

Transactional models appear to be most appropriate and applicable to healthcare settings. During transactional interactions, the communicating individuals assign meaning to each message, hopefully the intended meaning of the sender. Each interaction is unique, with unique realities common to each communicating individual, along with particular requirements and constraints. These realities, requirements and constraints may be internal or external to the communicators. Regardless of their origin, these realities influence the effectiveness of the interaction at the time. This indicates the need to explore the effect of these factors upon meaning and responses in order to achieve *mutual understanding* and effective communication (Fig. 1.1).

Mutual understanding requires a shared focus or mutual attention upon the messages during the interaction. Therefore, every communication act requires the active involvement of all communicators to listen to and understand all responses, and to understand the factors affecting those responses (Brill & Levine 2005; Hassan et al 2007; Levine 2012). This facilitates understanding

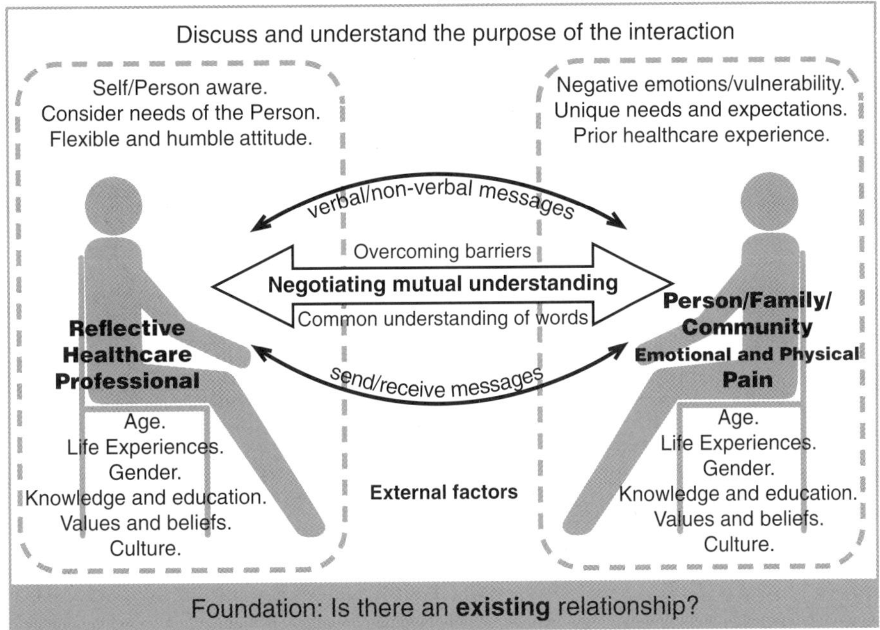

FIGURE 1.1
A model to guide communication in the healthcare professions.
Note: Person/s is used to describe all those relating to the healthcare professional during practice, including other employees and colleagues.

of all verbal and **non-verbal messages** between the sender and receiver. This resultant understanding enables individuals to overcome any **barriers** to effective communication; to be able to consider reactions (including feedback) and to provide appropriate responses. This encourages successful interactions and achievement of mutual understanding, thereby encouraging those communicating to trust their ability to effectively communicate (Stein-Parbury 2021). This strengthens the interaction, encouraging the sender and receiver to continue communicating. Therefore, understanding the internal and external realities, requirements and constraints relevant to each Person/s empowers communicators to achieve effective communication in healthcare.

The **model** presented here (Fig 1.1) acknowledges the effects of various internal and external factors upon the interacting individuals. It highlights the importance of achieving mutual understanding, despite barriers and consideration of the various factors affecting the outcome of every interaction (Table 1.1). Despite many of these factors being obvious, they are often overlooked or assumed, and thus require consideration/exploration.

Possible factors impacting effective communication

Possible factors common to both the sender and receiver

The realities common to each individual communicating may require accommodation to achieve shared understanding. Firstly, it is essential that all communicators understand the *purpose of the interaction*. Failure to understand the reason for the interaction may produce inappropriate

TABLE 1.1
Possible factors affecting communicating individuals

Factors common to all communicators	Possible internal factors	Possible external factors
Understanding the purpose of the interaction	Positive and negative emotions	Context: including surroundings, noise, temperature, light, phone
Age and thus abilities	Knowledge, education and understanding	Background and life experiences
Gender	Particular disorders and pain	Pre-existing relationship
Personality	Language, words and meaning	Privacy and confidentiality
Value, beliefs and culture	Ability – hearing and cognition	Time pressures

expectations of the interaction and inaccurate **assumptions** about meaning, thereby producing **misunderstandings** (see Chapter 18). Such misunderstandings can produce negative and undesired results. This highlights the need to achieve a common understanding about the purpose of each unique interaction. Other realities relevant to each communicator are *age* (this affects their level of understanding, possible education and thus knowledge), gender and personality. These can affect the type of communication and relevance of particular information. For example, when communicating with a young child, they may not understand particular words or be able to fulfil particular expectations, such as completing particular required documentation. Therefore, when interacting with a young child it is appropriate to adjust the communication style by avoiding the use of complex words or sentences. This adjustment of communication style facilitates mutual understanding for both the child and the healthcare professional. However, using the same simplistic language when interacting with an adolescent or adult may cause offence. The age of the Person/s seeking assistance may affect their range of life experiences and thus level of knowledge and understanding of the healthcare process, while the age of the healthcare professional may also affect their experience with life and the healthcare process.

Gender can also affect the focus and content of an interaction. For example, communicating with an adolescent female about personal hygiene requires particular details, not all of which would be appropriate for a male of the same age. A female Person seeking assistance may find it difficult to have a male healthcare professional assisting her, for example, with showering or other personal requirements. Age and gender will therefore require consideration when communicating and/or completing the healthcare process with particular age and gender groups.

Particular *personality* types, often with differing styles of communication, typically process information differently. Understanding and accommodating these differences will promote a shared understanding of all relevant information. Along with personality, every individual has particular **values** and **beliefs**, whether they are receiving or providing care. The healthcare professional typically values the healthcare process, being aware of their **role**, while valuing and believing in the importance of their role within the process. The Person/s may not share this awareness or belief. Their particular values and beliefs about health and maintaining health may not relate to those of the healthcare professional. For example, they may use particular **interventions** not typical of healthcare services, including acupuncture or particular elixirs. Some values and beliefs may or may not relate to their cultural **background**. Variations of **culture** within families and **social** groups can create particular values and beliefs and their unique interpretation and/or application of these values and beliefs within the healthcare process. For example, some cultures expect to provide meals for any family member when they are an inpatient; some expect to use traditional medicines for particular conditions. The particular values, beliefs and cultural backgrounds impact expectations of healthcare and thus all communication events within the healthcare process.

Possible factors internal to the Person/s, whether sender or receiver

The possible internal factors of the Person/s seeking healthcare assistance may vary depending on the individual. Many of these Person/s are experiencing sometimes quite overwhelming *negative emotions* (Riding et al 2017). The feelings of vulnerability, not always limited to the Person/s (Gulbrandsen 2018; Plotkin & Shocet 2018), because of the unknown and the associated fear of the unknown, can be debilitating, reducing the ability to process information and to effectively communicate.

- Suggest the possible emotions you might experience if requiring healthcare intervention.
- How might each group member express these emotions if they were the "Person/s"?
- How might you "manage" or respond to these emotions if you were the healthcare professional?

Previous experience with healthcare services can have either a negative or positive effect on Person/s. Negative experiences can increase the incidence of negative emotions when requiring healthcare. These experiences typically relate to ineffective communication (Hill 2015), producing negative expectations and negative emotions. Such emotions may vary depending on previous experiences and the knowledge of the interacting individuals.

Every individual has particular *knowledge* and associated levels of *understanding* affecting their ability to comprehend particular messages (Honeycutt & Milliken 2021). Thus, when practising as a healthcare professional, it is important to acknowledge and explore, where appropriate, the level of understanding and/or knowledge of the audience, whether relating to the Person/s, a family member or a colleague, for example, about a particular health profession or procedure. This may change the content and type of messages for all future interactions with these individuals.

A particular *disorder or condition* affecting an individual may also influence the success of the interaction. In some circumstances it may be essential to communicate only one idea or step at a time. For example, individuals experiencing extreme **pain** or who have limited cognitive ability or reduced affect may require adjustments in the communication style of the healthcare professional and in their manner of constructing and delivering messages.

The *language background* of the audience requires consideration to achieve mutual understanding (Fageeh 2011). Language background may also require an adjustment in the style of communicating (Liu et al 2023; see Chapters 9 and 16, and Section 4), along with possibly the need to simplify word choice.

The *ability* of each communicator may also affect understanding. When communicating with someone who has limited *hearing* ability, the use of verbal messages may be ineffective. There are many other methods of communicating that enable the effective sending and receiving of messages, regardless of hearing ability (see Chapters 10 and 11). As mentioned above, *cognitive* ability may also affect understanding of messages. In such cases, simple, one-point messages and/or visual methods of communication may facilitate understanding. Regardless of the cause of the variation in ability, the healthcare professional will need to adjust the methods of communicating to achieve mutual understanding.

A common understanding of words

Mutual understanding is essential for effective communication. Effective communication requires two or more people to focus on and discuss a topic of mutual interest; to have a mutual desire, intent or need to communicate about the topic, along with the opportunity to communicate and the means of communicating. It requires a shared understanding of the **context**, the words and non-verbal messages. Thus, if there is no common understanding of the spoken word, non-verbal cue or way of communicating, there will be no mutual understanding and thus no exchange of information, or effective communication (Nunan 2013). This potentially limits health outcomes and thus resultant satisfaction for all.

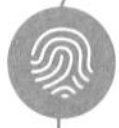

Consider the difference in meaning of the words below. Suggest how the different meanings might affect communication.

- State the different meanings of the following words: file, stand, form, compress, bracing, crutch and "a simple case".
- What factors might change the meaning an individual assigns to a word or combination of words?
- How can you ensure you and your audience achieve/share a common understanding?

Share and discuss your ideas with the large group.

Communication is **ineffective** without mutual understanding. Therefore, the sending and receiving of a message achieves nothing unless there is shared meaning and thus meaningful exchange of information. The specific purpose of communication for healthcare professionals is to share information and fulfil needs (see Chapters 3, 4 and 5). Mutual understanding requires the healthcare professional to explore and understand the experiences and perspectives of the other Person/s and their needs (Stein-Parbury 2021). This reflects Person-centred communication, thereby demonstrating a Person-centred approach (Australian Commission on Safety and Quality in Health Care [ACSQHC] 2011; Finney Rutten et al 2015). It also facilitates development of relevant and appropriate interventions and responses, thereby fulfilling identified needs. If words and non-verbal messages fail to establish mutual understanding, there is no appropriate information to guide an intervention, potentially limiting satisfactory fulfilment of needs. For example, if there is no connection (Hassan et al 2007; Horan et al 2011) and exchange of information with mutual understanding when needing a toilet or something in which to vomit, the results can be messy and indeed time-consuming.

An additional factor requiring consideration is whether or not to use *professional* **jargon**. The decision of how and when to use professional jargon requires the healthcare professional to understand and consider the experience and background of the Person/s (Haddad et al 2019). The use of healthcare professional terminology may be appropriate if the Person/s has a healthcare background and understanding of the particular healthcare profession. It may also be appropriate if they have previous experience with such terminology, but may cause confusion if they have no knowledge, understanding or experience of such terminology. When communicating with healthcare colleagues about related professional topics, use of non-professional terminology may cause confusion! When communicating as a healthcare professional, in order to avoid confusion it is important to consider and sometimes request information about the knowledge and experience of the audience. It is certainly beneficial to ensure understanding of all relevant terms and expectations.

Effective communication in healthcare requires a connection between the sender and receiver of messages, initially for the common purpose of exchanging information and achieving mutual understanding. It requires healthcare professionals to negotiate, continue discussion and validate understanding of needs and expectations during interactions until achieving mutual understanding, thereby ensuring appropriate interventions and satisfactory, meaningful outcomes.

Possible factors external to the sender and receiver

The words in the activity above (file, stand, etc) have meanings that might vary within the *context* (Nunan 2013). Thus, if asked for a "file" (e.g. *Pass that file please*) when there is no obvious folder with pieces of paper inside, the receiver of the request might search for other meanings of the word. Seeing a nailfile, they might assume that is the required file. In this case, the receiver of the message assumes the meaning because of the surroundings. Other contextual conditions potentially affecting effective communication include *noise* levels in the **environment**; *temperature,* whether too hot or too cold; *light* – sometimes too dark or too bright – and possible interruptions from *phones*. These aspects of context require consideration and adjustment in order to achieve mutual understanding, along with focused and effective communication.

There are other external factors affecting the meaning an individual might assign to a word. Someone who comes from a particular *background* (Haddad et al 2019) or who has had particular life *experiences* might assign a particular meaning to one word. For example, a carpenter would have a particular understanding of the word "file". Someone with a scientific or nursing background might assume the word "stand" means a structure used to hold or support something, while someone with a political background might assume it means to run for election. Someone with a military background might assume it means to resist an onslaught without retreating, while someone with another background or experience might believe it means to assume an upright position on both legs. In this case, it is the background and experience of the communicating individuals that affect the understanding of the particular word. The background or experience might be particular to a family, socioeconomic group or culture. All of these factors and more can vary the meaning of messages. It is important when communicating in healthcare professions, therefore, to consider relevant factors influencing the achievement of mutual understanding, effective communication and thus positive health outcomes.

A positive, pre-existing *relationship* or previous positive interactions between the sender and receiver will typically contribute to relaxed interactions and the achievement of mutual understanding when communicating. In contrast, previous negative interactions may require both communicators to overcome and hopefully replace the negative emotions with positive ones to achieve mutual understanding and effective communication. *Privacy* while interacting may contribute to positive experiences when communicating during the healthcare process. Privacy and assurances of **confidentiality** typically reassure service users, contributing to both their ability to understand and to follow any instructions (see Chapter 19).

A major external factor affecting many individuals around the world is *time pressure*. Both senders and receivers of messages often experience pressure relating to time. Increasing expectations upon both healthcare professionals and Person/s can create a focus on the next event, other needs or requirements. This has the potential to reduce the achievement of mutual understanding, with assumptions of meaning and receiver understanding being a reality when communicating.

All the identified factors in this model of communication have an impact on the effectiveness of communication. Therefore, when providing healthcare, it is important to consider and accommodate them to achieve mutual understanding, effective communication and both relevant and satisfying health outcomes.

Factors specific to the sender

Senders of messages often express their messages according to their own opinions, agenda, previous experience, needs or emotions at a given time. For example, senders often communicate their intended meaning using **emphasis** or stress on a particular word, rather than through the actual words (Crystal 2008).

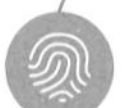

Consider:

- "I *do* think it *is* time those supplies were in the store" means: someone needs to put the supplies in the store now! And might mean: Can you do it now?
- "Have *you* seen that XXXXX?" means: I have asked everyone else – do you know? Or it could mean: You had it last, you must have it, or at least know where it is!
- It is often the emphasis on particular words that changes the intended meaning of a sentence.

Compare:

- *I want* a drink of water.
- I want a drink of *water*.

The emphasis changes the meaning of each statement. The first is a statement of a desire to have a drink of water and could mean: "you all have your drinks, and now I want mine!" The second indicates that the desired drink is water and nothing else. In each case, the emphasis indicates the particular desire of the individual sending the message. If the receiver fails to note the emphasis in the last sentence, for example, the sender of the message may not receive the desired drink.

Factors specific to the receivers or "audience"

In every communicative event someone receives a message or particular information. The *audience* is the person or group of people receiving the message or information. In healthcare professions, many people constitute the audience, including colleagues, Person/s, family members and Carers.

There are many factors influencing the effectiveness of communication and some of these factors are specific to the receiver/audience. When communicating as a healthcare professional, the potential impact of these audience factors upon communication mandates their consideration.

- List the possible people with whom a healthcare professional might communicate.
- For each person or group of people, list factors specific to that person or group that might affect their ability to understand a sent message.
- Choose a scenario from Section 4 that interests group members. Consider all the information about relating to both the male and female Person/s in that scenario. List possible factors specific to that scenario which could potentially affect communication.

It is not only the age, background and experiences of the receiver/audience that affect their levels of understanding. Receivers of messages often interpret them according to their own *opinions*, experience, *ideas, needs, current condition* (e.g. pain, discomfort, aphasia) and/or *emotions* at that given time. This may assist or adversely affect their understanding of the messages (see Chapters 7 and 8, and Section 4). Effective communication between a healthcare professional and the Person/s should be an exchange of facts, ideas, needs and emotions contributing to a therapeutic outcome (Paré & Lysack 2004; Seikkula & Trimble 2005). A healthcare professional considering and appropriately accommodating and/or adjusting to the opinions, perspectives, experiences, ideas, needs and emotions of the receiver, will usually promote mutual understanding, thereby achieving effective communication and satisfactory health outcomes.

Mr Mack is an elderly, obese man who lives at home. He is experiencing increasing difficulty showering himself. The healthcare professional assessing Mr Mack has known him for several years. This healthcare professional arranges for the installation of a grab rail in the shower and delivery of a standard shower chair with armrests to assist Mr Mack to shower safely. Mr Mack appears thankful. However, despite being grateful, when he tries to use the shower chair he discovers he is too large to sit in it comfortably and it does not fit well in the shower space. A year later, he falls while showering, fracturing his right hip. The healthcare professional wonders how this could happen if Mr Mack was using his shower chair.

- Suggest possible internal factors within Mr Mack that could affect the failure to achieve effective communication and feedback between Mr Mack and the healthcare professional.
- How might the healthcare professional accommodate these internal factors?
- Suggest possible internal and external factors affecting the healthcare professional potentially contributing to the ineffective communication relating to showering for Mr Mack.
- Suggest how to manage the internal factors affecting the healthcare professional in this and other possible scenarios.
- Suggest how to manage the external factors affecting the healthcare professional in this and other possible scenarios.
- Suggest how to manage all these factors affecting both Mr Mack and the healthcare professional to achieve mutual understanding.

Chapter summary

Effective communication occurs when people send, receive, process and successfully understand messages. Such communication produces mutual understanding, an essential requirement of communication in healthcare. There are both external and internal factors influencing mutual

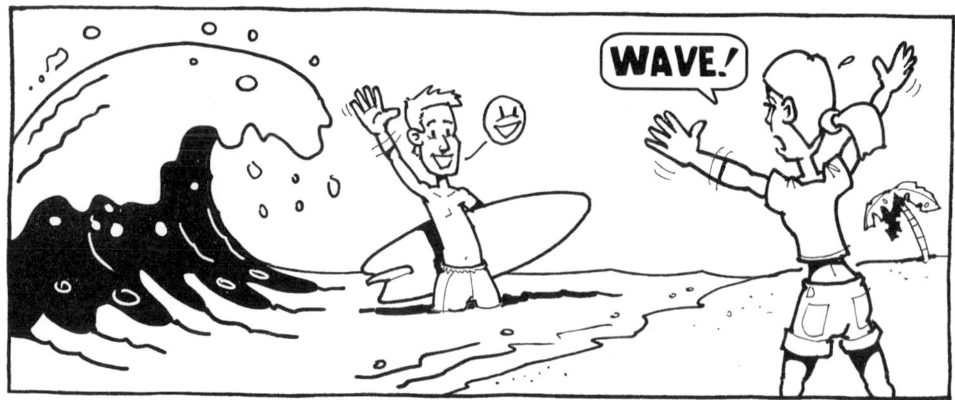

FIGURE 1.2
Mutual understanding is essential!
Courtesy Roger Harvey © Elsevier Australia.

understanding during information exchange. These factors may either facilitate or impede communication. The model presented in Fig. 1.1 acknowledges the effect of internal and external factors upon the interacting individuals. It highlights the importance of mutual understanding and consideration of the various factors impacting the outcome of all interactions. These factors occur in the environment (external) and in the sender and receiver (internal). A sound understanding and consideration of these factors contributes to effective communication and positive, satisfying health outcomes.

References

Australian Commission on Safety and Quality in Health Care (ACSQHC), 2011. Patient-centred care: Improving quality and safety by focusing care on patients and consumers. ACSQHC, Sydney.

Berlo, D., 1960. The process of communication: An introduction to theory and practice. Holt, Rinehart and Winston, New York.

Boggs, K., 2023. Interpersonal relationships: Professional communication skills for nurses, 9th ed. Elsevier, St Louis, MO.

Brill, N.I., Levine, J., 2005. Working with people: The helping process, 8th ed. Pearson, Boston.

Camerini, A.-L., Schulz, P.J., 2015. Health literacy and patient empowerment: Separating conjoined twins in the context of chronic low back pain. PLoS ONE, 10(2), e0118032.

Chung, H.C., Hsieh, T.C., Chen, Y.C., et al, 2018. Cross-cultural adaptation and validation of the Chinese Comfort, Afford, Respect, and Expect scale of caring nurse–patient interaction competence. Journal of Clinical Nursing, 27(17–18), 3287–3297.

Coad, J., Smith, J., Pontin, D., et al, 2018. Consult, negotiate, and involve evaluation of an advanced communication skills program for health care professionals. Journal of Pediatric Oncology Nursing, 35(4), 296–307.

Conroy, T., Feo, R., Boucaut, R., et al, 2017. Role of effective nurse–patient relationships in enhancing patient safety. Nursing Standard, 31(49), 53.

Cooper, A., Gray, J., Willson, A., et al, 2015. Exploring the role of communications in quality improvement: a case study of the 1000 lives campaign in NHS Wales. Journal of Communication in Healthcare, 8(1), 76–84.

Crystal, D., 2008. How language works. Penguin Books, London.

Duman, M., 2015. Better measures needed on the impact of health communication. Journal of Communication in Healthcare, 8(1), 3–4.

Fageeh, A.A., 2011. At crossroads of EFL learning and culture. Cross-cultural Communication, 7(1), 62–72.

Finney Rutten, L.J., Agunwamba, A.A., Greene, S.M., et al, 2015. Enabling patient-centred communication and care through health information technology. Journal of Communication in Healthcare, 7(4), 255–261.

Gilligan, T., Coyle, N., Frankel, R. M., et al., 2018. Patient–clinician communication: American Society of Clinical Oncology consensus guideline. Obstetrical and Gynecological Survey, 73(2), 96–97.

Graduate Careers Australia, 2016. Graduate Outlook 2016: A snapshot. Graduate Careers Australia, Melbourne.

Gulbrandsen, P., 2018. The possible impact of vulnerability on clinical communication: some reflections and a call for empirical studies. Patient Education and Counseling, 101(11), 1990–1994.

Haddad, A.M., Doherty, R.F., Purtilo, R.B., 2019. Health professional and patient interaction, 9th ed. Elsevier/Saunders, St Louis, MO.

Hall, J.A., Gulbrandsen, P., Dahl, F.A., 2014. Communication study: Physician gender, physician patient-centered behavior, and patient satisfaction: A study in three practice settings within a hospital. Patient Education and Counseling, 95(3), 313–318.

Hassan, I., McCabe, R., Priebe, S., 2007. Professional–patient communication in the treatment of mental illness: A review. Communication and Medicine, 4(2), 141–152.

Henderson, A., 2019. Communication for health care practice. Oxford University Press, Melbourne.

Hill, A., 2015. Delayed diagnosis of cancer in primary care: What do our complaints tell us? New Zealand Health and Disability Commission, April. Online. Available at: www.hdc.org.nz/.

Hill, A., 2011a. Consumer-centred care: seamless service needed. New Zealand Health & Disability Commission, August. Online. Available at: www.hdc.org.nz/.

Hill, A., 2011b. Recurring themes. Society of Anaesthetists Newsletter, Feb.

Honeycutt, A., Milliken, M.A., 2021. Understanding human behavior: A guide for health care providers, 10th ed. Cengage Learning, Boston, MA.

Horan, S.M., Houser, M.L., Goodboy, A.K., et al, 2011. Students' early impressions of instructors: understanding the role of relational skills and messages. Communication Research Reports, 28(1), 74–85.

Koponen, J., Pyööräälää, E., Isotalus, P., 2010. Teaching interpersonal communication competence to medical students through theatre in education. Communication Teacher, 24(4), 211–214.

Levett-Jones, T., 2020. The relationship between communication and patient safety. In: Levett-Jones, T. (ed.), Critical conversations for patient safety, 2nd ed. Pearson, Sydney, 2–13.

Levine, J., 2012. Working with people: The helping process, 9th ed. Pearson, San Antonio.

Levinson, W., Lesser, C.S., Epstein, R.M., 2010. Developing physician communication skills for Patient-Centered Care. Health Affairs, 29(7), 1310–1318.

Liu, S., Volcic, Z., Gallois, C., 2023. Introducing intercultural communication: Global cultures and contexts, 4th ed. Sage, London.

Lucas, B., Cooper, A., Wilson, A., 2021. The undervalued role of communication in healthcare improvement and its critical contribution to engaging staff and saving lives. Journal of Communication in Healthcare, 14(1), 5–7.

Moss, B., 2020. Communication skills in health and social care, 5th ed. Sage, London.

Nunan, D., 2013. What is this thing called language? 2nd ed. Palgrave Macmillan, Basingstoke.

Paré, D., Lysack, M., 2004. The willow and the oak: From monologue to dialogue in the scaffolding of therapeutic conversations. Journal of Systemic Therapies, 23, 6–20.

Pennebaker, J.W., Evans, J.F., 2014. Expressive writing: Words that heal. Idyll Arbor, Enumclaw.

Plotkin, J.B., Shocet, R., 2018. Beyond words: What can help first year medical students practice effective empathic communication? Patient Education and Counseling, 101(11), 2005–2010.

Prasad, V., Vandroos, A., Toomey, C., et al, 2013. A decade of reversal: An analysis of 146 contradicted medical practices. Mayo Clinic Proceedings, 88, 790–798.

Riding, S., Glendening, N., Heaslip, V, 2017. Real world challenges in delivering person-centred care: a community-based case study. British Journal of Community Nursing, 22(8), 391–396.

Rood, G., Elkin, K., 2014. Aged care – Right intervention, right time. New Zealand Health and Disability Commission, March. Online. Available at: www.hdc.org.nz/.

Rosen, D., 2014. Vital conversations: Improving communication between doctors and patients. Columbia University Press, New York.

Rucker, A., Windemuth, B., 2019. Utilising team strategies and tools to enhance performance and patient safety (TeamSTEPPS) to improve effective communication in long-term care settings. Journal of Post-Acute and Long-term Care Medicine, 20(3), PB 26.

Schramm, W., 1954. The process and effects of mass communication. University of Illinois, Urbana, IL.

Seikkula, J., Trimble, D., 2005. Healing elements of therapeutic conversations: dialogue as an embodiment of love. Family Process, 44, 461–473.

Shahid, S., Thomas, S., 2018. Situation, Background, assessment, recommendation (SBAR) communication tool for handoff in health care – A narrative review. Safety in Health, 4, 7.

Shannon, C., Weaver, W., 1949. The mathematical theory of communication. University of Illinois Press, Urbana, IL.

Stein-Parbury, J., 2021. Patient and person: Interpersonal skills in nursing, 7th ed. Churchill Livingstone Elsevier, Sydney.

Tamparo, C.D. & Lindh, W.Q., 2017. Therapeutic communication for healthcare professionals, 4th ed. Cengage Learning, Boston, MA.

Vanderhooft, J.E., 2021. Ineffective communication: The uninformed injured worker. Journal of Bone and Joint Surgery, 103(19), 1772–1776.

CHAPTER 2

The overarching goal of communication for healthcare professionals:
Person-centred Care

Chapter objectives

Upon completing this chapter, readers should be able to:

- demonstrate understanding of the relevance of the World Health Organization (WHO) International Classification of Functioning, Disability and Health (ICF) model for communication with a Person/s in healthcare
- demonstrate understanding of the overarching purpose of communication for the healthcare professional
- reflect upon and discuss the importance of each step required to fulfil the purpose of communication in healthcare: Person/Family-centred Care
- demonstrate every component of each step of the model of Person/Family-centred Care in healthcare practice.

The purpose of communication in healthcare is ultimately to facilitate the delivery of an appropriate, satisfactory and relevant service. This, therefore, requires healthcare professionals to achieve mutual understanding by communicating to facilitate positive, safe and satisfying service delivery for all (Horan et al 2011; Kuipers et al 2019; O'Kane 2020; Rosen 2014; Rucker & Windemuth 2019; Vanderhooft 2021). Such Person-centred Care and resultant service delivery also requires collaboration with the relevant Person/s (den Boer 2017; van der Meer et al 2018) through Person-centred communication (O'Kane 2020). This chapter explores the means of achieving this goal of Person-centred Care, to ensure optimal outcomes and thus satisfaction, along with the health and wellbeing for all Person/s relating within (remember this includes colleagues) and to healthcare services. Achieving this goal is founded on effective communication.

An international World Health Organization classification demonstrating the importance of effective communication

The International Classification of Functioning, Disability and Health (ICF) (World Health Organization [WHO] 2001), shown in Fig. 2.1, is a biopsychosocial classification highlighting the complex and multidimensional nature of health, and the factors affecting health and functioning (Allan et al 2006). It provides a common language for multidisciplinary or interprofessional communication in healthcare. The ICF classifies the "components of health", placing health on a continuum indicating that any limitation in functioning can disrupt health and wellbeing.

In addition, the ICF describes the importance of **participation** in six interrelated domains or life situations (Ewert et al 2004; Weigl et al 2004) relevant to all healthcare professions:

1. Communication
2. Movement
3. Learning and applying knowledge
4. Participation in general tasks and the demands of those tasks
5. Self-care and interpersonal interactions
6. Major life areas associated with work, school and family life.

The ICF classification encourages healthcare professionals to consider the factors affecting **function**, participation and a sense of wellbeing. It directs healthcare professionals to collaborate *with the Person* to overcome the challenges limiting participation in daily life. Why? Because participation positively affects health and wellbeing of both the Person/s and the healthcare professional (Jackson et al 2021; Kuipers et al, 2019; Mackenzie et al 2021; Sheppard & Broughton 2020; van der Meer 2018). The ICF directs healthcare professionals to develop holistic goals, not driven merely by assessment results, opinion or **physical** needs, but rather Person-centred and thus unique to the needs and goals of the unique individual (Trad 2013).

The ICF model indicates the importance of the domain of communication for facilitating participation and functioning in relevant activities and thereby significantly affecting health. It demonstrates that ineffective communication potentially limits intervention outcomes, thereby

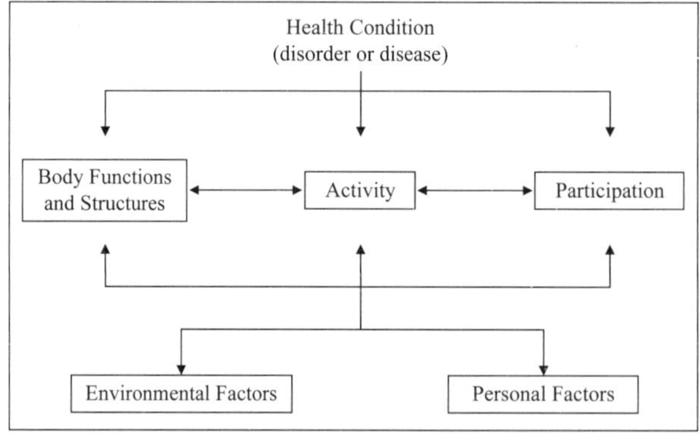

FIGURE 2.1
International Classification of Functioning, Disability and Health (ICF).
WHO 2001. Towards a common language for functioning, disability and health: ICF. The International Classification of Functioning, Disability and Health. WHO, Geneva, p. 9.

restricting functioning and disrupting health and wellbeing. It reminds healthcare professionals to acknowledge the importance of communication and a focus on the Person/s, for their satisfaction, health and a sense of wellbeing. It therefore encourages the healthcare professional to interact with each unique individual to encourage engagement in the act of communicating about their healthcare needs (Australian Commission on Safety and Quality in Health Care [ACSQHC] 2018; Klammer & Pöchhacker 2021; Larkins 2007; van der Meer et al 2018).

Official expectations for effective communication and Person-centred Care

It is not only the WHO that requires effective communication (ACSQHC 2018). Registration requirements for most healthcare professions in Australia and New Zealand include skills in effective communication. See the Australian Health Practitioner Regulation Agency (AHPRA) home page and consult the registration requirements for relevant healthcare professions. The *New Zealand Health Practitioners Competence Assurance Act 2003* (New Zealand Legislation 2003) consistently refers to the need for healthcare practitioners/professionals to communicate effectively in practice. Rights for healthcare consumers also repeatedly refer to the requirement for effective communication. Therefore, it is not merely the outcomes of effective communication, but also relevant peak organisations and legislations that mandate effective communication in healthcare.

A model to guide the overall purpose of communication for healthcare professions

Healthcare professions exist to provide specific services to individuals seeking their assistance. Regardless of the particular profession, communication is an essential requirement within their service. Mutual understanding between the individual seeking the service and the healthcare professional should be a characteristic of any meaningful interaction. It is vital to ensure positive outcomes. Mutual understanding (successful exchange, discussion and understanding of information) provides the foundation for the development of a therapeutic relationship between the individual and the healthcare professional. Developing this therapeutic relationship is the responsibility of the healthcare professional (Schwank et al 2018), therefore depending on demonstrations of respect and empathy (Kristensen et al 2022), and being worthy of trust, developing rapport and consistently listening effectively while collaborating to produce change. This therapeutic relationship should therefore ensure collaboration and the centrality of the individual or group needs and desires (van der Meer et al 2018) when formulating goals and interventions, thereby facilitating Person-centred, patient-centred, client-centred, Family-centred or community-centred Care (ACSQHC 2018; Broady 2014; Doherty & Thompson 2014; Haddad et al 2019; Harms 2015; Hebblethwaite 2013; Hoffman & Tooth 2017; Kuipers et al 2019; Mojta et al 2014; Parker & Sutherland, 2021; Rosen 2014; Stein-Parbury 2021; Trad 2013; WHO 2007) (see Fig 2.2).

The concept of **Person/Family-centred Care** as an underlying philosophy of healthcare (ACSQHC 2018; Liang et al 2023; WHO 2007) is globally the focus of discussion and publication in some healthcare professions. In other healthcare professions it is an assumed underlying philosophy rarely requiring discussion but guiding practice. Whereas in other professions it is neither an assumption nor a topic of discussion.

Please note, although inclusion of the family in goal setting and interventions may occur in various contexts of practice, the use of the word *family* applies particularly in practice involving children (Carvill & McLoughlin 2018). It is essential when working with children, but may

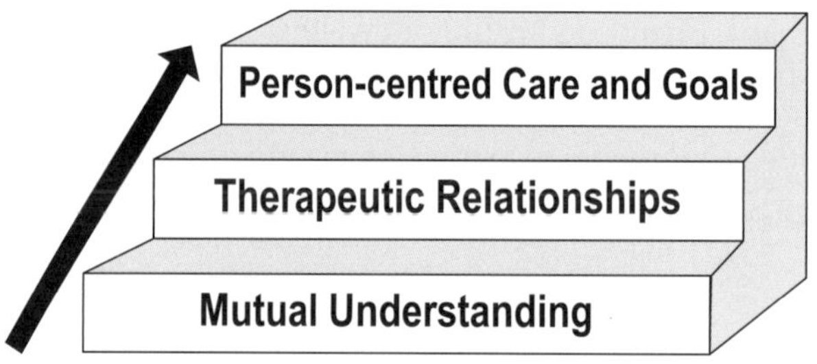

FIGURE 2.2
A model to guide Person/Family-centred Care.

significantly contribute to positive treatment outcomes in other practice contexts, depending on the desires of the Person and the dynamics of the family.

Person/Family-centred Care is a global expectation in health policy as a foundational requirement for healthcare (Grealish et al 2019). Therefore, always considering the unique needs of each healthcare consumer is respectful (Stoilkova-Hartman et al 2018). It requires a partnership between the healthcare professional and the Person/s seeking their services. This **collaborative partnership** exists to establish the needs and goals of the Person/s (Beesley et al 2017). It requires the healthcare professional to embed within the relationship relevant knowledge and skills, while allowing the Person to inform future interventions because of their unique needs and desires (Santana et al 2018; Stein-Parbury 2021). It enables the Person to achieve their goals with the assistance of the healthcare professional (Duncan 2021). Achievement of these goals **empowers** the individual to achieve positive outcomes, including meaningful participation and fulfilment in their daily lives.

Miss Brown, a 78-year-old woman, was admitted to a rehabilitation ward after experiencing a stroke. Initially she was drowsy, but happy and cooperative. After a few days she became distressed, refusing to be involved in any interventions or relate to anyone from the multidisciplinary team.

- How would you respond to Miss Brown?

First response: In response, many healthcare professionals on the team gently repeated that Miss Brown did not need to worry, she was all right now and everything would be OK. Some told her she could relax now, as everyone on the team was there to help her. One healthcare professional sympathetically said it must feel terrible suddenly finding yourself in hospital after a stroke, but that it would be OK in the end, so she should cheer up. She was also kindly told she simply needed to do as she was asked and she would eventually go home. This made Miss Brown sob.

- Are these responses healthcare professional-centred or Person-centred? Explain why.

Second response: One healthcare professional on the team took a different approach, using the components of mutual understanding with Miss Brown. This healthcare professional was able to establish that Miss Brown was very worried about her best friend and constant companion, Billy. Billy was her pet bird who needed daily food and water. This healthcare professional organised to bring Billy to the hospital. Miss Brown began seeing Billy every day and thus began enjoying her treatment and eventually returned home with Billy.

- Is this response healthcare professional-centred or Person-centred? Explain why and then explain the difference between the two responses.
- How do you think this healthcare professional established the cause of the distress for Miss Brown? What did the healthcare professional say or do to identify the cause?

Mutual understanding

Mutual understanding means that those communicating share a common understanding and meaning – all communicating individuals comprehend the verbal and non-verbal signals used during the interaction. In the healthcare professions, mutual understanding must mean more than simply understanding words.

Respect

A foundational factor contributing to mutual understanding, appropriate results and satisfaction in any healthcare profession is **respect** (Egan 2014; Egan & Reese 2019). Respect of self and other people is a fundamental and core value of healthcare professions (Auckland District Health Board 2016). In fact, some state it is an ethical requirement of healthcare (Sokol-Hessner et al 2018). It affects the beliefs that individuals have about themselves and others. It requires unconditional positive regard for self and other people, regardless of appearance, disability, weaknesses or failures, position or **status**, beliefs and values, cultural background, material possessions and/or socioeconomic level (Haddad et al 2019; Rogers 1967). Respect demonstrates that the healthcare professional values every individual (Beach et al 2017; Bridges et al 2021). It is the foundation of demonstrations of empathy or empathic reactions in a healthcare professional.

Empathy

As a healthcare professional, it is imperative to understand that every Person/s seeking care feels disconnected, disempowered and **vulnerable**. Many such individuals often feel unable to understand or manage the demands of their current situation (Butt 2021; Stein-Parbury 2021), possibly experiencing fear of the unknown elements of the situation. Plato, in ancient Greece, said:

> *"The highest form of knowledge is empathy, for it requires us to suspend our egos and live in another's world."*

Any vulnerable individual wants and needs to know that the healthcare professional desires to both appreciate and understand their life experiences and needs in order to provide meaningful assistance (Fitzpatrick et al 2014; Honeycutt & Milliken 2021; James 2023; Rosen 2014; Soto-Rubio & Sinclair 2018). Demonstration of this understanding in care will increase the ability of the Person/s to process any information (Householder & Wong 2011). It will also encourage commitment to and engagement in the intervention process (James, 2023; Rosen 2014). It is the responsibility of the healthcare professional to demonstrate this care and understand the helplessness and vulnerability of each individual. Direct, clear and accurate recognition of the *emotions* of the individual and expression of this understanding is known as **empathy** (Frankel 2017; Slade & Sergent 2022; Stein-Parbury 2021; Trad 2013) (see Chapter 13). This does not mean expressing similar emotions (sympathy), but accurately identifying, validating and accepting the reality of their emotions.

Draw a line down the middle of a page. Place the word "Empathy" at the top of one column and "Sympathy" at the top of the other column. Consider the above scenario about Miss Brown.

- Write responses to Miss Brown in each column that demonstrate both sympathy and empathy.
- Suggest ways in which the healthcare professional expressed empathy to discover the cause of the emotions dominating Miss Brown.

Davis and Musolino (2016) and Morse and Volkman (2010) state that expressing empathy to the vulnerable individual enables both humane and productive communication. There is also evidence indicating its contribution to the development of a positive relationship (James 2023). This manner of communicating therefore has a positive effect (Healey 2018; Tamparo & Lindh 2017) upon the participation of the individual in all activities associated with healthcare interventions (Fig 2.3). It is important to understand that statements like "I understand" or "You are OK" or "It will be alright" do not demonstrate empathy and are rarely reassuring.

- If you are feeling helpless and vulnerable, how do you feel when someone indicates they are interested in what you are feeling and attempts to understand and validate your experiences and feelings?
- What actions and/or words demonstrate that someone is interested?
- How might expressing such interest and care affect communication?

Appropriate expressions of empathy require both personal and professional skill. Such skill necessitates honest reflection about self, practice in expressing empathy, making time to practise, commitment to the expression of empathy and, in many cases, self-control on the part of the healthcare professional (Rosen 2014). It requires awareness of and respect for the feelings of the individual;

PEANUTS
NOW, YOU LISTEN TO ME, YOU STUPID BEAGLE..
THE DOCTOR IS IN
YOU CAME TO ME FOR HELP, AND YOU'RE GOING TO GET IT!
WE'RE GOING TO HAVE A GOOD DOCTOR-PATIENT RELATIONSHIP, OR I'M GOING TO SLUG YOU! DO YOU UNDERSTAND?
THE DOCTOR
IT'S NOT NECESSARY TO SALUTE...
THE DOCTOR IS IN

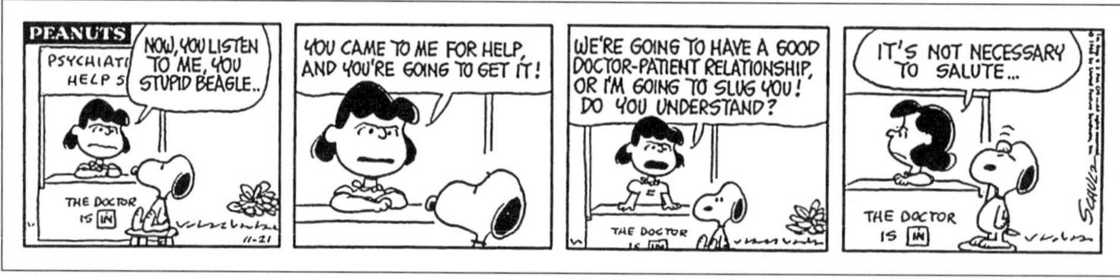

FIGURE 2.3
The doctor is IN.

being able to see and understand the world from their perspective and also respecting that perspective (Eriksen et al 2014). Appropriate expressions of empathy require the healthcare professional to make responsible choices about when, what and how they communicate. The healthcare professional also needs to be aware of and able to control, express and/or resolve their own negative emotions, without allowing them to affect the vulnerable individual (see Chapters 7 and 8). Appropriate expressions of empathy take little time or effort, potentially resulting in the individual believing they are the most important person for the healthcare professional at that moment. While expressions of empathy are beneficial in all areas of life, they are essential when practising as a healthcare professional (Egan 2014; Egan & Reese 2019; Foster & Yaseen 2020; Harms 2015; Honeycutt & Milliken 2021; Stein-Parbury 2021). They encourage the Person/s to have confidence in and trust the healthcare professional (Trad 2013). See Chapter 13 for a deeper exploration of expressing empathy.

Developing trust

Healthcare professionals must consider whether they will validate and acknowledge the experience, emotions and associated needs of the individual and, if so, at which point (Davis & Musolino 2016)? While such choices require skill, healthcare professionals must take every appropriate opportunity to recognise negative emotions by expressing empathy with those around them. Acceptance and validation of the emotions associated with the experience develops **trust**.

In small groups, discuss:

- How do negative emotions affect the ability to send, receive or understand messages?
- Why are positive feelings and reactions essential when communicating as a healthcare professional?
- From the perspective of the Person/s receiving healthcare, list the possible consequences of negative emotions either in the healthcare professional or in the Person/s.

Share these ideas with the entire/large group.

Acceptance and validation through expressions of empathy demonstrates respect. Respect is something all individuals appreciate. In combination with expressions of empathy it produces positive emotions, thereby facilitating the development of trust during an interaction (Bayne et al 2013). Effective communication encourages the development of trust. Trust is strengthened by particular behaviours. The behaviour of a healthcare professional worthy of trust will be open, humble, honest, predictable and reliable (O'Kane 2020). Interacting to engender trust is often an inherent requirement found in the codes of practice for particular healthcare professions (Mason & Morley 2009). Whether mandated or not, it is a characteristic of effective communication relevant to achieving mutual understanding. In combination, *respect, empathy* and *trust* are foundational for achieving the first step of Person/Family-centred Care and goals: *mutual understanding.*

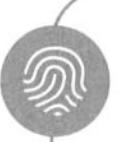

- What behaviours help you trust someone? Make a list of behaviours that indicate someone is trustworthy.
- Are these behaviours that you often demonstrate? Why? Why not?
- List ways of demonstrating them in your chosen healthcare profession.

A therapeutic relationship

Mutual understanding (respect, empathy and trust) facilitates the development of a therapeutic relationship. Therapeutic relationships require a positive connection between the Person/s and the healthcare professional (Eriksen et al 2014). This connection is known as **rapport**. Trust within the relationship facilitates development of rapport, thereby further engendering development of trust. This rapport or genuine connection can increase engagement in interventions (Crowden 2013), facilitate collaboration and motivate individuals to persevere in order to overcome their challenges, thereby potentially producing positive outcomes with the Person/s achieving their health-related goals (English et al 2022).

A therapeutic relationship requires independence not dependence. It demands a focus on the needs of the Person/s, not fulfilment of the needs of the healthcare professional. There may be consideration of strong and deep emotions along with genuine distress within the Person, but this consideration is *always* focused on the needs of the Person not the needs of the healthcare professional (Haddad et al 2019). A therapeutic relationship does not foster manipulation, nor does it desire to manipulate. In a therapeutic relationship the healthcare professional desires to listen effectively, while sharing their knowledge, skill, and, where required, comforting and supporting to facilitate health, function, wellbeing and satisfactory participation in life.

Chinese scholar Lao Tsu (700 BC), when answering the question *What should a therapist do?* (there were no healthcare professionals in 700 BC!) said:

Go to the people → Work with them
Learn from them → Respect them
Start with what they know → Build with what they are
And when the work is done, the task accomplished
The people will say "We have done this ourselves".

An essential component contributing to this therapeutic relationship is **effective listening** (see Chapter 11); listening that demonstrates focus on the needs/desires of the Person with respectful, compassionate consideration and, where possible, accommodation of those needs and desires. This will also contribute to a positive connection with the Person/s. Effective listening is an overarching aim of interpersonal communication in healthcare (Gehenne et al 2020; Golden et al 2020; Thistle & McNaughton 2015). The healthcare professional must invest the time to listen, validating and confirming understanding in every situation.

A therapeutic relationship, based on respect, using active listening, engenders trust and co-operation (Crowden 2013; Gehenne et al 2020), thereby encouraging a *collaborative partnership*. It does not control or dominate. A collaborative partnership is one in which the contribution of each individual (sharing of information) is essential to achieve a satisfactory and appropriate outcome. It facilitates involvement from an individual (the Person), who is intimately aware of his or her own needs, allowing their perspective to inform healthcare interventions. It does not assume the healthcare professional has all the required information to inform the relevant healthcare process. However, it does require contributions from the healthcare professional who has the knowledge, understanding and skill relevant to their profession to assist. It facilitates shared decision-making involving shared discussion of care plans (Golden et al 2020; Santana et al 2018). This *collaboration* provides the opportunity for the individual to be an agent of change in their own circumstances, ultimately enabling them to improve their health and increase their levels of function and participation in everyday life. It encourages the individual or family to face and overcome the relevant challenges (Murphy et al 2015) to achieve their goals.

Rapport, effective listening and *collaboration* are important components of therapeutic relationships, the second step in *Person/Family-centred Care and goals.*

Person/Family-centred Care and goals

The steps above contribute to a focus on the Person/s. They ensure the Person/s is the centre of the therapeutic relationship and intervention process (Ross et al 2015; van de Meer et al 2018). The characteristic of each step mandates that the healthcare professional should not place their own desires or values consciously or unconsciously upon the Person/s. Instead, these steps require investigation of the abilities, understanding, feelings, needs and desires of the Person/s, in order to establish and prioritise their personal goals for participation in their life. Each step has particular characteristics and skills, contributing to the achievement of the third step.

The previous steps will potentially provide the individual with feelings of **control** and thus increase *positive emotional responses*. These will empower an individual to continue to face and overcome sometimes seemingly overwhelming challenges restricting participation and function, thereby affecting their health and wellbeing. These *empowering* feelings will provide the motivation, support and strength to establish and achieve meaningful goals, thereby assisting in maintaining levels of motivation, effort and satisfaction within the Person/s (Riding et al 2017; Rosen, 2014). These communication events contribute to and increase *positive outcomes* (Lawn et al 2014) and satisfaction for both the Person/s and the healthcare professional (van der Meer et al 2018).

While the ultimate purpose of communication in healthcare may be to deliver a service or intervention, implementing this model can create experiences that facilitate function, empowering the Person/s to participate, thereby positively affecting their health and wellbeing. It potentially makes the delivery of any healthcare service a satisfying and positive experience for all (ACSQHC 2018).

Fig. 2.4 summarises the discussion in this chapter about the overall goal of communication for healthcare professionals and a model of Person/Family-centred Care.

Person/Family-centred Care and Goals
Positive Outcomes: satisfaction, health and wellbeing
Empowering: motivated to overcome barriers
Positive Emotions: from feelings of control
Therapeutic Relationships
Collaboration: able to be an agent of change
Effective Listening: focus and compassion
Rapport: positive/genuine connection
Mutual Understanding
Trust: predictable, reliable and worthy of trust
Empathy: validating their perspective
Respect: accepts and values the Person

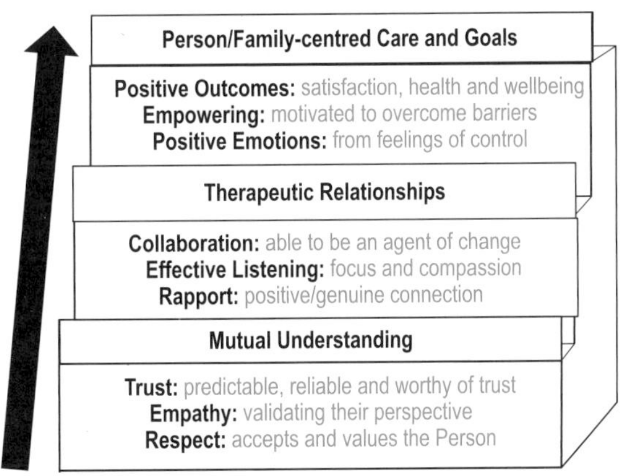

FIGURE 2.4
The components of a model to guide Person/Family-centred Care.

In small groups:

- Choose and read a scenario from Section 4. Discuss how to demonstrate respect, empathy and trust while developing rapport with this Person/s.
- Decide how you might develop rapport, collaboration and empowerment of this Person/s.
- Role-play effective communication in an initial interaction aimed at Person/Family-centred Care and goals with the "Person" from the scenario.
- Discuss the effectiveness of this interaction, considering the components of the model of Person/Family-centred Care.

Chapter summary

Person/Family-centred Care is mandated by governments and registration bodies around the world. When practising as a healthcare professional, Person/Family-centred Care is built upon mutual understanding, requiring respect, expressions of empathy and development of trust. It also requires therapeutic relationships, involving development of rapport, effective listening and collaboration with the Person/s. It has particular definite results, which not only empower, but also produce positive results and emotions. The model presented in this chapter can guide healthcare. If the healthcare professional demonstrates and achieves each step of the model, they can facilitate satisfaction for all involved in healthcare by achieving the overarching goal of communication for healthcare professionals: Person/Family-centred Care.

USEFUL WEBSITES

Communication, Person-centred Care and Person Rights in Healthcare

Australia

Australian Charter of Healthcare Rights: catalogue.nla.gov.au/Record/5249757

Australian Commission on Safety and Quality in Health Care: www.safetyandquality.gov.au

Australian Safety and Quality Framework for Health Care:

www.safetyandquality.gov.au/sites/default/files/migrated/Australian-SandQ-Framework1.pdf

For policy makers:

www.safetyandquality.gov.au/sites/default/files/migrated/ASQFHC-Guide-Policymakers.pdf

10 Tips for Safer Health Care:

www.safetyandquality.gov.au/sites/default/files/migrated/Tips-for-Safer-Health-Care-PDF-302KB.pdf

Top Tips for Safe Health Care:

www.safetyandquality.gov.au/publications-and-resources/resource-library/top-tips-safe-health-care

New Zealand

New Zealand Code of Health and Disability Consumer Rights:

www.hdc.org.nz/your-rights/about-the-code/code-of-health-and-disability-services-consumers-rights/

The Code and your rights: www.hdc.org.nz/your-rights/the-code-and-your-rights/

Impact of communication failure:

www.hdc.org.nz/media/5144/the-impact-of-communication-failures-march-2019.pdf

New Zealand Health Strategy Roadmap of Actions 2016:

www.health.govt.nz/system/files/documents/publications/new-zealand-health-strategy-roadmapofactions-2016-apr16.pdf

References

Allan, C.M., Campbell, W.N., Guptill, C.A., et al., 2006. A conceptual model for interprofessional education: The international classification of functioning, disability and health (ICF). Journal of Interprofessional Care, 20, 235–245.

Auckland District Health Board, 2016. Report on inpatient experience: Dignity and respect. ADHB, Auckland, New Zealand.

Australian Commission on Safety and Quality in Health Care (ACSQHC), 2018. Implementing the comprehensive care standard: Approaches to person-centred screening. ACSQHC, Sydney.

Bayne, H., Neukrug, E., Hays, D., et al., 2013. Communication Study: A comprehensive model for optimizing empathy in person-centered care. Patient Education and Counseling, 93(2), 209–215.

Beach, M.C., Branyon, E., Saha, S. 2017. Diverse patient perspectives on respect in healthcare: A qualitative study. Patient Education and Counseling, 100(11), 2076–2080.

Beesley, P., Watts, M., Harrison, M., 2017. Developing your communication skills in social work. Sage, London.

Bridges, C., Duenas, D.M, Lewis, H., et al., 2021. Patient perspectives on how to demonstrate respect: Implications for clinicians and healthcare organizations. PLoS ONE, 16(4): e0250999.

Broady, T., 2014. What is a person-centred approach? Familiarity and understanding of individualised funding amongst carers in New South Wales. Australian Journal of Social Issues, 49, 285–307.

Butt, M., 2021. Approaches to building rapport with patients. Clinic Med, 21(6), e662–663.

Carvill, A., McLoughlin M., 2018. Child and family centred care: A cultural perspective. In: Holland, K. Cultural awareness in nursing and health care. An introductory text, 3rd ed. Routledge, New York.

Crowden, A., 2013. Ethics and indigenous health care: Cultural competencies, protocols and integrity. In: Hampton, R., Toombs, M. (eds), Indigenous Australians and health: The wombat in the room. Oxford University Press, Melbourne.

Davis, C.M., Musolino, G.M., 2016. Patient practitioner interaction: An experiential manual for developing the art of healthcare, 6th ed. Slack, Thorofare, NJ.

den Boer, J., Nieboer, A.P., Cramm, J.M., 2017. A cross-sectional study investigating patient-centred care, co-creation of care, well-being and job satisfaction among nurses. Journal of Nursing Management, 25, 577–584.

Doherty, M. & Thompson, H. 2014. Enhancing person centred care through the development of a therapeutic relationship. British Journal of Community Nursing, 61, 502–507.

Duncan, E.A.S., 2021. Skills and processes in occupational therapy. In: Duncan, E.A.S. (ed.), Foundations for practice in occupational therapy, 6th ed. Elsevier, Edinburgh.

Egan, G., 2014. The skilled helper: A problem management and opportunity approach to helping, 10th ed. Brooks/Cole, Belmont CA.

Egan, G., Reese R.J., 2019. The skilled helper: A problem management and opportunity approach to helping, 11th ed. Cengage, Boston MA.

English, W., Gott, M., Robinson, J., 2022. The meaning of rapport for patients, families, and healthcare professionals: A scoping review. Patient Education and Counseling, 105(2022), 2–14.

Eriksen, K.A., Arman, M., Davidson, L., et al., 2014. Challenges in relating to mental health professionals: Perspectives of persons with severe mental illness. International Journal of Mental Health Nursing, 23(2), 110–117.

Ewert, T., Fuessl, M., Cieza, A., et al 2004. Identification of the most common patient problems with chronic conditions using the ICF checklist. Journal of Rehabilitation Medicine, 44(Suppl), 22–29.

Fitzpatrick, N., Breen, D.T., Taylor, J., et al., 2014. Parental satisfaction with paediatric care, triage and waiting times. Emergency Medicine Australasia, 26(2), 177–182.

Foster, A.E., Yaseen, Z.S., (eds), 2020. Teaching empathy in healthcare: Building a new core competency. Springer Nature Switzerland AG, Cham, Switzerland.

Frankel, R.M., 2017. The evolution of empathy research: Models, muddles and mechanisms. Patient Education and Counseling, 100(11), 2128–2130.

Gehenne, L., Lelorain, S., Anota. A., et al., 2020. Testing two competitive models of empathic communication in cancer care encounters: A factorial analysis of the CARE measure. European Journal of Cancer Care, 29(6), 13306.

Golden, S.E., Ono, S.S., Thakurta, S.G. et al., 2020. I'm putting my trust in their hands. A qualitative study of patients' views on clinician initial communication about lung cancer screening. Chest, 158(3), 1260–1267.

Grealish, L., Simpson, T., Soltau, D., et al., 2019. Assessing and providing person-centred care of older people with cognitive impairment in acute settings: Threats, variability, and challenges. Collegian, 26(1), 75–79.

Haddad, A.M., Purtilo, R.B., Doherty, R.F., 2019. Health professional and patient interaction, 9th ed. Elsevier/Saunders, St Louis, MO.

Harms, L., 2015. Working with people: Communication skills for reflective practice, 2nd ed. Oxford University Press, Melbourne.

Healey, K., 2018. The skilled communicator in social work: The art and science of communication in practice. Palgrave, London.

Hebblethwaite, S., 2013. "I think it could work but ...": Tensions between the theory and practice of person-centred and relationship centre care. Therapeutic Recreation Journal, 47(1), 13–34.

Hoffman T., Tooth L., 2017. Shared decision making. In: Hoffman, T., Bennett, S., Del Mar, C. (eds). Evidence-based practice across the health professions, 3rd ed. Elsevier, Sydney.

Honeycutt, A., Milliken, M.A., 2021. Understanding human behavior: A guide for healthcare providers, 10th ed. Cengage Learning, Boston, MA.

Horan, S.M., Houser, M.L., Goodboy, A.K., et al., 2011. Students' early impressions of instructors: Understanding the role of relational skills and messages. Communication Research Reports, 28(1), 74–85.

Householder, B.J., Wong, N.C.H., 2011. Mood state or relational closeness: Explaining the impacts of mood on the ability to detect deception in friends and strangers. Communication Quarterly, 59(1), 104–122.

Jackson, S.B., Stevenson, K.T., Larson, L.R., et al., 2021. Outdoor activity participation improves adolescents' mental health and well-being during the COVID-19 pandemic. International Journal of Environmental Research and Public Health, 18, 2506.

James, T.A., 2023. Building empathy into the structure of health care. Trends in Medicine, Harvard Medical School Postgraduate Education. Online. Available at: https://postgraduateeducation.hms.harvard.edu/trends-medicine/building-empathy-structure-health-care.

Klammer, M., Pöchhacker, F., 2021. Video remote interpreting in clinical communication: A multi modal analysis. Patient Education and Counseling, 104, 2867–2876.

Kristensen, T., Ejersted, C., Ahnfeldt-Mollerup., et al., 2022. Profiles of GPs with high and low self-reported physician empathy – personal, professional, and antibiotic prescribing characteristics. BMC Primary Care, (2022) 23, 243.

Kuipers, S.J., Cramm, J.M., Nieboer, A.P., 2019. The importance of patient-centered care and co-creation of care for satisfaction with care and physical and social well-being of patients with multi-morbidity in the primary care setting. BMC Health Services Research, 19(13) Open Access, doi.org/10.1186/s12913-018-3818-y.

Larkins, B., 2007. The application of the ICF in cognitive-communication disorders following traumatic brain injury. Seminars in Speech and Language, 28(4), 334–342.

Lawn, S., Delany, T., Sweet, L., et al 2014. Control in chronic condition self-care management: How it occurs in the health worker-client relationship and implications for client empowerment. Journal of Advanced Nursing, 70(2), 383–394.

Liang, H., Reiss, M.J., Isaacs, T., 2023. Factors affecting physicians' attitudes towards patient-centred care: A cross-sectional survey in Beijing. BMJ Open, 13, e073224.

Mackenzie, L., O'Toole, G. Gustafsson, L., 2021. Core business: Task, activity and occupation analysis. In: Brown, T., Bourke-Taylor, H., Isbel, S., et al. (eds), Occupational therapy Australia, 2nd ed. Routledge, Melbourne.

Mason, R., Morley, M., 2009. Trust: Can occupational therapists take it for granted? British Journal of Occupational Therapy, 72, 466–468.

Mojta, C., Falconer, M.K., Huebner, A.J., 2014. Fostering self-awareness in novice therapists using internal family systems therapy. American Journal of Family Therapy, 42, 67–78.

Morse, C.R., Volkman, J.E., 2010. An examination into the dyadic effects of mood in social interactions. Communication Research Reports, 27(4), 330–342.

Murphy, L., Wells, J.S., Lachman, P., et al., 2015. A quality improvement initiative in community mental health in the Republic of Ireland. Health Science Journal, 9(1), 1–11.

New Zealand Legislation, 2003. Health Practitioners Competence Assurance Act. Parliamentary Counsel Office, New Zealand. Online. Available at: www.legislation.govt.nz/act/public/2003/0048/latest/DLM203312.html

O'Kane, D., 2020. Communication in healthcare practice. In: Barkway, P. & O'Kane, D., Psychology for health professionals. Elsevier, Sydney.

Parker, D.M., Sutherland, C., 2021. The Person-centred frame of reference. In: Duncan, E.A.S. (ed.), Foundations for practice in occupational therapy, 6th ed. Elsevier, Edinburgh.

Riding, S., Glendening, N., Heaslip, V., 2017. Real world challenges in delivering person-centred care: A community-based case study. British Journal of Community Nursing, 22(8), 391–396.

Rogers, C., 1967. On becoming a person. Constable, London.

Rosen, D., 2014. Vital conversations: Improving communication between doctors and patients. Columbia University Press, New York.

Ross, H., Tod, A.M., Clarke, A. 2015. Understanding and achieving person-centred care: The nurse perspective. Journal of Clinical Nursing, 24 (9–10), 1223.

Rucker, A., Windemuth, B., 2019. Utilising team strategies and tools to enhance performance and patient safety (TeamSTEPPS) to improve ineffective communication in long-term care settings. Journal of Post-Acute and Long-term Care Medicine, 20(3), PB26, doi.org/10.1016/j.jamda.2019.01.097.

Santana, M.J., Manalili, K., Jolley, R.J., et al., 2018. How to practice person-centred care: A conceptual framework. Health Expectations, 21(2), 429–440.

Schwank, A., Carstesen, T., Yazdani F., et al 2018. The course of self-efficacy for therapeutic use of self in Norwegian Occupational Therapy students: A 10 month follow-up study. Occupational Therapy International, 2018, 2962747.

Sheppard, A., Broughton, M.C., 2020. Promoting wellbeing and health through active participation in music and dance: A systematic review. International Journal of Qualitative Studies on Health and Well-being, 15(1), 1732526.

Slade, S., Sergent, S.R., 2022. Interview techniques. StatPearls Publishing, Tampa, FL.

Sokol-Hessner, L., Folcarelli, P.H., Annas, C.L., et al., 2018 A road map for advancing the practice of respect in health care: The results of an interdisciplinary modified Delphi consensus study. The Joint Commission Journal on Quality and Patient Safety, 44, 463–476.

Soto-Rubio, A., Sinclair, S., 2018. In defense of sympathy, inconsideration of empathy and in praise of compassion: A history of the present. Journal of Pain and Symptom Management, 55(5), 1428–1434.

Stein-Parbury, J., 2021. Patient and person: Interpersonal skills in nursing, 7th ed. Churchill Livingstone Elsevier, Sydney.

Stoilkova-Hartman, A., Franssen, F.M.E., Augustin, I.M.L., et al., 2018. COPD patient education and support – achieving patient-centredness. Patient Education and Counseling, 101(11), 2031–2036.

Tamparo, C.D. & Lindh, W.Q., 2017. Therapeutic communication for healthcare professionals, 4th ed. Cengage Learning, Boston, MA.

Thistle, J.J., McNaughton, D., 2015. Teaching active listening skills to pre-service speech-language pathologists: a first step in supporting collaboration with parents of young children who require AAC. Language, Speech & Hearing Services in Schools, 46 (1), 44–55.

Trad, M., 2013. Teaching communication skills and empathy through engaged scholarship. Radiation Therapist ,22, 21–31.

van der Meer, L., Nieboer, A. P., Finkenflügel, H., et al., 2018. The importance of person-centred care and co-creation of care for the wellbeing and job satisfaction of professionals working with people with intellectual disabilities. Scandinavian Journal of Caring Sciences, 32(1) 76–81.

Vanderhooft, J.E., 2021. Ineffective communication: The uninformed injured worker. The Journal of Bone and Joint Surgery, 103(19), 1772–1776.

Weigl, M., Cieza, A., Anderson, C., et al., 2004. Identification of relevant ICF categories in patients with chronic health conditions: a Delphi exercise. Journal of Rehabilitation Medicine, 44 (Suppl), 12–21.

World Health Organization (WHO), 2007. People-centred health care: A policy framework. WHO, Geneva.

World Health Organization (WHO), 2001. International Classification of Functioning, Disability and Health. WHO, Geneva. Online. Available at: www.who.int/classifications/icf/en/.

CHAPTER 3

The specific goals of communication for healthcare professionals: 1 Introductions and providing information

Chapter objectives

Upon completing this chapter, readers should be able to:

- reflect upon the relationship between the overarching goal and the specific goals of communication for healthcare professionals
- state the role, types and purpose of introductions
- identify the characteristics of an effective introduction
- demonstrate skills in introductions
- reflect upon the importance of skills relating to providing information, including managing feedback
- demonstrate understanding that the two-way process of providing information requires organisation, relevant sequencing of information, timing and clarifying understanding
- reflect upon the process of providing and receiving constructive feedback.

The overarching goal of all healthcare professionals is to provide meaningful interventions reflecting Person/Family-centred Care. This requires mutual understanding, resulting in a therapeutic relationship. This goal should guide every interaction between healthcare professionals and the Person/s. There are, however, specific goals that also guide the communication of healthcare professionals. The specific goals may vary from one interaction to another. This chapter examines two of these goals:

1. making effective verbal introductions
2. effectively providing information, including providing constructive feedback.

Making introductions and providing information are two specific goals of communication for healthcare professionals. Many other goals for communicating fall within these two areas.

The second goal (Chapter 4), relating to the specific goals of communication in the healthcare professions, examines the skills of:

- effectively gathering information (by *interviewing* and using the related skill of *questioning*)
- effective comforting
- effective confronting.

The third goal, the focus of Chapter 5, relates to the skills of effective closure of services.

These skills require specific management to ensure appropriate outcomes for all individuals involved in an interaction, and thus are considered separately in Chapters 4 and 5.

It is also important to remember that the code of rights for all people seeking healthcare requires provision of and access to all information relevant to their care, along with effective communication about that care (Australian Commission on Safety and Quality in Health Care [ACSQHC] 2022; Health and Disability Commissioner [NZ] 2022). This is something that all healthcare professionals should remember when managing information relating to all their care (including communication) and interventions.

Making verbal introductions

In Person/Family-centred services, the initial purpose of every healthcare professional is to introduce *themselves*, their *role*, their workplace environment and their service. Introductions are a form of providing information (Slade & Sergent 2022), with many underestimating their significance and potential impact (Gillen et al 2018; Granger 2013). Introductions can establish a precedent for any future interactions with the individual; they "set the tone and the scene" (Gilleylen 2007; Harms & Pierce 2019). Introductions inform the individual who is listening about the healthcare professional performing the introduction, thereby establishing the reliability and trustworthiness of that particular healthcare professional (Eriksen et al 2014; Sanders & Burke 2014). Introductions also demonstrate respect for and interest in the listening individual and in the often-overwhelming and disempowering circumstances surrounding that individual (Gilleylen 2007; Granger 2013). Introductions should reassure the listening individual, allowing them to decide whether or not they will continue listening. They should produce a sense of confidence or a level of trust that motivates the listening individual to willingly invest in any future interactions (Eriksen et al 2014; Householder & Wong 2011).

In healthcare, the Person/s listening – whether they are the Person/s seeking assistance, a related person or a colleague – often feels vulnerable and helpless, creating confusion and reducing understanding (Golden et al 2020; Honeycutt & Milliken 2021). Person/s often feel unsure of and overwhelmed by their circumstances and the generally unknown environment surrounding healthcare professions. This may also be the situation for new colleagues (including colleagues unfamiliar with the particular context) and students.

Every introduction should reflect the essential characteristics of Person/Family-centred Care.

- What generally occurs during an introduction?
- What constitutes an effective introduction when you are in a new environment and do not know anyone?
- What does an effective introduction achieve for the healthcare professional and the Person?
- What should the healthcare professional introduce?

Remember: The Person/s you are assisting is feeling vulnerable and possibly disconnected from others and/or overwhelmed by their current life situation.

- Consider what you might need to know to feel less vulnerable if you were in their situation.
- Consider what would assist you to understand and remember all the information

Introductions are important. They affect the perceptions of the Person about the healthcare professional (Levett-Jones & Reid-Searl 2022). Introductions generally provide information to allow the speaker and listener to achieve mutual understanding and establish whether they share a common purpose (Holmes et al 2010). The vulnerable Person/s listening to a healthcare professional is certainly listening for answers. In their mind, they have often-unconscious questions they want answered about the talking healthcare professional (Harms & Pierce 2019), for example, *Who is this person? What do they want? What can they do to help me? Do they really want to help me? Can I trust them? Will they listen to me? Will they understand me and therefore help me? Will they really want the best for me? Will they want what I want? Are they worth listening to? Do I want to keep listening?*

The verbal message or actual words used may contribute to the answers of only two or three of the questions in the mind of each listener. In fact, during the introduction, the manner and non-verbal messages of the healthcare professional may provide the most powerful messages to the Person/s (Devito 2021; Turner et al 2010). As both verbal and non-verbal messages influence all interactions and future collaboration between the Person/s and the healthcare professional, as well as overall satisfaction (Rosen 2014), they must "send" the same message (Bevan et al 2011; Lawton 2011). For example, when introducing yourself, smiling at the Person/s and making eye contact can demonstrate concern for the Person/s, as well as establishing rapport (English et al 2022).

Introducing oneself and the associated role

Introducing oneself is simple; it is a statement of a name. *"Hi, I'm …"* is easy to say many times a day. Yet healthcare professionals often fail at this basic task. As a result, campaigns such as the "#hellomynameis campaign" (www.hellomynameis.org.uk/) begun by Doctor Kate Granger, in the UK encourage a focus on introducing oneself when functioning as a healthcare professional. Such introductions are more than courteous, they encourage a human connection between the healthcare professional and the Person requiring their assistance (Granger 2021). However, it can be challenging to introduce the role of a healthcare profession. A publicly well-known and well-understood healthcare profession may seem easy to introduce. It may even be tempting not to introduce such a healthcare profession. However, possible preconceptions or misconceptions may cause confusion (remember, vulnerability also causes confusion!) If the practitioner role changes in a particular setting (many healthcare professions have a different focus and thus aim in different contexts) or is relatively unknown and not clearly understood, the role requires clarification. In some circumstances, even with well-known healthcare professions, it can be reassuring to outline the role of the particular healthcare profession in the particular setting. This can be achieved using questions or a verbal or written explanation.

Some healthcare professions are unknown or commonly misconstrued in the public mind. In such cases, preconceptions can be equally challenging. It is important to use a clear and easy-to-understand explanation of the role of these professions (Lawton 2011; Staggers & Brann 2011), avoiding any potentially confusing descriptions in this explanation (Bevan et al 2011). It may be useful to include specific examples of the role of the particular healthcare profession in the specific setting or context. However, the use of practitioner or professional jargon may produce further confusion, while also potentially increasing their anxiety (English et al 2022; Khuan et al 2021) and reducing development of rapport (Maryville University, Nursing 2023). It may be important when **explaining** a role to understand the role of other healthcare professions, as this may assist in avoiding confusion about the role of this profession compared with that of other healthcare professions. When working with adults, a written explanation may address any misconceptions concerning the role of a particular healthcare profession. When working with some audiences, relevant illustrations may enhance a written introduction.

Failure to introduce a particular role, or at least to question and clarify understanding of the role, may result in a difficult-to-correct misunderstanding. More importantly, the Person/s requiring assistance may not receive the appropriate service, thereby limiting potential outcomes and possibly having legal implications.

- Write down the role of your healthcare profession.
- Introduce yourself and explain your role to:
  - someone from your healthcare profession. Do they understand you? Do they agree?
  - someone from another healthcare profession. Do they understand you? Do they agree? Discuss their perception of your healthcare profession.
- Do you need to adjust your explanation because of the above responses?

Introducing the unfamiliar environment

There is usually an element of uncertainty and anxiety for an individual entering an unfamiliar environment (Haddad et al 2019). New environments create questions about a number of things – the physical layout of the environment, the people in the environment, the emotional safety and predictability of the environment, the possible events and routines occurring within the environment, who to ask for a blanket, and, for some, survival within the new environment.

These questions and the overall goal of a healthcare professional determine the order of an environmental introduction. Thus, the first part of an environmental introduction is usually introducing the physical environment. Essential information for all newcomers to an unfamiliar environment includes the location of the toilet! In an inpatient setting, information relating to ward routines, including how to order meals, meal times, visiting hours and particular relevant events or procedures, can assist in reducing anxiety. Introducing the physical environment and related routines does not merely assist in the orientation of the Person/s, but also allows the healthcare professional and the Person/s to begin progressing through the steps facilitating Person/Family-centred Care.

Further information required for an environmental introduction will depend on the needs of the newcomer. If they indicate a need to know more about the events they can expect in the environment, then a verbal or written description of the typical events should follow the initial physical introduction. It may be more appropriate to provide a deeper explanation of possible events just before they occur, rather than when a person is new to an environment. Remember that the Person/s is vulnerable, even remembering a name may be difficult (Baverstock & Finlay 2020). Thus they may initially "miss" important information if too much information is provided in a new and unfamiliar environment. When people feel vulnerable what they remember may be selective; that is, they may only remember particular parts of the information and forget other, often significant, information (Morse & Volkman 2010).

- Have a group member explain a time when feeling vulnerable and anxious because of being in an unfamiliar environment affected their understanding and memory. Consider the importance of the information at the time.
- Discuss why such feelings might produce this reduction in cognitive function.
- Suggest when it is important that the healthcare professional compensate for the selective understanding of the Person/s.
- Suggest ways a healthcare professional might assist the Person/s to overcome selective understanding and memory

A verbal or written introduction of the other people or practitioners in the environment should follow the initial environmental introduction. It is important to find a suitable time to introduce these people, or at least arrange a time for such an introduction. It may be beneficial to provide a written description of the people they might encounter and their respective roles. Allowing a person to read such a document at their leisure facilitates understanding and may stimulate questions during future interactions.

If the newcomer exhibits anxiety of any kind, it may be necessary to demonstrate particular interest in their emotional safety and to explore the causes of their anxiety. This demonstrates respect and empathy (Davis & Musolino 2016; Klaber & Bailey 2019). It will also improve satisfaction, producing positive outcomes. Answering their questions or indicating interest in and care about their concerns also produces emotional safety. Such behaviour indicates to the Person/s the willingness of the healthcare professional to consider and address their concerns. Physical concerns are often easy to address; for example, perhaps they need a cup of something to drink or a blanket. Emotional concerns require more thought, self-awareness and time to address (Butt 2021). It is important at this early stage to spend time acknowledging their concerns and fears, and reassure them with relevant information to allay these fears (Stein-Parbury 2021). Statements such as *You'll be alright* and *You don't need to worry – we'll look after you here*, will not reassure them and they do not demonstrate respect or empathy. It is sometimes helpful to introduce a concerned and fearful Person to another Person with similar difficulties who has positive experiences associated with assistance from the particular healthcare profession or service. Consideration of emotional concerns during an initial introduction, regardless of time pressures, is important for establishing the new, unfamiliar environment as a safe and caring environment for future interactions.

Whether the healthcare professional first provides or gathers information in their initial interaction with the Person/s varies according to the needs of the Person/s and the context. It is essential to consider the factors affecting both providing and gathering information. The order chosen in this book reflects the reality that introductions provide information. It is not intended to suggest that one has greater significance than the other or that one should occur before the other. In reality, when attempting to understand the perspective of the vulnerable individual, the healthcare professional simultaneously provides and gathers information.

Providing information: a two-way process

A healthcare professional provides information to various people throughout the working day. This information takes two main forms – verbal and written – and generally has the purpose of

informing, **instructing** or **explaining**. When a healthcare professional informs, they provide information about roles in the healthcare service, possible events, procedures or situations – usually about what to expect. This information may empower the Person/s to act and react appropriately (Egan & Reese 2019). Instructions are directions about ways to successfully complete tasks or required procedures. Information or instructions will reassure the Person/s and/or create questions. If the information creates questions, then the healthcare professional responds with more information in the form of answers that inform, instruct or explain. The healthcare professional must respond to the needs of the Person/s by providing the required information and ensuring their understanding of that information. The provision of information is a two-way process requiring mutual understanding in order to achieve satisfactory outcomes.

Understanding information

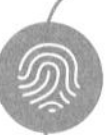

Consider a specific time when you received new information (e.g. listening to the person next to you introduce themselves or listening to the news). What made it easy to understand? What limited your understanding? Was your understanding related to words only or were there other factors?

- Divide a page into two, top to bottom. On one side list the factors that assisted your understanding and on the other side list those that limited your understanding.
- Using the information in this list, create a list of ways to effectively organise and present information about your healthcare profession to ensure understanding.
- Consider whether understanding the process or knowing the name of the next person (nurse, doctor, orderly and so forth) to assist them might encourage them and reduce their anxiety or stress? Suggest why.

Regardless of the reason for providing information, it is important to consider the factors that facilitate understanding. These factors fall into three main categories relating to the presentation and organisation of the information and environmental factors. Chapter 12 describes the environmental factors affecting understanding.

Before presenting information it is important to *prepare the listener*. Preparing the listener involves asking permission to provide the information at that time. It requires a clear statement of the purpose and significance of the information to be discussed during the interaction. This simple, respectful preparation potentially relaxes the Person/s, ensuring that they listen to and focus upon understanding the information. It is important to establish whether they know anything about the particular topic, event or procedure. Establishing their existing knowledge can provide an appropriate point at which to begin presenting the information. While demonstrating respect and developing trust, this provides an opportunity to establish the accuracy of their previous knowledge. This also potentially compensates for any changes in or development of information. Discussion of their existing knowledge may also develop interest and enhance concentration.

The presentation of information must be clear and consider the language needs and the physical, emotional, cognitive and spiritual needs of the Person/s (Householder & Wong 2011; Morse & Volkman 2010; O'Toole & Ramugondo 2018; Staggers & Brann 2011). It is important to ensure the Person/s is feeling well enough to concentrate, because if they feel unwell or tired they will understand and retain less. This is important if communicating potentially distressing information (Sweeny et al 2013). In such circumstances, making another time to present the information will be beneficial for all, increasing the likelihood of achieving effective communication.

To ensure effective communication, it is important to avoid overlaying the information with opinion, bias or uncertainty. For example, *I think you should ..., It is obvious you must ..., Have you thought about doing ...?, Maybe the procedure will be tomorrow*, and so on. While presenting information it is also important to avoid distractions. Present and explain one point at a time. State each point clearly and succinctly using precise language, while avoiding the use of words such as "here", "there", "thing", etc. However, a long, complicated and wordy presentation of each point is time-consuming and often results in the listener losing concentration (Devito 2021).

When presenting each point, healthcare professionals should focus on that point until they are sure the Person/s understands. It is often helpful to provide examples to illustrate or explain each point, thereby facilitating comprehension. If instructing, it may be beneficial to demonstrate the task while explaining each point. Reporting the experiences of another Person/s receiving assistance from the specific service or healthcare profession may also facilitate understanding; however, maintaining confidentiality is imperative (see Chapter 19). Repeating the important points can be appropriate and may enhance understanding. Take care, however, because repeating information may not be necessary and may negatively affect the reception of and response to the information.

Seeking an indication of their understanding may be more beneficial than repetition, and the use of specific questions will confirm their actual understanding. Careful observation of the non-verbal responses of the Person/s may also indicate their interest and understanding. When completing the presentation of the information, it is important to provide an opportunity for the Person/s to express their perception of the information, explore issues relevant to them and information related to their needs, as well as asking questions (Friess 2011). If giving instructions, close observation of the Person/s performing the task will demonstrate their understanding and ensure safe performance of the task.

Organising the information is equally important. Compiling the information into well-ordered points assists in achieving understanding. It may be appropriate to begin with the points that generally stimulate the most interest and then move to related but less motivating points (Holli & Beto 2023). Initially it is helpful to introduce the main point of the information and then to present the detail of each connected point. If presenting information about a procedure, it is important to present the points in order of each step to avoid confusion. It is also important to use language appropriate to the audience (Lawton 2011; Staggers & Brann 2011). When each point has been explained, it is important to finish with either a summary of the main point(s) or questions to establish understanding of each point. This repetition provides an opportunity to further process the information and to ask questions to clarify meaning.

Organising the information includes consideration of the *timing* of providing particular information. Providing detailed information about something that is 4 weeks away has limited relevance and meaning. Providing information about something that is immediate, however, will be both meaningful and relevant. Providing information in both verbal and written forms (with graphics) allows processing, answering of relevant questions and thus understanding. Research indicates that providing written information may enhance retention and compliance levels (Cinar et al 2013). The written form of any information must consider the above factors.

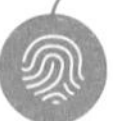

- Choose a procedure or routine typically used in your healthcare profession.
- Compile a clear and easy-to-understand written form about the procedure or routine with all required information.
- Read over your written information carefully and, if necessary, adjust it to make it easier to understand.
- Present your written explanation to someone who is NOT from your healthcare profession. Do they understand it? Together, discuss ways of refining and improving it.

In pairs:

- Select a scenario from Section 4. Read the provided information related to the chosen scenario. Consider factors affecting the understanding of the Person/s.
- In pairs, take turns introducing your profession to the Person from the chosen scenario. After each turn, evaluate the success of the introduction. Suggest how your partner might improve their introduction.

Providing constructive feedback

Feedback is the process of providing information to individuals about their behaviour. It includes information about the reaction of others to their behaviour (how they may affect others). It should assist individuals to decide if they should change particular aspects of their behaviour or maintain appropriate behaviour in order to achieve their goals.

There are two types of feedback – positive and constructive negative feedback. Positive feedback encourages the individual to continue their behavioural patterns, while constructive negative feedback encourages self-awareness, promoting the use of their strengths to produce change. Please note: the receiver of the feedback decides on the type of feedback given and their response. It is not possible for someone to make another individual respond in a particular manner. The receiver/responder alone is able to control their reactions!

Criteria for providing useful and constructive feedback

- Constructive feedback always describes the behaviour and its effect upon others, avoiding judgement or interpretation. It is important to avoid evaluative and judgemental language when providing feedback. This can be achieved by describing reactions to the particular behaviour using "I" statements: *I felt uncomfortable when ...*, or *I felt confused when ...* or *I felt compelled to accept your perspective, regardless of my own ...* Avoiding judgemental terms (inappropriate; dominating; aggressive; disrespectful; disruptive and so forth) potentially prevents a defensive response.
- It may be appropriate to respectfully ask the individual if they would appreciate some feedback about their behaviour, rather than imposing the feedback.
- Wherever possible, constructive feedback occurs at the earliest opportunity after the event. However, it is important to consider the readiness of the individual to receive it at that time, whether the presence of another individual constitutes support or threat and whether the particular place is appropriate for such feedback.

- Constructive feedback is specific, recounting behaviour during specific interactions. For example: *Earlier today when discussing appropriate interventions for Mr X, I felt you were not listening to the different suggestions. I felt forced to accept your ideas and if I did not accept your ideas, I would experience an "attack" from you. Your non-verbal behaviour suggested you were right and we were wrong.*
- Constructive feedback considers both the needs of the receiver and provider of the feedback. If the provider of the feedback fails to consider the needs and emotional capacity of the receiver at that time, the feedback may be ineffective, meeting only the needs of the individual providing the feedback. Consideration of the receiver determines the manner of expressing the feedback, along with maintaining the focus upon the individual receiving the feedback.
- Constructive feedback focuses on behaviour, which the receiver can adjust, and may include discussion of how to change the behaviour.
- Constructive feedback requires receiver validation of understanding of the feedback, thereby confirming mutual understanding.
- It may be more effective if several individuals provide the feedback. This can confirm that the effect of the behaviour is common to other individuals, not just the unique perspective of one individual.
- Constructive feedback must always be provided in a respectful, empathic manner, avoiding dogmatic and dominating verbal and non-verbal styles of communication.

Chapter summary

Introductions are crucial in establishing the quality and thus success of future interactions. Introducing oneself, the role of the particular healthcare profession and the environment is reassuring and important for Person/Family-centred practice, satisfaction and positive outcomes. Introductory information about a healthcare profession may be in verbal or written form. It must consider the needs of the Person/s hearing or reading the information. Effective introductions should demonstrate respect and empathy, establishing trust and the reliability of the healthcare

Hi. My name is Sam, I am ie beagan de fadhb agus ta me ag dtriabloid a dfhag
?
Hi. My name is Sam, I am going to be assisting you ta me ag dtriabloid a dfhag
I really hope things improve! I only understood some of that!
Hi. My name is Sam, I am going to be assisting you to decide upon and achieve your goals. But first let me tell you about this service ...
That makes me feel much better. Thank you

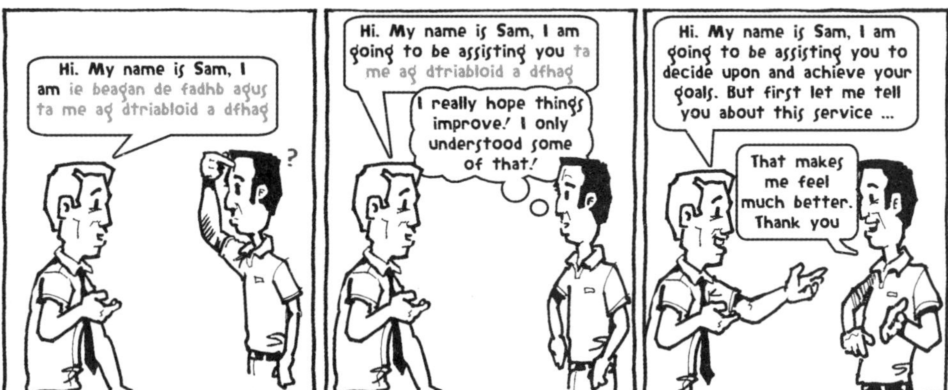

FIGURE 3.1
Quality introductions achieve better results.
Courtesy Roger Harvey © Elsevier Australia.

professional, achieving mutual understanding and a therapeutic relationship, ultimately resulting in meaningful and positive interventions. They are most effective when they prepare the Person/s listening, establish their current knowledge and previous experience, consider their needs, including emotional needs, and avoid the personal opinion or bias of the healthcare professional. They must also be clear (without the use of medical or professional jargon) and succinct, avoiding uncertainty, as well as being organised, ordered and "timed" with allocation of time to establish the understanding of the listening Person/s. The manner of presenting, organising and sequencing the relevant information (whether introducing, informing, instructing, explaining or providing feedback) has equal significance for satisfaction and positive healthcare outcomes.

REVIEW QUESTIONS

1. The ultimate goal of healthcare professions is:

   ____

2. Introductions establish the quality of future interactions and include introducing:

   i. ______________________________

   ii. ______________________________

   iii. ______________________________

3. Providing information about a healthcare profession can take two main forms:

   i. ______________________________

   ii. ______________________________

4. Providing information requires mutual understanding and may inform, instruct or explain. The manner of providing information should result in:

   i. ______________________________

   ii. ______________________________

5. When providing information there are important principles to follow, including consideration of at least seven points. List the points below.

   i. ______________________________

   ii. ______________________________

   iii. ______________________________

   iv. ______________________________

   v. ______________________________

   vi. ______________________________

   vii. ______________________________

References

Australian Commission on Safety and Quality in Health Care (ACSQHC), 2022. Australian charter of healthcare rights. ACSQHC, Sydney, Australia. Online. Available at: www.safetyandquality.gov.au/national-priorities/charter-of-healthcare-rights/

Baverstock, A., Finlay, F. 2020. Hello my name is .... Archive of Disease in Childhood: Education and Practice, 105(1), 63.

Bevan, J.L., Jupin, A.M., Sparks, L., 2011. Information quality, uncertainty, and quality of care in long-distance caregiving. Communication Research Reports, 28(2), 190–195.

Butt, M., 2021. Approaches to building rapport with patients. Clinical Medicine, 21(6), e662–663.

Cinar, F.I., Tosun, N., Akbaurak, N., et al., 2013. Comparison of the efficacy of written information vs verbal plus written information in rheumatic patients who receive colchicine treatment. Gulhane Medical Journal, 55(2), 94–100.

Davis, C.M., Musolino, G.M. 2016. Patient practitioner interaction: An experiential manual for developing the art of healthcare, 6th ed. Slack, Thorofare, NJ.

Devito, J.A., 2021. The interpersonal communication book, 16th ed. Pearson, Boston.

Egan, G., Reese R.J., 2019. The skilled helper: A problem management and opportunity approach to helping, 11th ed. Cengage, Boston MA.

English, W., Gott, M., Robinson, J., 2022. The meaning of rapport for patients, families, and healthcare professionals: A scoping review. Patient Education and Counseling, 105(2022), 2–14.

Eriksen, K.A., Arman, M., Davidson, L., et al., 2014. Challenges in relating to mental health professionals: Perspectives of persons with severe mental illness. International Journal of Mental Health Nursing, 23, 110–117.

Friess, E., 2011. Politeness, time constraints and collaboration in decision-making. Technical Communication Quarterly, 20(2), 114–138.

Gillen, P., Sharifuddin, S.F., O'Sullivan, M., et al., 2018. How good are doctors at introducing themselves? #hellomynameis. Postgraduate Medical Journal, 04/2018, 94, 1110.

Gilleylen, S.E., 2007. How to make a proper introduction. Washington Informer, Feb 10, 22–28.

Golden, S.E., Ono, S.S., Thakurta, S.G. et al., 2020. I'm putting my trust in their hands. A qualitative study of patients' views on clinician initial communication about lung cancer screening. Chest, 158(3), 1260–1267.

Granger, K., 2021. #Hellomynameis campaign. Online. Available at: www.hellomynamcis.org.uk/.

Granger, K., 2013. Healthcare staff must properly introduce themselves to patients. British Medical Journal (BMJ), 347, 15833.

Haddad, A.M., Purtilo, R.B., Doherty, R.F., 2019. Health professional and patient interaction, 9th ed. Elsevier/Saunders, St Louis, MO.

Harms, L., Pierce, J., 2019. Working with people: communication skills for reflective practice, 2nd Canadian ed. Oxford University Press, Ontario.

Health and Disability Commissioner (HDC, New Zealand), 2022. Code of health and disability services: Consumers' rights. The Health and Disability Commissioner, Auckland.

Holli, B.B., Beto, J.A., 2023. Nutrition counselling and education skills for dietetics professionals, 8th ed. Jones & Bartlett, Burlington, MA.

Holmes, G.N., Harrington, N.G., Parrish, A.J., 2010. Exploring the relationship between pediatrician self-disclosure and parent satisfaction. Communication Research Reports, 27 (4), 365–369.

Honeycutt, A., Milliken, M.A., 2021. Understanding human behavior: A guide for healthcare providers, 10th ed. Cengage Learning, Boston.

Householder, B.J., Wong, N.C.H., 2011. Mood state or relational closeness: Explaining the impacts of mood on the ability to detect deception in friends and strangers. Communication Quarterly, 59 (1), 104–122.

Khuan, L., Hahafiah, M., 2021. Nurses' opinions of patient involvement in relation to patient-centered care during bedside handovers. Asian Nursing Research, 11(2021), 216–222.

Klaber, R.E., Bailey, S., 2019. Kindness: An underrated currency. British Medical Journal, 367, l6099.

Lawton, B., 2011. What's in a name? Denotation, connotation, and "A boy named Sue". Communication Teacher, 25(3), 136–138.

Levett-Jones, T., Reid-Searl, K., 2022. The clinical placement. An essential guide for nursing students, 5th ed. Elsevier, Sydney.

Maryville University, 2023. Building patient rapport: A guide for nurses. Maryville University, St Louis, MO.

Morse, C.R., Volkman, J.E., 2010. An examination into the dyadic effects of mood in social interactions. Communication Research Reports, 27(4), 330–342.

O'Toole, G., Ramugondo, E., 2018. Occupational therapy and spiritual care. In: Carey, L.B., Mathisen, B.A., (eds), Spiritual care for allied health practice: A person-centred approach, Jessica Kingsley, London.

Rosen, D., 2014. Vital conversations: Improving communication between doctors and patients. Columbia University Press, New York.

Sanders, M., Burke, K., 2014. The "hidden" technology of effective parent consultation: A guided participation model for promoting change in families. Journal of Child and Family Studies, 23(7), 1289–1297.

Slade, S., Sergent, S.R., 2022. Interview techniques. StatPearls Publishing, Tampa, FL.

Staggers, S.M., Brann, M., 2011. Making health information clear and readable for the masses. Communication Teacher, 25(2), 94–99.

Stein-Parbury, J., 2021. Patient and person: Interpersonal skills in nursing, 7th ed. Churchill Livingstone Elsevier, Sydney.

Sweeny, K., Shepperd, J.A., Han, P.K.J., 2013. The goals of communicating bad news in health care: Do physicians and patients agree? Health Expectations, 16(3), 230–238.

Turner, M.M., Banaw, J.A., Rains, S.A. et al., 2010. The effects of altercasting and counter attitudinal behaviour on compliance: A lost letter technique investigation. Communication Reports, 23(1), 1–13.

CHAPTER 4

The specific goals of communication for healthcare professionals: 2 Questioning, comforting and confronting

Chapter objectives

Upon completing this chapter, readers should be able to:

- identify the role of interviewing and questioning to gather information in healthcare
- outline the appropriate manner of interviewing and questioning to gather information
- list the different types of questions, their purpose and their effect
- use appropriate questions to gather information
- reflect upon the significance of comforting during the healthcare process
- state the significance and characteristics of encouragement versus discouragement
- state the basis of, role of, and reasons for confronting.

The overarching aim of providing Person/Family-centred Care should guide every interaction. The specific purpose of effective communication for healthcare professionals is outlined in this book in three parts. The first part of the discussion, in Chapter 3, described introductions and providing information. The second part, in this chapter, examines the specific purposes of:

- effective interviewing and questioning to gather information
- effective comforting – encouraging versus discouraging
- effective confronting of unhelpful attitudes and beliefs.

The third part, in Chapter 5, explores closure of interactions and services.

Interviewing and questioning to gather information

A healthcare professional gathers various types of information from many sources throughout the working day. Gathering information is an essential component of Person/Family-centred Care (Giroldi et al 2015), more often using technology for gathering and managing information

(Dyb et al 2021; Mamta & Gupta 2021). Studies have identified particular instruments for exploring the gathering of information in various healthcare settings (Beal et al 2022; Herout et al 2018). There are various skills for gathering information in healthcare (Brata et al 2015). Such skills develop with practice and reflection. However, there are particular important considerations to be made when gathering information. These include noting the possible responses and emotions of the Person/s providing the information, the effect of the environment upon these responses, and the possibly sensitive nature of the required information (Avraam et al 2022).

The most common method for a healthcare professional to gather information through personal interaction is either a formal or informal interview (Slade & Sergent 2022). The interviewing process in healthcare usually begins with a more formal setting – the initial interview. This type of interview seeks to gather both general and specific information about the Person/s and the factors affecting them. Whether or not it is an initial interview, it is reassuring for the Person/s (the interviewee) to know the purpose of the interview (Holli & Beto 2023). Therefore, taking the time to explain the reason for each interview is a way of demonstrating respect and care for the interviewee(s), thereby developing a therapeutic relationship, potentially allaying fears and increasing satisfaction. Regardless of the particular healthcare profession or the purpose of the interview, the question is the major communication style used to gather information.

Questioning: the method

A question is a method, and, in common with most methods, it requires practice to develop skill in successfully using this method. The skill of asking questions to gather the maximum amount of desired information in the required time is valuable in all resource-stretched and time-scarce healthcare professions. It is important to know the purpose of questioning, types of questions, what information they typically gather and the effect that particular questions may elicit in the Person/s. This knowledge assists healthcare professionals in deciding what question types to use or to avoid when gathering information.

Why use questions?

In the healthcare professions, using questions does more than gather information. Questions serve several purposes in contributing to Person/Family-centred care. Initially, questions assist the healthcare professional to demonstrate respect and empathy, and develop trust and rapport (Beesley et al 2017; Giroldi et al 2015). The right question at the correct time encourages the Person/s to relax and develop confidence in the healthcare professional, and may assist them to recognise the interest of that practitioner (Devito 2021). Secondly, the right question can encourage either or both verbal or non-verbal communication (Honeycutt & Milliken 2021). Questions can facilitate exploration of, and elaboration about, particular areas, thereby providing additional relevant information (Davis & Musolino 2016). Questions also establish mutual understanding; they **clarify** whether the Person/s understands the healthcare professional and whether the healthcare professional understands the Person/s. Finally, regardless of the type of question, the ultimate goal of questioning is to gather information. This information will create a clear understanding of the needs and desires of the Person/s, allowing the healthcare professional to collaborate to establish and fulfil relevant goals (Preston et al 2018). This increases satisfaction with the process and the care, producing positive outcomes.

Types of questions and the information they gather

There are two main types of questions – closed and open questions.

Closed questions

Closed questions elicit discreet information that is short and definite (Beesley et al 2017; Boggs 2023; Harms & Pierce 2019), typically being used in time-pressured circumstances. They are often recognised as questions that have a yes or no answer. For example, *Is the pain sharp? Did you use the splint? Are you comfortable? Were you able to walk today? Is your workstation appropriate for your needs? Are you taking your medication?*

In Person/Family-centred Care, after an introduction the first question should be a closed one to seek the permission of the Person/s to ask some questions. For example, *Is it all right if I ask you some questions?* Such a question demonstrates respect, a desire to empathise (Davis & Musolino 2016) and an indication that the Person/s may have control over the events directly relating to them. After asking this initial question it is best to use open questions until there is trust and adequate levels of rapport.

When communicating with people who do not have English as their native language, it is important to remember that there are different ways of answering particular kinds of closed questions that can cause confusion. In English, the question, *It doesn't hurt, does it?* requires a yes if it hurts or a no if it does not hurt. In some languages such a question requires the opposite answer – yes indicates it does not hurt, while no indicates it does hurt. This difference in responses provides a warning for healthcare professionals; it indicates that the use of particular types of closed questions with individuals from non-English-speaking backgrounds requires careful clarification and negotiation to establish mutual understanding. It may be tempting to use closed questions with such people because they require minimal spoken language. However, in such circumstances it may be more productive to use simply worded, explicit questions; for example asking, *Where does it hurt*? rather than *Does it hurt?*.

When communicating with people from a non-English-speaking background it may also be tempting to rely on movements of the head to indicate yes or no. This can also create confusion, as different cultures use shaking and nodding of the head to mean different things. Thus it is important for healthcare professionals, when attempting to establish mutual understanding, to be aware of the possible confusion potentially relating to this type of non-verbal communication.

Some closed questions require specific and discreet information, rather than yes or no (Beesley et al 2017). For example, *Where does it hurt most? How long did you wear the splint? What do you think will make you comfortable? What made it possible for you to "take a walk" today? What aspect of your workstation (e.g. desk, chair, computer) causes the most discomfort or pain? What medications do you take? What time do you usually take your medication?* Some such questions might follow a basic "yes" or "no"(closed) question or they might replace them.

Another form of closed questioning requiring discreet or specific information is the multiple-choice question. Multiple-choice questions can be useful if people are unable to provide specific answers. Instead, the healthcare professional uses their knowledge of the specific situation to provide possible answers. These answers can assist the Person/s to clarify their thoughts and thus provide an appropriate answer (Stein-Parbury 2021). *Would you describe the pain as burning, sharp, dull, gripping, pressing, in a particular place or moving?* is one example of a multiple-choice question. However, avoid including too many choices!

Think of an issue that is specific to your healthcare profession and create a multiple-choice question about this issue. (If relevant, you may use the question in the text about pain, splinting, comfort, workstation or medication; if not, devise a relevant and appropriate question.)

Use the question with a friend to test its clarity and effect. Explain any terms specific to your profession, if necessary.

In all closed questions there is only one answer, which is short, definite and clear. The question does not require elaboration or descriptive detail. Closed questions can be useful when the healthcare professional requires particular types of information. They are sometimes the most appropriate questions to ask in particular situations, for example, in Emergency or if a Person is in extreme pain or is short of breath. Such questions demand little of the Person; they can save time and provide the exact answer without the complications of too much thought or too many words. In some situations it may be important to repeat the answer for the Person/s, potentially confirming mutual understanding.

Open questions

Open questions are the other main type of question. There is no succinct or wrong or right answer to an open question. These questions give the Person/s answering control over the interview, allowing the healthcare professional to listen, observe and learn (Beesley et al 2017; Harms & Pierce 2019). Open questions are useful when the required information is not discreet, potentially needing thoughtful discussion of either memory, elaboration, opinion, detail and/or sometimes description of experiences and feelings. Open questions can be less threatening because they allow the Person/s answering the ability to control the information they provide, therefore, being more appropriate in the beginning of an interaction. Open questions are useful when there is a need to explore or elaborate on a particular subject (Devito 2021). They are also useful when changing the subject or when gathering information from a sensitive or defensive Person/s. Open questions may begin with *How ...?* and *What ...?*, but can also begin with phrases such as *Tell me about ...*

Change the following closed (some are leading – see next page) questions into open ones.

1. Do you feel angry?
2. How many children do you have?
3. Did you make yourself comfortable?
4. Did you follow your exercise regimen carefully?
5. Is your workstation comfortable?
6. Does taking your medication make you feel ill?

Questions that probe

Questions that probe usually seek more information about a particular topic (Stein-Parbury 2021). They should encourage the Person/s to provide more detail about the information already provided. The subject of a probing question usually arises from information provided during the interaction, beginning with phrases such as: *Can you tell me more about ...? What happened before ...? What were you thinking when ... happened? How did you feel about ...?* The answers to probing questions provide specific detail about situations, people, events, thoughts and feelings. They can provide deeper insight into the Person/s, their supports and needs and, often, their feelings.

Probing questions may also arise from non-verbal messages, often relating to and reflecting specific emotional responses. Such questions can explore the apparent emotional needs of the Person/s; for example, *You appear unhappy; what are you feeling? Why are you feeling angry?*

However, such questions must be used with care. If the healthcare professional is able to explore and resolve the emotional needs of the Person/s, such questions can be effective and appropriate. However, if the training of the particular healthcare professional does not include managing emotions, it will be more appropriate to ask if the Person/s would like to explore their emotions with a trained healthcare professional. If they indicate "yes", then the healthcare professional can introduce the Person to the appropriate healthcare professional.

Probing questions can also change the focus or return the focus to an earlier point in the conversation (Stein-Parbury 2021). A probing question is useful if the healthcare professional requires information about something different to the current focus, or if the healthcare professional requires additional information about a previous point. Overuse of probing questions may create a negative response in the Person/s, as probing questions can produce the feeling of interrogation (Harms & Pierce 2019). It is important to be aware of the responses of the Person/s (both verbal and non-verbal) and react to fulfil both the general and specific goals of communication in the healthcare professions.

Questions that clarify

Questions that clarify usually seek understanding rather than information (Stein-Parbury 2021). If the Person/s gives information that is unclear or may be interpreted in several ways, the healthcare professional can ask for clarification or an explanation (Devito 2021); for example, *What did you mean when you said …? Can you explain what happened …? Do you mean …?* Either the Person/s or the healthcare professional can use questions that clarify particular points. Such questions are important in order to achieve mutual understanding and avoid misunderstandings (Haddad et al 2019). Any lack of understanding or incomplete meaning may result in assumptions potentially limiting the possible outcomes of the interventions.

Overuse of questions to clarify meaning may have a negative effect on the interaction. They may suggest that the healthcare professional is not able to understand or make himself or herself understood to the Person/s. It is important in such situations to listen effectively and to demonstrate respect and empathy, rather than frustration, while attempting to establish mutual understanding.

Questions that "lead"

Leading questions direct the response of the listener. They are not Person-centred, do not allow the Person/s control and usually do not elicit honest responses. A vulnerable Person/s will often answer a leading question according to the cues in the question suggesting the desired answer to the question. For example, *It's a beautiful day, isn't it?* leads the listener to agree and say, *Yes, beautiful*, or *Oh, it's a bit hot, isn't it?* leads the listener to agree that it is hot, regardless of their actual feelings. Leading questions such as these do not necessarily have a negative effect (Haddad et al 2019). If the subject of a leading question is external to the Person/s, their actions and needs, then the effect can be positive, creating a link between the healthcare professional and the Person/s. When used, such questions do not seek important information and thus are not threatening; they are a verbal recognition of the presence of the Person/s.

However, if used to gather important information, leading questions are not always positive. A healthcare professional who uses leading questions will limit the development of trust and the accuracy of the gathered information. For example, questions such as *You weren't drinking alcohol while you were on this medication, were you?* or *You're all right, aren't you?* or *That didn't hurt so much, did it?* or *We covered how to care for your back and I know you understand the importance of caring for your back, so I know you didn't try to move furniture, did you?*

usually direct the Person/s to the required answer of *No, I was not drinking, Yes I'm all right, No, that was OK,* and *No, I did not move furniture,* regardless of the truth. It is best to avoid leading questions (Beesley et al 2017) if the healthcare professional seeks to encourage an honest relationship based on respect, trust and non-judgement, as well as relevant and satisfactory outcomes.

In groups of four:

- divide a page vertically in two. On one side list the types of questions and on the other side list the emotions you might feel if you were in a situation where you felt vulnerable
- explain why and discuss how you might act as a healthcare professional to overcome these responses.

The skill of questioning depends upon another beneficial skill – listening (see Chapter 11). However, a successful interview involves more than skill in questioning and listening. It also involves appropriate timing of questions, the use of appropriate non-verbal messages, the use of silences, appropriate closure and, most importantly, a focus on the vulnerable Person/s.

Comforting: encouraging versus discouraging

Comforting can be a valuable means of developing a therapeutic relationship. The vulnerable and sometimes disconnected Person/s often share their anxieties and negative emotions with healthcare professionals. The healthcare professional has knowledge of their particular healthcare service and understands what that service offers, while the Person/s typically does not have that knowledge or understanding. The healthcare professional also possesses knowledge about conditions and the consequences of those conditions, which may also be unknown to the Person/s. This knowledge may make it difficult for the healthcare professional to understand the concerns, anxieties and negative emotions of vulnerable individuals. However, it is this knowledge that dictates careful and respectful management of all interactions between the healthcare professional and the Person/s (Egan 2014; Egan & Reese 2019). The healthcare professional is responsible for ensuring the comfort of the Person/s to encourage, affirm and empower them to continue with meaning, purpose and quality in their life. This will ensure positive outcomes (Mjaaland et al 2011). Remember that such Person/s may also include a colleague new to the service or a student.

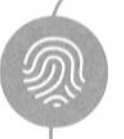

- Consider a time when you were feeling anxious or negative about something – perhaps an examination or a job interview, or feedback from an assignment.
- Did you share your feelings with anyone? How did they respond? How did you feel after they responded? Was it the way they responded that provoked your feelings?
- How might understanding reactions and feelings to negative events assist you as a healthcare professional?

The way a healthcare professional responds to expressions of anxiety or negative emotions either encourages, affirms and empowers, or discourages, trivialises and dismisses that Person/s and their anxieties or emotions (Devito 2021). This indicates the responsibility of the healthcare professional to always respond with respect and empathy.

Characteristics of encouragement and discouragement

Table 4.1 outlines the characteristics of encouraging and discouraging responses to expressions of negative emotions.

TABLE 4.1
Characteristics of possible responses to expressions of negative emotions

Encouraging responses	Discouraging responses
Focus attention on the Person/s and acknowledge their emotions (*You seem to be feeling ...*). Indicate that in this situation such emotions are appropriate and common (*It is OK to feel like this and it is something other people feel ...*). Indicate (without a detailed description) that the healthcare professional has some understanding because of a similar experience (*Mmm, I remember feeling that way when I had ...*). Ask for clarification of the emotions and the cause (*Are you feeling ...? Can you explain how you are feeling?*).	State that there is no need to feel the emotions. (*No need to worry, we'll look after you. Lots of people have this – we have a good success rate*). Acknowledge the emotions, but change the subject (*Yes it is common to feel afraid of this. Did you bring the ...?*). Interrupt, to avoid hearing the expression of such emotions. Totally ignore the expressions of emotions.

Classifying responses to negative emotions

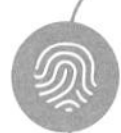

Consider each response to the following expressions of anxiety and decide whether it is encouraging or discouraging.

1. Person: I am really worried about this surgery.

   Healthcare professional (HcP): You don't need to worry. Dr Super is a great surgeon and it is a routine procedure.
2. Person: I don't know how I will cope at home.

   HcP: Don't worry, you'll be OK. There's lots of help available.
3. Person: I don't like hospitals – my Dad died in one.

   HcP: No wonder you don't like hospitals! That must have been difficult. Do you want to tell me about it?
4. Person: Boy, we are busy today. Two new people have just arrived. I don't think I will get everything done.

HcP: The quicker you get over that feeling the better. It is always the same here – busy, busy!

5. Person: I am just not coping here – I can't do this.

   HcP: You're feeling overwhelmed. Mmm (watching as the person struggles to complete a task and then gives up) ... that can be difficult. What are you struggling with most?

6. Person: I am angry. I need that report for the appointment tomorrow and it's not ready.

   HcP: I understand your anger. I am not too impressed either – it was supposed to be ready today. What time is the appointment? Maybe it can be delivered there tomorrow before the appointment.

How would you typically respond to each of these statements? Change the discouraging, trivialising and dismissive responses to encouraging, affirming and empowering responses.

It is obvious from the examples above that the easiest and shortest way to respond to negative emotions has a discouraging effect. It may seem appropriate to the healthcare professional because they have both relevant knowledge and previous experience, but such responses rarely satisfy the needs of the anxious or negative individual. Empathic listening; that is, listening with the intent to understand and "hear" the Person/s, will assist in responding appropriately to the needs of the Person/s. However, healthcare professionals are often busy, therefore often responding in a manner that requires minimal time or effort. When communicating with an anxious or negative Person/s, however, it is important to express respect, empathy and interest, when responding. Such a response is an investment that ultimately saves time, developing a therapeutic relationship, improving satisfaction and increasing positive outcomes. Responding in this manner is not always easy as the healthcare professional has knowledge and understanding overriding the negative emotions. It is important, however, to respond in a **non-judgemental** way to indicate the value and equal **status** of the vulnerable Person/s. People often feel vulnerable when discussing an area in which they have no expertise. Responses demonstrating a superiority of knowledge without sharing that knowledge will only discourage and may appear dismissive. A dismissive response does not acknowledge the emotions – whether logical or illogical – of any Person/s. Producing encouraging, affirming and empowering responses is sometimes difficult, It is however, essential to maintain Person/Family-centred Care.

Practising encouraging responses

Role-play each scenario in pairs, taking turns to be the healthcare professional (who responds encouragingly) and the Person. Compare the responses and note the different effects of the responses. List encouraging, affirming and empowering responses.

Person 1: You are worried about your family because you are the person who always prepares their meals and now you have a broken shoulder.

Person 2: You are angry and frustrated because you have not improved in the way the doctor said you would after the surgery on your back. The doctor has not answered your questions, nor given any explanation for your lack of improvement.

Person 3: Your child is in the final stages of leukaemia. You are emotionally exhausted and worried about being able to remain emotionally calm and supportive to your spouse and family as you watch him die.

Person 4: You have had your leg amputated because of a car accident. You cannot see how you can go back to work – you are a roof tiler. You are worried about your finances.

Person 5: You are a national sports star and you have recently had a relatively minor knee injury. You are worried that your coach will replace you while you are recovering.

Person 6: You are tired, frustrated and desperate because your 79-year-old husband fell more than 20 hours ago – he is in extreme pain, has been left to lie on a trolley for all that time and no-one seems interested in examining him.

Person 7: You have been experiencing homelessness for a few months, and today is the anniversary of your father's death. You are depressed and exhausted.

In the busy life of a healthcare professional it is important that all words are **comforting** to encourage and empower those seeking assistance, reinforcing mutual understanding and the therapeutic relationship.

Confronting unhelpful attitudes or beliefs

Sensitive confrontation requires the healthcare professional to demonstrate respect and develop trust, thereby improving service outcomes. Many individuals who seek the assistance of healthcare professionals express **attitudes** and beliefs, potentially restricting their communication, recovery and participation. The healthcare professional can challenge the Person/s to examine these attitudes and beliefs by appropriately and sensitively **confronting** them (Egan & Reese 2019). In some cases, confronting involves sensitively disagreeing with the Person/s (Honeycutt & Milliken 2021). If expressed sensitively and with empathy, confrontation or challenge can facilitate new perspectives, thoughts and behaviours in many individuals (Egan & Reese 2019; Stein-Parbury 2021), thereby improving the effectiveness of communication. Confrontation provides an opportunity to highlight the discrepancies or inconsistencies apparent in the life or environment of the individual (Holli & Beto 2023). It can empower individuals to face those discrepancies, patterns of thought and actions requiring change, thereby potentially adjusting them to facilitate improved communication, recovery and increased participation (Levine 2014).

Only experienced healthcare professionals should attempt to confront attitudes or beliefs. If an inexperienced healthcare professional is concerned about the attitudes and beliefs of a particular Person/s, it is advisable to develop a therapeutic relationship with that Person/s and discuss any responses with a healthcare professional experienced in confronting or challenging. Egan (2014) states that the healthcare professional must "earn the right to challenge". This statement indicates the significance of the therapeutic relationship when confronting individuals. Any confrontation or challenge must arise from a developed therapeutic relationship; one demonstrating respect and rapport. If there is genuine mutual understanding with freedom from judgement and an established therapeutic relationship, confrontation may increase the likelihood of positive communication and satisfactory health outcomes.

Levine (2014) and Egan (2014) agree that any confrontation or challenge must be specific and relate to a particular behaviour, attitude or belief. Generally, judgemental and intimidating confrontation of the Person/s will damage rather than empower. Statements such as: *You are your own worst enemy – you depress yourself* will only discourage them. However, asking a question relating to a particular idea or belief (e.g. *Do you think it is true that your life is terrible? Can you think of anything that was good yesterday?*) might challenge the individual about the belief limiting their functioning, perhaps encouraging them to think differently about their life and/or management of their ideas and beliefs about themselves. It is important to avoid underestimating the power of confrontation to promote radical change in thought patterns (Sluzki 2010). A positive change in thought patterns can increase interest, communication, participation and recovery.

When confronting, it is important that the healthcare professional uses non-verbal messages that reinforce rather than contradict the verbal message. If the voice, face or hands of the speaker contradict the spoken words, this inconsistency will produce confusion and negative emotions in the listener (Burrus & Willis 2020), rendering the confrontation ineffective.

Confrontation should not judge or criticise, blame or threaten. It should *not* provide the opportunity for the healthcare professional to express anger or frustration (Levine 2014). Nor should confrontation or challenge ever be direct and assertive, because strength of expression may become a barrier potentially disempowering the Person/s (Egan 2014; Egan & Reese 2019). Instead, tentative and sensitive expression will allow the Person/s to confront the attitude or belief, thus potentially facilitating the required changes in thought and actions. Confrontation is about respect and understanding to encourage and strengthen the vulnerable Person/s to embrace changes in thoughts and behaviours.

A student healthcare professional has failed an assessment task, receiving a third of the possible marks. Very distressed and near to tears, they express belief that they just cannot do the course – that they are "dumb" and cannot learn anyway.

The lecturer feels there was limited application to the assessment task, but has noticed that the general attitude and manner of the student suits the healthcare professions. The lecturer makes a choice about how to respond.

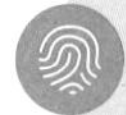

Imagine you are the lecturer in the above scenario.

- What is your response?
- Will you judge them? Write down how and why.
- Will you encourage them? Write down how and why.
- Will you confront and challenge them? Write down how and why.

In groups of four, assign two people to observe and scribe, and two to play the following roles. Continue acting the role-play until there is some kind of closure.

Person 1: You are the lecturer. Respond to the distressed student. Choose how you will respond before the role-play begins.

Person 2: You are the distressed student. Talk to the lecturer. You feel that the mark for your assignment simply reinforces that you cannot successfully complete this healthcare course. You did very well during professional placement, but you cannot do the academic work.

- Discuss the effect of the interaction – the reactions and resultant feelings. How did the lecturer respond? Did the response encourage the student to begin to change their beliefs about him/herself? Did the non-verbal behaviours support the words?
- Repeat the role-play and the discussion with different people in the different roles.

It is challenging for healthcare professionals to confront the attitudes or beliefs of another Person/s, but, if performed appropriately, confrontation produces positive outcomes. The willingness of healthcare professionals to challenge themselves, thereby increasing self-awareness, enhances the ability to confront (Egan & Reese 2019). If healthcare professionals are comfortable with confronting and challenging their own attitudes and beliefs, they will be more able to understand the needs of the Person/s they seek to confront. Confrontation in the healthcare professions is not something that necessarily occurs every day. However, when appropriate, confrontation enhances and produces effective communication, participation and recovery.

- In groups of three, choose a scenario from Section 4 from the Person/s experiencing strong emotions. Consider all the information relating to the Person/s in that scenario and role-play the situation. One person assumes the role of the Person/s, another the healthcare professional with the third person assuming the role of observer.
- Practise questioning, comforting and, if appropriate, confronting.
- Take turns completing the role-play, with different people taking different roles.
- After completing each interaction, discuss the elements of the interaction that successfully demonstrated questioning, comforting and confronting. Consider how to improve expertise in each of these communicative skills.

Chapter summary

Healthcare professionals commonly gather information using an interview. Questions are a typical feature of interviews. Appropriate questions potentially assist the development of trust and rapport, establishing mutual understanding and a therapeutic relationship. Person/s seeking care typically feel vulnerable. Therefore, the healthcare professional must consider the emotions of the Person/s and their possible responses. They must also consider the effect of the environment upon those responses, especially if discussing sensitive information (see Chapter 12). It is important to explain the purpose of the interaction and to use the relevant type of questions, closed or open, for the situation. The healthcare professional is also responsible for responding appropriately to negative emotions in order to comfort the Person/s, as well as to encourage and empower them. Confronting behaviours, attitudes and beliefs restricting the involvement of the Person/s can facilitate improved participation and recovery. However, confronting requires experience, effective listening, non-judgemental and appropriate non-verbal responses, along with tentative expression of those responses. In addition, to effectively use confrontation, a healthcare professional must confront their own attitudes and beliefs. Regardless of individual responses, interviewing and questioning to gather information in the healthcare professions aims to produce relevant Person/Family-centred interventions and positive outcomes.

You're my two O'clock, aren't you? How long did you say you have been wetting the bed?
Oh. I am so embarrassed ... how could you ask me that here?

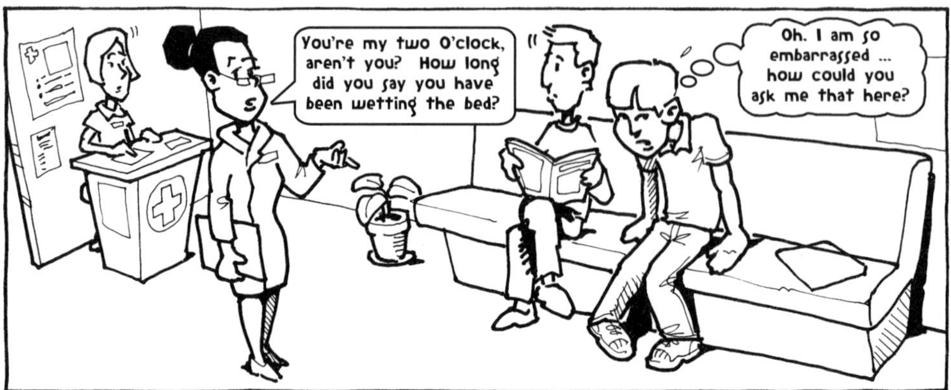

FIGURE 4.1
There is always a right time and place!
Courtesy Roger Harvey © Elsevier Australia.

REVIEW QUESTIONS

1. When gathering information, the healthcare professional must consider three major factors:

   i. ______________________________

   ii. ______________________________

   iii. ______________________________

2. State five results of questions.

   i. ______________________________

   ii. ______________________________

   iii. ______________________________

iv. ______________________________

v. ______________________________

3. There are two main types of questions – closed or open.

   List five features of closed questions.

   i. ______________________________

   ii. ______________________________

   iii. ______________________________

   iv. ______________________________

   v. ______________________________

   List five features of open questions.

   i. ______________________________

   ii. ______________________________

   iii. ______________________________

   iv. ______________________________

   v. ______________________________

4. Encouraging and discouraging responses have particular characteristics. List three characteristics of encouraging responses.

   i. ______________________________

   ii. ______________________________

   iii. ______________________________

5. Confrontation challenges attitudes and beliefs, potentially producing positive results. It requires:

   i. ______________________________

   ii. ______________________________

   iii. ______________________________

   iv. ______________________________

6. What must a healthcare professional confront in themselves in order to confront a Person/s effectively?

___

___

___

7. How would a healthcare professional effectively confront the abovementioned list?

___

___

___

References

Avraam, D., Jones, E., Burton P., 2022. A deterministic approach for protecting privacy in sensitive personal date. BMC Medical Informatics and Decision Making, 22, 24.

Beal, S.J., Dynan, L., Patzke, A., et al., 2022. Impact of automated information sharing on health care delivery to youths in foster care. Journal of Pediatrics, 249, 111–113.

Beesley, P., Watts, M., Harrison, M., 2017. Developing your communication skills in social work. Sage, London.

Boggs, K., 2023. Interpersonal relationships: Professional communication skills for nurses, 9th ed. Elsevier, St Louis, MO.

Brata, C., Marjadi, B., Schneider, C.R., et al., 2015. Information-gathering for self-medication via Eastern Indonesian community pharmacies: A cross-sectional study. BMC Health Services Research, 15(1), 1–11.

Burrus, A.E., Willis, L.B., 2020. Professional communication in speech-language pathology. How to write, talk and act like a clinician, 4th ed. Plural, San Diego, CA.

Davis, C.M., Musolino, G.M., 2016. Patient practitioner interaction: An experiential manual for developing the art of healthcare, 6th ed. Slack, Thorofare, NJ.

Devito, J.A., 2021. The interpersonal communication book, 16th ed. Pearson, Boston.

Dyb, K., Berntsen, G.R., Kvam, L., 2021. Adopt, adapt, or abandon technology-supported person-centred care initiatives: Healthcare providers' beliefs matter. BMC Health Services Research, 21, 240.

Egan, G., 2014. The skilled helper: A problem management and opportunity approach to helping, 10th ed. Brooks/Cole, Belmont CA.

Egan, G., Reese R.J., 2019. The skilled helper: A problem management and opportunity approach to helping, 11th ed. Cengage, Boston MA.

Giroldi, E., Veldhuijzen, W., de Leve, T., et al., 2015. Communication Study: "I still have no idea why this patient was here": An exploration of the difficulties GP trainees experience when gathering information. Patient Education and Counseling, 98, 837–842.

Haddad, A.M., Purtilo, R.B., Doherty, R.F., 2019. Health professional and patient interaction, 9th ed. Elsevier/Saunders, St Louis, MO.

Harms, L., Pierce, J., 2019. Working with people: Communication skills for reflective practice, 2nd Canadian ed. Oxford University Press, Ontario.

Herout, J., Dobre, J., Plew, W., et al., 2018. Gathering information in healthcare settings: A tool to facilitate on-site work. Proceedings of the Human Factors and Ergonomics Society Annual Meeting, 62(1), 600–604, DOI:10.1177/1541931218621137.

Holli, B.B., Beto, J.A., 2023. Nutrition counselling and education skills for dietetics professionals, 8th ed. Jones & Bartlett, Burlington, MA.

Honeycutt, A., Milliken, M.A., 2021. Understanding human behavior: A guide for healthcare providers, 10th ed. Cengage Learning, Boston.

Levine, J., 2014. Working with people: The helping process, 9th ed. Pearson, San Antonio.

Mamta, M., Gupta, B.B. 2021. An attribute-based keyword search for m-Health networks. Journal of Computer Virology and Hacking Techniques, 17, 21–36.

Mjaaland, T.A., Finset, A., Jensen, B.F., et al., 2011. Physicians' responses to patients' expressions of negative emotions in hospital consultations: A video-based observational study. Patient Education and Counseling, 84, 332–337.

Preston, J., Galloway, M., Wilson, R., et al., 2018. Occupational therapists and paramedics for a mutually beneficial alliance to reduce the pressure on hospitals: A practice analysis. British Journal of Occupational Therapy, 81(6) 358–362.

Slade, S., Sergent, S.R., 2022. Interview techniques. StatPearls Publishing, Tampa, FL.

Sluzki, C.E., 2010. The pathway between conflict and reconciliation: Coexistence as an evolutionary process. Transcultural Psychiatry, 47(1), 55–69.

Stein-Parbury, J., 2021. Patient and person: Interpersonal skills in nursing, 7th ed. Churchill Livingstone Elsevier, Sydney.

CHAPTER 5

The specific goals of communication for healthcare professionals: 3 Effective conclusions of interactions and services: Negotiating closure

Chapter objectives

Upon completing this chapter, readers should be able to:

- identify the importance of effective conclusions
- outline the features of effective conclusions
- effectively prepare for conclusions
- discuss concluding or closure in four different circumstances: after a single (one only) interaction; a session among many; services after a period of care and due to a life-limiting illness.

The provision of Person/Family-centred Care includes the specific goals of effectively introducing and providing information (Chapter 3); gathering information through effective questioning, comforting and confronting (Chapter 4); and thirdly, effectively concluding or finalising interactions and services. Effective concluding or finalising is the focus of this chapter, which explores:

- the importance of effective conclusions
- features of effective conclusions
- preparing for conclusions
- concluding or finalising in four different circumstances: after a single (one only) interaction; a session among many; services after a period of care and due to a life-limiting illness.

The importance of effective conclusions

Service access and individual interactions both regularly conclude, or "come to an end", in healthcare. Despite this, there is limited consideration, discussion or guidance regarding this aspect of communication. Effective conclusions contribute to the collaborative therapeutic relationship, thereby demonstrating respect and encouraging ongoing empowerment (Pagano 2015). They also encourage positive emotions and ongoing future use of healthcare services (James 2023). Careful planning, attention, compassion and understanding are essential aspects of effective conclusions in healthcare (Thompson 2021; Waran et al 2016). Finalising interactions, sessions and services requires as much preparation as interviews for the healthcare professional and the Person. This contributes to the appropriate use of the allocated time (Moss 2020), potentially ensuring the achievement of relevant, meaningful healthcare goals and Person-centred Care.

There are various reasons for **conclusions** or finalising services, including: achievement of the purpose of the single interaction; use of the allocated time for the session; achievement of the particular preformulated goals; use of all allocated funding; completion of the allocated treatment plan timeframe; limited Person and healthcare professional time; unplanned or expected death of the Person and/or change in staffing, just to list a few! Some of these are planned and others imposed by external factors. Regardless of the reason for **closure**, it is essential that the healthcare professional prepares themselves and the Person for the conclusion of their service (Beesley et al 2017). An effective and appropriate conclusion of healthcare interactions and services enhances Person-centred Care by reinforcing positive experiences, making such conclusions a necessary aspect of effective communication in healthcare (Tamparo & Lindh 2017).

Features of effective conclusions or finalising

Effective conclusions in healthcare require planning from the beginning of each interaction (Moss 2020). They also relate to the processes associated with the particular healthcare profession. Consideration of these processes will provide signals for the healthcare professional to prepare the Person for conclusion of the particular interaction or their overall services. At the beginning of the healthcare process, the healthcare professional would *introduce* themselves and their role to the particular Person/s (Chapter 3). They would either *ask* or assume permission to relate to the Person/s, depending on the circumstances causing the interaction. They would then provide an *explanation* for relating to or contacting the Person/s. This explanation encourages the Person to engage in the discussion, motivating them to interact (Woodcock Ross 2016). The content of the ensuing conversation and resultant interventions would then depend on the gathered information, the focus of the particular healthcare profession, and the needs and desires of the Person/s. It would also depend on the particular reason for the intervention for the Person and the expected outcome of the initial interaction. Effective *outcomes* of every interaction would require all aspects of effective communication, including, but not limited to: respect; effective listening; questioning; consideration of non-verbal messages; summarising and clarifying the plans for that Person/s. These are some of the important components of the foundation for effective conclusions. However, summarising and clarifying are essential aspects of effective conclusions.

When concluding, there are various important steps for effective conclusions, as mentioned above, requiring aspects of effective communication. These include summarising and clarifying. Summarising and clarifying definitely contribute to mutual understanding and avoidance of unsatisfactory outcomes. Whether separately or together, they provide opportunity for the Person and the healthcare professional to achieve mutual understanding and thus effective communication.

Summarising contributes to the achievement of mutual understanding. Effectively gathering information and summarising it indicates to the Person/s that the healthcare professional has been listening and has understood them. This also provides opportunity for the Person/s to correct any misconceptions (Lister et al 2021). Summarising requires listing the key or important points from the discussion or document, and rephrasing them in a clear, succinct and concise form. This provides an overview of the content of the discussion or document. The summary of the interaction or discussion is always shorter than the original. An effective summary should assist in clarifying the meaning of the major points from the interaction (Healy 2018).

Summarising can assist the Person/s to remember those important points. It can facilitate remembering the overall content of the interaction, rather than only focusing on one or two points (Henderson 2019). A healthcare professional can create the summary or they may ask the Person to summarise what they understand from the discussion or document. This could lead to clarifying their understanding. If the interaction includes provision of documents, highlighting the important points in the text, may empower the Person/s to understand the content of the summary document. This would then guide the process of summarising the discussion of the document.

Clarifying also contributes to achieving mutual understanding (Beesley et al 2017; Haddad et al 2019), thereby encouraging the therapeutic relationship and the achievement of positive outcomes. Clarification typically means to explain the meaning of either a particular message or the overall message, to ensure demonstration of understanding of all messages (Stein-Parbury 2021). Therefore, clarifying any messages requires consideration of the intended meaning of the message. Thus when clarifying, the healthcare professional attempts to provide a clear explanation of that meaning of any sent or received messages. They seek to remove any confusion or ambiguity. It can include outlining the content of the discussion, along with formulated goals and future plans. Questions may be used to clarify understanding (Chapter 4); this can occur towards the end of the interaction and/or session (Friess 2011; Moss 2020). Whether using questions or summarising, clarifying seeks to empower the Person/s with clear understanding of all messages.

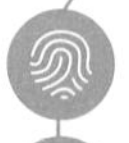

- Choose two paragraphs of text from this chapter and create a summary.
- In groups of four, each person presents the summary of their chosen text. Each group member compares each summary with the original text to ensure they have the same meaning. Where necessary, clarify the meaning of each summary.

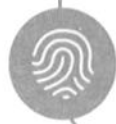

- According to feedback, rewrite your summary clarifying where necessary.

Conclusions include non-verbal messages. They typically signal the end of the interaction. This sometimes includes particular body movements and/or facial expressions. It is important to remember that conclusions require appropriate non-verbal cues to support any verbal messages (Holli & Beto 2023; Moss 2020; Pagano 2015).

- List the specific non-verbal cues that might indicate a conclusion or ending.

An important feature of effective conclusions is providing the contact details of the healthcare professional or relevant services. This allows the Person/s to contact the healthcare professional or service if requiring further information or intervention. Perhaps an equally important component of effective conclusions is the healthcare professional remembering the *purpose* of the interaction. This enables the healthcare professional to make decisions about managing the content of the session, in order to complete all necessary tasks and to achieve the goals for that session (Moss 2020).

Preparing to conclude or finalise

Some endings will have more significance than others, depending on the investment of the healthcare professional and the Person in the therapeutic relationship, and sometimes the length of time of providing or receiving healthcare. Regardless of the significance of the therapeutic relationship, there can be a tendency for individuals enjoying an experience to want to avoid the conclusion or end of the experience. Shulman (2016) suggests this tendency to avoid conclusions is a reality in Western society. Despite this tendency to avoid or not "face" closure or conclusions, there are individuals from any society who prefer continuity and familiarity in life. This can be especially true when experiencing often unexpected challenges in life. In such situations, individuals often avoid change. These realities indicate the importance of managing conclusions in a positive and effective manner, to encourage and empower the Person in managing their health and their everyday functioning.

- What have your reactions been to conclusions of various kinds, including: enjoyable interactions and positive experiences; significant relationships; meaningful events; particular enjoyable stages in your life?
- How have you managed your reactions when an occurrence or the experience of closure has been negative, causing you distress or trauma?

- As a group, discuss and
  - list possible ways to effectively manage the emotions potentially related to concluding or ending a "one-off" meaningful interaction
  - suggest factors that might contribute to positive conclusions or closure in healthcare
  - list possible ways to effectively manage the negative emotions potentially related to concluding or ending the therapeutic relationship, so the healthcare professional and the Person/s regain control of their emotions, accepting the closure without feelings of judgement or rejection
  - list possible ways to effectively manage negative emotions potentially related to concluding or ending the therapeutic relationship for the healthcare professional.

It is important for the healthcare professional to consider how to successfully manage any conclusions or goodbyes. Preparing to "say goodbye" and effectively end the services, whether after a single interaction or a series of sessions is a vital aspect of Person-centred Care and effective communication.

Concluding initial meetings, single face-to-face or telephone interactions

When connecting for the first time or expecting only one interaction, the healthcare professional would initially introduce themselves. If it is not a pre-made appointment, they would need to ask if the time is convenient for a discussion with the Person/s. They would also ask permission to discuss their particular healthcare role and any other relevant aspects of the healthcare process applicable to their particular healthcare profession. During an initial or single interaction it would be important to establish the existing knowledge of the Person and to explore any previous experiences with healthcare services and sometimes their understanding of the particular healthcare profession. It would also be important to establish their understanding of the reason for the particular interaction. Sometimes such sessions result in questions the healthcare professional is unable to answer, or in requests requiring solutions outside the scope of the particular healthcare professional. In such circumstances, the healthcare professional may need to advise the Person that they will be referred to another relevant practitioner who will contact them in the future. In such situations, that healthcare professional must provide relevant information in a referral to the appropriate practitioner.

Completing or finalising the interaction and discussion would include all aspects of effective communication, with constant awareness of non-verbal messages. It would be important to indicate when there are between 5 and 10 minutes before the end of the session. Before concluding, it is important to ask if the Person would like to make any further comments or ask any questions (Friess 2011), saying something such as: *I have to go in a few minutes. Is there anything else you would like to discuss before I go?*

After hearing their comments, clarifying their understanding and/or answering their questions, the healthcare professional should summarise the discussion. The summary should include clarification of any future plans or requirements. Before finishing the interaction or session, the healthcare professional should provide their contact details, thereby providing opportunity for the Person to contact them with any further thoughts or questions. When finishing the interaction, the healthcare professional should thank them for their time and contribution to the session. It can be important to indicate enjoyment of the interaction and pleasure at the possibility of meeting them in the future. Remember that particular non-verbal cues signal the conclusion of the interaction.

Concluding individual treatment sessions

It is common in healthcare to provide multiple treatment sessions to one Person or to groups of individuals. Such sessions are either scheduled appointments or allocated times in a day or week. At the beginning of a period of care, it is important to collaboratively establish the purpose of the care, and thus relevant goals, and a plan to achieve these goals. This encourages goal formulation for each session. At the beginning of each session, reminding the Person of the focus of the particular session and then at the end, if appropriate, the achievements from the session, provides an encouraging conclusion to the session. However, regardless of the progress, whenever close to concluding, it is important to signal the time for the conclusion of the session. *We have 10 minutes before the end of this session* informs both the Person and the healthcare professional of the remaining time, thereby suggesting the possible focus of the final 10 minutes. This time warning facilitates achievement of a positive conclusion. A focus on achievements also promotes a positive end of the session. This potentially encourages the Person to have positive thoughts about any future sessions or interactions with health services.

Concluding provision of healthcare services after a period of care

There are various reasons for the conclusion of healthcare services. Typically the stabilising of a condition and/or recovery from a condition due to interventions, and/or the death of a person due to a life-limiting illness, signals the pending conclusion of services. Therefore, after a period of healthcare with a particular service, a positive end or conclusion of these services is important. Conclusions or final interactions are often challenging for both the Person and the healthcare professional (Egan & Reese 2019). They may be associated with a sense of loss, rather than being a positive event, thereby creating painful emotions. If the particular healthcare experience has been an encouraging and empowering one, concluding or finishing may produce regret and a sense of loss, for both the Person and the healthcare professional. If the Person or carer has relied on the therapeutic relationship for a sense of wellbeing, there is the potential to increase the difficulty of concluding services. Some Person/s may withdraw emotionally, while others may express their negative emotions, sometimes creating challenges for the healthcare professional.

Conclusions may become more difficult due to the need to finish because of time or funding constraints. This may produce emotional distress for the Person/s from being unable to achieve their planned goals. In such situations, it is important to allow time for the Person to regain control of their emotions. If unresolved emotions continue and the healthcare professional must leave, where possible, it may be important to introduce someone else to manage these emotions. If this is not possible, it will be important to contact the Person or carer later that day or the next day to discuss their emotional state – to enquire about their current emotional state.

Regardless of the individual reactions to concluding services, expressions of appreciation (Holli & Beto 2023) and encouragement about achievements and progress, from the healthcare professional (Moss 2020; Nelson-Jones 2016) may facilitate management and possibly resolution of the negative emotional responses because of concluding the service.

Introducing the reality of an approaching completion of services may include such statements as: *When we first met, we planned to have 8 weeks of interventions, so that means in 2 weeks you will have your last session. Is there anything particular you want to consider or explore in the remaining two sessions?* or, *We now have two sessions before you finish with this service. What do you want to achieve in these two sessions?* Such questions not only prepare the Person for the conclusion of their healthcare services, they also allow the Person to collaboratively prioritise their concerns and/or needs in the final two sessions. It may also promote discussion of their progress and the challenges they have overcome during the period of care. Reviewing progress, along with acknowledging and highlighting the achievements before concluding services can be empowering, promoting resilience and meaningful engagement in life.

- Suggest how to express appreciation of the contribution of the Person/s and/or carer to the interaction after one interaction with the healthcare professional.
- Suggest how to express appreciation of the contribution of the Person/s to the interaction after 2 months of receiving healthcare from a particular healthcare professional.

Concluding services due to a life-limiting illness

Concluding services or endings need to be positive. This may be challenging if the conclusion is sudden or "out of the control" of the healthcare professional. The occasional, temporary disruption in services due to illness or absence of the Person/s or healthcare professional may cause negative emotional responses. Such occurrences require particular management to avoid lasting negative responses and to ensure Person-centred Care and continuation of trust, along with ongoing commitment to attending and/or intervention strategies. However, concluding can be challenging and sometimes confronting when assisting a Person/s preparing to "say goodbye" due to a life-limiting illness causing death. In such circumstances an Indigenous Person/s will prefer to die in the location of their birth (Eckermann et al 2010). This can be difficult for any city-based health service. However, ensuring their return to Country is imperative, thereby ensuring the wellbeing and satisfaction of the individual and their community (Waran et al 2016).

These types of end-of-life conclusions typically, but not always, occur when the Person experiences a progressive incurable disease in palliative care settings (Palliative Care Australia 2018). The Australian Palliative Care Standards (2018) indicate that effective communication and mutual understanding of the Person is mandatory in such care. Any services or care for such Person/s, facing the end of their life must also be absolutely Person/Family-centred and age-appropriate. The care must respond to and accommodate the values, needs and priorities of the Person, their family and/or carers. It must contribute to the quality of life for the Person as they experience their conclusion or the end of their life. Such care affirms life, while also recognising death as an inevitable part of life (Ministry of Health New Zealand 2001; Palliative Care Australia 2018). Such care potentially reduces the challenges of conclusions and endings in such circumstances, although it will not necessarily remove them.

Effective communication is an essential component of end-of-life care (Henderson 2019). This requires collaboration and awareness of the effects of the condition and any interventions upon the life of the Person. Pain and symptom management are also essential in such care (WHO 2020). Conclusions in these situations require preparation for either rapid or sudden closure, depending on the functioning of the individual Person and stage of the disease. The healthcare professional must also consider the cultural background of the Person and their family, to allow the Person to live and die well according to their own cultural expectations (Anderson et al 2021; Entwistle et al 2018). Each culture has particular practices related to death and dying. It is important that end-of-life conclusions consider and accommodate these practices, while continuing to maintain the dignity of the Person throughout the process (Pringle et al 2015). In addition to considering the relevant cultural practices, it is essential to also integrate the psychological and spiritual aspects of healthcare into these conclusions (WHO 2020). Such conclusions must also consider the expectations and needs of family and relevant carers, providing appropriate support to assist the family to manage the loss of their family member. Bereavement counselling may be beneficial for family members and in some cases, the healthcare professional.

When a healthcare professional experiences closure in these circumstances, it is essential they not only prepare for the death of the Person, but also effectively manage their own emotional response and possible bereavement relating to the permanent conclusion of this therapeutic relationship.

Components of effective conclusions

1. Verbally notifying the Person/s of the approaching conclusion of the session or of care.
2. Summarising the overall content of the session or of their care.
3. Allow time for discussion and questions to clarify any confusion.
4. Identifying and discussing the achievements and effects of the healthcare process.
5. Expression of enjoyment of relating to and providing care for the Person.
6. Expression of appreciation of the contribution the Person made to their care process.
7. Provision of contact details for the healthcare professional and /or relevant services.

Person-centred Care informs and therefore empowers the Person/s to feel positive about taking control of their health needs and their quality of life. Healthcare professionals are required to provide open, complete and timely information to patients about their treatment throughout the period of care (NSW Health 2011). This includes discussion and preparation of concluding that care.

- Choose one type of conclusion and a scenario from Section 4. Consider the details of the scenario and role-play a session relevant to your healthcare profession, ensuring an effective conclusion at the end of the role-play.
- Discuss the effect of the conclusion for the Person and consider how to adapt or change it for future conclusions.

Chapter summary

Prior to concluding, regardless of the type of ending, it is important to ensure that the Person understands all messages and processes used during the interactions and what to expect or do in the future. This may take the form of asking them to summarise the content of the discussion or their perceptions of their improvement or their understanding of future expectations. It may also include an opportunity for the Person to make any comments about their experience of the healthcare process with the particular healthcare professional. During the concluding process, the healthcare professional must closely observe both their own non-verbal messages and those of the Person to evaluate their actual level of understanding and to ensure some level of emotional resolution and comfort. It is also important to provide opportunity for them to ask questions to ensure their comfort, and understanding of both their unique but relevant issues, and their satisfaction with the process. It may also be important to indicate appreciation of all interactions with the Person and, if appropriate, of their contribution to all interactions. Often it may be beneficial to provide written summaries of all relevant information, especially if relating to ongoing requirements relating to their healthcare. If concluding services after months of interventions, it may be important to ensure they have relevant contact details. This will allow them to contact the healthcare service if requiring assistance in the future.

1 Advise when they will finish
2 Summarise content of their care
3 Discuss and clarify all
4 Outline results or effects of care
5 Indicate enjoyment of assisting them
6 Be thankful for their participation
7 Provide contact details
I must remember these things; this is the second-last session for Jack.
Thanks for seeking my assistance. It has been a pleasure working with you. Here are my contact details if you need anything.
Thanks.

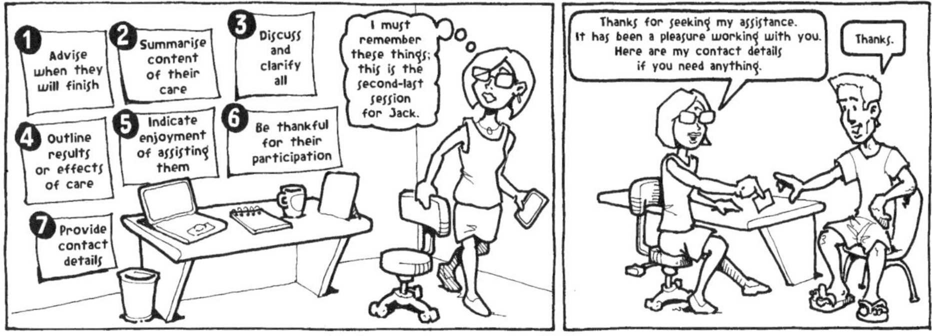

Figure. 5.1
Ensuring achievement of effective conclusions.
Courtesy Roger Harvey © Elsevier Australia.

REVIEW QUESTIONS

1. What are three essential aspects of conclusions?

   i. ______________________________

   ii. ______________________________

   iii. ______________________________

2. Suggest five reasons for the importance of effective conclusions in healthcare.

   i. ______________________________

   ii. ______________________________

   iii. ______________________________

   iv. ______________________________

   v. ______________________________

3. What can effectively preparing the Person/s for conclusion of services achieve for that Person?

   i. ______________________________

   ii. ______________________________

   iii. ______________________________

   iv. ______________________________

4. What are five features of effective conclusions for healthcare professionals?

   i. ______________________________

   ii. ______________________________

   iii. ______________________________

   iv. ______________________________

   v. ______________________________

5. In your own words, create a definition of summarising.

____

____

____

6. Outline appropriate methods of preparing to conclude an interaction or intervention process.

   i. ______________________________

   ii. ______________________________

   iii. ______________________________

   iv. ______________________________

   v. ______________________________

   vi ______________________________

7. What are the components of closure when assisting a Person who is preparing to die?

   i. ______________________________

   ii. ______________________________

   iii. ______________________________

   iv. ______________________________

   v. ______________________________

   vi ______________________________

   - Suggest how a healthcare professional might assist family members of a dying Person.

____

____

____

References

Anderson, N.E., Robinson, J., Moeke-Maxwell, T., et al., 2021. Paramedic care of the dying, deceased and bereaved in Aotearoa, New Zealand. Progress in Palliative Care, 29(2), 84–90.

Beesley, P., Watts, M., Harrison, M., 2017. Developing your communication skills in social work. Sage, London.

Eckermann, A., Dowd, T., Chong, E., et al., 2010. Binaŋ Goonj: Bridging cultures in Aboriginal health, 3rd ed. Elsevier, Sydney.

Egan, G., Reese R.J., 2019. The skilled helper: A problem management and opportunity approach to helping, 11th ed. Cengage, Boston MA.

Entwistle, V.A., Cribb, A., Watt, I.S., et al., 2018. "The more you know, the more you realise it is really challenging to do": Tensions and uncertainties in person-centred support for people with long-term conditions. Patient Education and Counseling, 101(2018), 1460–1467.

Friess, E., 2011. Politeness, time constraints and collaboration in decision-making. Technical Communication Quarterly, 20(2), 114–138.

Haddad, A.M., Purtilo, R.B., Doherty, R.F., 2019. Health professional and patient interaction, 9th ed. Elsevier/Saunders, St Louis, MO.

Healy, K, 2018. The skilled communicator in social work: The art and science of communication in practice. Palgrave, London.

Henderson, A., 2019. Communication for health care practice. Oxford University Press, Melbourne.

Holli, B.B., Beto, J.A., 2023. Nutrition counselling and education skills for dietetics professionals, 8th ed. Jones & Bartlett, Burlington, MA.

James, T.A., 2023. Building empathy into the structure of health care. Trends in Medicine, Harvard Medical School Postgraduate Education. Online. Available at: postgraduateeducation.hms.harvard.edu/trends-medicine/building-empathy-structure-health-care.

Lister, S., Hofland, J., Grafton, H. et al. (eds), 2021. The Royal Marsden Hospital manual of clinical nursing procedures, student edition, 10th ed. Wiley-Blackwell, Chichester.

Ministry of Health, 2001. The New Zealand palliative care strategy. MOH, Wellington. Online. Available at: www.health.govt.nz/our-work/life-stages/palliative-care/palliative-care-strategy-2001.

Moss, B., 2020. Communication skills in health and social care, 5th ed. Sage, London.

Nelson-Jones, R., 2016. Basic counselling skills: A helper's manual, 4th ed. Sage, London.

NSW Health, 2011. Your healthcare, rights and responsibilities: A guide for NSW health staff. NSW Health, Sydney.

Pagano, M.P., 2015. Communication case studies for health care professionals: An applied approach, 2nd ed. Springer, New York.

Palliative Care Australia, 2018. National palliative care standards, 5th ed. Australian Government, Department of Health, Canberra.

Pringle, J., Johnston, B., Buchanan, D., 2015. Dignity and patient-centred care for people with palliative care needs in the acute hospital setting: A systematic review. Palliative Medicine, 29(8), 675–694.

Shulman, L., 2016. The skills of helping individuals, families, groups and communities, 8th ed. Cengage, Boston, MA.

Stein-Parbury, J., 2021. Patient and person: Interpersonal skills in nursing, 7th ed. Churchill Livingstone Elsevier, Sydney.

Tamparo, C. D. & Lindh, W. Q., 2017. Therapeutic communication for healthcare professionals, 4th ed. Cengage Learning, Boston, MA.

Thompson, N., 2021. People skills, 5th edition. Palgrave Macmillan, Basingstoke.

Waran, E., O'Connor, N., Zubair, M.Y. et al., 2016. "Finishing up" on country: Challenges and compromises. Internal Medicine Journal, 46(9), 1108–1111.

Woodcock Ross, J., 2016. Specialist communication skills for social workers: Developing professional capability, 2nd ed. Palgrave Macmillan, London.

World Health Organization (WHO), 2020. WHO definition of palliative care. Online. Available at: www.who.int/cancer/palliative/definition/en/.

SECTION 2

Achieving effective communication by developing awareness within the healthcare professional

CHAPTER 6

Awareness of and the need for reflective practice in healthcare communication

Chapter objectives

Upon completing this chapter, readers should be able to:

- demonstrate understanding of the importance of reflection for the healthcare professional
- state the difference between reflective and reflexive practice
- list their own personal responses to experiencing and resolving negative emotions
- reflect on their personal functioning and management of negative emotions and events when communicating
- demonstrate understanding of the significance of changes in thoughts, behaviours and interventions resulting from reflection
- identify the steps of a reflective cycle relevant to healthcare professionals.

Effective communication requires an understanding of how and why an individual responds to the people around them, and how and why those people respond or react to that individual. It requires critical awareness of "self", both strengths and weaknesses (Bolderston 2020), along with personal values and beliefs (Williams 2022), as well as awareness of the effects of personality and communication styles upon interactions (see Chapters 7 and 8). Effective communication also requires an understanding of the effect of aspects of the self, the "Person" and the environment upon the outcomes of all interactions. **Reflection** promotes understanding of these aspects (Bassot 2020; Karnieli-Miller 2020). It also facilitates consideration of how to accommodate these aspects for future interactions, to continue demonstrating respect and acceptance (Moss 2020) and to improve care (Bourget-Murray et al 2022; Dean 2020). Awareness of self also promotes awareness of the benefits of reflection. This prompts the question: *Which should be considered first – awareness of self or reflection?* In this book, reflection is seen as providing the foundation upon which to build awareness of self, including personal biases and stereotypes, awareness of others, listening skills, non-verbal cues and the impact of relevant contexts.

PLEASE NOTE: It is important here to distinguish between the healthcare professional "reflecting back" their perceptions of the feelings of the Person/s and the self-reflection of the healthcare professional.

Reflection about self, life and healthcare is a circular process using experience, knowledge and theory to understand, guide and inform thoughts, action, emotional responses and resultant professional care (Ceo-DiFrancesco et al 2020; Hitchiner 2010; Johnston & Paley 2013; Smith-Lickess et al 2022). The increased self-awareness from reflection provides the basis for critically evaluating actions and beliefs to implement positive change. Reflection ultimately facilitates the transformation of the individual healthcare professional, thereby transforming the thoughts and actions of that individual to consistently achieve positive results during practice (Bassot 2020; Ceo-DiFrancesco et al 2020). It increases learning about personal strengths and shortcomings or areas for improvement, thereby producing a deeper understanding of "self" (Bolderston 2020; Davis & Musolino 2016; Dean 2020; Levett-Jones et al 2018).This enables the self-aware healthcare professional to use these individual strengths to overcome any professional shortcomings (Bassot 2020).

This understanding and resultant transformation empowers the healthcare professional to focus on the needs of others (Ceo-DiFrancesco et al 2020). Reflection raises awareness of those factors contributing to the self-maintenance essential for healthcare professionals (Dean 2020; Mann 2008). It also contributes to continuing professional development (Beesley et al 2017; Moss 2020), assisting development of skills and effectiveness when designing interventions and communicating during care (Egan & Reese 2019). Reflection also potentially provides methods for improving care and developing new understanding of healthcare processes (Edmondson 2022; Wieczorek et al 2018), thereby producing increased satisfaction with that care (Tregoning 2015).

In addition, within the competency standards or guidelines for practice, various healthcare professions in Australia mandate reflection and **critical reflective practice** relating to the feelings, beliefs and aspects of healthcare practice and healthcare outcomes to consistently improve healthcare (midwifery, nursing, occupational therapy, paramedics, podiatry and speech pathology) (Box 6.1). These professions apparently consider self-reflection to be important for developing the knowledge and skills of individual healthcare professionals within the healthcare process. The standards for dietitians, medical doctors, midwives, nurses, podiatrists and speech pathologists link reflection to lifelong learning. The standards prepared for dietitians, oral health/hygienists, social workers and surgeons use the concept of "critical thinking or analysing" or being "critically reflective" of all aspects of their care to inform that care. The Medical Council (Australia 2023) expects its doctors to reflect upon activities to continually improve knowledge, skills and attitudes to achieve professional learning and competence. The Physiotherapy Standards link self-reflection to the quality of care (Australian Physiotherapy Association 2011). The Podiatry Standards mention the use of a reflective journal to achieve the outcomes associated with reflection (Australian and New Zealand Podiatry Accreditation Council 2014). These support the importance of reflective practice for healthcare professionals.

The "what" of reflection: a definition

Beyond the expectations of particular healthcare professions, there is evidence indicating that reflection provides connection with, awareness of and clarity about unconscious emotional processing

BOX 6.1 Particular professional competency standards, practice guidelines or practice frameworks

Dietitians: Dietitians Association of Australia, 2021. National Competency Standards for Dietitians in Australia. Dietitians Association of Australia, Canberra.

Doctors (Medical): Medical Board of Australia, 2023. Building a Professional Performance Framework. AHPRA, Melbourne.

Midwives: Nursing and Midwifery Board of Australia, 2018. Midwife Standards for Practice. AHPRA, Melbourne.

Nursing: Nursing and Midwifery Board of Australia, 2021. Registered Nurse Standards for Practice. AHPRA, Melbourne.

Occupational therapy: Occupational Therapy Board of Australia, 2018. Australian Occupational Therapy Competency Standards (AOTCS) 2018. Occupational Therapy Board of Australia, Melbourne.

Oral health: Australian Dental Council, 2016. Professional Competencies of the Newly Qualified Dental Hygienist, Dental Therapist and Oral Health Therapist. Australian Dental Council, Melbourne.

Paramedics: Paramedics Australia, 2021. Professional Capabilities for Registered Paramedics Paramedicine Board, AHPRA.

Kaunihera Manapou Paramedic Council New Zealand, 2020. Standards of Cultural Safety and Clinical Competence for paramedics.

Physiotherapy: Australian Physiotherapy Association, 2011. Standards for Physiotherapy Practices (8th ed., amended 2014).

Podiatry: Podiatry Board of Australia, 2022. Professional Capabilities for Podiatry AHPRA, Melbourne.

Podiatrist Board of New Zealand, 2021. Podiatry Competence Standards.

Social work: Australian Association of Social Workers, 2013. Practice Standards. Australian Association of Social Workers, Canberra.

Speech pathology: Speech Pathology Australia, revised 2011, updated 2017. Competency-based Occupational Standards for Speech Pathologists. Speech Pathology Australia, Melbourne.

Surgeons: Royal Australasian College of Surgeons, 2020. Nine RACS Competencies. Royal Australasian College of Surgeons, Sydney.

(Bassot 2020; Egan & Reese 2019; Taylor 2011; Tregoning 2015; Wilkins 2014). Self-reflection occurs when individuals examine their attitudes and reactions to an interactive experience. It reveals causes of negative emotional responses, facilitating understanding of these reactions. It allows resolution of these causes and, ultimately, changes in thought, and thus behaviour, in preparation for more positive responses in similar, future interactions (Parker 2015). The process of reflection usually clarifies some parts of an interaction, potentially allowing the fading or removal of other parts (Fig. 6.1).

Boud and Walker (1991) suggest that reflection is the basis of knowledge. Reflection for the healthcare professional is certainly the basis of self-knowledge. It provides knowledge of strengths and of areas for improvement, encouraging professional development (Beesley et al 2017;

Levett-Jones et al 2018; Neville 2018). Communication in healthcare can become self-expression without reflection. This indicates the difficulty of achieving effective healthcare communication without reflection. Some view reflection as the process of revisiting experiences in order to understand them, thereby encouraging different responses during future interactions. When reflection results in changes in behaviour over time to manage similar situations with greater satisfaction, this is known as reflective practice (Boud et al 1987; Gibbs 1988; Gustafson & Fagerberg 2004; Mantel & Scragg 2019; Stein-Parbury 2021; Wilkins 2014). Furthermore, consideration of how the *self* and *research* affect and are affected by particular events is known as reflexivity (Finlay & Gough 2003; Mantel & Scragg 2019). Current discussion of reflexivity often highlights the ability to simultaneously reflect and interact throughout an interactive experience (Beesley et al 2017; Henderson 2019). Perhaps the most effective healthcare professionals are both **reflective** and **reflexive**.

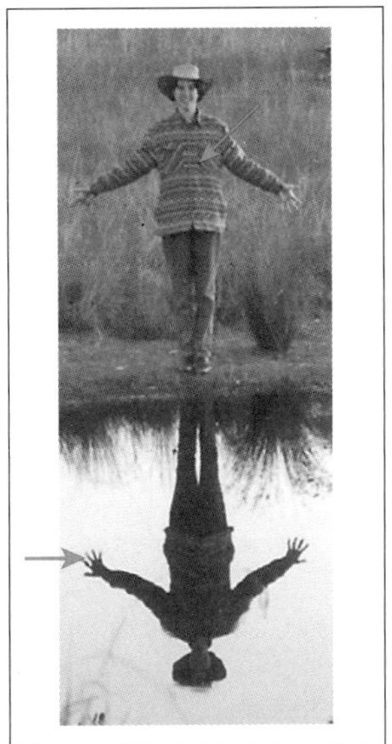

FIGURE 6.1
Some things become clearer when reflecting and others fade.

Reflection for a healthcare professional consists of thoughtful and often critical consideration of self, particular events, experiences and responses occurring during previous interactions or times of decision-making (Harms & Pierce 2019). Such reflection promotes understanding of the motives, thoughts, attitudes, emotions and associated reactions occurring during those interactions or while making those decisions. Reflection is not always an individual process, often occurring within a social context or an interprofessional team (Boud 2010; Dean 2020). In fact, research has indicated that it can be beneficial for healthcare professionals to reflect with colleagues in order to understand their experiences when providing care (Flanagan et al 2020), as well as when discussing quality care, and evaluating and/or developing particular interventions (Wieczorek et al 2018).

Regardless of the context, reflection facilitates clearer understanding of the causes of the negative reactions that can occur during interactions. Reflection highlights areas requiring conscious attention and further exploration, often resulting in acceptance and resolution of the causes of negative reactions. This resolution then facilitates behavioural change and thus effective communication during future interactions. Particular individuals react differently to reflecting, and factors such as personality, age and gender can influence understanding of and commitment to reflection. Because reflection promotes informed and controlled thought, and thus potentially more effective behaviour, practising reflection has potential benefit for all healthcare professionals, regardless of personality, age or gender.

For healthcare professionals, reflection is about careful, deliberate and critical consideration of events and their causes that occur during interactions in healthcare. It does not provide a formula for thoughts or behaviours, or a "one-answer-fits-all" solution, but it does provide insight and understanding, thereby leading to adjustment of thoughts and behaviour while providing healthcare (Parker 2015).

The "why" of reflection: reasons for reflecting

Reflection is an important means of learning about attitudes, experiences and self. It provides information to promote improved performance when communicating with others. It allows healthcare professionals to repeat actions, reactions and interventions that achieve positive results, or to change reactions or interventions to avoid negative effects (Levett-Jones et al 2018). Reflection provides healthcare professionals with awareness of their individual abilities (Bassot 2020). It also highlights limitations in their abilities and skills. Thus, through reflection, healthcare professionals can focus on improving those skills that will increase their emotional control and therefore facilitating effective communication and Person/Family-centred Care.

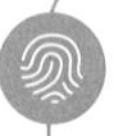

Identifying strengths through reflection

- List at least five things you know you perform well.
- List five things in which you would like to improve your performance.
- Ask someone who knows you well to make a similar list outlining what you perform well.
- Ask this person, *Do you know how I will react to your list?* Was their expectation of your reaction correct?
- Compare both lists. Are they similar? Consider the list of the person who knows you well and explore why you might agree or disagree with their list.

Reflection allows healthcare professionals to understand the "chaos" that is sometimes evident during interactions (Haddad et al 2019; Stein-Parbury 2021). It indicates that individuals are responsible for their own reactions and emotions, whether the individual is the healthcare professional or the Person/s. Reflection reveals that no-one can actually make another person feel particular emotions or make them react in a particular way. It indicates that feelings and emotional responses come from within the individual, usually originating from previous life experiences. Reflection releases the healthcare professional, allowing them to understand that they are not the cause of emotional responses in others, and that the other person is not the cause of the emotional responses of the healthcare professional. It provides the understanding that individuals behave and respond in particular ways because of underlying, unconscious and usually internal causes. This realisation encourages the tolerance and understanding that promotes unconditional positive regard of individuals, regardless of the situation (Haddad et al 2019; Rogers 1967). It also highlights the relevance and importance of reflection for healthcare professionals.

Understanding personal responses

1. When you have a negative emotional response to an interactive event, what is your usual reaction? Do you say or think, *They/It made me feel really bad?* Is this your typical response?
2. If so, have you ever explored the reasons why you respond in this manner in particular circumstances?
3. Have you ever thought that negative emotions are your responsibility?
4. Have you ever thought, *I make a choice about how I will feel* during an interaction?
5. Have you ever wondered about the other person and what caused them to relate in that particular way?

6. Can you see the benefit of considering the above perspectives? That is, that:
   i. your attitudes and reactions are your responsibility and you may need to explore your reactions and resolve the causes
   ii. a negative interaction may reveal more about the other person than it does about you and thus their reactions are not your responsibility.
7. Reflect on the benefits of understanding that you are responsible for your own reactions to situations – that you cannot make anyone feel a particular emotion and nor can others make you feel emotions. You alone control your responses; you alone can choose how you will feel and react.

Reflection offers the individual an understanding of their **dominant** or **primary personal needs**, allowing them the opportunity to fulfil that need outside of their work environment. If healthcare professionals seek fulfilment of their most pressing need within their professional life, not only will they experience disappointment but they will focus on themselves thereby failing to provide Person/Family-centred Care and appropriate interventions. It is important to remember that individuals are responsible for their emotional responses and for how they fulfil their most pressing need/s.

Reflection assists in developing understanding that the value of an individual does not come from the perspective of others, or the role they have in society, or the car they drive or the clothes they wear and so forth. It highlights the reality that awareness of individual value is derived from understanding and respecting the "self". Reflection can contribute to an individual acknowledging and accommodating their shortcomings while also recognising and accepting their own value and worth.

Reflection also provides understanding, not only to increase self-control, but also to promote self-honesty, self-awareness, self-acceptance and, ultimately, self-respect. If healthcare professionals are able to practise these they will be more able to demonstrate **honesty** and respect towards others, along with awareness and acceptance of the vulnerable individuals seeking healthcare (Haddad et al 2019). Self-awareness promotes the overall goal of every healthcare profession – effective communication to achieve successful Person/Family-centred interventions and satisfactory Person-centred outcomes (Devenny & Duffy 2014).

In addition, reflection is important when learning about unfamiliar cultural contexts (Ceo-DiFrancesco et al 2020). It provides an understanding about the culture of the healthcare professional compared with the unfamiliar culture. This understanding can facilitate appropriate behaviour and positive communicative interactions to ensure effective communication with individuals from other cultures (see Chapter 16).

The above discussion presents many reasons for healthcare professionals to practise reflection. These reasons definitely enhance communication and healthcare practice outcomes.

Reflection upon barriers to experiencing, accepting and resolving negative emotions

There is a longstanding argument about the reality of the role of the unconscious in determining behaviour. The concept of an unconscious mind with power to influence behaviour can cause discomfort and thus some people prefer to avoid discussing the possible role and the effect of a subconscious in everyday life (Murphy 2019; Murray et al 2009). The idea of "invisible" processes affecting an individual is unnerving; however, psychologists do suggest the existence of unconscious mental processes occurring outside the awareness of the individual affecting behaviour (Murphy 2019). Indeed, there is substantial scholarly discussion about the definition, name and use of unintentional or unconscious barriers or responses to experiencing, accepting and resolving the reality of negative emotions (Blackman 2004; Cramer 2000, 2018, 2020; Egan & Reese 2019; Hentschel et al 2004; Murphy 2019; Tamparo & Lindh 2017).

Defences (American Psychiatric Association 2022), adaptive mental mechanisms (Vaillant 2000), commonly known as **defence mechanisms** or unconscious responses, assist the individual to unconsciously avoid uncomfortable emotions, thoughts, information or desires by removing them from the conscious mind. These responses are one method of managing otherwise difficult thoughts and emotions. Every individual unconsciously uses these responses to avoid experiencing negative or anxiety-provoking emotions. Some responses are a form of deception (Smith 2007); they allow the individual to continue behaving in a particular way, regardless of the outcome of their behaviour. Others are simply ways of "coping with life" at a particular time; to maintain self-esteem and self-respect, and, as such, are successful coping mechanisms encouraging mature functioning. For example, individuals experiencing grief may use denial for a time to facilitate completion of funeral arrangements, adjustment and acceptance. While processing grief does not usually require prolonged use of denial, denial in the short term can be an effective response. Overuse of particular responses, however, limits self-awareness and constructive management of negative emotions. It also affects the harmony within the individual, limiting personal development and change (Egan & Reese 2019).

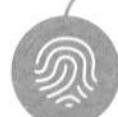

Exploring your emotional responses

1. How comfortable are you with considering your emotional responses? Do you find it easy or do you prefer to avoid consciously experiencing emotions?
2. Do you think that feeling emotions is a sign of weakness? If so, why?
3. Do you think *your* emotional responses are less important? If so, why are the feelings of others more important than your feelings?
4. OR do you believe *your* emotions are more important than the emotions of others?
5. Do you find that your emotions dominate your actions? If so, suggest reasons for this.
6. Do you think you really do *not* have emotional responses? If so, it is important to remember that everyone feels. Take time to consider why you stop yourself from feeling negative emotions.
7. Are the thoughts identified by answering these questions true? For example, is it true that the feelings of others are more important than your feelings? Or that your feelings are more important than those of other people? Where do these ideas originate?

Unconscious responses can be important for survival in particular situations – they may allow a person to continue functioning in extremely challenging circumstances (Murray et al 2009). Continual use of such responses by individuals will, however, habitually disconnect them from reality, sometimes distorting reality and limiting their ability to achieve effective communication and thus appropriate care. Over-reliance on particular responses reduces the ability to consider and choose possibly appropriate options or responses during difficult interactions.

Recognition of the habitual use of particular responses allows an individual to understand their behaviour, facilitating choice and control during difficult interactions.

Description and categorisation of these responses have occurred for many years. Cramer (2000, 2018, 2020) suggests there is a continuum of maturity influencing the use of these responses. The ability of the individual to function as a mature adult indicates the use of the mature responses. These include altruism, sublimation, suppression, anticipation and **humour**. They are temporary, adult ways of managing particular emotions However, they are essential for maintaining positive mental health (Vaillant 2000). Children often demonstrate use of the *immature* responses, which are childish ways of managing negative emotions. These include projection, fantasy, hypochondriasis, passive aggression and "acting out". The use of immature responses typically decreases as people develop into adulthood. The movement along the continuum usually indicates less self-deception.

The commonly used responses and possible definitions are outlined in Table 6.1.

TABLE 6.1
Commonly used responses to negative emotions or events and definitions

Category	Possible responses	Description
Psychotic	Denial	The person refuses to accept the truth about something (e.g. refuses to believe particular news).
Immature	Projection	Unacceptable feelings, thoughts and inadequacies, unwanted characteristics and inappropriate desires are attributed to another person (e.g. I am unconsciously angry with you, but I convince myself you are angry with me – that it is your fault, not my emotion). Such individuals commonly blame others for uncomfortable situations.
	Fantasy	The person ignores the real world, creating an imaginary world that fulfils their needs not met by reality. The fantasy relieves the discomfort of life. The individual does not usually insist on or act on the fantasy. For example, children may have a special imaginary friend.
Neurotic	Displacement	Strong feelings about one person are unhealthily redirected onto another (e.g. after a disagreement with a supervisor, the person goes home and shouts at their roommate or kicks the dog).
	Repression	Unconscious removal of painful or anxious memories from conscious thought. This usually occurs during childhood. Repression has a powerful influence on behaviour and can be destructive.
	Reaction formation	Conscious thoughts and emotions are the opposite of the actual unconscious wishes and emotions (e.g. the person really likes another person, but consciously believes they do not like that person).
	Isolation of affect (intellectualisation)	Excessive use of conscious thought to deny uncomfortable emotions or events. The person may focus on details to avoid emotions (e.g. intellectualisation allows someone to organise a funeral without being overwhelmed by emotion).

Continued

TABLE 6.1
Commonly used responses to negative emotions or events and definitions—cont'd

Category	Possible responses	Description
Mature	Sublimation	Strong unacceptable desires and emotions are rechannelled into personally and socially acceptable channels (e.g. aggressive impulses are channelled into a game of squash).
	Suppression	The person makes a semiconscious decision to ignore a thought, idea or wish momentarily. They return to it later.
	Humour	This subtle and elegant defence occurs when least expected and permits the expression of emotions without discomfort or paralysis to relieve emotional tension. It does not deny pain or seriousness – it simply allows expression and improves life.

Adapted from Vaillant 1995, p. 36.

Every individual uses these responses in some form at some time to continue functioning in life (Honeycutt & Milliken 2021). However, habitual use of such responses causes maladaptive behaviour. Individuals demonstrating obvious maladaptive behaviour (e.g. some forms of psychosis) usually employ immature responses.

- Consider individually each of the responses in Table 6.1. List behaviours that indicate use of each. How might you recognise these? Can you think of someone you know who regularly uses any of these? Can you explain their use?
- Consider those responses *you* have used in life. Why did you use them? Why did you stop using them?
- If you still use such responses, how will this affect your communication as a healthcare professional? Do you need to seek assistance from a psychologist or counsellor to reduce the use of such responses, as they are blocking your ability to experience, accept and resolve particular emotions?

Consideration of the responses that individuals regularly use can assist the healthcare professional or the Person/s to overcome barriers to experiencing particular emotions, thereby facilitating change in thoughts and behaviours, and thus in healthcare outcomes. Awareness of typical responses can empower individuals to "face" the reality of their situation, thereby negotiating required changes in their typical responses and in their behaviour. With such awareness, healthcare professionals can learn to appropriately manage both expected and unexpected challenging situations in order to communicate effectively and to provide consistent Person/Family-centred Care.

Healthcare professionals who reflect are able to identify the reasons for their negative reactions during interactions and, as a result, potentially resolve the causes of these reactions. They are potentially able to improve their skills in managing emotional responses (of themselves and others) that control and negatively influence their communication. Such healthcare professionals are able to use their skills of reflecting to observe and recognise emotions and/or their possible causes, in those around them and thus validate and clarify these emotions and/or their possible causes, thereby facilitating effective communication.

The "how" of reflection: models of reflection

So how does one reflect? Reflection is not just about exploring ideas and thoughts. Effective reflection requires writing or recording the content of the reflective process. This not only increases self-learning, but it also provides a record to allow future identification of professional learning and achievements, along with changes in managing emotions and functioning within the healthcare process. Beginning self-reflection in this manner can empower the healthcare professional to routinely reflect during interactions (Edmondson 2022), thereby improving the communication and events within the interaction. It is often not difficult to consider some past interactions – the more pleasant ones usually do not pose questions, just positive memories, happiness and pleasure. However, the difficult or painful ones often leave an individual feeling uncomfortable and wondering why they or others behaved in that way. To remove any guilt associated with such interactions, an individual will sometimes wish to re-experience the events for an opportunity to react differently. Alternatively, individuals may feel hurt and resentful because of the actions or words of another during an uncomfortable interaction. The purpose of reflection is to empower the healthcare professional by providing information about how to react appropriately, and thus (i) avoid regret and guilt; or (ii) understand, accept and forgive, rather than continuing to feel hurt and resentful as a result of the experience.

A model of reflection is a useful tool when attempting to answer the question of how to reflect. A model guides an individual through a process, explaining how to effectively complete the process. There are various models to facilitate reflection. When beginning the process of reflection, using a model can assist in developing skills in critical self-reflection. It is important to choose a model suited to the personality, thought processes and **learning styles** of the particular healthcare professionals. Some may think that the process of reflection does not require directions or a plan because it simply requires the individual to ask and answer questions of themselves. While this may be true in some cases, other people find it difficult to establish which questions to ask and to determine the exact focus of those questions. Sometimes thoughts lack clarity when accompanied by uncomfortable emotions. The use of a model to guide reflection can clarify and resolve those emotions by providing a focus for possible questions. Such focus facilitates appropriate answers for understanding any communicative interaction, being particularly beneficial when considering uncomfortable or challenging interactions. The information in the following paragraphs is adapted from an article by Boud and Walker (1990).

Reflection upon an interaction requires description of the interaction by returning to it through thought, verbal expression, written expression or some combination of all three (Koshy et al 2017). As mentioned earlier, writing reflections increases learning, providing the opportunity to identify change in the future. When recording reflections, consideration should be given to the individuals involved in the interaction and *all* the known information about each person (e.g. knowledge of and past experience in relating to these individuals). Examining the process of a previous interaction can guide the healthcare professional to understand its outcome. This understanding, together with other information (e.g. whether they appear happy, tired, hurried, preoccupied), is something most people relate to and absorb unconsciously when beginning an interaction. The appearance of the person, their non-verbal behaviour or perhaps an environmental factor (e.g. the threat of rain can cause preoccupation), provides this information. Consciously considering such information assists when reflecting on an interaction.

- When reflecting upon negative interactions, list the factors (e.g. age, knowledge, experience, emotional state) affecting the interaction and required skills when relating to the "Person". First consider the healthcare professional, then the Person/s and then a colleague.
- Choose and consider a scenario from Section 4. Identify a list of factors that the healthcare professional would need to consider when interacting with the Person/s in that scenario.

Reflection should also involve consideration of the expectation and intention of each interacting person. It should establish whether the intent of each person was clear initially and throughout the interaction, and whether everyone in the interaction had the same expectation, purpose or intention. If there were differences in the intention of each person, consideration could be given to the way in which this variation influenced the outcome of the interaction. Reflection should involve consideration of a method for clarifying intent in future interactions. Consideration of how an individual or the healthcare professional was feeling before the interaction (i.e. were there related or unrelated events causing negative emotions before the interaction that may have adversely and unconsciously affected their intent?) is important and may explain differences in expectation, purpose or intention.

Reflection should consider the events that occur during and factors affecting the interaction or intervention, including actions, words, non-verbal behaviour and environmental factors. A person who is an effective reflector makes the choice to reflectively explore relevant interactions or interventions. They begin by identifying an appropriate experience – one that they repeatedly "return to" after the event. They then describe the experience and all relevant details of the interaction or intervention. They explore the details of and reactions or results associated with the experience, considering the reason for each detail, factors affecting the outcome of each detail and the overall consequence of the interaction or intervention. Sometimes the overall result is positive despite negative events during the experience; while answers to questions relating to each "event" within an interaction or intervention are important, it is the overall result that must guide future interactions or interventions. After exploring the details of the experience and identifying their role in the outcome of the experience an effective reflector uses the insight about the event to establish goals for future similar interactions or interventions. After establishing these goals, they will develop strategies and action plans to ensure achievement of these goals in future interactions or interventions. This may change or reinforce aspects of their care, for all future communication. These steps suggest a model to encourage the healthcare professional to use their knowledge, skills and experience to develop and consistently provide effective healthcare (Fig. 6.2).

Managing an unexpected change in intention

Edith is a 76-year-old mother of three, who lives alone. She has been falling regularly lately, and her last fall caused her to fracture her neck of femur. As Edith has indicated that she feels unsafe living alone, a family meeting to discuss her future living arrangements has been organised for today. One of her daughters has been happy to talk about Edith living with her, so the team is confident that this meeting will be positive with an agreeable outcome for all family members. The daughter who is happy to have Edith live with her arrives a little earlier to spend time with her mother, and during that time Edith experiences bowel incontinence. Because of her embarrassment, Edith has been successfully hiding this problem from her daughter. The daughter, while not showing her mother, has a strong emotional reaction to this event. A nurse cleans up the floor and Edith just in time for the meeting. The other children arrive feeling confident because they know their sister is happy to have their mother live with her; they have no idea of the "accident" that just happened before the meeting.

- Suggest the possible interprofessional team members who should be present for such a meeting.
- Decide how the negative emotion of the daughter might unconsciously affect her responses in the meeting. Remember that her intent was positive, but she has had no time to process the event or her emotions, nor does she have any idea of the support services available for her mother, herself and her immediate family.
- Discuss the possible effects this negative emotion might have on the events during the meeting and on the people interacting throughout the meeting. Remember that all members of the family are present, including Edith.

Reflection should also include exploration of the necessity or suitability of each "experience" or intervention. While negative events are sometimes necessary to produce positive outcomes, they require skilful management and experienced personnel consistently monitoring both interaction and intervention outcomes. Some situations require discussion with the significant others of the Person. These can result in the expression of strong emotions that initially appear negative; however, the expression of these emotions with appropriate management of these emotions may result in positive interventions and resolution of negative emotions.

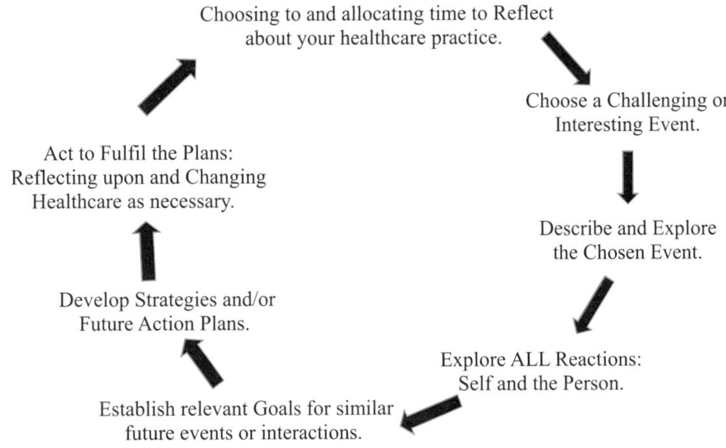

FIGURE 6.2
A healthcare-related model to guide reflective care.

When the healthcare professional is responsible for the negative results of events, they should reflect on the causes of these events and, if appropriate, how to avoid unnecessary events in future interactions. It is important to examine the causes and reactions of all the interacting individuals, including the healthcare professional, to avoid repetition of negative events during similar experiences.

Reflection should consider the emotional responses of all interacting individuals. These emotional responses may or may not be expressed verbally during an interaction. They may simply be non-verbal responses requiring exploration and understanding to guide future interactions and, perhaps, interventions. The cause of these responses should be considered and support or suggestions provided for resolution of these responses. Sometimes this support requires referral to another appropriate healthcare professional. No healthcare professional has *all* the answers for every Person/s, and this reality should guide healthcare professionals when communicating with everyone involved in and relating to the healthcare professions.

Johns (1993, 2022) provides a model to assist the process of reflection. He states reflection must be done to achieve depth of understanding, not merely an exercise to "go through the process". Although similar to the Boud and Walker model (1990), Johns expresses the steps differently, including additional factors for possible consideration. The following considers both the earlier and later model of structured reflection (Johns 2022):

1. Describe the experience and any important contributing factors.
2. Consider the possible causes of the reactions, including the above-mentioned contributing factors and the perspectives of the purpose of the interaction.
3. Consider the significant background information relating to the environment and each individual in the interaction, and how this may have affected the interaction.
4. Consider the aims of each action and the possible reasons for the actions or reactions.
5. Consider the consequences of the actions, including the feelings of each individual.
6. Consider why possible alternative actions were not chosen and the possible consequences of such actions.
7. Consider the resultant learning and how to change reactions in the future.

These seven points adapted from the Johns model, provide a sound basis for reflection about interactive experiences, either while practising as a healthcare professional or in daily life. Remember it is important to consider the evidence base for appropriate care, the ethical requirements of that care, the personal beliefs and values of the healthcare professional and any relevant experience of care provisions and the results.

1. When events become unsatisfactory, what questions are beneficial? Consider an uncomfortable event you remember, preferably a recent one (e.g. with teachers, family members, fellow workers, or an accident, perhaps in a carpark). Use the following questions to guide your reflection about that event.
   - What was the purpose of the communicative interaction?
   - What was I feeling before the interaction?
   - Was I preoccupied? Was I focused?
   - Do I have a fundamental bias relating to this person or situation? Do I have a past negative history when communicating with the person or in similar situations? If so, why? How might I resolve this negative history?

- When did this interaction begin to deteriorate or "go wrong"?
- Was the trigger one or more of the following?
  - Something that was said?
  - Something that happened before?
  - Something the person was already feeling?
  - Non-verbal? From who?
  - Something else? If something else, identify the trigger.
- How do I feel in response to this event? What is the cause(s) of these emotions?
- What could I have done differently?
- What do I do now?
- What do I need to do in relation to the other person?
- What do I need to do within myself to ensure positive interactions in the future?

2. Do these questions assist you to isolate and highlight those factors that could promote a more comfortable and satisfactory interaction next time?
3. What other questions could assist you to change your patterns of thought and actions to ensure positive reactions and outcomes that produce effective communication?

Reflection is a process that, although challenging, does not have to be tedious. It takes commitment and varying amounts of time – the time typically decreases with practice. Writing in a **journal** or professional case files and sipping an enjoyable drink may assist the process of reflecting. Other people may assist if they are willing to honestly explore the reasons for any negative responses. The benefits of reflection are many for both the Person/s and the healthcare professional (Thompson 2021).

The result of reflection: achieving self-awareness

Reflection is the primary method of achieving self-awareness. It reveals the reality of the unique characteristics of each individual, thereby promoting understanding of self and others. It has the potential to create a new awareness and provide direction for constructive use of that awareness to establish the truth about the self and related events (Taylor 2011). This truth allows the individual to employ different methods of relating, reacting and behaving (Backus & Chapian 2014). Reflection promotes control of responses to ensure positive interactions. Thus reflection can promote change in future responses during all interactions, thereby contributing to the effectiveness of the communication.

Reflection is a process through which the individual considers and learns from positive and negative experiences. The individual considers the meaning of their experiences and why the experiences have that particular meaning. This consideration facilitates understanding of the inadequacy, fear or vulnerability of the inner-self that manipulates and directs thoughts and responses during interactive experiences (Murphy, 2019). These inadequacies and fears often cause negative and regrettable events during interactions and healthcare processes (Backus & Chapian 2014). The process of reflection facilitates understanding of the action required to overcome the inadequacies, fears or vulnerabilities manipulating the reactions of individuals when communicating and interacting. This understanding can increase the effectiveness of healthcare communication.

Chapter summary

Reflection facilitates awareness of factors impacting on the effectiveness of communication. It can increase self and other awareness, thereby transforming the thoughts and actions of the healthcare professional to achieve effective communication and positive healthcare outcomes. Reflection explores the reasons for the responses during interactions and interventions, along with the resultant feelings about the experiences. Reflection also encourages identification of ways to change any negative responses or results while providing care. It should involve reflexivity: examining the self and personal responses to events and experiences. The use of a model relevant to the needs and thought processes of the reflecting individual, can guide reflection to achieve increased self-awareness and control of negative responses, thereby improving healthcare. Such models suggest describing the events during the interaction or intervention, identifying the intentions of the people interacting and considering the factors (self, person and environment-related factors) contributing to the responses during the healthcare process. Reflection requires commitment, allocation of regular time to reflect in written form, particular equipment (dedicated password-protected computer file or notebook and pen) and honest consideration of the causes of any negative results of communicative interactions within healthcare.

I cannot do anything useful ...
Why worry about reflection?
I need to understand ...

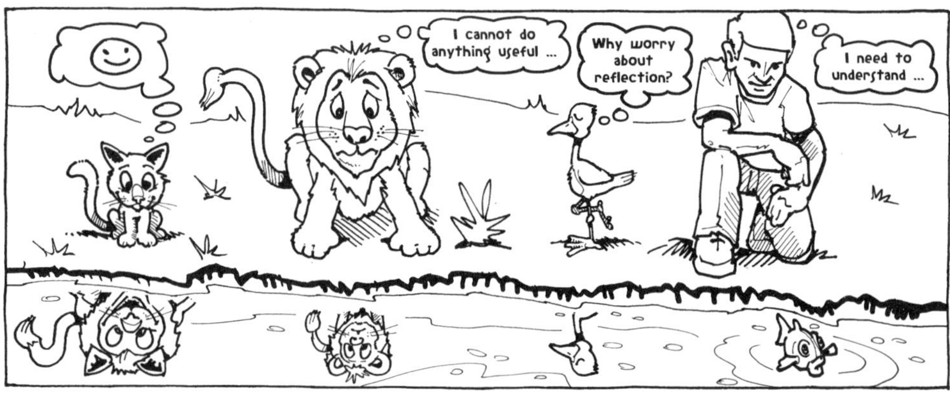

FIGURE 6.3
Reflection can identify areas requiring change.
Courtesy Roger Harvey © Elsevier Australia.

REVIEW QUESTIONS

1. Reflection is thoughtful exploration and consideration of the ________________ of experiences and ________________ during those experiences.

2. What is reflexive practice?

____

____

____

____

3. What does reflection encourage when considering future events within interactions in healthcare?

____

____

____

____

4. State three reasons why everyone uses barriers or particular responses to negative emotions.

   i. ____

   ii. ____

   iii. ____

5. What is the purpose of a model of reflection?

____

____

____

____

6. What five actions are beneficial when reflecting regardless of the particular model of reflection?

   i. ____

   ii. ____

   iii. ____

   iv. ____

   v. ____

References

American Psychiatric Association, 2022. Diagnostic and statistical manual of mental disorders, 5th ed., text revision. (DSM–5–TR). APA, Washington DC.

Australian and New Zealand Podiatry Accreditation Council, 2014. Podiatry Competency Standards for Australia and New Zealand (rev.). Australian and New Zealand Podiatry Accreditation Council, Melbourne.

Backus, W., Chapian, M., 2014. Telling yourself the truth, repackaged ed. Bethany, Ada, MI.

Bassot, B., 2020. The reflective journal, 3rd ed. Macmillan Education International, London.

Beesley, P., Watts, M., Harrison, M., 2017. Developing your communication skills in social work. Sage, London.

Blackman, J.S., 2004. 101 Defenses: How the mind shields itself. Brunner-Routledge, New York.

Bolderston, A., 2020. Continuing professional development: Reflective practice. Journal of Medical Radiation Sciences, 67(1), 96.

Boud, D., 2010. Relocating reflection in the context of practice. In: Bradbury, H., Frost, N., Kilminster, S., et al. (eds), Beyond reflective practice: New approaches to professional lifelong learning. Routledge, Abingdon.

Boud, D.J., Walker, D., 1991. Experience and learning: Reflection at work. Deakin University, Melbourne.

Boud, D.J., Walker, D., 1990. Making the most of experience. Studies in Continuing Education, 12 (2), 61–80.

Boud, D., Keogh, R., Walker, D., 1987. Reflection: Turning experience into learning. Routledge, Oxon. (Digital 2005).

Bourget-Murray, J., Page, P., Penn-Barwell, J., 2022. What's important: Postoperative debriefings and surgical team communication. Journal of Bone and Joint Surgery, 104(2), 201–202.

Ceo-DiFrancesco, D., Dunn, L.S., Solorio, N. 2020. Transforming through reflection: Use of student-led reflections in the development of intercultural competence during a short-term international immersion experience. The Internet Journal of Allied Health Sciences and Practice, 18(2), Article 8.

Cramer, P., 2020. Psychodynamic perspective of defense mechanisms. In: Carducci, B.J., Nave, C.S. (eds), The Wiley encyclopedia of personality and individual differences: Models and theories. John Wiley & Sons, Hoboken, NJ.

Cramer, P., 2018. The development of defense mechanisms during the latency period. Journal of Nervous and Mental Diseases, 206(4), 286–289.

Cramer, P., 2000. Defense mechanisms in psychology today: Further processes for adaptation. American Psychologist, 55(6), 637–646.

Davis, C.M., Musolino, G.M., 2016. Patient–practitioner interaction: an experiential manual for developing the art of healthcare, 6th ed. Slack, Thorofare, NJ.

Dean, E., 2020. How to harness your Covid-19 experience for reflective practice, Nursing Standard, 35(6), 67–69.

Devenny, B., Duffy, K., 2014. Person-centred reflective practice. Nursing Standard, 28(28), 37–43.

Edmondson, W., 2022. Transformative learning for Aboriginal and Torres Strait Islander health practice. In: Edmondson, W., Williams, R., (eds), Burda-Burda Balayi health professionals and Indigenous health: Working at the interface. Oxford University Press, Melbourne.

Egan, G., Reese R.J., 2019. The skilled helper: A problem management and opportunity approach to helping, 11th ed. Cengage, Boston MA.

Finlay, L., Gough, B. (eds), 2003. Reflexivity: A practical guide for researchers in health and social sciences. Blackwell, Oxford.

Flanagan, E., Chadwick, R., Goodrich, J., et al., 2020. Reflection for all healthcare staff: A national evaluation of Schwartz Rounds. Journal of Interprofessional Care, 34(1), 140–142.

Gibbs, G., 1988. Learning by doing: A guide to teaching and learning methods. Further Education Unit, Oxford Polytechnic, Oxford, UK.

Gustafson, C., Fagerberg, I., 2004. Reflection: The way to professional development? Journal of Clinical Nursing, 13, 271–280.

Haddad, A.M., Purtilo, R.B., Doherty, R.F., 2019. Health professional and patient interaction, 9th ed. Elsevier/Saunders, St Louis, MO.

Harms, L., Pierce, J., 2019. Working with people: Communication skills for reflective practice, 2nd Canadian ed. Oxford University Press, Ontario.

Henderson, A., 2019. Communication for health care practice. Oxford University Press, Melbourne.

Hentschel, U., Smith, G., Draguns, J.G., et al. (eds), 2004. Defense mechanisms: Theoretical, research and clinical perspectives. Elsevier, Amsterdam.

Hitchiner, J.J., 2010. A reflection on reflection. Midwifery News 58, 36–37.

Honeycutt, A., Milliken, M.A. 2021. Understanding human behavior: A guide for healthcare providers, 10th ed. Cengage Learning, Boston.

Johns, C., (ed.), 2022. Becoming a reflective practitioner, 6th ed. Wiley Blackwell, Hoboken, NJ.

Johns, C., 1993. Professional supervision. Journal of Nursing Management, 1, 9–18.

Johnston, J., Paley, G., 2013. Mirror mirror on the ward: Who is the unfairest of them all? Reflections on reflective practice groups in acute psychiatric settings. Psychoanalytic Psychotherapy, 27(2), 170–186.

Karnieli-Miller, O., 2020. Reflective practice in teaching of communication skills. Patient Education and Counseling, 103(10), 2166–2172.

Koshy, K., Limb, C., Gundogan, B., Whitehurst, K., et al., 2017. Reflective practice in health care and how to reflect effectively. International Journal of Surgery Oncology, 2(6) e20.

Levett-Jones, T., Reid-Searl, K., Bourgeois, S., 2018. The clinical placement: An essential guide for nursing students, 4th ed. Elsevier, Sydney.

Mann, K.V., 2008. Reflection: Understanding its influence on practice. Medical Education, 42(5), 449–451.

Mantel, A., Scragg, T., 2019. Reflective practice in social work, 5th ed. Sage, London.

Moss, B., 2020. Communication skills in health and social care, 5th ed. Sage, London.

Murphy, J., /revised by McMahan, I., 2019. The power of your subconscious mind. Simon & Schuster, UK.

Murray, S.A., Kendall, M., Carduff, E., et al., 2009. Use of serial qualitative interviews to understand patients' evolving experiences and needs. British Medical Journal, 338, b3702.

Neville, P., 2018. Introducing dental students to reflective practice: A dental educator's reflections. Reflective Practice, 19(2), 278 – 290.

Parker, Z., 2015. Breaking the pattern: From reactive to reflective practice. International Journal of Therapy and Rehabilitation, 22(2), 58–59.

Rogers, C., 1967. On becoming a person. Constable, London.

Smith, D.L., 2007. Why we lie: The evolutionary roots of deception and the unconscious mind. St Martin's Press, New York.

Smith-Lickess, S.K., Stefanic, N., Shaw, J., et al, 2022. What is the effect of a low literacy talking book on patient knowledge, anxiety and communication before radiation therapy starts? A pilot study. Journal of Medical Radiation Sciences, 69(4), 463–472.

Stein-Parbury, J., 2021. Patient and person: Interpersonal skills in nursing, 7th ed. Churchill Livingstone Elsevier, Sydney.

Tamparo, C.D., Lindh, W.Q., 2017. Therapeutic communication for health care professionals, 4th ed. Cengage Learning, Boston MA.

Taylor, B.A., 2011. Reflective practice for healthcare professionals, 3rd ed. Open University Press, Milton Keynes.

Thompson, N., 2021. People skills, 5th ed. Palgrave Macmillan, Basingstoke, UK.

Tregoning, C., 2015. Communication skills and enhancing clinical practice through reflective learning: A case study. British Journal of Healthcare Assistants, 9 (2), 66–69.

Vaillant, G.E., 2000. Adaptive mental mechanisms: Their role in a positive psychology. American Psychologist, 55, 89–98.

Vaillant, G.E., 1995. The wisdom of the ego. Harvard University Press, Cambridge, MA.

Wieczorek, C.C., Nowak, P., Frampton, S.B., et al., 2018. Strengthening patient and family engagement in healthcare – the New Haven recommendations. Patient Education and Counseling, 202(8), 1506–1513.

Wilkins, D., 2014. Reflective practice (key themes in health and social care). British Journal of Social Work, 44(3), 787–788.

Williams, R., 2022. Cultural safety frameworks: Principles into Practice. In: Edmondson, W., Williams, R., (eds), Burda-Burda Balayi health professionals and Indigenous health: Working at the interface. Oxford University Press, Melbourne.

CHAPTER 7

Awareness of self to enhance healthcare communication

Chapter objectives

Upon completing this chapter, readers should be able to:

- recognise the importance and benefits of self-awareness for a healthcare professional
- state some of their own values, motives, characteristics and abilities
- list the values, characteristics and abilities that benefit a healthcare professional
- demonstrate understanding of their own basic dominating relationship need(s)
- recognise the effect of conflict between needs and values
- reflect upon their listening and speaking abilities
- appreciate the relevance of differences in personality for effective communication.

Self-awareness: an essential requirement

Self-awareness or understanding "self" equips individuals to manage life (Henderson 2019). It also equips relevant individuals for an effective career as a healthcare professional. Self-awareness allows a person to know and understand him- or herself (Di'Angelo 2020). It empowers individuals to know how they will react in any situation, assisting them to understand why they react as they do in those situations (Australian Health Practitioner Regulatory Authority [AHPRA] & National Boards 2022; Egan & Reese 2019; Johns 2017). Self-awareness increases self-understanding, potentially resulting in increased understanding and control of emotions, thoughts and behaviours (Devito 2021; Henderson 2019; Siraj et al 2013). It allows the individual to be effectively self-conscious, being able to balance the demands of the interaction while being simultaneously aware of their internal thoughts and reactions (Egan & Reese 2019; Johns 2017). This understanding resulting from reflective self-awareness assists healthcare professionals to effectively empathise (Butt 2021; Edmondson 2022), and thus achieve effective care, resulting in satisfying outcomes (Lawn et al 2014; Rasheed 2015; Rasheed et al 2019).

Self-awareness potentially enables the individual to use this understanding to achieve positive interactions, resulting in effective communication and positive healthcare outcomes. Moss (2020) suggests that self-awareness of personal emotional states increases the ability of healthcare professionals to recognise and respond appropriately to the needs of others. Stein-Parbury (2021) and Rasheed and colleagues (2019) state that self-awareness is essential for developing a therapeutic relationship, thereby promoting open, honest and genuine healthcare professionals unafraid to be caring human beings. Self-awareness potentially facilitates unconditional positive regard for others without prejudice, judgement or negativity (Rogers 1967). Healthcare professionals who increase their self-awareness will consistently experience positive outcomes from their interactions (Shih et al 2009; Younas et al 2020).

Becoming self-aware is a continual journey requiring commitment and perseverance (Fathima et al 2020; Taylor 2011). When embarking on the journey towards self-awareness, it is important to remember that even the most self-aware individuals sometimes experience negative interactions. For many individuals, the level of self-awareness varies, and thus they may regularly experience negative outcomes when interacting at different times. Such times are inevitable and should motivate those committed to self-awareness to persevere in their attempts to achieve awareness and control of self. Self-awareness allows healthcare professionals to respond to the needs of the Person/s, rather than responding to their own needs. This response ultimately facilitates the desired outcome of any interaction with a healthcare professional: effective communication and Person/Family-centred Care, resulting in appropriate and effective interventions, along with positive outcomes.

The benefits of achieving self-awareness

While achieving self-awareness is sometimes uncomfortable, there are many resultant benefits. Self-awareness allows healthcare professionals to recognise, know, understand and resolve their own emotional needs. It frees healthcare professionals to choose how to react rather than reacting to fulfil unconscious emotional needs at any given time. It promotes recognition of personal strengths and understanding of areas requiring development or improvement (Davis & Musolino 2016). Self-awareness provides understanding of the inadequacies and fears that unconsciously manipulate and direct thoughts and responses while interacting (Murphy 2019). This understanding facilitates greater control while relating, decreasing regrets about interactions (Shih et al 2009). The greatest benefit of self-awareness is self-respect, facilitating acceptance, confidence and valuing of self (Shealy et al 2019). Self-acceptance empowers healthcare professionals to value and respect others regardless of the situation or reason for their need for interventions (Davis & Musolino 2016). Reflection is a key component for achieving self-awareness. There are also various management tools; for example, 360-degree feedback. This is anonymous feedback given by colleagues that can increase the level of self-awareness (Richardson 2010) and improve performance (Awdishu et al 2018).

In this chapter, the reader is encouraged to begin the journey of practising self-awareness. This chapter seeks to demonstrate, for both the healthcare professional and those around them, the benefits of self-awareness for achieving effective communication.

Beginning the journey of self-awareness

In order to become self-aware, it is essential to commit to achieving self-awareness. A reflective journal is a helpful learning tool when developing self-awareness (Beesley et al 2017; Moss 2020). Recording answers to questions and thoughts while reflecting assists in highlighting information and learning about self (Bassot 2020). It is helpful to revisit a reflective journal at later times as a reminder of the growth and change achieved from a commitment to becoming self-aware.

Answering questions about "self" is essential for achieving self-awareness. Honest answers to such questions inform individuals, empowering them to choose appropriate responses and behaviours when communicating (Henderson 2019). Answering questions about personal characteristics and related abilities begins the process of understanding "self" – or becoming self-aware – and self-regulating (Siraj et al 2013).

Part 1

- Make a list of things you enjoy doing. Of those things, what do you do well? What do you not do well?
- Make a list of things you dislike doing. Of those things, what do you do well? What do you not do well?
- Do you like the things you naturally perform well? Is this because you perform them well?
- Do you dislike things you perform poorly? Why?
- List the characteristics and abilities that assist your performance in these activities.
- List the characteristics and abilities that limit your performance in these activities.

Part 2

- Make a list of all the things you feel you do well and those you feel you do not do well, whether or not you enjoy doing them.
- Share this list with someone who knows you well and ask if they agree. If they disagree, ask them for examples to demonstrate their understanding of what you do well and what you do not do well.
- Does this interaction change the way you see your abilities?
- Are you able to believe their understanding of your abilities?
- Why or why not?

Sometimes an individual has the characteristics and abilities to perform an activity well, but past experiences and negative emotions have clouded their knowledge and understanding of those characteristics and abilities. In such situations, some people, when told they do not perform an activity well, decide to practise that activity until they do perform it well. Many activities can be conquered with practice (e.g. riding a bicycle; playing basketball; creating a chair from timber; writing assignments, presentations and reports; conducting relevant assessments; teaching; managing others; providing leadership and communicating). Other people, when told they cannot perform something well, withdraw from performing that activity, thereby never conquering it. Such decisions might not be significant where the ability is something that is not essential to quality of life (e.g. knitting or washing a car). However, some abilities (e.g. communication and self-control) are necessary for daily life, thus requiring perseverance to improve skills in those activities. There are particular characteristics that individuals develop because of personality and experience potentially promoting the development of abilities. An awareness of self provides information about those characteristics, thereby promoting thoughtful control to enhance communication.

- Are there characteristics that you do not demonstrate well that you feel you need to develop to become an effective healthcare professional (e.g. patience or flexibility or confidence when communicating with strangers or making decisions without assistance)?
- What can you do to develop these characteristics and the associated abilities?

Individual values

All people have values affecting their thoughts and actions (Williams 2022). A value is the measure of worth, importance or usefulness of something or someone (Banks 2020). Values develop while experiencing life. They originate from families, friends, teachers, the media, religious leaders and caregivers (Haddad et al 2019). Values influence thoughts, motivation, desires, dreams, decisions and actions. They contribute to the development of particular characteristics and thus abilities or inabilities. If an individual values handmade garments, they may persevere to learn knitting or sewing. If they do not, they may never begin the process of testing their abilities in either knitting or sewing. If an individual values respect of self and others when interacting, they interact to both demonstrate and expect respect (Harms & Pierce 2019). Values can provide stability when experiencing emotionally and/or morally challenging situations in practice. Accurate self-awareness of values can guard against self-doubt during such experiences. This indicates the importance of awareness of personal values (Kay 2018) and, where possible, awareness of the values of the Person/s to ensure appropriate responses and actions.

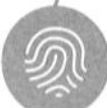

What do I value?

Make a list of what is important to you. The items on the list may be objects (e.g. car, phone, computer), specific people (e.g. son, sister, father, partner), characteristics (e.g. perseverance, organised, aggression), states of being (e.g. health, wellbeing, safety), or particular activities (e.g. shopping, travelling, volunteering).

Why do I value these?

- Consider the items on the list and decide why you value them. One reason might be the way they make you feel, while another reason may be that your family or friends think these things are important.
- Have your values changed over time? Consider each one on your list and state how they have changed and what caused the change.

Exploring and sharing the reasons for valuing

In groups of four:

- Share your listed values and the reasons why you value them.
- List any common values among the members of the group.
- List any of these values that are essential for a healthcare professional.

Is a healthcare profession an appropriate choice?

There are particular values, characteristics and abilities that facilitate effective practice in the healthcare professions. It is important to be aware of these values, characteristics and abilities. This awareness assists in verifying the choice to become a healthcare professional. Some individuals pursue a career in a healthcare profession because someone they admire is a healthcare professional or because they are sure of employment upon completion of their studies. These individuals may be seeking a career that does not suit their interests, values or abilities. Other individuals pursue a career in a healthcare profession because they are aware of the role, the values and the required characteristics and abilities of the profession, and feel they meet the necessary requirements.

Others may not pursue a career in the healthcare professions because they lack awareness that their interests, values, characteristics and abilities are well suited to such a career. Still others do not pursue a career in the healthcare professions because it does not provide the economic return they desire or because it is too consuming of time and emotions. The reasons for the choice to become a healthcare professional usually indicate the values of that individual.

Values of a healthcare professional

The overall purpose of healthcare professions focuses on supporting the health and wellbeing of the Person/s or others. Sometimes this overall purpose focuses on individuals, and at other times on individuals within the context of a family or community. If people are the central focus of all healthcare professions, it seems appropriate to assume that all healthcare professionals must value and appreciate people (Shih et al 2009). If healthcare professionals do not value and appreciate people and their associated needs, they can potentially produce inappropriate and ineffective interactions and interventions.

- Together, define “health”. Does your healthcare profession value health? How does your healthcare profession demonstrate this value?
- Now define “quality of life”. Does your healthcare profession value quality of life? How does your healthcare profession demonstrate this value?
- Now define “wellbeing”. Does your healthcare profession value wellbeing? How does it demonstrate this in practice?

In groups of the same healthcare profession:

- list and define other values of your healthcare profession
- suggest other healthcare professions that share these values.

It is important that healthcare professionals value both themselves and others (Boggs 2023; Rasheed 2015). Demonstrations of respect, expressions of empathy and development of trust indicate the desire of the healthcare professional to understand and assist people. It is important that healthcare professionals value the therapeutic relationship by developing rapport using collaboration and listening to empower. In combination, these essential factors of all healthcare promote Person/Family-centred Care. It is also essential that healthcare professionals value the knowledge and skills specific to their profession and those of other healthcare professions. If these values are not important to an individual, that individual should not become a healthcare professional.

Characteristics and abilities that enhance the practice of a healthcare professional

While particular healthcare professions require specific interests and abilities, there are underlying characteristics and associated abilities that benefit individuals in all healthcare professions. The questions on the previous pages highlight some of these characteristics and abilities. Completion of the following activity should assist in highlighting abilities suited to healthcare professional practice, along with the presence of these abilities in the reader.

Am I suited to a healthcare profession?

Stage 1

Answer the following questions and list characteristics or events that validate your answer.

- Do I generally enjoy relating to people?
- Do I enjoy relating to people who are different to me, regardless of the differences?
- Do I enjoy relating to people who require assistance?
- Am I able to relate to people who are expressing strong negative emotions?
- Can I generally think clearly when others are expressing negative emotions?
- Do I generally enjoy communicating with people?
- Am I an effective and appropriate communicator?
- Am I typically empathic when relating to others?
- Do I enjoy creative problem-solving?
- Do I enjoy empowering people to assist themselves?
- Do I enjoy encouraging people?
- Do I enjoy assisting in solving problems with other people?
- Do I enjoy challenges?
- Am I generally patient with myself and others?
- Am I an active and effective listener?
- Do I usually attempt to understand myself and other people?
- Am I emotionally flexible? (able to control emotions according to the needs of the context)

Stage 2

- Consider the questions in Stage 1 and name the characteristics and/or abilities highlighted in the questions. Does your healthcare profession value these? Decide whether all health-care professions value these characteristics and abilities.

Stage 3

Do you feel you exhibit these characteristics and abilities?

- Which ones do you feel you perform well?
- What has contributed to your development of these characteristics and abilities?
- Which ones do you feel you do not perform well?
- What has limited your development of these characteristics and abilities?
- What can you do to develop those characteristics and abilities you feel you do not perform well?

Personal unconscious needs

There are unconscious needs that every individual has which contribute to "inabilities" or limitations in relationships (Stein-Parbury 2021). These unconscious needs create typical ways of relating. They affect the characteristics and outcomes of relationships. This reality indicates the importance of healthcare professionals being aware of the basic needs that dominate ways of relating and their expectations of relationships. There are three basic human relationship needs:

1. the need to be accepted and valued – to have a "place", feel special and know that others care (Honeycutt & Milliken 2021; Levine 2012)
2. the need to be in control
3. the need for affection and affirmation (Stein-Parbury 2021).

All humans have these needs. At different times, individuals long to feel valued for who they are, as they are – to feel accepted and special. This need may express itself through relationships in which that individual is always fulfilling the needs of others and "doing" for others, regardless of whether or not the other can "do" it for themselves. These people find it difficult to say no when asked to assist. Some people have a predominant need for control, and thus will limit involvement in relationships and unpredictable situations. This need expresses itself in relationships with others who are happy to do exactly what the person requires, in the exact manner. These people find it difficult to enter situations involving risk-taking or change. Other individuals predominantly seek affection and affirmation in relationships. They consistently seek relationships that affirm whatever they do or want. These people crave affirmation and fear rejection, therefore often finding it difficult to say "no". While everyone experiences these needs, some people have a consistently dominant area of need influencing all their relationships and interactions. The dominant need of individuals may vary according to the events in their lives at a particular time. It is important for individuals who choose a career in a healthcare profession to know which of these needs typically dominate their relationships, and the situations that might trigger this unconscious need.

- Discuss each basic human relationship need listed above and suggest the effects of each need on the communication and relationships of healthcare professionals.
- Consider how these needs might affect individuals seeking healthcare and suggest how a healthcare professional might manage each of these needs in the Person/s seeking care.
- For each need, state specific actions that reflect the basic need. How might these actions relate to your particular healthcare profession?

Awareness of the dominant area of personal need(s) allows the healthcare professional to make choices to fulfil the needs of the Person/s rather than fulfilling their own needs. Answering particular questions (see following page) may assist in highlighting which basic human relationship need typically dominates ways of relating in different individuals.

Reflecting upon answers to these questions is important for healthcare professionals. Such reflection increases self-awareness and control of thoughts and emotional reactions. It also decreases the fulfilment of personal needs while practising as a healthcare professional, thereby increasing the ability to achieve effective communication and focus on fulfilling the needs of the Person/s.

Conflict between values and needs

When practising as a healthcare professional, it is possible to assist people who demonstrate detrimental habits resulting from conflict between personal values and relationship needs. In such circumstances it is the responsibility of the healthcare professional to provide non-judgemental assistance. Self-awareness of the personal values and needs of the healthcare professional promotes self-control and positive understanding of the Person/s. Self-awareness potentially frees the healthcare professional to make the choice to provide non-judgemental assistance. Considering their own experiences of conflict between personal values and needs reminds the healthcare professional of the difficulties associated with this conflict, thereby facilitating greater tolerance and genuine understanding of those seeking healthcare.

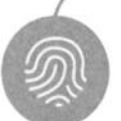

1. Answer each question with *yes, no* or *sometimes*. In reality, the three basic human relationship needs will be true for everyone some of the time (Stein-Parbury 2021). However, these questions ask for the *usual* tendency you experience. Remember that honest answers will increase your self-awareness, potentially empowering you to overcome the "inabilities" or limitations associated with relating because of a predominant need.
   - Do I have a well-defined physical comfort zone that I do not enjoy leaving?
   - Do I have a well-defined emotional comfort zone that I do not enjoy leaving?
   - Do I have a well-defined social comfort zone that I do not enjoy leaving?
   - Do I usually feel there is only one answer to a problem and one way to do tasks? Or that there is only one place to keep certain things?
   - Do I usually feel I must have the answer to every situation and problem?
   - Do I only enjoy relating to people who need my help?
   - Do I often feel I am the only person who can solve certain problems?
   - Do I define myself by doing things for other people who need me?
   - Do I often feel I must fix a problem?
   - Do I often feel I must do something to make things better and to "rescue" people?
   - Do I only feel OK if I am helping people?
   - Do I usually respond strongly to any critical comment about me?
   - Do I find that other people often act in ways that are inappropriate or annoying?
   - Do I find it easy to see the negative rather than the positive aspects of a person?
   - Do I stop relating to people when I experience a difficult interaction with them?
   - Do I find it easy to form negative ideas about people who are different to me?
   - Do I find it easy to have ideas about a person because of their appearance?
   - Do I find it difficult to say no to requests for help?
   - Do I usually want other people to take care of me?
   - Do I often worry about whether people like me or not?
   - Do I feel most content when people do exactly what I want?
   - Do I feel better when people are telling me I am great?
2. Classify each question into the three basic human needs. Some may fulfil two needs.
3. Consider your answers to the questions and decide which basic need(s) typically dominate(s) your way of relating.
4. Write down what you could do to control this need(s) in order to ensure that you, as a healthcare professional, are able to meet the needs of others.

In small groups of no more than three:

1. Agree on the classification of the needs represented in each question.
2. Match the following characteristics to one or more of the basic human needs: controlling, self-focused, inflexible, need-to-be-needed, scheming, rigid, selfish, cold, calculating, self-absorbed, manipulative, stubborn, attention-seeking, judgemental, intolerant, perfectionist.
3. List any other characteristics that would represent one or more of the basic human needs.
4. Discuss the possibility that there may be gender differences in the experience and expression of these needs. Give examples of the possible differences.
5. Explore factors potentially producing gender differences and decide how this might affect healthcare.
6. Decide how knowledge of basic human needs affects a healthcare professional.

In situations where someone has developed a detrimental habit (such as alcoholism, overeating, self-harming or drug abuse) because their dominant need has overcome their values, the healthcare professional should not express either verbal or non-verbal judgement. It is important to remember that the Person/s is feeling vulnerable and insecure and possibly disempowered. The healthcare professional seeks to empower people to achieve change, and a judgemental response will only discourage rather than empower. Awareness of personal values and needs, and the possible conflict between the two, is important for all healthcare professionals. This awareness assists them to understand the existence of the detrimental habit resulting from such conflict. Awareness of the existence and experience of conflict between values and needs can assist healthcare professionals to overcome any of their own detrimental habits, assisting them to overcome those habits.

Perfectionism as a value

The value of "**perfectionism**", or always being right in actions and words, may override the need for affection and affirmation. Individuals who value perfectionism may value being right above everything else. When experiencing being wrong, they cannot recognise positive elements of interactions. For such individuals, the value of perfectionism overcomes the need for and often the ability to receive affection and affirmation (Backus & Chapian 2014). Individuals who value perfectionism can develop the detrimental habit of constantly telling themselves that whatever they say or do is not good enough, regardless of the often-exceptional quality of the attempt. Consistent affirmation, affection and repeated truth about the quality of the attempts are required to overcome this detrimental habit.

This value of perfectionism results in some individuals finding it difficult to complete and submit something (e.g. a written assignment or medical records). It can also result in individuals redoing the same thing repeatedly, despite their skill in the task and the adequacy of their initial attempt. Other individuals may perform a task, but only see the imperfections, regardless of the overall quality of the result. For other individuals, the overriding value of perfectionism can mean they do not complete something as well as they are able to because they feel they will not do it well enough – they will not reach perfection. When individuals refuse to do something because they believe they will not achieve an appropriate level of perfection, they may not be able to admit their feelings of inadequacy.

Negative self-talk can result in an individual refusing to attempt something with anyone else present, despite their competence in the activity. Perfectionism may mean that the individual is constantly planning future tasks – making lists of things to do and ways to complete those things – in an attempt to remember everything or to mentally prepare to "perfectly" complete the tasks. It can also mean those people find it difficult to believe or accept any form of affirmation about the quality of their performance.

Self-awareness of personal communication skills

Some individuals are effective communicators from birth, others develop skills through life experiences, and others make conscious efforts to become effective communicators. Effective communicators are able to express themselves clearly, listen effectively, while observing all non- verbal messages. They are committed to understanding the needs of their "audience" and producing messages to negotiate mutual understanding. If the audience does not demonstrate understanding, effective communicators take turns at communicating and negotiating to guarantee mutual understanding and thus effective communication. They listen carefully, responding to facilitate further positive and effective communication.

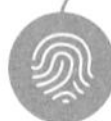

- Do you enjoy communicating verbally? Why do you think this is so?
- Do you usually listen when communicating verbally? Why do you do this?
- Do you usually talk? Why do you do this? What do you usually talk about?
- Which do you prefer – listening or talking? Why is this so?
- Do you ask questions about the other person to continue the communication?
- Do you often request clarification?
- Do you let others ask questions or speak rather than you talking?
- Do you usually finish a verbal interaction feeling satisfied?
- Do you often feel dissatisfied after a communicative interaction?
- Do you enjoy communicating if you feel unmotivated to communicate?

In providing answers to the questions above, many people may note that their role when communicating varies depending on the topic and the people communicating. This is often true and may indicate that the individual is an effective communicator, typically responding appropriately to any topic, audience, situation or context. Alternatively, it may indicate an uncertainty when communicating that could benefit from reflection and conscious efforts to develop skills in effective communication. If the honest answers to these questions were predominantly *yes*, this could indicate skill in listening and speaking, while answers of predominantly *no* could indicate lack of skill or confidence in either. A healthcare professional must demonstrate skill and confidence when communicating to facilitate excellence in practice and the achievement of Person/Family-centred goals and Care (Younas et al 2020). This may require commitment and perseverance to deliberately explore personal values and often along with the values of colleagues and employers. This will facilitate understanding of the diversity of implied values, resulting in improved communication in multi-disciplinary contexts (Eaton & Mason 2019).

Self-awareness of skills for effective listening

Full attention is not always necessary for effective communication in personal situations. For a healthcare professional, however, effective listening requires full attention, skill and often practice (see Chapter 11). Listening must be adapted to the particular individual and the context (Devito 2021). It requires active engagement with the person and their message (Devito 2021; Myers & Krepper 2020). The listener indicates active engagement through appropriate non-verbal cues (see Chapter 10). Effective listening requires understanding of more than the words being spoken; it also requires understanding of the expressed emotions. Effective listening is an essential skill for a healthcare professional because it demonstrates empathy, respect and trustworthiness. Effective listening is characteristic of a therapeutic relationship promoting Person/Family-centred goals and Care. Everyone, however, is guilty of ineffective listening at particular times. Understanding the reasons for ineffective listening empowers the healthcare professional to overcome those reasons, and, whenever necessary, practise effective listening.

Self-awareness of skills for effective speaking

Self-awareness can assist an individual to identify the characteristics and abilities that enable **effective speaking** skills. Some people demonstrate interest in others with ease and **efficacy**. Such individuals demonstrate this interest naturally when communicating, whether speaking or listening. They typically demonstrate an engaging enthusiasm for their topic and their listeners, thereby promoting understanding. Some individuals have a natural ability to effectively interpret non-verbal cues in messages, while others must learn the meaning of such cues from experience. Some are naturally observant, noticing relevant aspects of individuals and relevant aspects of situations or environments. Some can intuitively understand the abilities and needs of those around them, while others must ask for information concerning those abilities and needs. Some people can think quickly and respond appropriately regardless of the situation, while others must compensate for lacking this ability with various strategies to achieve effective communication. All these skills assist in achieving effective communication when interacting. It is important that individuals know and understand their spoken abilities. Such understanding allows the healthcare professional to either practise the skill of speaking or employ strategies to facilitate effective speaking when communicating.

Skills producing effective speaking include personal abilities; familiarity and comfort with the topic; experience; skill in **interpreting** non-verbal behaviours; and skill in perceiving and understanding the characteristics of each Person/s. It is important for healthcare professionals to be aware of this complexity when developing skills in speaking. Effective speaking requires demonstration of interest and enthusiasm for both the topic and the "audience". It requires skill in, as well as knowledge and understanding of, the particular topic. Studying to become a particular healthcare professional potentially provides this skill, knowledge and understanding. Effective speaking requires understanding of the non-verbal behaviours affecting the presentation and meaning of spoken words. It also requires understanding of the listening individual(s) or the audience.

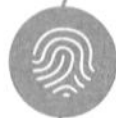

Write down your answers to the following questions:

- What factors encourage you to demonstrate interest and enthusiasm for a subject when speaking or interacting?
- What do you usually do to indicate this interest and enthusiastic focus?
- What encourages you to demonstrate interest and enthusiasm towards the person/people (audience) listening?
- What would you do to demonstrate interest and focus on each individual person?
- How do you demonstrate interest and enthusiasm through your words?
- How do you demonstrate interest and focus through your non-verbal behaviour?

In groups, discuss answers to these questions:

- What can healthcare professionals do to demonstrate interest and enthusiastic focus?
- What might assist them in this demonstration?
- What factors might limit this demonstration? How could they overcome these factors?
- Choose a scenario from Section 4 that the group finds *uninteresting*.
- Discuss ways to demonstrate interest and enthusiastic focus for the Person/s in this scenario.

A genuine interest in and enthusiasm for the topic, the Person/s and their health journey is important. Such interest and enthusiasm should produce a desire in the healthcare professional to understand and engage with the Person/s and the relevant information about them. This desire and the resultant knowledge should promote the use of appropriate words and sentence structures to facilitate Person/s and healthcare professional understanding. The use of appropriate non-verbal behaviour will further facilitate Person/s understanding and, ultimately, mutual understanding. Interest and enthusiastic focus on behalf of the healthcare professionals, in turn, creates an interest within the Person/s. These emotions encourage the Person/s to engage with the healthcare professionals, potentially assisting in developing and maintaining consistent concentration. They create a desire to know and understand the presented information, enhancing effectiveness in communication and resultant interventions.

Healthcare professionals typically use culturally unique and specific language and behaviours. These are an important aspect of the culture and identity of each health profession. It is therefore important to recognise that the average Person/s is unfamiliar with this language and method of communicating (Boggs 2023). They will also not understand the related behaviours or actions or their purpose. Using this language and these behaviours can be both alienating and disempowering for the Person/s. Therefore, one of the key skills for healthcare professionals is to adapt their communication to each Person/s to ensure mutual understanding, maximum engagement and empowerment. In contrast, healthcare professionals may use medical terminology with individuals from their health profession and other healthcare professionals to ensure the accuracy of their communication and thus interventions for the Person/s. It is important to accommodate the abilities and understanding of the current "audience" when communicating as a healthcare professional.

Personality and resultant communicative behaviours

Over the centuries there have been many descriptions of human personality types affecting communication. The ideas of Hippocrates (460–370 BC) led to the description of four basic temperaments: sanguine, choleric, melancholic and phlegmatic (Arikha 2007; Kagan 1998). The ideas of Plato (approximately 428–347 BC) led to the development of four descriptors: artisan, idealist, guardian and rationalist (Keirsey 1998). The ideas of the Hellenistic philosophers led to the development of the following descriptions of personality: idealist, traditionalist, hedonist and rationalist (Long & Sedley 1987). In the early twentieth century, Carl Jung (1941) pursued theories of the collective unconscious, archetypes and personality types (Berger 2006). In the mid-twentieth century, Oscar Ichazo from Bolivia suggested the Enneagram of personality, which identifies nine types: reformer, helper, achiever, individualist, investigator, loyalist, enthusiast, challenger and peacemaker (Riso & Hudson 2000). Later in that century, Isabel Briggs Myers and her mother Katharine Briggs began exploring the Jungian theories to explain differences in personality; this resulted in the Myers-Briggs Type Indicator (MBTI) (Briggs & Myers 1975). Wilson (2010) suggested social styles of relating: analytical, driver, amiable and expressive. These are only a few of the ways of describing human personality. Understanding of the basic **personality preferences** and combinations thereof, regardless of the system, assists healthcare professionals to understand their own communicative behaviour and that of others. Particular tendencies determined by personality produce particular characteristics and thus variations in managing communicative interactions. These characteristics predict a preference for relating in a particular manner within particular situations, and may predict a different style in other circumstances.

An awareness of the different personality types assists with the understanding of differences in styles of communicating. Some personality types enjoy working with people and are better communicators than others; others are task-oriented and prefer to work alone. Individuals can generally adjust their personality tendencies while communicating if they possess well-developed skills in self-awareness. Knowledge and awareness of individual tendencies can assist individuals to make the required adjustments and to recognise, understand and accept different tendencies in others. Healthcare professionals can use this knowledge of differences in the Person/s or colleagues to achieve effective communication and appropriate interventions.

Chapter summary

Self-awareness or understanding of "Self" is important and beneficial for all healthcare professionals. It requires commitment, time, reflection and a sense of humour. Self-awareness sometimes feels uncomfortable. However, it allows the healthcare professional to identify their personal values and abilities (along with communication preferences and skills) and to acknowledge and control their thoughts (including negative self-talk) and negative emotions while communicating. It facilitates positive attitudes; honest, open interactions consistently promoting beneficial outcomes, while interacting within the diversity experienced when practising as a healthcare professional.

Self-awareness assists healthcare professionals to be aware of their basic primary relationship needs and how to control those needs when providing healthcare. It also facilitates awareness of personal listening and speaking preferences. Self-awareness facilitates acceptance of people with different, sometimes opposite values, abilities and personalities allowing the healthcare professional to relate with understanding rather than judgement. The results of self-awareness when working in a healthcare profession outweigh the challenges. It enhances effective communication and Person/Family-centred Care, thereby producing positive outcomes.

Effective communicators talk and act like people. Not like Gorillas.
Hurry up. Tell me what I want to know.

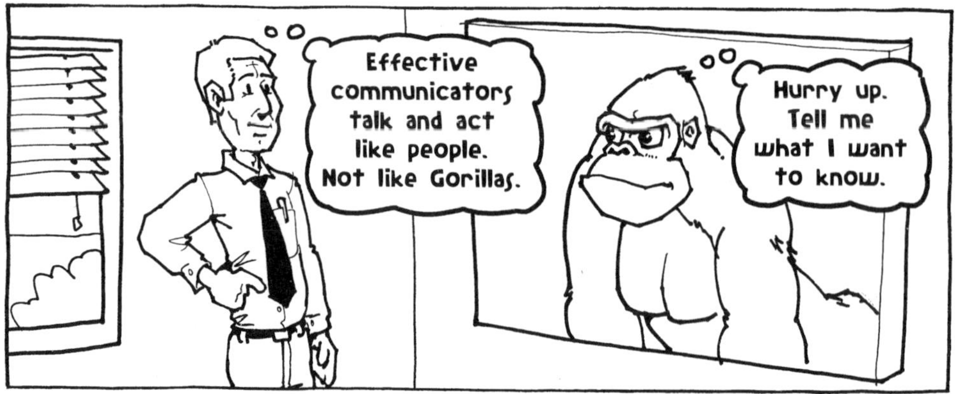

FIGURE 7.1
An effective communicator knows when they communicate like a gorilla!
Courtesy Roger Harvey © Elsevier Australia.

REVIEW QUESTIONS

1. What four actions does self-awareness allow the healthcare professional to perform?

    i. ____________________

    ii. ____________________

    iii. ____________________

    iv. ____________________

2. What are three unconscious primary needs that manipulate people?

    i. ____________________

    ii. ____________________

    iii. ____________________

3. Why is it beneficial for a healthcare professional to understand the existence of conflict between needs and values?

____

____

____

____

4. How does perfectionism affect people?

____

____

____

____

5. How might an understanding of the variations in personality assist a healthcare professional?

____

____

____

____

6. What does self-awareness achieve for the healthcare professional in practice?

____

____

____

____

References

Arikha, N., 2007. Passion and tempers: A history of the humours. HarperCollins, New York.

Australian Health Practitioner Regulation Authority (AHPRA) & National Boards, 2022. Code of Conduct. AHPRA, Sydney.

Awdishu, L., Zheng, A., Granas, A.G., et al., 2018. 360-degree feedback model to enhance interprofessional learning (Version 1). MedEdPublish, 7, 154.

Backus, W., Chapian, M., 2014. Telling yourself the truth, repackaged ed. Bethany, Ada, MI.

Banks, S., 2020. Ethics and values in social work, 5th ed. Red Globe Press, London.

Bassot, B., 2020. The reflective journal, 3rd ed. Macmillan Education International, London.

Beesley, P., Watts, M., Harrison, M., 2017. Developing your communication skills in social work. Sage, London.

Berger, A.A., 2006. 50 ways to understand communication. Rowan & Littlefield, Oxford.

Boggs, K., 2023. Interpersonal relationships: Professional communication skills for nurses, 9th ed. Elsevier, St Louis, MO.

Briggs, K., Myers, I.B., 1975. The Myers-Briggs type indicator. Consulting Psychologist Press, Palo Alto, CA.

Butt, M.F., 2021. Approaches to building rapport with patients. Clinical Medicine (London), 21(6), e662–663.

Di'Angelo, R., 2020. Who is Phoenix? Journal of Medical Ethics, 46(11),753–754.

Davis, C.M., Musolino, G.M., 2016. Patient–practitioner interaction: An experiential manual for developing the art of healthcare, 6th ed. Slack, Thorofare, NJ.

Devito, J.A., 2021. The interpersonal communication book, 16th ed. Pearson, Boston.

Eaton, G., Mason, P., 2019. Values: What are they worth in paramedicine? Canadian Paramedicine, 42(1), 18–19.

Edmondson, W., 2022. Transformative learning for Aboriginal and Torres Strait Islander health practice. In: Edmondson, W., Williams, R. (eds), Burda-Burda Balayi health professionals and Indigenous health: Working at the interface. Oxford University Press, Melbourne.

Egan, G., Reese, R.J., 2019. The skilled helper: A problem management and opportunity approach to helping, 10th ed. Cengage, Boston MA.

Fathima, F., Chantal, C., Thavanesi, G., 2020. Using life story on the journey to self-awareness with patients in a wellness program at a mental health care facility. Occupational Therapy in Mental Health, 36(4), 353–372.

Haddad, A.M., Purtilo, R.B., Doherty, R.F., 2019. Health professional and patient interaction, 9th ed. Elsevier/Saunders, St Louis, MO.

Harms, L., Pierce, J., 2019. Working with people: Communication skills for reflective practice. 2nd Canadian ed. Oxford University Press, Ontario.

Henderson, A., 2019. Communication for health care practice. Oxford University Press, Melbourne.

Honeycutt, A., Milliken, M.A., 2021. Understanding human behavior: A guide for healthcare providers, 10th ed. Cengage Learning, Boston.

Johns, C., 2017. A reflective framework for clinical practice. In C. Johns (ed.), Becoming a reflective practitioner. Wiley & Sons, UK.

Jung, C.G., 1941. The development of personality. Routledge, London.

Kagan, J., 1998. Galen's prophecy: Temperament in human nature. Basic Books, New York.

Kay, N.S. 2018. Self-awareness in personal transformation. In: Neal, J. (ed.) Handbook of personal and organizational transformation. Springer, Fayetteville, AR.

Keirsey, D., 1998. Please understand me II: Temperament, character and intelligence. Prometheus Nemesis Books, Delmar.

Lawn, S., Delany, T., Sweet, L., et al., 2014. Control in chronic condition self-care management: How it occurs in the health worker–client relationship and implications for client empowerment. Journal of Advanced Nursing, 70 (2), 383–394.

Levine, J., 2012. Working with people: The helping process, 9th ed. Pearson, San Antonio.

Long, A.A., Sedley, D.N., 1987. The Hellenistic philosophers, vol. 1. Cambridge University Press, Cambridge.

Moss, B., 2020. Communication skills in health and social care, 5th ed. Sage, London.

Murphy, J., /revised by McMahan, I., 2019. The power of your subconscious mind. Simon & Schuster, UK.

Myers, K.K., Krepper, R., 2020. Nurses' active empathic listening behaviours from the voice of the patient. Nursing Economics, 38(5) 267–275.

Rasheed, S.P., 2015. Self-awareness as a therapeutic tool for nurse/client relationship. International Journal of Caring Sciences, 8(1), 211–216.

Rasheed, S.P., Younas, A., Sundus, A., 2019. Self-awareness in nursing: A scoping review. Journal of Clinical Nursing, 28(5–6), 762–774.

Richardson, R.F., II, 2010. 360-degree feedback: Integrating business know-how with social work values. Administration in Social Work, 34(3), 259–274.

Riso, D.R., Hudson, R., 2000. Understanding the Enneagram: The practical guide to personality types. Houghton Mifflin, Chicago.

Rogers, C., 1967. On becoming a person. Constable, London.

Shealy, S.C., Worrall, C.L., Baker, J.L., et al., 2019. Assessment of faculty and preceptor development intervention to foster self-awareness and self-confidence. American Journal of Pharmaceutical Education, 83(7), 1534–1546.

Shih, F., Lin, Y., Smith, M.C., et al., 2009. Perspectives on professional values among nurses in Taiwan. Journal of Clinical Nursing, 18(10), 1480–1489.

Siraj, H.H., Salam, A., Hani Azmina, C.M.N.A., et al., 2013. Self awareness and reflective skills in the promotion of personal and professional development of future medical professionals. Education in Medicine Journal, 5 (4), 29–33.

Stein-Parbury, J., 2021. Patient and person: Interpersonal skills in nursing, 7th ed. Churchill Livingstone Elsevier, Sydney.

Taylor, B.J., 2011. Reflective practice for healthcare professionals, 3rd ed. Open University Press, Milton Keynes, UK.

Williams, R., 2022. Cultural safety frameworks: Principles into practice. In: Edmondson, W., Williams, R., (eds), Burda-Burda Balayi health professionals and Indigenous health: Working at the interface. Oxford University Press, Melbourne.

Wilson, L., 2010. The social styles handbook: Find your comfort zone and make people feel comfortable with you. Nova Vista Publishing, Portland.

Younas, A., Rasheed, S.P., Sundus, A., et al., 2020. Nurses' perspectives of self-awareness in nursing practice: A descriptive qualitative study. Nursing and Health Sciences, 22(2), 398–405.

CHAPTER 8

Awareness of how personal assumptions affect healthcare communication

Chapter objectives

Upon completing this chapter, readers should be able to:

- understand and recognise personal assumptions and associated stereotypical judgements
- account for the effect of stereotypical judgement upon communication
- examine some of their personal stereotypical prejudices and expectations
- demonstrate the importance of communicating without judgement
- describe the characteristics of a healthcare professional who communicates without judgement
- explain how to overcome tendencies to assume, stereotype and judge
- develop strategies that promote non-judgemental communication.

Personal assumptions can negatively affect communication. Such assumptions and underlying biases, potentially originating from values and beliefs, may produce stereotypical, value-laden judgements of and **prejudice** towards particular types of individuals and groups (Abdou et al 2016; Levine 2012). The values and beliefs of an individual, although often invisible, provide the foundation for assumptions and biases, and ultimately discrimination, in healthcare (Johnson & Withers 2018; Thompson 2020). This can affect the quality of care and resultant healthcare outcomes. Therefore, it is important for all healthcare professionals to be aware of and understand their thoughts, reactions and characteristics possibly resulting in biases and judgements. These often-irrational biases develop over time from significant others or parental models (Honeycutt & Milliken 2021). These assumptions (sometimes false) and biases create stereotypical judgements (Edmondson 2022). Value-laden, stereotypical judgements often occur because of appearance or some observable behaviour or characteristic creating stereotypical expectations (Abdou & Fingerhut 2014; Clement et al 2015; Haddad et al 2019; Loch et al 2014). Communicating without judgement occurs when the healthcare professional *avoids* making a **judgement** about a Person/s regardless of differences, appearance, socioeconomic status and circumstances (Johnson & Withers 2018; Passi 2018). This requires understanding and control of the factors contributing to those biases and judgements.

Stereotypical judgements may be positive or negative. For example, if being able-bodied and fit are considered positive attributes, a judgement stating that surfers are able-bodied and fit is positive. However, this statement may not always be true. Similarly, if violence and terrorism are considered negative attributes, a judgement stating that all Muslims condone violence and terrorism is negative. However, this statement is definitely not true. A **stereotype** is a fixed impression about an individual or group (Devito 2021; Eckermann et al 2016) that may have some connection with reality due to the appearance of similarities within the individual or group. A stereotype in itself may initially be beneficial because it provides a framework from which to commence communicating (Eckermann et al 2016). However, a negative stereotype producing prejudice and judgement (Liu et al 2018) can dominate all communication with an individual or group, causing detrimental outcomes. They can limit the possibility of relating to more than the stereotype (Holliday et al 2021). This potentially produces discrimination, thereby compromising any learning about the individual and the development of a therapeutic relationship. This ultimately compromises the quality of care.

Reasons to avoid stereotypical judgement when communicating

Assumptions, biases, prejudice and resultant stereotypical judgements can negatively affect communication. They may result in conflict, misunderstandings and communication breakdown, and therefore poor health outcomes (Abdou et al 2016). They may also affect expressions of empathy and the therapeutic relationship (Sloane & Petra 2021). These are good reasons why healthcare professionals should avoid prejudice-based stereotypical judgements (Egan & Reese 2019). However, there are additional reasons to avoid stereotypical judgements. Stereotypical attitudes often develop from limited information (ignorance) or misinformed assumptions (Holliday et al 2021; Levine 2012), thus producing incorrect judgements (Borden 2018) and discrimination (Beesley et al 2017; Moss 2020). In addition, relating to someone through a stereotype potentially reduces the Person/s to something that is less than who they are; that is, to the confines of the stereotype. Therefore, the healthcare professional is not allowing the Person/s to have thoughts, opinions and habits different from the stereotype. It is also possible that the stereotype is based on an unconscious belief about an "in" group and a subordinate "out" group (Bowe et al 2014). This suggests that the beliefs or culture of the individual making the stereotypical judgement are the standard for evaluating the "other" Person/s or culture (Higginbottom et al 2014; Paternotte et al 2015; Sandín-Vázquez et al 2014; Sloane & Petra 2021). Stereotypical judgement usually occurs unconsciously and thus has serious implications for healthcare professionals (Johnson & Withers 2018). If unconscious, prejudice and possible resultant stereotypical judgements will unknowingly influence the communication of the healthcare professional, with potentially unpleasant results (Moss 2020) and the possibility of compromising interventions.

Although a stereotypical judgement may benefit the individual holding the stereotype, by justifying their own characteristics, values or behaviours, it produces lenses that negatively affect communication. Therefore, a stereotypical judgement creates barriers when communicating

(Clement et al 2015; Cook et al 2014; Phelan et al 2015) and when providing care. The first barrier occurs if there exists a preconceived or fixed idea about the individual or their group (Brochu et al 2014; Moss 2020). This idea will limit the ability to hear or experience anything that is different from the constructs of the stereotype. The second barrier limits the possibility of relating to particular qualities or abilities within the individual if those qualities contradict the stereotype. In such cases, the stereotypical judgement may not allow the individual to be unique or different to the stereotype. For example, a young healthcare professional can be as competent as an older one, but a stereotypical judgement may not allow them to be considered competent. Alternatively, an elderly person may lead a very active life despite the stereotypical judgement that elderly people are frail and dependent (Christman 2014). If such stereotypical judgements occur, all communicators experience limited negotiation of meaning and mutual understanding – if such judgements do occur, there will be limited success in communication. More importantly, while these barriers limit the possibility of effective communication, they also limit the potential to achieve Person/Family-centred Care and positive intervention outcomes.

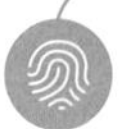

Explore your prejudice

- What are your honest answers to the following questions?
  - Are you willing to be close friends with someone from any other culture or religious group?
  - Are you willing to have a long-term romantic relationship with someone from another culture, political party or religious group?
  - Are you willing to choose to talk to someone who "lives on the street" (is homeless) when you are out shopping?
  - Are you willing to allow people who are obviously different to you to have value and credibility?
- Are you able to answer the questions above with a definite yes? If not, are you able to determine the reason for your uncertainty and the source of any of your biases?
- What can a healthcare professional do to overcome any unconscious tendency to prejudice or stereotypical judgements?

Adapted from Devito 2019

Stereotypical judgement relating to roles

Stereotypical judgements often lead to expectations of particular behaviour within particular roles. This is potentially as detrimental as applying a stereotype to the characteristics of an individual or group (Cook et al 2014). Expectations of particular behaviour from an individual in the role of an administration assistant, for example, are beneficial whenever that individual behaves according to those expectations. If an individual expects an administration assistant to make their favourite hot drink every morning, but the administration assistant does not consider that activity part of their role, there will be potential disappointment and maybe frustration in one individual and anger in the other. Understanding stereotyping facilitates consideration of what behaviour a healthcare professional expects from the Person/s (Phelan et al 2015; Thompson 2020) and what the Person/s might expect from a particular healthcare professional role.

- What behaviour represents an "ideal" Person/s? (For example: focused, compliant, attentive, trusting ...) Answer this question alone, making a list of your expected behaviours. Use your expectations, not those of other healthcare professionals.

1. Discuss the individual lists within a group and together agree upon a list.
2. How would these expectations affect the reactions to, and communication with, someone who does not behave according to these expectations?
3. How can a healthcare professional ensure they allow the Person/s to be unique and thus fulfil their unique needs, regardless of the particular role of the healthcare professional?

Expectations of a healthcare professional

Many individuals have stereotypical attitudes affecting their expectations of people and situations. While parental and societal influences contribute to the creation of these attitudes, experience will also influence them. An individual who has a negative experience with one healthcare service or healthcare professional may generalise this experience to expect similar experiences from all healthcare professionals (Holliday et al 2021). It may take only one negative experience with a particular healthcare professional to create the expectation that all individuals from that healthcare profession will be identical (Harms & Pierce 2019). Such negative experiences can encourage the Person/s to be defensive and sometimes aggressive when relating to all healthcare professionals. It is the responsibility of the healthcare professional to communicate **without** assumptions, stereotypical judgements or expectations. This avoids reinforcing any pre-existing negative stereotypes, an important aspect of healthcare.

A young mother brings her 3-year-old child who has Down Syndrome to a speech pathologist for assistance with oral communication. At home, the child verbalises and communicates. However, in the clinic the child is nervous and overwhelmed by the situation, so does not communicate or respond in any way. The healthcare professional assumes the child cannot verbalise and, not listening to the mother, provides strategies to manage a non-verbal child.

- Discuss honestly in a group how you would respond if you were the mother.
- Can group members explain the response of the speech pathologist?

The mother, upset and infuriated, never returns to that speech pathologist and takes some time to seek the assistance of another.

This healthcare professional demonstrated stereotypical judgements that negatively affected the vulnerable mother for some time. This response was not conducive to fulfilment of Person/Family-centred Care, certainly limiting communication and positive outcomes.

An "ideal" healthcare professional demonstrates differing behaviours and communicative qualities according to the needs of the individual and the requirements of the particular situation. The following list highlights the characteristics and behaviours of an **ideal healthcare professional** that will affect the quality of their communication and ultimately their care.

An ideal healthcare professional should be:

- reflective and self-aware (Dossey et al 2015; Haddad et al 2019; Harms & Pierce 2019; Rasheed et al 2019)
- knowledgeable about and skilled in their healthcare profession (Stein-Parbury 2021)
- empathic and non-judgemental (Doohan & Saverman 2015; Rasheed et al 2019)
- respectful and caring (Levine 2012; Egan & Reese 2019)
- warm, compassionate and genuine (Harms & Pierce 2019)
- open and humble (Devito 2021; Sloane & Petra 2021)
- willing to be human and supportive, often with emotions and sometimes through **touch** (Dossey et al 2015; Harms & Pierce 2019)
- concerned about others and accepting of differences (Johnson & Withers 2018)
- honest and sensitive (Devito 2021).

- If you have sought assistance from a healthcare professional, what were your expectations? Is there anything else to add to the above list?
- Do the characteristics in the above list assist in the creation of a healthcare professional who communicates without stereotypical judgement? Explain how and why.

People sometimes expect specific physical characteristics of an individual in a particular role. For example, some people seeking assistance refuse to see a young healthcare professional. They believe a young healthcare professional cannot possibly have enough experience to be competent, and therefore will only see a healthcare professional over a particular age. Some young healthcare professionals take special care to appear older in order to combat this stereotypical expectation. Some mature-aged recent graduates find this overwhelming, despite appearing older, as recent graduates often require time to develop confidence in their professional identity and skills.

Some people apply gender stereotypes to particular healthcare professional roles. In such cases, a Person/s may insist on receiving assistance from a healthcare professional of a particular gender, if they believe that only a female/male should fulfil that role. For example, some people believe that nurses or massage therapists should be female and medical specialists or physiotherapists should be male.

If a Person/s holds any stereotypical expectations, this can affect the development of trust and rapport, thereby affecting any subsequent communication. Overcoming the stereotypical expectations of others requires perseverance and sound, effective professional care. Similarly, if a healthcare professional holds stereotypical expectations of the Person/s there are usually comparable consequences. Overcoming personal stereotypical judgement in the healthcare professional requires careful, self-aware vigilance and tolerance in order to maintain respectful, non-discriminatory and **non-judgemental** attitudes, thereby producing effective communication (Brochu et al 2014; Coleman et al 2014; Moss 2020; Rasheed et al 2019) and quality care.

Developing attitudes to avoid stereotypical judgement

Most individuals have unconscious values and beliefs (Murphy 2019) creating unconscious biases, prejudice and stereotypical judgements. Many biases develop when a parent or significant other expresses a particular sentiment (consistent with their values and beliefs), which the child then adopts (Honeycutt & Milliken 2021), often with more conviction than the parent. Such convictions create stereotypical judgements, which, when superimposed upon information and behaviour, increase the complexity of any interaction, creating barriers to effective communication. Honest evaluation of current values and beliefs causing **bias** and prejudice is essential in healthcare professionals to avoid stereotypical judgements and to achieve effective communication and Person/Family-centred Care (Devito 2021; Egan & Reese 2019; Levine 2012).

Honest evaluation of values and prejudice

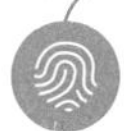

Read the following points and write down your immediate and honest response to each of these groupings. Avoid trying to explain or change your thoughts – simply write down the thoughts that immediately come into your mind. Be honest with yourself!

- What are your attitudes or bias towards:
  - an individual who is obese?
  - an individual with an intellectual disability?
  - an individual who smokes?
  - an individual with a criminal record?
  - an individual who buys their clothes from a second-hand clothing store?
  - an individual who has a hearing impairment?
  - an individual who has a speech impairment?
  - an individual who is homeless or lives on the street?
  - an individual who self-harms?
  - an individual who is Muslim? (Did you know there are various types of groupings within the Muslim faith?)
  - an individual who is a Christian?
  - an individual with a different sexual orientation to you?
- Are there any other "groups" of people that elicit a negative stereotypical response in you? Consider this and explain why.
- Consider how your thoughts and reactions will affect your ability to communicate without stereotypical judgement if providing healthcare to anyone from these groups.

It is essential to overcome the biases and/or prejudices that create stereotypical judgements in order to avoid negatively influencing interactions with different individuals (Honeycutt & Milliken 2021). Self-awareness is essential to overcome these biases (see Chapters 6 and 7). Seeking exposure to or joining activities with particular groups or people who are different with an open and accepting attitude is also beneficial in this process (Haddad et al 2019; Hill 2010). Such exposure will allow the development of perceptions based upon positive experiences. This will provide information about similarities, as well as differences. Exposure to particular groups or people will reveal that there are many variations within any grouping, thereby potentially reinforcing the uniqueness of every individual, regardless of their ethnicity or their departure from societal norms. An example of a common stereotypical judgement from many Westerners is that Asians are all the same. In reality, there are many different countries in Asia and within those countries there are multiple ethnic groups and variations within these groupings. It takes exposure and willingness to perceive and accept the differences (tolerance) to understand that Asians are definitely not all the same. If the healthcare professional finds it difficult to expose himself or herself to differences and accept those differences, it can be beneficial to explore the basis of the attitudes of those healthcare professionals who regularly communicate without judgement (Thompson 2020). Discussion of how the non-judgemental individual achieves this may assist a healthcare professional who is struggling to overcome stereotypical judgements that are negatively affecting their communication.

It is important for healthcare professionals to understand and accept those around them, despite the differences. In order to avoid judgemental communication, healthcare professionals will benefit from being aware of their personal stereotypical attitudes – and from seeking experiences that will change those attitudes (Hill 2010). It is beneficial for healthcare professionals to be flexible and willing to regularly evaluate their personal opinions and attitudes (Devito 2019, 2021). When reacting with a negative attitude based upon a stereotypical prejudice, it is important that healthcare professionals should strive to overcome that judgement. An awareness of the personal assumption and/or bias producing the judgement facilitates potential change in that assumption and/or bias and ultimately acceptance of the "different" individual or group. Learning to celebrate differences is an important skill for every healthcare professional.

Stereotypical judgement will limit any perception of the **worth** or value of an individual or their opinions. The judging person will find reasons why that particular individual does not have value or worth. For example, thoughts such as *They will be lazy because they are overweight* or *They will be unreliable because they smoke – they'll always be off smoking*, limit the ability to acknowledge any hardworking or reliable behaviour from that individual. Alternatively, thinking *Oh, that new staff member can't even speak clearly, obviously they don't know what they are talking about*, limits the possibility of acknowledging the benefits of that individual and their possible contribution to the team and to healthcare.

Stereotypes and biases prompt judgement of an individual because of outward appearances or behaviour (e.g. age, gender, skin colour, clothing, jewellery, tattoos, religious grouping, nationality, political party or particular behaviours), rather than perceptions of their personal attributes and value. In the healthcare professions, this tendency can result in the labelling of people. The overweight individual is "lazy", the individual who smokes is "unreliable", and the individual who cannot speak properly is "dumb". While labels may reflect something, in reality they are unhelpful and dehumanise the individual, removing them from emotions and value. It is common to hear statements such as *The knee in Room 407* or *the cardiac arrest just referred* within some healthcare professions and, while understandable from many perspectives, such statements are unhelpful and unnecessary. They certainly reduce the Person/s to a diagnosis rather than being a valuable individual with a range of needs.

- What labels did you or another student have at school?
- How did these labels make you or the other student feel?
- What are the implications of these feelings (whether negative or positive) for healthcare professionals?
- How do these implications highlight the responsibility of the healthcare professional to avoid labelling or stereotyping?

A bias restricts the ability to understand a person, their thoughts and actions. The presence of bias and stereotypical judgement in a healthcare professional does not allow the healthcare professional to view the individual as they actually are (more than their appearance, socioeconomic status or behaviour and so forth), therefore seriously restricting the ability to demonstrate empathy, acceptance and a sense of equality. This also has the potential to affect the intervention and resultant health outcomes.

Overcoming the power imbalance: ways to demonstrate equality in a relationship

Non-judgemental thoughts and behaviours promote respect, acceptance and **thus equality**. The understanding that each individual is vital and important (Honeycutt & Milliken 2021) assists with achieving equality when communicating. It is important to remember that healthcare professionals are in a position of power because of their knowledge and familiarity with their role and the particular healthcare service. This understanding emphasises the need to express acceptance and avoid communicating a sense of superiority. Flexibility and humility are key characteristics (Devito 2021), contributing to the construction of equality in relationships in all healthcare services. In addition, if differences stimulate stereotypical judgements, there are particular responses that promote equality when communicating (see Table 8.1).

Non-judgemental communication requires conscious awareness of consistent thoughts and repeated responses, to avoid stereotypical judgements in communication. It requires self-awareness and tolerance to promote acceptance and respect for the Person/s, regardless of the challenges. Non-judgemental communication has many positive outcomes and rewards.

TABLE 8.1
Promoting equality when communicating as a healthcare professional

Do	Do not
• acknowledge the person. • acknowledge what they say, regardless of your agreement with the statements. • acknowledge cultural differences and learn about those differences. • adjust practice to accommodate cultural differences. • be tolerant of differences. • consider similarities.	• make demands (e.g. *Get that done now*); instead make polite requests and ask relevant questions. • assume because of appearance or action. • make "should" or "must" statements (e.g. *You must do these exercises or keep to that diet*) – they imply judgement and non-compliance. • interrupt – this suggests your ideas are more important than those of others. • focus on the differences.

Adapted from Devito 2019.

Consider the scenarios in Section 4.

- Are there one or more that elicit a stereotypical judgement in you? If so, can you identify why?
- How might you overcome this tendency to stereotypical judgements if relating to such a Person/s?

Chapter summary

Personal assumptions resulting in stereotyping refers to biases that develop over time and create prejudice and discrimination towards certain people or groups. Communication based upon stereotypical judgements, developing from personal assumptions, limits the possibility of relating to the whole Person/s, potentially resulting in misunderstandings. It is important for healthcare professionals to develop attitudes of unconditional positive regard for all Person/s seeking their assistance. Resolving personal assumptions to produce non-judgemental communication is the key to overcoming the inherent power imbalance in the relationship between the healthcare professional and the Person/s. It is essential when aiming for Person/Family-centred Care and effective communication.

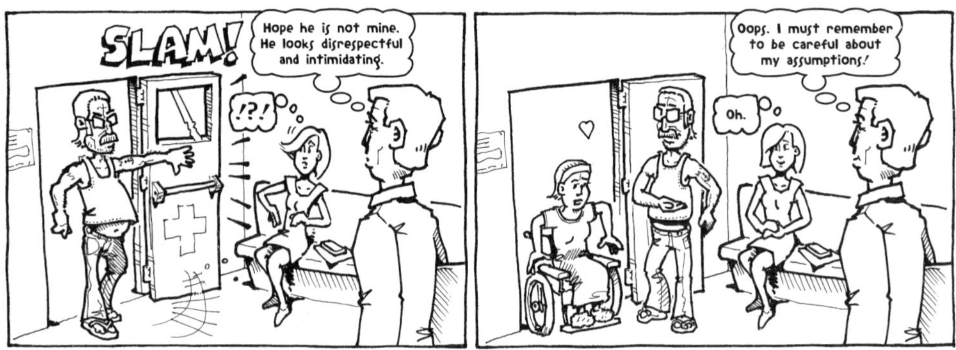

FIGURE 8.1
Assumptions can form a barrier.
Courtesy Roger Harvey © Elsevier Australia.

REVIEW QUESTIONS

1. Define "stereotype" and give an example of a positive and a negative stereotype.

2. Give three reasons why it is important for healthcare professionals to avoid communicating stereotypical judgement.

   i. ____

   ii. ____

   iii. ____

3. What communication barriers can stereotypical judgement produce?

   i. ____

   ii. ____

4. Identify the characteristics of a healthcare professional that are most closely related to effective communication skills. Explain why and how.

   ____

   ____

   ____

   ____

5. Suggest three ways a healthcare professional can avoid stereotypical judgement.

   i. ____

   ii. ____

   iii. ____

6. List five behaviours (some of which are communicative) to overcome the power imbalance in the relationship between the healthcare professional and the Person/s seeking assistance. Give original examples of each behaviour.

   i. ____

   ii. ____

   iii. ____

   iv. ____

   v. ____

References

Abdou, C.M, Fingerhut, A.W., Jackson, J.S., et al., 2016. Healthcare stereotype threat in older adults in the health and retirement study. American Journal of Preventive Medicine, 50(2), 191–198.

Abdou, C.M., Fingerhut, A.W., 2014. Stereotype threat among black and white women in health care settings. Cultural Diversity and Ethnic Minority Psychology, 20(3), 316–323.

Beesley, P., Watts, M., Harrison, M., 2017. Developing your communication skills in social work. Sage, London.

Borden, E., 2018. Looking within: Using cultural humility in communications. Oncology Nurse Advisor, Jan/Feb, 28–30.

Bowe, H., Martin, K., Manns, H., 2014. Communication across cultures: Mutual understanding in a global world, 2nd ed. Cambridge University Press, Melbourne.

Brochu, P.M., Pearl, R.L., Puhl, R.M., et al., 2014. Do media portrayals of obesity influence support for weight-related medical policy? Health Psychology, 33(2), 197–200.

Christman, A., 2014. Communicating with elderly patients. Radiologic Technology, 85(5), 580–582.

Clement, S.S.O., Graham, T., Maggioni, F., et al., 2015. What is the impact of mental health-related stigma on help-seeking? A systematic review of quantitative and qualitative studies. Psychological Medicine, 45(1), 11–27.

Coleman, R., Major, L.H., 2014. Ethical health communication: A content analysis of predominant frames and primes in public service announcements. Journal of Mass Media Ethics, 29(2), 91–108.

Cook, J.E., Purdie-Vaughns, V., Meyer, I.H., et al., 2014. Intervening within and across levels: A multilevel approach to stigma and public health. Social Science and Medicine, 103, 101–109.

Devito, J.A., 2021. The interpersonal communication book, 16th ed. Pearson, Boston.

Devito, J.A., 2019. The interpersonal communication book, 15th ed. Pearson, Boston.

Doohan, I., Saveman, B-I., 2015. Need for compassion in prehospital and emergency care: A qualitative study on bus crash survivors' experiences. International Emergency Nursing, 23(2), 115–119.

Dossey, B.M., Keegan, L., Barrere, C.C., 2015. Holistic nursing: A handbook for practice, 7th ed. Jones & Bartlett, Sudbury MA.

Eckermann, A., Dowd, T., Chong, E., et al., 2016. Binaŋ Goonj: Bridging cultures in Aboriginal health, 4th ed. Elsevier, Sydney.

Edmondson, W., 2022. Transformative learning for Aboriginal and Torres Strait Islander health practice. In: Edmondson, W., Williams, R., (eds), Burda-Burda Balayi health professionals and Indigenous health: Working at the interface. Oxford University Press, Melbourne.

Egan, G., Reese R.J., 2019. The skilled helper: A problem management and opportunity approach to helping, 11th ed. Cengage, Boston MA.

Haddad, A.M., Purtilo, R.B., Doherty, R.F., 2019. Health professional and patient interaction, 9th ed. Elsevier/Saunders, St Louis, MO.

Harms, L., Pierce, J., 2019. Working with people: Communication skills for reflective practice, 2nd Canadian ed. Oxford University Press, Don Mills, Ontario.

Higginbottom, G.M.A., Safipour, J., Yohani, S., et al., 2014. An ethnographic study of communication challenges in maternity care for immigrant women in rural Alberta. Midwifery, 31(2), 297–304.

Hill, T.E., 2010. How clinicians make (or avoid) moral judgements of patients: Implications of the evidence for relationships and research. Philosophy, Ethics, and Humanities in Medicine, 5, 11–24.

Holliday, A., Kullman, J., Hyde, M., 2021. Intercultural communication: An advanced resource book for students, 4th ed. Routledge, New York.

Honeycutt, A., Milliken, M.A., 2021 Understanding human behavior: A guide for healthcare providers, 10th ed. Thomson Delmar, New York.

Johnson, R., Withers, M., 2018. Cultural competence in the emergency department: Clinicians as cultural learners. Emergency Medicine Australasia, 30, 854–856.

Levine, J., 2012. Working with people: The helping process, 9th ed. Pearson, San Antonio.

Liu, S., Volcic, Z., Gallois, C., 2018. Introducing intercultural communication: Global cultures and contexts, 3rd ed. Sage, London.

Loch, A.A., Guarniero, F.B., Lawson, F.L., et al., 2014. Stigma toward schizophrenia: Do all psychiatrists behave the same? Latent profile analysis of a national sample of psychiatrists in Brazil. BMC Psychiatry 13(1), 1–10.

Moss, B., 2020. Communication skills in health and social care, 5th ed. Sage, London.

Murphy, J., /revised by McMahan, I., 2019. The power of your subconscious mind. Simon & Schuster, UK.

Passi, N., 2018. Looking forward, looking back: An Indigenous trainee perspective. Emergency Medicine Australasia, 30, 862–863.

Paternotte, E., van Dulmen, S., van der Lee, N., et al., 2015. A systematic review of effective intercultural communication in mental health. Patient Education and Counseling, 98(4), 420–445.

Phelan, S.M., Burgess, D.J., Yeazel, M.W., et al., 2015. Impact of weight bias and stigma on quality of care and outcomes for patients with obesity. Obesity Reviews, 16(4), 319–326.

Rasheed, S.P., Younas, A., Sundus, A., 2019. Self-awareness in Nursing: A scoping review. Journal of Clinical Nursing, 28(5), 762–774.

Sandín-Vázquez, M., Larraz-Antón, R., Río-Sánchez, I., 2014. Immigrant patient care inequalities: The importance of the intercultural approach. Procedia – Social and Behavioral Sciences, 132, 277–284.

Sloane, H., Petra, M., 2021. Modeling cultural humility: Listening to students' stories of religious identity. Journal of Social Work Education, 57(1), 28–39.

Stein-Parbury, J., 2021. Patient and person: Interpersonal skills in nursing, 7th ed. Elsevier, Sydney.

Thompson, N., 2020. Anti-discriminatory practice: equality, diversity and social justice, 7th ed. Palgrave Macmillan, London.

CHAPTER 9

Awareness of the whole "Person/s" for healthcare communication

Chapter objectives

Upon completing this chapter, readers should be able to:

- reflect upon who, in practice, constitutes the Person/s for a healthcare professional
- consult relevant information about the Person/s to ensure effective communication
- consider the physical aspects and associated needs of the Person/s when communicating
- recognise the significance of the sexual aspect and needs of the Person/s in practice
- understand the impact of and accommodate the cognitive skills of the Person/s
- relate to the possible implications of the social needs of the Person/s
- reflect upon the need to relate to the spiritual aspects and needs of the Person/s.

Effective communication with a Person/s requires understanding and consideration of various aspects of that individual, or whole-person care. However, before discussing these aspects, it is necessary to explore important elements of communication to assist the healthcare professional when communicating with the Person/s.

Who is the Person/s?

Before beginning, it is important to reiterate who constitutes the Person/s for the healthcare professional. As mentioned earlier in the book, this perspective indicates that the "Person/s" includes both those seeking healthcare, as well as other healthcare professionals (colleagues) and supporting staff providing relevant assistance (Bayne et al 2013). Those seeking assistance include the individual requiring direct intervention, along with the carers, guardians, families, friends, neighbours, and, in some cases, relevant community members. Healthcare professional colleagues include individuals from many healthcare professions. Some of these healthcare professionals may form an inter-professional team within the particular health service, while others may contribute to fulfilling the needs of the Person/s from outside the service. Supporting staff are found in every health service and provide essential services to both healthcare professionals and service seekers. These Person/s include those who answer the phone and those who clean the floors and toilets. Their contribution is vital. Therefore, it is important to recognise their contribution as an equal part of the service of any healthcare profession.

Relevant information about the Person/s

Gathering relevant information about the Person/s is important. Some information will be more relevant to particular healthcare professionals than to others. For example, knowing the dominant hand of the individual seeking assistance is particularly relevant for specific healthcare professions, whereas for others it is irrelevant. There are other types of information about the Person/s that are important regardless of the healthcare profession. It is beneficial to know the abilities, age and gender of the Person/s, because this can guide the expectations, practice and communication style of the healthcare professional. For example, knowing their particular abilities might facilitate adjustment of expectations; knowing the age of the Person/s allows the healthcare professional to adapt their language level and equipment, while knowing their gender might guide the focus of the conversation (Brito et al 2011).

- Discuss how it feels when a message is too simple or too complex.
- Suggest non-verbal messages that indicate someone finds the message too simple or too complex.
- Suggest how to ensure you choose appropriate words for the particular Person/s.

When communicating with the Person/s it is important to know the reason they are seeking care, and, where applicable, the cause, condition/s or diagnosis creating their need/s. It is important to know what they expect from the service of the particular healthcare profession and to know the goals they want to achieve through intervention. It may be important to know their previous experience with the healthcare professions because this information may explain particular reactions. It may also be important to know their background and perhaps their interests. There are usually relevant forms specific to healthcare services, providing a basis for questions to gather the required information. This type of information, while necessary, is not the focus of this chapter. The major focus of this chapter is the often unseen aspects of the Person/s and associated needs, particularly their emotional, **sexual**, cognitive, social and **spiritual** needs. Although perhaps considered obvious, the noticeable physical needs of the Person/s also require brief consideration as they may guide the reaction of the healthcare professional.

Defining the *whole* "Person"

The consideration of the "Person" in the healthcare professions requires consideration of the **whole Person** (see Chapter 13). This means attending to more than the physical (Falkenheimer 2018; Morris et al 2016). The "whole" Person is a dynamic system in which every aspect of the individual simultaneously affects and interacts with the other aspects. The whole Person contains five fundamental aspects: the physical, including the sexual aspect; the emotional; the cognitive; the social, including cultural; and the spiritual aspect (Levine 2012). The dynamic interaction of these aspects influences, and may determine, skills in communicating and interacting. It is important for healthcare professionals to consider the needs associated with the interplay of all aspects of the Person/s (Hansen et al 2016). Consideration of the most obvious aspect of the Person/s while neglecting the less obvious aspects limits the potential outcomes of the intervention. Please note: it is not the responsibility of individual healthcare professionals to fulfil the needs of every aspect of the Person/s. However, being aware of the possible impact of particular aspects of the Person/s upon recovery can highlight the need to refer them to a relevant healthcare profession for fulfilment of the relevant need at a particular time. It is important to remember that these aspects exist as a dynamic whole. They are mutually dependent and mutually affect each other (Burkhardt 2015).

The most obvious aspect of an individual is usually the *physical* one, because it is immediately noticeable. It includes the body of the Person/s, the functioning of their internal organs and their external body parts. However, the other aspects of this dynamic system often become obvious during repeated interactions with the healthcare professional. Recognition and willingness to discuss the *sexual* aspect or needs of an individual may be essential in some healthcare professions. Sexual dysfunction can affect the overall functioning of the individual; ignoring it can limit the health and wellbeing of the individual. In some cases, unconditional acceptance of the sexual preference of the individual is important for positive outcomes. As mentioned above, ignoring the less obvious aspects of the individual can adversely affect the outcomes of interventions.

The *emotional* or **psychological aspect of the individual** may not be immediately obvious, but may dominate the Person/s seeking healthcare. Whether or not obvious, the emotional aspect of the Person/s is part of every individual (Burkhardt 2015). It is important to explore and address the issues causing the emotional distress, either directly or by referral to the appropriate healthcare professional or service (sometimes a chaplain). Resolution of emotional distress allows the Person/s to focus on the relevant health-related goals, rather than the dominating emotions.

As the healthcare professional continues to relate to each individual, the *cognitive* aspect of that Person/s may become more obvious if there is difficulty or ease in processing information. This aspect includes thought processes, learning, problem-solving, memory and so forth. In such cases, lack of ability or desire to collaborate is not always resistance. It may arise from lack of understanding because of decreased cognitive ability or limited language skills. In contrast, some cognitively able individuals may disengage from therapeutic interventions because of boredom. Both levels of **cognition** require the healthcare professional to adjust the interventions to produce positive outcomes.

The previous *social* experiences and/ or *cultural* background of the individual inform the social aspect of the Person/s. They may be the least obvious and often the most significant aspect affecting expectations and outcomes. Experiences of previous social interaction may affect the response of the Person/s to particular interactions with healthcare professionals. Cultural norms can also influence interactions; thus awareness of cultural norms is essential when relating to people from different cultures (see Chapters 16 and 17). An important aspect that can dominate the individual is the *spiritual* aspect. This aspect of the individual provides meaning for self, life and the universe (Cobb et al 2014; Moosavi et al 2019). It is central to the existence of individuals, incorporating and, for some, transcending all other aspects (van der Riet & Pitt 2020). It involves beliefs and moral values, possibly including relating to the world at a spiritual level. Many healthcare professionals neglect this aspect, but it may influence the motivation and interest of the Person/s and thus the outcomes of any healthcare professional intervention (Morris et al 2016; van der Riet & Pitt 2020).

While it is possible to focus upon one aspect of the whole Person/s, dividing the whole into parts for analysis can be problematic (Blaszko Helming et al 2020; Harms & Pierce 2019) because each aspect exists in an intricate and sometimes delicate relationship with the other aspects. Analysis of one aspect is often useful and transformative. Such analysis, however, should always consider the effects of the other aspects (Bateman 2014).

There are times during life when one particular aspect may dominate the dynamic system of the whole individual. The demands of life at that time, or the particular choices made by the individual, result in the Person/s giving greater priority to a particular aspect of their whole more often than the other aspects. For example, the physical aspect of an elite athlete may dominate their focus and functioning because of the requirement for physical training. A student is required to use the cognitive aspect regularly, thus the cognitive aspect may prescribe their focus and functioning. A grieving individual may experience extreme emotional stress, so the psychological aspect of a grieving individual may dominate their functioning. An individual who chooses to be a monk or nun usually makes choices based upon the spiritual aspect. The need for social acceptance during adolescence may mean that the social aspect of the adolescent drives their existence at that stage in life. These realities are important aspects of every individual. They may require consideration when providing healthcare.

All of the above aspects of an individual contribute to the functioning and performance of the Person/s. Consideration and sometimes accommodation of each aspect of the individual while practising as a healthcare professional is potentially beneficial for the individuals seeking assistance. It enhances the development of the therapeutic relationship, thereby contributing to Person/Family-centred Care and thus the results of the overall intervention.

- List the various healthcare professions that may also provide assistance to any Person/s you might assist. Consider both government and non-government medical and alternative healthcare services. Do not forget that the Person/s might have needs related to feet, teeth, joints or various other needs that healthcare professionals outside the traditional medical model are best qualified to fulfil.

Physical aspects of the Person/s

A Person with obvious physical needs, who is seeking the assistance of a healthcare professional, may or may not require specific action from them. Someone in a wheelchair may require a clear passage to a particular destination or may feel more comfortable if the healthcare professional sits to interact with them rather than standing over them.

Some obvious physical characteristics of the Person/s may communicate particular information. For example, the shape of their eyes and face, the colour of their skin; their clothing and so forth. It is important that healthcare professionals are aware of their personal reactions to these characteristics. It may appear possible to assume the socioeconomic background of an individual by their designer clothing or the amount and type of jewellery they wear. However, it is important to remember that this vulnerable Person/s is seeking to present a particular image and that their clothing may in fact be an attempt to present a non-existent state. Assuming the socioeconomic background of a smelly "other" with dirty and cheap clothing is equally dangerous. It is important that healthcare professionals avoid making assumptions because of the appearance of the Person/s and remember to relate equally to each individual regardless of physical characteristics.

It is sometimes possible to assume the cultural and religious background of an individual because of their clothing; once again, however, it is necessary to proceed with care when assuming anything about someone because of their appearance. Respect and professional training in the healthcare professions can guide appropriate responses to the physical appearance and physical needs of the Person/s, empowering healthcare professionals to respond appropriately to those needs regardless of particular physical aspects. This response has the potential to empower the Person/s seeking assistance.

Sexual aspects of the Person/s

People are sexual beings regardless of their culture or gender. Note that sexuality here is not synonymous with gender. Individuals usually have sexual organs, and while these may determine their gender, they do not necessarily determine their ability to discuss and relate to their sexuality. The sexual aspect of individuals refers to their particular reproductive organs and the responsibilities associated with the use of those organs (Honeycutt & Milliken 2021), as well as their sexual preference. Particular healthcare professions may or may not relate to the sexuality or sexual functioning of the individual. All healthcare professionals, however, may need to respond *without* verbal or non-verbal judgement to possible differences in their sexual preference and the sexual preference of the Person/s seeking their assistance.

Amy is 14 years old with an intellectual disability. She has recently begun menstruating and her mother has found it difficult to teach her how to manage this change in her body from the perspectives of both hygiene and sexual activity.

1. How would you feel if you were asked to assist Amy to manage the sexual changes in her body and ensure safe sexual activity in the future?
2. Write a list of the things you would find difficult in this situation and how you might overcome these difficulties.

- Discuss possible strategies for assisting Amy and her mother to manage the emotional and sexual aspects of this situation.

Some individuals find it difficult to explicitly discuss or consider their own sexuality and gender preferences. Such individuals may or may not find it difficult to relate to the sexual aspect of another Person/s. This is true both for some healthcare professionals and some individuals seeking assistance.

Peter/Peta is a 25-year-old with paraplegia. He/she is about to begin sleeping with his/her partner for the first time since his/her accident. You have an excellent relationship with Peter/Peta, with many things in common – similar age and interests, same gender, etc. He/she indicates fear about his/her sexual abilities since the accident and asks you for assistance about how to approach having intercourse with his/her partner. The doctor says Peter/Peta should be able to function sexually, but has given no other guidance or reassurance.

- Discuss how you might feel if the Person/s asked you this question.
- Discuss the possible ways of responding to empower Peter/Peta.
- Are you aware of relevant services to support Peter/Peta? How would you source appropriate services to support Peter/Peta.

Certainly some healthcare professionals within the scope of their practice would not usually expect to consider the sexual aspect of a Person/s. However, if a particular healthcare professional develops a safe therapeutic relationship with a Person/s, that Person/s may wish to discuss their sexual concerns with that healthcare professional. This discussion may or may not feel comfortable, but if managed appropriately it may empower the Person/s to seek qualified assistance, thereby empowering them to fulfil their sexual needs.

Emotional aspects of the Person/s

Validation

Validation of emotions is important for the Person/s, who sometimes feels overwhelmed, but typically feels vulnerable and uncertain when consulting a healthcare professional. Validation confirms the existence of their negative emotions, potentially allowing them to acknowledge and accept the existence of these emotions. Acknowledging the legitimacy of the negative emotions is often difficult for the Person/s because they may feel confused and ungrateful at that time (see the scenario about Eric later in this chapter). The process of validation requires the healthcare professional to recognise the emotional cues of the Person/s and accurately name those emotions. These emotional cues are often communicated non-verbally and thus require sensitive and respectful validation. This process, if performed sensitively, generally releases the Person/s to acknowledge those emotions with greater acceptance and less confusion. The Person/s often feels more able to express, understand and control their emotions after validation. It is important to note that validation does not indicate whether the emotions are reasonable or appropriate; it simply states the existence of the emotions. Healthcare professionals indicate unconditional positive regard by: (i) separating themselves from their values and judgements (Rogers 1967); (ii) recognising the emotion in the Person/s; and (iii) expressing awareness of the emotion – usually by asking a question relating to the particular emotion, but sometimes with non-verbal cues.

- In groups of six or seven, choose five of the following emotions: happy, frustrated, excited, sad, devastated, unhappy, disappointed, confused, bored, sleepy, depressed, guilty, embarrassed, rejected, helpless, irritated, angry, ashamed, insecure.

- Choose one of the five emotions. Have each member of the group simultaneously non-verbally express the chosen (same) emotion.
- Consider the variations in the ways of non-verbally expressing each emotion.
- Repeat this until the group has expressed all the five chosen emotions.
- How might a healthcare professional compensate for the variations in the meaning of non-verbal communication?

Clarification within validation

It is important to recognise that each individual has a unique communication style. Recognition and understanding of the communication style of the individual ensures positive communication outcomes. Accurate validation of emotions cannot occur without this recognition of individual communication styles (Hall et al 2014). Different cultures, different social groups and different families increase the variations in communication styles. Therefore, in recognition of these variations, healthcare professionals might request clarification of their perceptions rather than assume they have accurately recognised the emotional cues of the Person/s. For example: *Are you OK? You seem upset/unhappy.* A request for clarification of the perception of the emotion is appropriate before recognising and validating an emotion. A question indicates the interest of the healthcare professional in the Person/s, allowing that Person/s to decide if they will acknowledge or deny the presence of the emotion. If acknowledgement of the emotion follows, the healthcare professional has the opportunity, if appropriate, to empathise and explore the emotion with the Person/s. If denial of the emotion follows, then the healthcare professional has "lost nothing" and is learning about the communication style of that individual.

In such situations, it may or may not be appropriate to pose another question asking the Person/s to name their strongest current emotion (it may be beneficial to create a multiple-choice question, by listing possible emotions for them). The healthcare professional must decide whether to pursue the presence of the emotional cues or to leave the Person/s to consider the question alone. The question may begin the exploration process of the emotions for the Person/s amid their confusion and fear, allowing verbal exploration later.

Many healthcare professionals will experience the expression of strong emotions from the Person/s and/or they may experience such emotions themselves. It is unwise to ignore or deny these emotions (Davis & Musolino 2016). Recognition and validation of strong emotions in the Person/s or healthcare professional is necessary, potentially beginning the journey of acknowledgement and possible resolution. This acknowledgement and resolution within the Person/s or healthcare professional facilitate understanding and control of often overwhelming emotions. This resolution can potentially improve the therapeutic relationship, the focus of interventions and related health outcomes (Bogaert 2020; James 2023).

Accurate validation of emotions requires skill. It may require the healthcare professional to clarify their perception of the emotions to facilitate honest communication. However, recognition and validation encourages the Person/s to honestly admit and consider the existence of their emotions. Accurate recognition of emotions either allows discussion and related action to resolve the cause or, if necessary, referral for assistance to resolve these emotions.

Eric, a 28-year-old, and Mandy, his wife of six months, wait quietly in a private room for someone to tell them the results of his tests. To fill the time and stop thinking the worst, they talk about the work they are doing on the house they have just bought and their future plans to travel and have a family.

The specialist doing the tests was highly recommended, so they feel confident. He finally comes into the room reading some papers. He smiles quietly and looks up. The tests are all clear. Eric and Mandy visibly relax. The specialist does not notice this, however, because he is not convinced that the results are accurate. He suggests more tests just to be sure of the diagnosis. He feels his hunch is right, considering the symptoms that Eric has been experiencing, and just wants to confirm this.

A few weeks later Eric and Mandy sit in the same room with a feeling of déjà vu. This time they are not trying to avoid thinking about anything – they feel tired and afraid.

When the pathology report arrives, the doctor and three other healthcare professionals rush into the room. This time the specialist has a big smile on his face. He excitedly says he was right; these tests have confirmed his hunch and Eric does have the chronic degenerative condition he has suspected from the symptoms. *I was right!* he says repeatedly.

Eric and Mandy are crushed – they have no idea of the implications of the condition, but they know their plans will need major changes. Their faces express devastation.

The specialist stops smiling and looks at them, surprised. He simply says, *You should be happy; it could have been worse – you have at least 10 good years.*

Stunned, Eric and Mandy thank the specialist for his perseverance in the search for a diagnosis. Eric is feeling completely confused and afraid; Mandy is horrified and devastated. Eric does not want to seem ungrateful, but this is not his idea of something to celebrate or something to smile about, and he is in shock. In the confusion he thinks these feelings must be inappropriate considering the response from the specialist – and then he notices the tears rolling down the face of the healthcare professional who had spent time with them when they first arrived at the health service; the one who knows they are newly married with wonderful plans for the future.

Eric in his mind thanks that healthcare professional because it indicates that his feelings are appropriate – he is allowed to feel terrible – and he bursts into tears.

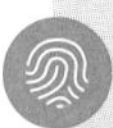

- Consider this scenario from the perspective of Eric and Mandy.
- Consider this scenario from the perspective of the specialist – remember the times you have been preoccupied with something or excited about something and have not noticed the feelings of the people around you.
- Consider this scenario from the perspective of the healthcare professional who had the courage to cry.
- Whose perspective do you find easiest to understand?
- What does this mean about your ability to demonstrate empathy?

1. Using the above thoughts, discuss the responsibility of the healthcare professional to focus on the needs of the Person/s, regardless of the feelings or thoughts of the healthcare professional.
2. List the reasons why this is the case.
3. What can a healthcare professional do to "survive" the process of sharing the perspective of hurt and often fearful people in order to express empathy on other occasions?
4. List actions or behaviours that will assist the healthcare professional to express empathy when communicating with the Person/s around them.

Adapted from Northouse & Northouse 1998

Cognitive aspects of the Person/s

Cognitive ability is the ability to process, store and retrieve information using reasoning, interpretation, intuition, perception, problem-solving, learning and memory. Cognitive events are conscious thoughts (Holli & Beto 2023) that the individual has in an attempt to process and understand received information. It is important that the healthcare professional and the Person/s possess basic cognitive abilities to negotiate mutual understanding and produce effective and emotionally comfortable interactions (Lamothe et al 2014). It is also important to understand that when feeling vulnerable, the individual may experience temporary deterioration in their cognitive processing skills.

An important cognitive ability is the ability to *concentrate* or attend throughout the communicative interaction. Understanding the limits of the attention span of the Person/s – whether their cognitive skills are developing (children) or declining (ageing adults) – is important because it allows the healthcare professional to adjust their communication as necessary. It is important that all communicating individuals *understand* that their words and non-verbal behaviours send particular messages and have *consequences*. Children (who are still developing their cognitive abilities) and individuals with limited cognitive abilities often find it difficult to understand the idea of cause and effect (Haddad et al 2019). For example, the individual who thinks they have lost their meal tray because they did not exercise enough care does not understand explanations about the cause and effect that resulted in the removal of the meal tray (i.e. completing mealtime and cleaning up at the end of the mealtime). Healthcare professionals have a responsibility when communicating with such individuals to communicate with understanding and skill. It is imperative that healthcare professionals adapt their manner of communicating according to the cognitive ability of the Person/s, continually making adjustments according to their observations of the effects of their communication upon that Person/s.

When communicating with children, it is important to remember that they have different cognitive skills at different ages (Berk 2022). Piaget and Inhelder (1958) and Piaget (1968) present a model of the stages of cognitive development (see Table 9.1). Although there is discussion about the accuracy of the timing of these stages, it does appear that children develop cognitive skills as they grow and experience their world. Variations can occur because individual children may demonstrate well-developed cognition at a particular age, while other children may not, despite apparently similar intelligence and experience. Adults with diminishing cognitive skills may revert to demonstrating cognitive abilities typical of these earlier stages. It is important to adjust communication styles according to the cognitive abilities of each Person/s.

When communicating with people who have limited cognitive abilities or a disorder affecting their comprehension of language, it is important for healthcare professionals to use short and simple sentences and, wherever possible, non-abstract words. This will maximise comprehension. There is no need to speak loudly unless they also have a hearing impairment.

If someone does not understand what is being communicated, regardless of the reasons for the lack of comprehension, they will cease listening. In such situations, it is less possible to negotiate meaning and mutual understanding. Interpreting the non-verbal cues related to potential comprehension is sometimes useful, but may be unreliable in many situations. To confirm adequate comprehension, the healthcare professional should ask the Person/s to repeat, in their own words, the meaning they ascribe to the delivered message.

Remember that emotional states may restrict cognitive functioning, regardless of the considered cognitive abilities of the individual. Consideration of and attention to the emotional state of

TABLE 9.1
The four stages of cognitive function from the Piagetian cognitive development model

Stage and typical age	Expected skills
Sensorimotor stage Birth to 2 years	Explores the world using their senses and movement typical of their developmental stage. Understands object permanence. Experiences stranger anxiety if without familiar company. Egocentric, focusing on their own needs. Limited understanding of cause and effect.
Preoperational 2 to 6 years	Developing language skills with increasing vocabulary. Pretend play. Egocentricity indicates they are unable to consider perspectives other than their own. However, they believe everyone views the world using their perspective, including their idea of right and wrong; they focus on obeying rules, often self-created rules. They think that inanimate objects can move, experience emotions and pain. Use words and pictures to represent things.
Concrete operations 7 to 11 years	Are able to be rational and logical. If they can manipulate an object they can apply logic to it. Begin to understand things may be different to the appearance. Able to imagine different scenarios. They also understand that even when things change, they can be the same = reversibility; however, they require concrete evidence of this. The blocks are the same even if they are arranged differently or a parent is the same, even when they appear different because of a haircut or wearing new clothing.
Formal operations 12 years–adulthood	They are able to speculate about various perspectives, having abstract logical thought by 16 years. They are able to imagine possibilities without symbolic images. They can problem-solve using deductive reasoning and evaluate validity without concrete evidence. Potential for mature moral reasoning.

Piaget & Inhelder 1958; Piaget 1968

the Person/s may increase their ability to concentrate, thereby improving the potential for effective communication.

Some individuals have limited but stable cognitive abilities – they are neither developing nor deteriorating. Most of these individuals have reached a particular level of cognitive functioning that is below the typical level of their age. Individuals with an intellectual disability are representative of this group, and they may require the use of particular methods of communication to achieve effective communication (see Chapter 10). Another group of individuals who may experience difficulty communicating are those who have a disorder related to the autism spectrum disorder (American Psychiatric Association 2022). Other individuals who may experience communication difficulties include those with head injuries, sensory impairments, learning disorders, specific language disorders and some physical disabilities, including cerebral palsy.

Individuals with limited verbal skills may communicate using certain behaviours, such as biting, hitting, kicking, pushing, spitting, screaming, crying, laughing, withdrawing, touching, smiling, smelling, reaching, physically guiding, head banging/butting, absconding from a particular situation, cuddling, undressing in public and many more. If an individual has severe difficulties communicating verbally, resorting to such behaviours may be the only manner of expressing their feelings at the time.

It is important for the healthcare professional to accommodate and appropriately manage difficult behaviours while implementing strategies to establish appropriate communicative behaviours for such individuals.

Social needs of the Person/s

Humans often seek social interaction. The extent and enjoyment of social interactions may vary according to personality type, but most typically functioning individuals seek the company of other humans at some point during every day (Levine 2012). Individuals who feel vulnerable and fearful may desire the company of people they trust. In such situations, the Person/s may not want to actively interact – they may simply desire the presence of a friendly, caring individual. In the busy world of the healthcare professional, they may be unable to meet this demand (Hillen et al 2014). It is important to accommodate this social need despite the time-scarce nature of practice. Trained volunteers may be able to fulfil this need for human company.

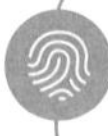

- If a Person/s seeking your assistance is lonely and often monopolises your time because of this loneliness, how might you assist this Person/s?

Many individuals have their needs for social contact met through the ownership of an animal. Underestimating the significance of the relationship with a long-term pet is unwise when assisting any individual, regardless of age or gender. A vulnerable Person/s may feel their pet is their only reliable and supportive social relationship, making acknowledgement of the pet essential.

John lives alone in a dark, cluttered room. His best friend is a bottle of cheap alcohol. He has recently experienced back pain and has come to an alternative health service for assistance. While he has plenty of money and clothes, he usually wears the same clothes that show little evidence of laundering. John rarely showers, so people leave the waiting room whenever he attends for treatment. John does not feel that anyone cares about him, so he does not care about himself.

Sam, the osteopath who treats John, is pleasant but distant. He usually works as quickly as possible and says very little while treating John. After treating John, he sterilises everything and thoroughly disinfects his hands.

Adrian, the cleaner, has lost the ability to smell and often works close to John when he is there, chatting as he cleans. He regularly asks John how he is going and how he is feeling. John has come for treatment for several weeks and Adrian has learnt a lot about John in that time. Adrian makes it his business to clean the waiting room whenever John is there, regularly expressing empathy towards John, and once bringing him some homemade cooking (Adrian's wife is a great cook). After a few weeks, John begins to attend appointments smelling fresh and in clean clothes.

1. Why do you think John looks forward to attending the health service?
2. Why do you think Sam reacts the way he does to John?
3. What do you think Adrian has learnt about John? Use your imagination.
4. Why do you think John is clean and in fresh clothes after he has been attending for several weeks?

Spiritual aspect and needs of the Person/s

Please note: Discussion of the spiritual aspect of the Person/s has been placed last, due to its underlying role in every individual and therefore its importance for every individual.

Every individual has a spiritual aspect. Some consider the spiritual aspect of an individual to be the core and pivotal aspect (Ronaldson 2014). This aspect of a Person/s determines the focus of their lives and dictates what is valuable and meaningful to them (Booth & Kaylor 2018; van der Riet & Pitt 2020; White 2006). It determines notions of self and the place of the individual in life. It can refer to the "things" that renew, the "things" that bring comfort and lift the spirit, as well as inspiring and encouraging "things". The spiritual aspect relates to the beliefs and values motivating and sustaining individuals (Hess & Ramugondo 2014; Moosavi et al 2019; O'Toole & Ramugondo 2018). As such, it is the basis for explanations about the meaning and purpose of the events of life. Consideration of spirituality is an important element of healthcare and can benefit the health and wellbeing of both healthcare professionals and the Person/s (Ano & Pargament; 2013; Ford et al 2012; Koenig et al 2023; Mthembu et al 2017; Schroeder et al 2016; White 2006). An individual may or may not be consciously aware of this aspect of their daily existence. It is an aspect of an individual that some prefer to keep private and may avoid discussing in any social context. Spirituality is often unconscious, but may become conscious when an individual feels vulnerable. At such times, this vulnerable, overwhelmed Person/s may seek to discuss their spiritual dimension.

In the past 20 years there has been a growing interest in spirituality and religion among many of the healthcare professions (Mathisen & Carey 2018). Despite the growing awareness of spirituality and the effect of this aspect on health and wellbeing (Booth & Kaylor 2018; Koenig et al 2023), many healthcare professionals fail to recognise and accommodate the spiritual aspects of the Person/s. Phelps and colleagues (2012) and Maley and colleagues (2016) indicate that consideration of spiritual needs is essential for holistic care (see Chapter 13). Failure of healthcare professionals to recognise the importance of spiritual issues may be a major source of distress for particular individuals. If spiritual issues are important to the Person/s, they require recognition and attention (Koenig 2018; O'Toole & Ramugondo 2018). Some cultures are constantly aware of a spiritual existence; thus the spiritual aspect for individuals from such cultures will be very significant. If the Person/s expresses needs with spiritual implications, it is important that the healthcare professional acknowledges and addresses those needs rather than ignoring them, regardless of the spiritual beliefs of the healthcare professional.

You have been assisting an elderly Asian man for several weeks. He appears to benefit from seeing you and there is indication of rapport between you. He attends regularly, but demonstrates limited progress. Through an interpreter, he indicates he is too tired to implement your suggestions, except during your treatment sessions. Empathic questioning reveals that he cannot sleep because every night the spirits of his previous wives, who died some years ago, torment him.

Regardless of your spiritual beliefs, you know this man would improve quickly if he had the energy to implement your suggestions outside your treatment sessions.

- List possible appropriate actions to assist this man.
- Consider the implications of not accommodating the spirituality of someone who kneels daily for prayer, if that Person has had a total hip replacement. (You will need to know the precautions relating to hip replacements when discussing this case.)

There are many ways of addressing the spiritual needs and concerns of the Person/s. It is important to remember that no healthcare professional has all the answers and it is acceptable to indicate this reality to the Person/s. Regardless of the personal beliefs of the healthcare professional, it is important to identify whether the Person/s requires an individual who understands their spiritual, religious or philosophical beliefs and, if necessary, connect them with such a spiritual specialist. Acknowledging the beliefs and values of the Person/s can motivate and sustain them in difficult situations.

When assisting someone for whom spirituality is significant, it is important to:

1. demonstrate respect for the Person/s and their ideas of spirituality
2. recognise the source of spiritual support for the Person/s and as required, allow access to that form of support
3. understand when the Person/s may be experiencing spiritual distress and behave in a manner that acknowledges and attempts to alleviate the distress.

Spiritual functioning affects the value the Person/s assigns to their body, their spirit, their emotions, their thoughts and those around them. It may affect their reaction to the suggestions and intervention of the healthcare professional (Sohl et al 2014). It may limit or encourage the cooperation of the individual seeking healthcare and that of their family. Ignoring the spiritual aspect, even when that aspect is obvious, is often detrimental to effective communication.

Spiritual issues may not appear relevant to the practising healthcare professional; however, if the Person/s considers them relevant, they require specific attention. Such attention will contribute to positive outcomes and is therefore a necessary consideration of the healthcare professional.

Chapter summary

Healthcare professionals relate to various Person/s in everyday practice. These Person/s include those seeking their assistance, healthcare professional colleagues and various support staff who maintain both the daily work schedule and the working environment. When communicating with the Person/s, it is important to establish the reason they are seeking assistance, their current condition and their expectations of the particular healthcare profession. The various aspects of the Person/s require consideration in daily practice. These aspects are the physical (including sexual), emotional, cognitive, social (including cultural) and spiritual aspects of the Person/s. They interrelate within a dynamic system; each contributing to the overall functioning of the

Person/s. Consideration of these aspects while interacting promotes effective communication, Person/Family-centred Care and positive healthcare outcomes.

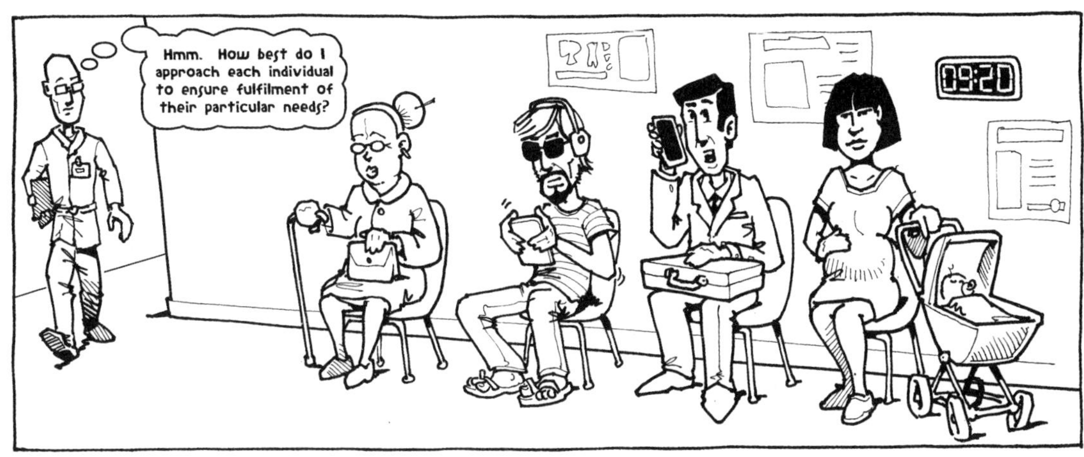

FIGURE 9.1
Awareness of the Person/s can be challenging, but is worthwhile.
Courtesy Roger Harvey © Elsevier Australia.

REVIEW QUESTIONS

1. What are the potential effects of failure to recognise each aspect of the whole Person/s?

____

____

____

____

2. Physical aspects of the Person/s may appear obvious. Suggest reasons why they might not always be reliable.

____

____

3. What are the components of the sexual aspects of a Person/s?

4. What might assist in meeting the emotional needs of the Person/s?

5. How can a healthcare professional accommodate the communication needs of a Person/s with limited cognitive skills?

6. What can affect the social aspect of a Person/s and how can a healthcare professional accommodate this aspect?

7. Why should a healthcare professional acknowledge the spiritual aspect of a Person/s and what are the potential benefits of acknowledging this aspect?

____

____

____

____

References

American Psychiatric Association (APA), 2022. Neurodevelopmental disorders. In: American Pyschiatric Association. Diagnostic and statistical manual of mental disorders, 5th edition, text revision (DSM-5-TR). APA, Washington DC.

Ano, G.G. & Pargament, K.I. 2013. Predictors of spiritual struggles: An exploratory study. Mental Health, Religion and Culture, 16(4), 419–434.

Bateman, S.D., 2014. Improving the holistic wound care experience and integrating an education regimen. Wounds UK, 10(2), 70–79.

Bayne, H., Neukrug, E., Hays, D., et al., 2013. A comprehensive model for optimizing empathy in person-centered care. Patient Education and Counseling, 93(2), 209–215.

Berk, L., 2022. Infants, children and adolescents, 9th ed. Sage Publications, Thousand Oaks, CA.

Blaszko Helming, M.A., Shields, D.A., Avino, K.M., et al., 2020. Dossey and Keegan's holistic nursing: A handbook for practice, 8th ed. Jones & Bartlett, Burlington, MA.

Bogaert, B., 2020. Need for patient-developed concepts of empowerment to rectify epistemic injustice and advance person-centred care. Journal of Medical Ethics, 47(12), e15.

Booth, L., Kaylor, S., 2018. Teaching spiritual care within nursing education. Holistic Nursing Practice, 32(4), 177–181.

Brito, R., Waldzus, S., Sekerdej, M., et al., 2011. The contexts and structures of relating to others: How memberships in different types of groups shape the construction of interpersonal relationships. Journal of Social and Personal Relationships, 28(3), 406–432.

Burkhardt, P., 2015. Holistic and integrative nursing understanding our roots. Beginnings, 35(1), 5–33.

Cobb, M., Puchalski, C.M., Rumbold, B. (eds), 2014. Oxford textbook of spirituality in health care. Oxford University Press, Oxford.

Davis, C.M., Musolino, G.M., 2016. Patient–practitioner interaction: An experiential manual for developing the art of healthcare, 6th ed. Slack, Thorofare, NJ.

Falkenheimer, S.A., 2018. PRIME: Partnership in international medical education: An oral history of the development of an international network in whole person medicine and whole person teaching. Ethics and Medicine, 34(2), 87–102.

Ford, D., Downey, L., Engelberg, R., et al., 2012. Discussing religion and spirituality is an advanced communication skill: An exploratory structural equation model of physician trainee self-ratings. Journal of Palliative Medicine, 15(1), 63–70.

Haddad A.M., Purtilo, R.B., Doherty, R.F., 2019. Health professional and patient interaction, 9th ed. Elsevier/Saunders, St Louis, MO.

Hall, J.A., Gulbrandsen, P., Dahl, F.A., 2014. Communication study: Physician gender, physician patient-centered behavior, and patient satisfaction: A study in three practice settings within a hospital. Patient Education and Counseling, 95(3), 313–318.

Hansen, E., Walters, J., Howes, F., 2016. Whole person care, patient-centred care and clinical practice guidelines in general practice. Health Sociology Review, 25(2), 157–170.

Harms, L., Pierce, J., 2019. Working with people: communication skills for reflective practice, 2nd Canadian ed. Oxford University Press, Ontario.

Hess, K. Y., Ramugondo, E., 2014. Clinical reasoning used by occupational therapists to determine the nature of spiritual occupations in relation to psychiatric pathology. British Journal of Occupational Therapy, 77(5), 234–242.

Hillen, M.A., de Haes, H.C.J.M., Stalpers, L.J.A., et al., 2014. How can communication by oncologists enhance patients' trust? An experimental study. Annals of Oncology, 25 (4), 896–901.

Holli, B.B., Beto, J.A., 2023. Nutrition counselling and education skills for dietetics professionals, 8th ed. Jones & Bartlett, Burlington, MA.

Honeycutt, A., Milliken, M.A., 2021. Understanding human behavior: A guide for healthcare providers, 10th ed. Cengage Learning, Boston.

James, T.A., 2023. Building empathy into the structure of health care. Trends in Medicine, Harvard Medical School Postgraduate Education. Online. Available: postgraduateeducation.hms.harvard.edu/trends-medicine/building-empathy-structure-health-care

Koenig, H.G., 2018. Religion and mental health: Research and clinical applications. Elsevier, New York.

Koenig, H.G., VanderWeele, T.J., Peteet, J.R.. 2023. Handbook of religion and health, 3rd ed. Oxford University Press, New York.

Lamothe, M.B., Boujut, E., Senasni, F., et al., 2014. To be or not to be empathic: The combined role of empathic concern and perspective taking in understanding burnout in general practice. BMC Family Practice, 15(1), 15–30.

Levine, J., 2012. Working with people: The helping process, 9th ed. Pearson, San Antonio.

Maley, C.M., Pagana, N.L., Velenger, C.A., et al., 2016. Dealing with major life events and transitions: A systematic literature review on and occupational analysis of spirituality. American Journal of Occupational Therapy, 70(4), 7004260010.

Mathisen, B. A., & Carey, L.B., 2018. Epilogue: allied health and spiritual care. In: Carey, L.B. & Mathisen, B.A. (eds). Spiritual care for allied health practice: A person-centred approach. Jessica Kingsley Publishers, London.

Moosavi, S., Rohani, C., Borhani, F., et al., 2019. Factors affecting spiritual care practices of oncology nurses: A qualitative study. Support Care Cancer, 27(3), 901–909.

Morris, A., Biggerstaff, D., Lycett, D., 2016. Capturing whole person care. Journal of Renal Care, 42(2), 71–72.

Mthembu, T. G., Wegner, L., Roman, N.V., 2017. Exploring occupational therapy students' perceptions of spirituality in occupational therapy groups: A qualitative study. Occupational Therapy in Mental Health, 33(2), 141–167.

Northouse, L.L., Northouse, P.G., 1998. Health communication: Strategies for health professionals, 3rd ed. Pearson Education, Michigan.

O'Toole, G., Ramugondo, E., 2018. Occupational therapy and spiritual care. In: Carey, L.B., & Mathisen, B.A. (eds). Spiritual care for allied health practice: A person-centred approach. Jessica Kingsley Publishers, London.

Phelps, A., Lauderdale, K., Alcorn, S., et al., 2012. Addressing spirituality within the care of patients at the end of life: Perspectives of patients with advanced cancer, oncologists and oncology nurses. Journal of Clinical Oncology, 30(20), 2538–2544.

Piaget, J., 1968. Six psychological studies. Vintage, New York.

Piaget, J., Inhelder, B., 1958. The growth of logical thinking: From childhood to adolescence. Basic Books, New York.

Rogers, C., 1967. On becoming a person. Constable, London.

Ronaldson, S., 2014. Spirituality in palliative care nursing. In: O'Connor, M., Lee, S., Aranda, S. (eds), Palliative care nursing: A guide to practice, 3rd ed. Ausmed, Melbourne.

Schroeder, J., Bracket, A., Buechler, C., et al., 2016. Widow(er)hood: Finding meaning through spirituality. American Journal of Occupational Therapy, 70(4), 7011510193.

Sohl, S.J., Borowski, L.A., Kent, E.E., et al., 2014. Cancer survivors' disclosure of complementary health approaches to physicians: The role of patient-centered communication. Cancer 121(6), 900–907.

van der Riet, P., Pitt, V., 2020. Communicating with people about their spiritual needs. In: Levett-Jones, T. (ed.), Critical conversations for patient safety, 2nd ed. Pearson, Sydney.

White, G., 2006. Talking about spirituality in healthcare practice: A resource for the multi-professional healthcare team. Jessica Kingsley, London.

CHAPTER 10

Awareness of the effects of non-verbal communication for the healthcare professional

Chapter objectives

Upon completing this chapter, readers should be able to:

- explain and give examples of non-verbal communication
- discuss the significance of non-verbal communication
- examine the benefits of non-verbal communication
- list and explain the results of non-verbal communication
- recognise and synthesise the components of non-verbal communication
- recognise types of communication for those who cannot use spoken words
- state the basic requirements for the use of alternative communication devices.

Non-verbal communication is, as the name implies, communication occurring in addition to or without words. It encompasses the environment, appearance, manner and style of communicating, and the internal values of the people communicating (Haith-Cooper 2014; Higginbottom et al 2014; Holli & Beto 2023). It contributes to creating positive first impressions with the Person/s, thereby developing a connection and potentially trust.

Non-verbal communication includes the behaviours that accompany words (Beesley et al 2017; Burrus & Willis 2020; Moss 2020). It conveys emotional and relational information (Henderson 2019; Henry et al 2012). It often relates to expressions of pain (Rowbotham et al 2014). Crystal (2007) states that even though non-verbal messages carry meaning, they are less flexible and adaptable than verbal modes of expression. While this may be true, non-verbal cues significantly influence the meaning of a sent message (sometimes communicating more than 80 per cent of the meaning), thereby potentially making them more important than the spoken words (Chan 2013; Egan & Reese 2019; Stevenson 2014).

There are various components of non-verbal communication (see Table 10.1). **Body language** is the general name given to non-verbal cues. Body language includes gesture, facial expression, and actions indicating focus or preoccupation, posture, eye contact, touch, gait and clothing (Myers et al 2020; Patel 2014; Stein-Parbury 2021). However, there are other non-verbal elements of speech relating to the voice. The technical name for non-verbal characteristics

TABLE 10.1
Components of non-verbal communication

Component		Sub-component	Positive and negative aspects
Environment		Disturbances	Limited privacy
		Arrangement, organisation and type of furniture	Colour and height
		Lighting	Lit to ensure safety and comfort
Body language		Body position	Position of arms while standing Position of head, arms, trunk and legs while sitting
		Facial expression	Forehead: frowns and eyebrows Mouth: smiles, tight, pursing
		Eye contact	Eyes regularly focusing on the eyes of the Person Eyes gazing over their shoulder Eyes avoiding contact
		Gestures	Use of fingers, hands, or entire upper limb
		Proximity (personal space)	Distance between individuals when sitting or standing Standing while the Person is sitting
Voice	Prosodic features	Volume	Hearing or not hearing the message
		Pitch	Height of the sound may cause distress
		Rate/Speed	Too fast or too slow
	Paralinguistic features	Emphasis on particular words	Changes the meaning
		Pauses	Can create discomfort May indicate thinking
		Tone	Can indicate distress or importance Can communicate displeasure

of the voice is suprasegmental features. There are two types of suprasegmental features: prosodic and paralinguistic. The **prosodic features of the voice** include volume, **pitch** and rate of speech, which combine to create the unique "rhythm" of a language. The **paralinguistic features of the voice** (also called paralanguage) use other vocal effects to convey meaning; they include emphasis, timely pauses and tone, as well as laughing, whining, moaning and other non-verbal sounds. Suprasegmental vocal characteristics, along with body language, can change meaning, and thus are worthy of recognition and examination when considering non-verbal communication.

The significance of non-verbal communication

Mehrabian (2009) and Patel (2014) indicate that words carry a small proportion of the meaning of a message. The **suprasegmentals** of a message and body language deliver most of the meaning. However, it is impossible to separate verbal and non-verbal messages (Chan 2013; Knapp et al 2021; Tregoning 2015). It is essential then that the non-verbal cues support rather than contradict the verbal messages. If the voice or face is preoccupied (Gorawara-Bhat et al 2013) or upset and the words contradict this message, the Person/s will experience confusion rather than empathy (Rosen 2014). They may, in fact, assume the healthcare professional is not interested in them or their needs (Burrus & Willis 2020). In short, body language and the spoken words must send the same message (messages of respect, warmth and acceptance) to avoid misunderstanding and negative outcomes. Consistency between verbal and non-verbal messages improves the satisfaction of the Person/s (Henry et al 2012; Rosen 2014), thereby achieving effective communication (Henderson 2019). This indicates that healthcare professionals must use both verbal and non-verbal forms of communication consciously and with care, regardless of the relative significance of either, in delivering the meaning (Knapp et al 2021; Moss 2020). It is also important to remember that both the Person/s and the healthcare professional are using and interpreting non-verbal communication throughout every interaction. Additionally, there will be different responses particular to and different for each individual (Allen 2021). Thus, understanding non-verbal messages may require questions to validate any interpretation of non-verbal communication.

The benefits of non-verbal communication

Skill in interpreting and using non-verbal behaviour potentially increases the attraction, popularity and psychosocial wellbeing of an individual. However, skilful use of non-verbal behaviours can also increase the likelihood of being able to manipulate other people. Thus, individuals who are skilful in using non-verbal communication can be influential in assisting and supporting, as well as in deceiving, other people. Healthcare professionals must take care to use their non-verbal messages to achieve effective and honest communication (Allen 2021).

The effects of non-verbal communication

Non-verbal behaviour often regulates or refines verbal communication (Beesley et al 2017; Egan & Reese 2019; Moss 2020). It can:

- substantiate or reiterate the meaning of the words (Moss 2020). For example, yelling *Yeah!* at a football game is often reiterated by throwing arms up in the air or jumping up and down)

- contradict or complicate the meaning of the words (Beesley et al 2017). For example, stating *I am OK* with a faltering voice and quivering lip may indicate the opposite meaning to the words
- reinforce or accentuate the meaning of the words. For example, saying *No thanks,* along with specific non-verbal gestures, tone of voice and body positions, such as covering a cup with a hand, makes the message very clear
- influence the response of the Person/s, regardless of words. For example: avoiding eye contact may indicate a desire to evade interaction, or holding up a hand may indicate a need to stop an interaction
- decrease anxiety and facilitate expression of opinions, feelings and concerns (Beesley et al 2017)
- express feelings (den Hertog & Niessen 2021; Knapp et al 2021).

Skilful and appropriate use of non-verbal messages for healthcare professionals communicates respect, acceptance, openness and empathy, along with confidence in their communication and professional skills (Burrus & Willis 2020).

In groups, explore the following.

Non-verbal communication can achieve positive and negative results.

- List the positive and negative results of non-verbal behaviours.
- Consider the results from the perspectives of both parties – the sender and the receiver.
- How might a healthcare professional ensure their non-verbal and verbal messages send the same message?
- How can a healthcare professional ensure their non-verbal messages send appropriate messages, even when they are feeling negative or pressured?

The components of non-verbal communication

Environment

The environment clearly communicates the level of interest in, and care for, the Person/s (Levine 2012; see Chapter 12). Seating arrangements in a cosy room that promote appropriate levels of connection communicate careful attention to the needs of those using the room. Healthcare professionals who focus on the interaction rather than being distracted by responding to every other event in the service (e.g. answering the telephone) deliver specific messages potentially developing trust and producing positive outcomes (Beesley et al 2017; Moss 2020).

Body language

Body language is a component of communication worldwide. There are particular rules for the use of body language that vary from culture to culture. The interpretation of body language must consider the context and the particular circumstances of the communicating people (Chan 2013; Levine & Ambady 2013). For example, someone waving both arms above their head may mean more than "hello"; they may mean "take care, danger near". The position of the body or body posture when sitting, or arms when standing, can also potentially communicate particular emotions. Folded arms might suggest particular negative emotions (disinterest, frustration or defensiveness) or they might suggest the individual is more comfortable with folded arms. The physical appearance and the apparent care the healthcare professional has taken with their appearance communicates particular messages. Conscious consideration of those messages assists the healthcare professional to communicate respect, equality and acceptance.

Facial expression

Facial expressions can be powerful additions to words and generally express emotions. As such, they are an essential element of social interactions (Beesley et al 2017; Nazarko 2015; Smith & Grant 2014). Facial expressions can convey messages without the use of words (Haddad et al 2019). Some individuals have expressive faces, while others rarely use their faces to express their emotions. Some comedians are excellent examples of people who, when performing, rarely use facial expressions to communicate their emotions (i.e. the classic "deadpan" delivery). Individuals with expressive faces must take care not to demonstrate emotions they regret when communicating during practice. Healthcare professionals should consciously use and control facial expressions to express respect, empathy and attention (Beesley et al 2017; den Hertog & Niessen 2021; Tregoning 2015). They should also remember that interpreting facial expressions may be difficult. In such circumstances, asking the Person/s for confirmation of understanding of their facial expressions is necessary.

- Do you regularly use your face to express your emotions?
- How successfully do you express your emotions using your face?

1. Each member of the group chooses an emotion (e.g. happy, sad, embarrassed, tired, angry, frustrated, disgusted, anxious, confused, peaceful, lonely, bored, sleepy, interested). Do not tell anyone in the group your chosen emotion.
2. Each person uses their face to express their chosen emotion.
3. The other group members write down the name of the person and the emotion they are expressing on a piece of paper.
4. When everyone has expressed their emotion, check the interpretations of the emotion. How many were incorrect? How could you vary your facial expression to more accurately express the emotion? How many variations of the same emotion were there?
5. What are the implications for a healthcare professional if different people assume different emotions from similar facial expressions? Or similar emotions from different facial expressions?

It is important to understand there are cultural variations in the use of facial expression to convey messages (Beesley et al 2017; Levine & Ambady 2013). These variations include both how the face is used and the meaning of particular facial expressions.

Eye contact

There are specific cultural variations in the use of eye contact. Eye contact in some cultures signals interest and attention (Montague & Asan 2014), while avoiding eye contact can indicate the opposite (i.e. disinterest). However, in some cultures, avoiding eye contact with particular individuals is a sign of respect. Nevertheless, eye contact can regulate turn-taking in an interaction. It can indicate the nature of the relationship between the communicating people. Using eye contact can assist the healthcare professional to assess the feelings or functioning of the Person/s while communicating (Gorawara-Bhat et al 2013; Montague & Asan 2014; Moss 2020; Nazarko 2015).

Some Aboriginal and Torres Strait Islander peoples may communicate discomfort or pain by turning their heads to avoid any possibility of eye contact. Some cultures have different rules or beliefs about eye contact relating to gender, age and status, and may avoid eye contact in particular situations.

Individually consider and reflect:

- What does eye contact mean for you?
- How do you use it?
- How might you manage a situation when the Person uses eye contact differently to you?

In groups of not more than four discuss:

- What might affect the willingness of someone to have eye contact with another individual?
- How can a healthcare professional manage this?

Gesture

Gestures vary from individual to individual and convey attitudes, feelings and ideas. They do not necessarily require words. Gestures can use the entire upper limb or one finger; using an arm to wave or a finger to wave conveys very different meanings. Folded arms can communicate lack of openness or unhappiness; a tapping foot along with folded arms communicates impatience, and looking at a watch while tapping a foot with folded arms has a different meaning again (i.e. "hurry up" anger). In these cases, the action clearly communicates the meaning without words.

Understanding subtle as well as obvious gestures is essential for effective communication (Haddad et al 2019; Henderson 2019). When working with people from different cultures, it is appropriate for a healthcare professional to state the conventions of gesture in their own culture and ask for the convention in the culture of the Person/s seeking assistance. For example, the healthcare professional might say *When we do this, it means this; what does it mean to you?* Asking such a question of the Person/s will assist understanding and build rapport.

- Choose five common gestures (e.g. waving, particular movements of the head). Do they have the same meaning every time they are used? If not, explore the factors that change the meaning.

If gestures can change meaning within a single culture due to context, it is inappropriate to assume that the gestures of one culture have the same meaning in another culture. Specifically asking about the meaning of particular gestures in the relevant culture is often conducive to the development of the therapeutic relationship.

Personal space or proximity

The use of **personal space** or proximity while interacting is important. It communicates interest and, in some cultures, the nature of the relationship. In some South Pacific cultures, the authority figure must always be at a higher level than others. Generally, however, wherever possible, it is important to attempt to communicate on the same physical level with the Person/s. That is, if they are sitting it is beneficial to explore how the healthcare professional can sit as well.

The distance between two interacting people communicates interest in the interaction and can indicate the intimacy of the relationship. The comfortable distance between standing individuals while relating varies from country to country. Cultural differences can result in individuals from a country with a smaller acceptable personal space "chasing" individuals from a country with a larger acceptable personal space around a room, as the first steps into the personal space of the second and the second moves away. Until they realise what is causing the constant movement, they will both experience discomfort during the interaction; one because they are standing too far apart and the other because they are too close to the other person. In such circumstances the healthcare professional can change the context, perhaps choosing to sit to communicate, or they may discuss the differences in proximity in order to achieve mutual understanding about proximity or personal space. It is important during all interactions to use relevant non-verbal communication techniques, such as gestures, tone of voice, and, where appropriate, eye contact, in order to communicate interest and to reassure the Person/s.

Suprasegmentals: prosodic features of the voice

Volume

The **volume of a voice** refers to whether the voice is loud or soft. Some individuals have voices that seem loud, even when the person thinks they are speaking softly. Such voices are distinctive and can often be heard clearly from a distance or among other noises. Different situations require changes in volume depending on the context and the environmental noise conditions. Some individuals lower their volume when they are nervous, while others will raise their volume when nervous. Using appropriate volume is very important when speaking with a Person/s because this demonstrates the characteristics of a caring healthcare professional. Many Aboriginal and Torres Strait Islander peoples speak with a low volume when discussing personal or important information and may be uncomfortable with loud volume in such situations (Australian Government Department of Health and Ageing 2014).

Pitch

Pitch refers to the frequency of the voice, which makes the voice sound high or low. Pitch changes the style of expression and communicates feelings. Variations in pitch change meaning and may give greater force or intensity of feeling to spoken words (Crystal 2007). In some cultures, variations in pitch can also indicate the opinion of the speaker. Pitch falls or rises, depending on the starting point of the voice. Various languages use falling or rising pitch to indicate meaning. For example, changes in pitch can mean the difference between a statement and a question. In some South Pacific groups, however, raising the pitch at the end of a sentence is a common feature of the language and does not indicate a question.

Rate

The speed or rate of speaking also affects comprehension. Different communities and cultures use particular rates of speaking, and most people within those communities adopt the rate that represents the norm. Some cultures value rapid speech, while others consider slow speakers to be competent speakers (Devito 2021). Within a particular culture, however, some people naturally speak more quickly or slowly than the majority. Speaking in public or in situations that create negative emotions may affect the speed of speaking; in turn, this may limit the ability of the listener to concentrate, which will decrease their understanding.

It is important for healthcare professionals to be aware of situations that potentially affect the rate of their speech, and to consciously adjust their rate in these situations to ensure adequate comprehension. Another situation that might require an adjustment in speech rate is when the healthcare professional is communicating with someone who has limited skills in the language of the healthcare professional. In this situation, using a slower than usual speech rate may facilitate understanding for the listener.

- Has anyone ever asked you to change your speed of speaking?
- Are there particular circumstances that make you speak more quickly or more slowly? What are these circumstances? How might you always ensure appropriate speed?
- List possible emotions that might affect the speed of speaking.
- Discuss the idea that the rate of speaking changes the understanding of spoken words.
- Decide whether speed is the only voice characteristic affecting understanding. Suggest others.

Suprasegmentals: paralinguistic features of the voice

Volume, pitch and rate combine to create rhythm while speaking. However, there are other important non-verbal characteristics of speech.

Emphasis

Emphasis is a characteristic of the voice that can be used to change meaning. Emphasis refers to the stress placed on words within phrases or sentences. When used skilfully, it is a powerful communication tool. However, care must be taken when using emphasis to communicate meaning, because it can easily produce negative effects in addition to positive effects. *You did* ***what?*** stresses the action and can have a positive or negative meaning. ***You*** *did what?* stresses the person and again may indicate disbelief that has a positive or a negative meaning.

In groups of three, complete this activity.

- Have a group member say each of the following statements. Then change the *emphasis* to indicate a change in meaning. In some cases, the emphasis may give the phrase the opposite meaning.
- Decide what each statement means with different emphases.
- Indicate where to place the emphasis to change the meaning.

1. Well that's a nice shirt.
2. You're so clever.

3. Have you finished yet?
4. Well do you want a cup of tea?
5. That colour really suits you.
6. Well that was good wasn't it?

Pauses

Pauses when speaking occur within sentences, as well as in conversations. They provide opportunities for taking a breath or for "looking up" from papers, if referring to notes. They provide opportunities for thinking in both the speaker and the listener. Pauses allow the speaker to compose their next sentence and the listener to process, understand and perhaps consider any questions they might want to ask the speaker. A speaker may pause in response to non-verbal cues given or not given by the listener. Such a pause allows the speaker to decide whether to clarify the words or to ask if the listener requires clarification, or, in some cases, to ask whether they are hearing and understanding. Respectful pauses or silences can be empowering for the Person/s. Such pauses require the healthcare professional to focus completely on the Person – on both the verbal and non-verbal aspects of their message, continuing to engage by either nodding the head or vocalising (*mmm*) to indicate focused listening.

Different cultures view pauses or silence differently (Beesley et al 2017). Some interpret them negatively, while others consider them essential when attempting to become familiar with an unknown individual. Sometimes, for some people, pauses of over 10–15 seconds may create feelings of discomfort. It is important to observe the non-verbal message of the Person/s during pauses of abnormal length as they may be processing rather than not engaging. In some Aboriginal and Torres Strait Islander cultures, pauses and silence facilitate communication and information-processing (Eckermann et al 2013; Harms & Pierce 2019). In these cultures, short pauses of less than several minutes can feel uncomfortable.

Pauses associated with vocalisation (e.g. *ah* or *um*) may communicate uncertainty (Devito 2021) or a level of incompetence. It is best for healthcare professionals to avoid such vocalised pauses. It is important for healthcare professionals to communicate confidence when speaking, whether through words, non-verbal cues or silence, because this assists the listener to trust and feel confident in the accuracy of the message. However, Person/s may require time to reflect on or process some questions. This may be true for Person/s with cognitive deficits due to medication or medical conditions, or if experiencing extreme pain or extreme emotions.

It is important to remember that during any interaction non-verbal messages are communicating something. Therefore, it is essential for the healthcare professional to consider what their non-verbal messages are communicating, to ensure they reinforce all spoken messages.

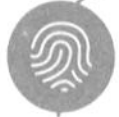

1. How do you respond to *pauses* in conversations?
2. How do you feel if you have verbally shared something personal and there is a pause with no response?
3. What do you do in such situations?

In groups of no more than five, consider the following:

1. How should you respond if someone has shared something personal with you and you simply have to stop, process and consider before responding?
2. Is a pause or silence appropriate when someone has asked a question and is waiting for a response? Why or why not?
3. Is a pause an appropriate response when you do not know what to say or how to respond? Why or why not?
4. What might be an appropriate response if you need time to consider your answer?
5. What might be an appropriate response if you do not have an answer?
6. Suggest situations when a pause might occur or be required for a healthcare professional.
7. Suggest strategies to manage these situations.

Tone

Emphasis and tone may occur together. Tone is associated with quality of voice, and it is the manner of expressing words that typically indicate feelings, attitudes or thoughts about a particular topic. Tone is usually expressed through changes in pitch, volume or duration of a word. The tone of voice can be used to change meaning in particular circumstances. Tone of voice usually affects the entire utterance, unlike emphasis, which usually affects a few words.

Tone can communicate a range of messages to the Person/s. The use of a quieter or softer tone can convey reassurance, empathy or validation. In some circumstances, healthcare professionals may need to use increased volume and stronger tones to indicate warning, urgency or to reinforce particular boundaries or limitations. In some situations, if increasing the urgency of the message (e.g. if enforcing boundaries or restrictions), the tone must change from a quieter tone, suggesting a request or suggestion, to a firmer often louder tone to convey the importance of the meaning of the statements or questions.

While non-verbal behaviours are powerful communicators of various emotions and ideas, it is easy to misunderstand them. It is therefore essential to validate perceptions of non-verbal messages because these vary from individual to individual and from culture to culture. Requests for validation allow the Person/s to either state or deny the emotions and ideas they are experiencing at that moment. They sometimes remind the Person/s of the power of their non-verbal messages, and encourage them to take responsibility for their non-verbal behaviours and the associated emotions or ideas.

Different individuals use non-verbal cues in different ways. Some use them consciously, while others use them unconsciously. Many individuals have been surprised while watching themselves on video to see the non-verbal use of their body or voice. Unconscious hair-twirling, arm-crossing, upper lip-stroking or nail-biting while concentrating may be habits so unconscious that the person is surprised when they see themselves doing them. Healthcare professionals must learn to observe and interpret non-verbal messages, but must also be aware of their own non-verbal behaviours (Beesley et al 2017; Henderson 2019). They should use non-verbal messages to communicate their exact meaning. This mandates that the words and the non-verbal messages have the same meaning.

In groups, discuss the following and report to the entire class.

- Consider how to express RESPECT using non-verbal messages.
- Consider how to express EMPATHY using non-verbal messages.
- Consider how to express TRUSTWORTHINESS using non-verbal messages.

Communicating with the Person/s who has limited verbal communication skills

When communicating with the Person/s who finds verbal communication difficult, it is necessary to use devices and forms of communication that do not rely on verbal transmission. **Augmentative and alternative communication (AAC)** refers to systems of communication for people who find speaking difficult or are unable to speak. Such communication systems may assist in reducing frustration levels and thus decrease the use of disturbing behaviours to communicate.

Augmentative and alternative forms of communication include the use of symbols, aids, strategies and techniques to transmit and receive messages through either electronic or non-electronic means (Beukelman & Mirenda 2013; Moss 2020). **Augmentative communication** refers to non-verbal forms of communication that *highlight* the spoken word through simultaneous gestures or signs (e.g. finger-spelling, key word signing [e.g. Makaton], sign language [e.g. Auslan, ASL]), or by pointing to objects or pictures. **Alternative communication** uses forms of communication to *replace* the spoken word (e.g. an electronic device using visual communication software or electronic voice generation).

Individuals who experience difficulty communicating because of physical or cognitive limitations may rely on AAC to transmit and receive information. The use of AAC will assist such individuals to interact socially and engage in the activities of their choice. Such individuals can use one or a combination of several forms of AAC to process and understand information as well as express themselves. Some individuals use AAC until speech develops, or to supplement attempts at vocalisation. For others, AAC is a permanent means of communication that can assist comprehension and self-expression.

Successful use of AAC requires competence in the dominant language of the environment, social competence in the expected norms of communication, competence in operating the particular system, and an ability to compensate for the ignorance of communication partners who are unfamiliar with the particular system. Understanding the norms of personal interaction and communication are necessary for effective communication. They include knowing when to speak, when to listen, what to discuss with particular individuals in specific situations and how to discuss or interact. Most individuals absorb these norms as they "grow up" in a particular culture or society and use them skilfully yet unconsciously whenever interacting.

Augmentative and alternative forms of communication are often visual in nature. (Any individual who finds it difficult to process auditory information may benefit from using visual forms of communication.) Visual forms of communication are useful because they are concrete and do not usually require abstract thought. They are also stable, lasting longer than the spoken word. The use of a symbol or sign resembling a real object also makes accurate assumptions possible for the person receiving the message.

If possible, it is beneficial for AAC devices to be flexible and portable, allowing the individual to use them in a variety of situations. Such devices are generally individualised to the needs, wants and emotions of the particular individual. Augmentative and alternative forms of communication can function to give directions, provide single-step pictures for completion of activities, or facilitate choices of activities. They can take many forms, for example:

- a community request card containing a picture of a particular type of burger and can of drink
- a noticeboard containing a pictorial representation of the schedule for the day
- a "chat book" introducing an individual who communicates regularly with a variety of people – the book might include pictures of their likes and dislikes, family, hobbies, social experiences and the events of the previous week
- a pictorial shopping list displaying pictures of the goods needed for the next week
- an activity choice board or book allowing an individual to choose the activity they would prefer to perform after completion of the current activity
- a pictorial representation of a particular health profession procedure or relevant object
- using mobile phone applications (apps) to translate speech into text.

These are the less technical forms of AAC. However, such systems can also take the form of electronic devices that may provide vocalisation in addition to visual forms of messages.

Healthcare professionals will find AAC systems to be useful when relating to the Person/s who has difficulty communicating using spoken words. They encourage self-expression and often increase independence. AAC creates a connection with those around the individual by increasing the likelihood of communicative exchanges.

- Consider four scenarios in Section 4: The Adolescent, the Older adult, People who are older and ageing, and the Person experiencing a hearing impairment.
- What form of non-verbal communication will be important when communicating with the Person/s in each scenario?

Chapter summary

Non-verbal communication refers to communication without words, and it is often more important than spoken words when deciding the meaning of a message. There are two main elements of non-verbal communication. The first is body language, which includes facial expression, eye contact, gesture and proximity. The other element is the suprasegmental features of the message, which refers to the non-verbal characteristics of the voice; they include volume, pitch, rate, emphasis, pauses, tone and non-verbal sounds, such as laughing or moaning.

Communicating with the Person/s sometimes requires the healthcare professional to communicate using alternative forms of communication, including electronic devices or graphic representations of actions or objects. In all interactions, however, non-verbal communication can have negative and positive results. It is therefore important that non-verbal messages complement verbal messages. Healthcare professionals must be aware of the variations in meanings of non-verbal cues and of their personal manner when using the elements of non-verbal communication. It is also important to remember that effective communication includes both verbal and non-verbal messages, with non-verbal messages contributing substantially to the meaning.

Tell me how you feel today.
You are not interested. I'm not telling you anything!
Tell me ... how do you feel today?
You seem interested; I think I can trust you!

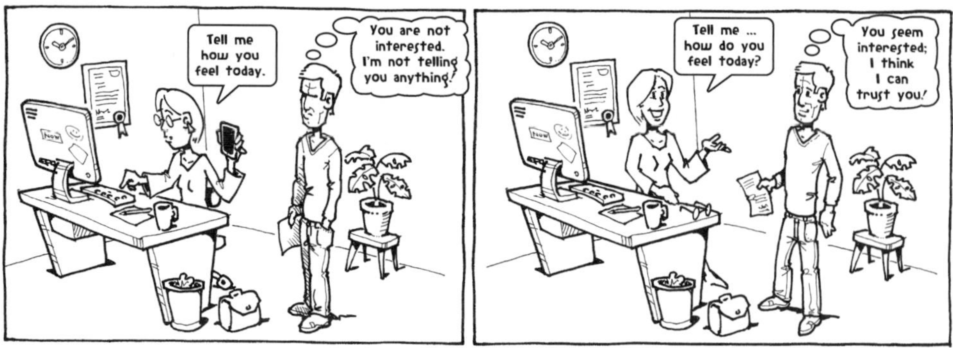

FIGURE 10.1
The power of non-verbal messages.
Courtesy Roger Harvey © Elsevier Australia.

REVIEW QUESTIONS

1. What are the three major components of non-verbal communication?

   i. ______________________________

   ii. ______________________________

   iii. ______________________________

2. What are the possible effects of non-verbal communication?

____

____

____

____

3. Give three examples of two of the three components of non-verbal communication.

   Component 1:

   i. ______________________________

   ii. ______________________________

   iii. ______________________________

   Component 2:

   i. ______________________________

   ii. ______________________________

   iii. ______________________________

4. Choose one aspect of the environment and explain how a healthcare professional might use that aspect to achieve positive results when communicating.

   ____

   ____

   ____

   ____

5. Choose two forms of body language and explain how a healthcare professional might use those forms to achieve positive results when communicating.

   ____

   ____

   ____

   ____

6. Explain how a healthcare professional might use two forms of the prosodic features of the voice to achieve positive results when communicating.

   ____

   ____

   ____

   ____

7. Explain how a healthcare professional might use two forms of the paralinguistic features of the voice to achieve positive results when communicating.

References

Allen, D., 2021. The step to take to support nervous or anxious patients. Nursing Standard, 36(2), 35–37.

Australian Government Department of Health and Ageing, 2014. Providing culturally appropriate palliative care to Indigenous Australians. Commonwealth of Australia, Canberra (The Mungabareena Aboriginal Corporation assisted in the preparation of this resource kit).

Beesley, P., Watts, M., Harrison, M., 2017. Developing your communication skills in social work. Sage, London.

Beukelman, D.R., Mirenda, P., 2013. Augmentative and alternative communication: Supporting children and adults with complex communication needs, 4th ed. Brookes, Baltimore.

Burrus, A.E., Willis, L.B., 2020. Professional communication in speech-language pathology. How to write, talk and act like a clinician, 4th ed. Plural, San Diego, CA.

Chan, Z.C.Y., 2013. A qualitative study on non-verbal sensitivity in nursing students. Journal of Clinical Nursing, 22(13/14), 1941–1950.

Crystal, D., 2007. How language works. Penguin Books, London.

den Hertog, R., Niessen, T., 2021. Taking into account patient preferences in personalised care: Blending types of nursing knowledge in evidence-based practice. Journal of Clinical Nursing, 30, 1904–1915.

Devito, J.A., 2021. The interpersonal communication book, 16th ed. Pearson, Boston

Eckermann, A., Dowd, T., Chong, E., et al., 2013. Binaŋ Goonj: Bridging cultures in Aboriginal health, 4th ed. Elsevier, Sydney.

Egan, G., Reese R.J., 2019. The skilled helper: A problem management and opportunity approach to helping, 11th ed. Cengage, Boston, MA.

Gorawara-Bhat, R., Dethmers, D.L., Cook, M.A., 2013. Physician eye contact and elder patient perceptions of understanding and adherence. The Science of Health Communication, 92(3), 375–380.

Haddad, A.M., Purtilo, R.B., Doherty, R.F., 2019. Health professional and patient interaction, 9th ed. Elsevier/Saunders, St Louis, MO.

Haith-Cooper, M., 2014. Mobile translators for non-English speaking women accessing maternity services. British Journal of Midwifery, 22(11), 795–803.

Harms, L., Pierce, J., 2019. Working with people: Communication skills for reflective practice, 2nd Canadian ed. Oxford University Press, Ontario.

Henderson, A., 2019. Communication for health care practice. Oxford University Press, Melbourne.

Henry, S.G., Fuhrel-Forbes, A., Rogers, M.A.M., et al., 2012. Association between nonverbal communication during clinical interactions and outcomes: A systematic review and meta-analysis. Patient Education and Counseling, 86, 297–315.

Higginbottom, G.M.A., Safipour, J., Yohani, S., et al., 2014. An ethnographic study of communication challenges in maternity care for immigrant women in rural Alberta. Midwifery, 31(2), 297–304.

Holli, B.B., Beto, J.A., 2023. Nutrition counselling and education skills: A practical guide, 8th ed. Jones & Bartlett, Burlington, MA.

Knapp, M., Hall, J., Horgan, T. G., 2021. Nonverbal communication in human interaction, 9th ed. Wadsworth, Boston, MA.

Levine, C.S., Ambady, N., 2013. The role of non-verbal behaviour in racial disparities in health care: Implications and solutions. Medical Education, 47(9), 867–876.

Levine, J., 2012. Working with people: The helping process, 9th ed. Pearson, San Antonio.

Mehrabian, A., 2009. Non-verbal communication. Aldine Transaction Publishers, Piscataway, NJ.

Montague, E., Asan, O., 2014. Dynamic modeling of patient and physician eye gaze to understand the effects of electronic health records on doctor–patient communication and attention. International Journal of Medical Informatics, 83(3), 225–234.

Moss, B., 2020. Communication skills in health and social care, 5th ed. Sage, London.

Myers, K.K., Krepper, R., Nibert, A., et al., 2020. Nurses' active empathic listening behaviours from the voice of the patient. Nursing Economics, 38(5) 267–275.

Nazarko, L., 2015. Top-quality communication skills remove obstacles to communicating with people with dementia. British Journal of Healthcare Assistants, 9(2), 60–65.

Patel, D.S., 2014. Body language: an effective communication tool. Journal of English Studies, 9(2), 90–95.

Rosen, D., 2014. Vital conversations: Improving communication between doctors and patients. Columbia University Press, New York.

Rowbotham, S., Wardy, A.J., Lloyd, D.M., et al., 2014. Increased pain intensity is associated with greater verbal communication difficulty and increased production of speech and co-speech gestures. PLoS One, 9(10), 1–6.

Smith, S., Grant, A., 2014. Facial affect recognition and mental health. Mental Health Practice, 17(10), 12–16.

Stein-Parbury, J., 2021. Patient and person: Interpersonal skills in nursing, 7th ed. Churchill Livingstone Elsevier, Sydney.

Stevenson, F., 2014. Achieving visibility? Use of non-verbal communication in interactions between patients and pharmacists who do not share a common language. Sociology of Health and Illness, 36(5), 756–771.

Tregoning, C., 2015. Communication skills and enhancing clinical practice through reflective learning: A case study. British Journal of Healthcare Assistants, 9(2), 66–69.

CHAPTER 11

Awareness of listening to facilitate Person/s-centred communication in healthcare

Chapter objectives

Upon completing this chapter, readers should be able to:

- define effective listening
- explain the importance of listening in Person/s-centred communication
- identify and accommodate the benefits of active listening
- discuss the concept of listening barriers and their effect upon communication
- discuss the characteristics of effective listening
- explore and examine cultural variations that affect listening
- understand the importance of appropriate disengagement.

The fundamental purpose of the healthcare professions – to provide relevant and effective healthcare – mandates Person/s-centred communication. The skill of achieving Person-centred Care or placing the Person/s at the centre of communicative interactions, can also be beneficial in everyday relationships (Adler & Proctor 2017; Bodie et al 2013; Devito 2021; van Dulmen 2017). Achieving Person/s-centred communication can be challenging (Moss 2020). However, it is essential for effective healthcare (Gilligan et al 2018). There is evidence of the relationship between effective listening and effective healthcare (Beesley et al 2018; Bodie et al 2018; Henderson 2019). There is also evidence of the relationship between listening and empathy (McKenna et al 2022), both of which are valued by the Person/s and healthcare providers. These are essential for a positive therapeutic relationship (Myers et al 2020, Slade & Sergent 2022). In addition, active listening contributes to achievement of effective communication (Mendes 2020). Some consider listening to be a necessary attribute for healthcare (Brown et al 2020), despite the tendency to overlook its role in the provision of care (King 2022). Listening is a widely used communication skill in life to develop connections with and understanding of others

(Jennings 2017; Umphrey & Sherblom 2018). Individuals listen every day – some more effectively than others. Considering the amount of time people spend listening each day, it is interesting that effective listening often requires practice and conscious effort. Effective listening is an "art", thereby reinforcing the need to practise and apply conscious effort (Gelinas 2018). The increase in electronic communication is decreasing "face-to-face" interactions and thus the amount of **active listening**. This potentially affects the quality and effectiveness of listening, indicating the need to practise and sometimes apply conscious effort to achieve effective listening.

- What is listening? List the necessary abilities to achieve effective listening.
- How do you know when someone is listening to you? What non-verbal and verbal behaviours indicate they are listening?
- How can you establish whether the listener has understood you?

Effective listening, as well as skills in speaking, reading and writing, are useful for any person to facilitate communication in general life, but are essential for a healthcare professional (Egan & Reese 2019; Harms & Pierce 2019; Holli & Beto 2023; Honeycutt & Milliken 2021; Krupa et al 2016; McKenna et al 2022; Moss 2020; Stein-Parbury 2021).

Defining effective listening

Effective listening requires all the components of Person/Family-centred Care. To listen effectively, a healthcare professional must understand what listening involves and how to perform it during their daily practice (Keller et al 2014). Effective listening requires the healthcare professional to consciously focus completely on the Person/s and visibly "tune in" (often known as *attending* listening) (Egan & Reese 2019; King et al 2012; Mann 2020; Moss 2020). It also demands demonstration of an understanding of the words and emotions communicated by the Person/s, along with all non-verbal messages. It necessitates expression of this understanding to the Person/s in both verbal and non-verbal forms – often referred to as "*reflecting* back" the messages expressed by the Person/s (Devito 2021, 2019). This is different from reflective listening, which requires the healthcare professional to attempt to hear and comprehend the perspective of the Person/s and to demonstrate this comprehension to the Person using both verbal and non-verbal messages (Jennings 2017).

Effective listening may also require the use of questions to *clarify* the accuracy of the perceptions of the healthcare professional (see Chapter 4). Effective listening then requires the healthcare professional to validate the expressed emotions to demonstrate awareness of their existence and accurate understanding of those emotions (Burrus & Willis 2020; see Chapter 10). Such listening facilitates effective and meaningful services and thus positive and effective outcomes (Thistle & McNaughton 2015).

Requirements of effective listening

Effective listening is an obligation of every healthcare professional. It requires the healthcare professional to:

- prepare themself to listen by removing any distractions and ensuring there are no interruptions (Stein-Parbury 2021)

- where possible, organise the physical environment (including furniture) to create equality and safety
- where possible, organise the setting to minimise distractions and interruptions (Moss 2020)
- adjust to all situations and needs regardless of the strength of the emotions and the severity of the need (Devito 2021)
- where possible, demonstrate physically their interest by the position of their body and their gestures, so they are visibly "tuned in" to the Person/s (Egan & Reese 2019)
- listen with their whole self (Davis & Musolino 2016) by using not only their observational and social skills, but also their emotional and cognitive skills, and sometimes their spiritual skills
- consciously focus all their attention fully on the Person/s (Holli & Beto 2023; van Dulmen 2017)
- seek areas of interest and relevance to their role to assist their continued focus and to develop the therapeutic relationship and appropriate outcomes (McKenna et al 2022)
- carefully observe all non-verbal messages of the Person/s (Bodie et al 2018)
- make conscious choices about which non-verbal messages are appropriate in response to the Person/s (Burrus & Willis 2020)
- consciously communicate interest and commitment to the Person/s through the use of verbal sounds and non-verbal cues (Thistle & McNaughton 2015)
- explore the meaning of all verbal and non-verbal messages (Devito 2019, 2021) by either paraphrasing or questioning (see Chapters 4 and 10)
- avoid stereotypical assumptions about the Person/s and the meaning of all their messages (Henderson 2019)
- avoid interrupting
- communicate the importance of the contribution of the Person/s to the process (Al-Momen et al 2015; Beesley et al 2018; Stein-Parbury 2021)
- consider cultural variations in listening (Harms & Pierce 2019) and associated non-verbal messages.

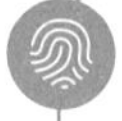

- Consider your skill in the listed requirements of effective listening.
- Divide a page into two. Label one side "Competent" and the other "More effort".
- Identify which of the listed actions you feel competent to perform and perhaps perform automatically when listening.
- Identify those you feel require more conscious effort.
- Share this list with someone who knows you well and ask them to comment on your allocation.
- Consider how to develop skills in the identified areas requiring effort.

Results of effective listening

Effective listening definitely improves outcomes, while also increasing the satisfaction of both the Person/s and the healthcare professional (Kawamichi et al 2015). However, it also enables the healthcare professional, and ultimately the Person/s, to:

- *relax*, share and explore relevant information, thereby increasing the knowledge and potential insights of the healthcare professional and the Person/s

- carefully *observe* the non-verbal messages, note their significance at the time and, if appropriate, validate those messages and sometimes diffuse emotions that may otherwise negatively dominate interactions
- *connect* and engage with (and often enjoy) different perspectives and emotions. It is often the non-verbal messages that encapsulate the less obvious and often primary needs at the time. Observations of these non-verbal messages offer the opportunity to validate and to collaborate in an equal partnership
- develop *trust* and *understanding* by unravelling the complexity of the needs. The understanding of the gathered information may reduce the occurrence of unnecessary events and the likelihood of difficulties, while ultimately increasing the possibility of meaningful and satisfactory outcomes
- *design* and develop relevant goals and interventions based on the information gathered through the collaborative relationship (Thistle & McNaughton 2015).

When listening effectively, the above points closely interact to produce mutual understanding, a therapeutic and/or collaborative relationship and Person/Family-centred Care.

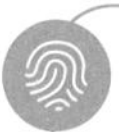

- Divide a page into two. On one side, list the first word of each result of effective listening: “Relax”, “Observe”, “Connect”, “Trust and understanding” and “Design”.
- On the other side, consider the 16 points listed in the requirements of effective listening and classify them according to which ones contribute to relax, observe, connect, trust and understanding, and design. Some of them may contribute to more than one result.
- How might you ensure you relax, observe, connect, trust and understand, and design whenever listening to a Person/s during practice?

Benefits of effective listening

Effective listening benefits the healthcare professional and the Person/s, as it ultimately improves intervention outcomes (King et al 2012). The healthcare professional who listens effectively is able to make appropriate decisions influencing the quality of care. When a healthcare professional is committed to effective listening, the Person/s seeking care feels valued and has more confidence (worthy of trust) in the healthcare professional because of their demonstrated listening skills (Bodie et al 2015; Henderson 2019). Thus, the therapeutic relationship develops appropriately because of these effective listening skills (Egan & Reese 2019; Gelinas 2018; King et al 2012; Stein-Parbury 2021; Thistle & McNaughton 2015). In addition, effective listening increases the probability of achieving mutual understanding and therefore mutually established, *relevant* goals.

Barriers to effective listening

Awareness of the **barriers** to effective listening prepares healthcare professionals to avoid potential hazards that might negatively affect the listening process (King 2022). There are various external and internal factors potentially negatively impacting effective listening (see Chapters 7, 8 and 12). The *external* (environmental) factors are important and not always obvious. Consideration of external interferences (Stein-Parbury 2021) – including noise levels, temperature, distractions and unrelated activity in the space allocated for the interaction – and adjustments where possible, will contribute to the understanding of the listener, enhancing their confidence (Umphrey & Sherblom 2018). A healthcare professional who continues listening instead of answering a telephone or pager indicates commitment to the needs of the Person/s, encouraging trust and the development of a therapeutic relationship (King 2022).

An effective listener attends to the *internal* "noise" of their emotions before listening, thereby ensuring their ability to listen, regardless of their own needs. A listener who is not psychologically prepared to listen because they are preoccupied with their own thoughts and emotions may misunderstand messages (Moscato et al 2007). Alternatively, a listener who is focused on their own ideas and assumptions may also fail to listen carefully if they attempt to predict what they will hear (Haddad et al 2019) because of preconceived assumptions or judgements (see Chapter 8).

Listening skills vary according to context and life events at any given time. Individuals may have habitual inner barriers affecting their ability to listen (Gordon 2004; see Chapter 8). These barriers fall into three major categories: (i) judging; (ii) ignoring the needs; and (iii) stipulating the solution. Overcoming these barriers is essential for a healthcare professional, as they significantly limit the effectiveness of listening. Certainly, everyone needs to "rest their brain" when listening in order to regain concentration. However, the questions listed below are not about those times of rest, but rather focus on *regularly* employed habits potentially restricting or enhancing listening effectiveness.

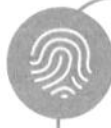

What do you typically do when listening? Answer the following questions *honestly*.

1. Do you concentrate totally on the person and their messages?
2. Do you allow yourself to think of things you have to do later?
3. Do you attempt to understand everything the person is communicating?
4. Do you sit quietly without responding verbally or non-verbally?
5. Do you attempt to identify the main point of the verbal communication?
6. Do you often interrupt?
7. Do you wait for the person to complete their message before responding?
8. Do you avoid eye contact while listening?
9. Do you keep an open mind and avoid judgement about the person or topic?
10. Do you try to "double-guess" or "read the mind" of the person speaking?
11. Do you focus on the other person regardless of how you are feeling?
12. Do you change the subject if the person begins expressing negative emotions?

Typically answering *yes* to the above odd-numbered questions and *no* to the even-numbered questions indicates effective skills in listening. Answering *yes* to any of the even-numbered questions indicates a need to practise listening to ensure more effective communication. Similarly, answering *yes* to some odd and some even questions also indicates a need to practise and improve listening skills. Remember individual skills in listening can vary; however, all healthcare professionals benefit from developing effective listening skills.

Most individuals at different times use barriers that limit the effectiveness of their listening (Gordon 2007). These barriers may be a protective device used during a particular interaction or they may be a learnt habit. The explanation for the use of barriers is irrelevant, because if they are used at all they limit the effectiveness of listening. It is important that healthcare professionals are aware of barriers to listening. They must be especially aware of the barriers they typically use themselves, in order to limit their use of such barriers when listening to individuals seeking their assistance.

The *language* of the listener may hinder the effectiveness of the communication if the healthcare professional has limited ability in the language of the Person/s (Keller et al 2014). Mutual understanding requires both communicators to have some level of competence in a common language. Effective listening is impossible without a common language.

In groups of no more than four, read the following list of barriers to listening and individually write your definition for each. Then discuss the definitions and as a group agree on a definition for each barrier. Together, think of an example of each barrier.

Interrupting	Intimidating
Monopolising	Placating
Rehearsing	Reassuring
Switching off	Breaking confidences
Partial listening	Advising
Mind-reading	Judging
Being right	Interrogating
Changing the subject	Language

Allow time for each group member to consider the answers to the following questions. Then as a group, discuss the answers.

- Of these barriers, which ones have you experienced when you have been communicating with someone?
- Have you experienced any of them regularly?
- What is the major emotion you experience when someone uses a listening barrier while you are speaking?
- List reasons why people would use these barriers to avoid listening.
- Do you sometimes use any of these barriers to listening? Why do you use them?
- Do you use one/some of them regularly?
- Are there particular circumstances in which you use these barriers or are they a habit?
- If you use barriers to listening in particular circumstances, describe the circumstances that prompt you to use the barrier(s). Explain why. How could you avoid their use?
- Brainstorm ways to overcome habitual use of a barrier to listening.
- List circumstances that might tempt a healthcare professional to use any of these listening barriers.
- Suggest ways to avoid using any of these barriers with people who require assistance.

If healthcare professionals desire to demonstrate honest, open and empathic communication with the Person/s, it is essential that they recognise **listening barriers** and the circumstances promoting their use. It is important to realise that both the healthcare professional and the Person/s may use these barriers.

There may be other barriers to listening in the healthcare professions, including the Person/s who is unable to produce speech (Burrus & Willis 2020) or an inability because of cultural norms affecting listening (Beesley et al 2018). A practising healthcare professional may encounter such barriers in practice and should take appropriate action to overcome the barriers and achieve effective communication.

Reasons for the use of barriers to listening

There are many reasons for the use of listening barriers, some of which are reasonably positive explanations for the use of a barrier. These might include:

- excitement over something being said
- preoccupation with a difficult situation
- busyness
- tiredness
- greater knowledge of the situation than the speaker
- genuine interest in the topic
- a desire to further understand the communication messages
- a desire to compose words carefully to avoid misunderstanding or hurt
- a need to communicate something urgently (e.g. a spider on the speaker!)
- a desire to share knowledge and understanding of the topic.

There are also negative explanations for the use of each listening barrier:

- An individual who finds a topic boring or not personally relevant may interrupt, "switch off", listen partially or change the subject.
- An individual who feels insecure and intimidated may monopolise, intimidate or interrogate during an interaction.
- An individual may rehearse a statement in their mind instead of listening because they want to correct the speaker about an error.
- When being right motivates a person, they might use several additional listening barriers, including attempting to mind-read.
- If mind-reading proves incorrect, an individual who feels they know more than the speaker might use advising or interrupting as a way of avoiding listening.
- An individual who feels someone is attacking them, might respond by judging the individual or attempting to intimidate or placate the person to stop them from continuing the perceived attack.
- An individual who finds the expression of negative emotions difficult, might placate or reassure without any real attempt to listen and understand the speaker.
- An individual who wishes to change the subject or redirect the attention from the speaker to the listener, may share confidential information about someone else.

All of these barriers to listening restrict the possibility of developing real Person-centred understanding, effective communication and positive intervention results.

Preparing to listen

Effective listening requires preparation and awareness of the factors contributing to interested and efficient listening. Sometimes the need for effective listening requires consideration and gathering of the required objects relevant to the discussion (e.g. diagnosis details, educational material). Systematic preparation of the necessary external and internal factors guarantees positive outcomes for the listening process.

Cultural expectations change the requirements for effective listening

Some skills associated with active listening may not be appropriate in some cultures, for example, eye contact. In some cultures, the age and gender of the speaker will affect the expectations of the listener. A factor that is considered important for effective communication in one cultural context is often inappropriate or unimportant in another culture. For example, the use of direct questions facilitates sharing of information in many Western middle-class contexts, while in some Indigenous cultures direct questions are offensive. In such Indigenous cultures, information may be shared through storytelling while performing activities together (see Chapter 17).

The principle of SAAFETY (see Table 11.1) reminds the healthcare professional of the necessary factors for preparing to listen and stresses the importance of a sense of safety for the Person/s when communicating with healthcare professionals.

TABLE 11.1
SAAFETY: Principles of preparing to listen for the healthcare professional

S	Schedule an interpreter, if required, to ensure effective communication.
A	Arrange your mind to enable complete focus and concentration on the Person/s.
A	Arrange the seating in a culturally appropriate way and remove physical barriers.
F	Familiarise yourself with the history and/or culture of the Person/s.
E	Environmental factors affect effective listening. Remove all distractions and reduce noise or activity. Check their comfort (including temperature). Ensure privacy.
T	Time dedicated to the Person/s, if necessary with a relevant community member and/or interpreter, is important.
Y	Why listen? Clarify and understand the purpose of the interaction.

In pairs:

- find someone you do not know well. Ask them to tell you about their fondest memory of school.
- before preparing to listen, consider the principle of SAAFETY (Table 11.1).
- listen carefully – ensure that they:
  - describe the environment at the time of the event
  - state who was present during the event
  - describe every action during the event
  - describe and explain the reactions of each person during the event
  - explain why it is their fondest memory.
- If the individual does not include these five factors, ask questions that will encourage them to provide this information.
- Make a verbal summary of the content of the description and have the individual verify the accuracy of your listening.

Characteristics of effective listening

Effective listeners use all of their knowledge and skills to understand and respond appropriately to the Person/s. They use active listening in preference to passive listening. Passive listening does not encourage continued interaction because the listener fails to engage with the speaker or the verbal or non-verbal content of their message. Active listening facilitates comprehension of all the messages of the Person/s (Rogers & Farson 1957) and is a core skill in effective listening.

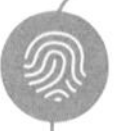

- Consider your usual style of listening. Are you naturally an active or passive listener? What conditions encourage you to listen actively?
- List the situations in which you adopt passive listening.
- How could you change your listening to active listening in these situations?

Effective listening, in common with all skills, requires commitment and practice. As mentioned above, it has particular characteristics and produces particular results. It also requires the healthcare professional to constantly avoid particular thoughts and actions. A healthcare professional aiming to be an effective listener should *always* avoid:

- stereotyping the Person/s, regardless of their appearance or skill in communicating (Haddad et al 2019)
- judging – this imposes personal values and beliefs onto the Person/s
- advising the Person/s, even if they request advice
- taking extensive notes while listening
- losing concentration because of thoughts about external matters (e.g. the next appointment, or what to have for dinner)
- interrupting with thoughts/opinions or ideas, instead of allowing the Person/s to finish
- a closed mind when listening (Holli & Beto 2023)
- double-guessing the meaning by making assumptions (Devito 2021)
- over-identification – this can interrupt the ability to remember and problem-solve (see Chapter 19)
- changing the focus to yourself, regardless of the similarity of experiences (see Chapter 9)
- negative and non-supportive non-verbal behaviours (see Chapter 10)
- passive disengagement while listening, regardless of your interest in the subject (see discussion below).
- Consider each point listed above and suggest behaviours that demonstrate each point.
- List ways to ensure you consistently avoid doing any of these when listening as a healthcare professional.

For more than 20 years the SOLER model (see Table 11.2) has highlighted the major non-verbal methods for communicating solidarity with the Person/s (Egan & Reese 2019). This model is an excellent guide for the use of non-verbal communication while listening in some sectors of Western society. However, the SOLER model does not necessarily accommodate cultural variations and expectations while listening (see Chapters 16 and 17).

TABLE 11.2
SOLER: A model of active listening for the healthcare professional

Sit	Sit to facilitate ease of sight and interaction between yourself and the Person/s. The orientation in space indicates an interest in and a commitment to the Person/s that communicates *I am here for you*.
Open posture	Assume a posture and facial expressions that communicate focused interest and openness to the Person/s. Avoid crossed arms because this may not indicate involvement and availability.
Lean towards the Person/s	Lean towards the Person/s slightly when listening to them. This will occur naturally if you are interested in the Person/s.
Eye contact	Use eye contact to indicate interest in the Person/s. When listening to a Person/s with a visual impairment, communicate interest by facing the Person/s as though they can see you. In cultures that consider eye contact rude there are other methods of communicating interest. Investigate these methods to assist you to communicate interest and concern to such Person/s.
Relax	Relax in order to assist development of trust and to encourage the Person/s to relax. Avoid loss of concentration through thoughts about unrelated things while listening – this is interpreted as lack of interest and is easily communicated to the listener/Person/s.

Adapted from Egan 2014.

Disengagement

Effective listening requires understanding of the importance of the process of **disengagement**, or satisfactorily concluding the interaction (see Chapter 5). Effective disengagement reinforces to the Person/s the level of interest and care from the healthcare professional. It requires time to ensure that everyone has understood the content of the interaction and the implications for the future. It therefore requires verbally summarising the content of the discussion and the need for any future actions. Particular non-verbal cues indicate disengagement; however, they can vary across cultures. As mentioned in Chapter 5, it may be necessary to explicitly state that the interaction is near completion.

- Choose a scenario from Section 4 that you feel will require effective listening.
- List particular characteristics of effective listening that you feel will assist interactions with the Person/s in this scenario.

Chapter summary

Person/s-centred communication cannot occur without effective listening. This requires active listening skills. Effective listening is beneficial for the healthcare professional, the

Person/s, the therapeutic relationship and the potential outcomes. It is important that healthcare professionals are aware of the requirements, results and characteristics of effective listening, along with the barriers to effective listening. An effective listener is aware of personal listening barriers and ways to overcome these when communicating and relating. They must also understand how to prepare to listen effectively and what to avoid when preparing to listen or when listening. Healthcare professionals must consider the cultural variations governing expectations for effective listening, as well as the need for appropriate disengagement. These elements of effective listening contribute to effective Person/Family-centred Care in any healthcare profession.

Oh, you mean I don't have to walk around while listening?
No. You have to use your non-verbal cues to communicate interest and care.
Oh - you mean like looking at the Person, leaning towards them, responding with interest ...and focusing on the Person?
Yes. If you listen actively, you are not bored and wishing you were somewhere else.
Okay. So the Person is the focus - not my thoughts and desires.
Yes, that's right.

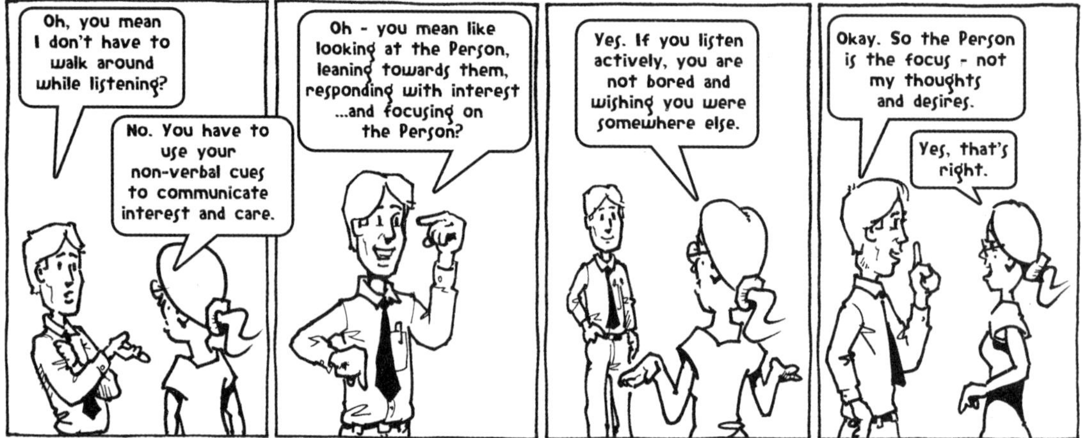

FIGURE 11.1
Active listening requires focus.
Courtesy Roger Harvey © Elsevier Australia.

REVIEW QUESTIONS

1. What is a basic characteristic of effective listening?

2. What abilities are required to listen effectively?

____

____

____

3. What are the benefits of active listening?

____

____

____

4. List six characteristics of effective listening and give examples of each.

   i. ____

   ii. ____

   iii. ____

   iv. ____

   v. ____

   vi. ____

5. List six actions a healthcare professional should avoid when listening.

   i. ____

   ii. ____

   iii. ____

   iv. ____

   v. ____

   vi. ____

6. Suggest ways that cultural expectations might change the requirements for effective listening.

___

___

___

7. How does effective disengagement contribute to Person/s-centred communication?

___

___

___

References

Adler, R.B., Proctor, R.F., 2017. Looking out, looking in, 15th ed. Cengage Learning Boston, MA.

Al-Momen, R.K., Al-Battal, S.M., Mishriky, A.M., 2015. Teaching communication skills in family medicine: A qualitative study. International Journal of Medical Science and Public Health, 4(1), 56–60.

Beesley, P., Watts, M., Harrison, M., 2018. Developing your communication skills in social work. Sage, London.

Bodie G.D., Gearheart C.C., Denham J.P., et al., 2013. The temporal stability and situational contingency of active-empathic listening. Western Journal of Communication, 77(2), 113–138.

Bodie G.D., Keaton S.A., Jones S.M., 2018. Individual listening values moderate the impact of verbal person centeredness on helper evaluations: A test of the dual-process theory of supportive message outcomes. International Journal of Listening, 32(3), 217–319.

Bodie, G.D., Vickery, A.J., Cannava, K., et al., 2015. The role of "active listening" in informal helping conversations: Impact on perceptions of listener helpfulness, sensitivity, and supportiveness and discloser emotional improvement. Western Journal of Communication, 79, 151–173.

Brown, T., Yu, M-L., Etherington, J., 2020. Are listening and interpersonal communication skills predictive of professionalism in undergraduate occupational therapy students? Health Professions Education, 6(2020), 187–200.

Burrus, A.E., Willis, L.B., 2020. Professional communication in speech-language pathology. How to write, talk and act like a clinician, 4th ed. Plural, San Diego, CA.

Davis, C.M., Musolino, G.M., 2016. Patient practitioner interaction: An experiential manual for developing the art of healthcare, 6th ed. Slack, Thorofare, NJ.

Devito, J.A., 2021. The interpersonal communication book, 16th ed. Pearson, Boston.

Devito, J.A., 2019. The interpersonal communication book, 15th ed. Pearson, Boston.

Egan, G., 2014. The skilled helper: A problem management and opportunity approach to helping, 10th ed. Brooks/Cole, Belmont CA.

Egan, G., Reese R.J., 2019. The skilled helper: A problem management and opportunity approach to helping, 11th ed. Cengage, Boston MA.

Gelinas, L. 2018. Listening as a caring competency. American Nurse Today, 13(10), 4.

Gilligan, T., Coyle, N., Frankel, R.M., et al., 2018. Patient–clinician communication: American Society of Clinical Oncology consensus guideline. Obstetrical & Gynecological Survey, 73(2), 96–97.

Gordon, J. (ed.), 2007. The Pfeiffer book of successful conflict management tools. [electronic resource]. Wiley, Hoboken.

Gordon, J. (ed.), 2004. Pfeiffer's classic activities for interpersonal communication. Pfeiffer, San Francisco.

Haddad, A.M., Purtilo, R.B., Doherty, R.F., 2019. Health professional and patient interaction, 9th ed. Elsevier/Saunders, St Louis, MO.

Harms, L., Pierce, J., 2019. Working with people: Communication skills for reflective practice, 2nd Canadian ed. Oxford University Press, Ontario.

Henderson, A., 2019. Communication for health care practice. Oxford University Press, Melbourne.

Holli, B.B., Beto, J.A., 2023. Nutrition counselling and education skills: A practical guide, 8th ed. Jones & Bartlett, Burlington, MA.

Honeycutt, A., Milliken, M.A., 2021. Understanding human behavior: A guide for healthcare providers, 10th ed. Cengage Learning, Boston.

Jennings, A., 2017. Utilizing standardised patients to teach motivational interviewing to Gerontology health care providers. Journal of Gerontology and Geriatric Research, 6(1), 385.

Kawamichi H., Yoshihara K., Sasaki A.T., et al., 2015. Perceiving active listening activates the reward system and improves the impression of relevant experiences. Social Neuroscience, 10(1), 16–26.

Keller, A.O., Gagnon, R., Witt, W.P., 2014. The impact of patient–provider communication and language spoken on adequacy of depression treatment for US women. Health Communication, 29(7), 646–655.

King, G., 2022. Central yet overlooked: engage and person-centred listening in rehabilitation and health-care conversations. Disability and Rehabilitation, 44(24), 7664–7676.

King, G.A., Servais, M., Bolack, L., et al., 2012. Development of a measure to assess effective listening and interactive communication skills in the delivery of children's rehabilitation services. Disability and Rehabilitation, 34 (6), 459–470.

Krupa, T., Kirsh B., Pitts, D., Fossey, E., (eds), 2016. Bruce and Borg's psychosocial frames of reference: Theories, models and approaches for occupation-based practice, 4th ed. Slack, Thorofare, NJ.

Mann, D., 2020. Gestalt therapy: 100 key points and techniques, 2nd ed. Routledge, Taylor & Francis, London.

McKenna, L., Brown, T., Oliaro, L., et al. 2022. Listening in health care. In: Worthington DL, Bodie GD, (eds). The handbook of listening. John Wiley & Sons, New Jersey.

Mendes, A., 2020. Communication in care: The importance of soft skills. Nursing and Residential Care, 22(9), doi: 10.12968/nrec.2020.22.9.4.

Moscato, S.R., Valanis, B., Gullion, C.M., et al., 2007. Predictors of patient satisfaction with telephone nursing services. Clinical Nursing Research, 16 (2), 119–137.

Moss B., 2020. Communication skills for health and social care, 5th ed. Sage, London.

Myers, K.K., Krepper, R., Nibert A., Toms R. 2020. Nurses' active empathic listening behaviours from the voice of the patient. Nursing Economics, 38(5), 267–275.

Rogers, C.R., Farson, R.E., 1957. Active listening. University of Chicago, Chicago.

Slade, S., Sergent, S.R., 2022. Interview techniques. StatPearls Publishing, Tampa, FL.

Stein-Parbury, J., 2021. Patient and person: Interpersonal skills in nursing, 7th ed. Churchill Livingstone Elsevier, Sydney.

Thistle, J.J., McNaughton, D., 2015. Teaching active listening skills to pre-service speech–language pathologists: A first step in supporting collaboration with parents of young children who require AAC. Language, Speech and Hearing Services in Schools, 46(1), 44–55.

Umphrey L.R., Sherblom J.C., 2018. The constitutive relationship of listening to hope, emotional intelligence, stress, and life satisfaction. International Journal of Listening, 32(1), 24–48.

van Dulmen, S., 2017. Listen: When words don't come easy. Patient Education and Counseling, 100(11), 1975–1978.

CHAPTER 12

Awareness of the effects of different environments upon healthcare communication

Chapter objectives

Upon completing this chapter, readers should be able to:

- recognise the physical factors within the environment that influence communication, the quality of the healthcare service and the outcomes of that healthcare
- recognise the factors contributing to the creation of the emotional environment
- identify the benefits of acknowledging and accommodating the emotional environments of all relevant people to ensure Person/Family-centred Care
- justify the importance of considering the cultural environment of both the particular healthcare service and the individuals in their healthcare service
- appreciate that there are varying sexual environments and understand that the sexual environment can influence responses during healthcare service delivery
- demonstrate understanding of various social environments and their influence on the individuals in healthcare services
- state the benefits of being aware of and understanding the spiritual environments of the individuals in healthcare services.

Individuals develop in many types of environments, including physical, social, emotional, sexual, cultural and spiritual environments. These environments interact to form a dynamic system determining the development and expectations of each individual when communicating. These expectations therefore influence the prospects and outcomes of communicative interactions. Such environments initially include the physical and social settings within the family home, the local community and the school. These physical and social environments provide the setting for other environments (Pati et al 2014), particularly emotional, cultural, sexual and spiritual environments. This chapter focuses upon increasing awareness of the effect of various environments upon healthcare communication.

- Divide a page in half, top to bottom. On one side, list the factors that have assisted your ability to achieve understanding within particular environments, and on the other side, list those that have limited your comprehension (e.g. noisy, emotionally tense or spiritually unfamiliar environments). Consider the aspects of your whole person, as well as cultural and financial aspects.

In groups:

- compare your individual lists, and combine all elements to devise a single list.
- using the combined list, describe the environment/s that best assist in achieving mutual understanding when providing or receiving information. Consider the perspectives of the healthcare professional and the Person/s.

There are unique factors affecting the responses during and after the results of interactions. Some of these factors are age, gender, social expectations, economic status, cultural norms, sexual preferences, attitudes, experience, level of education, professional knowledge and associated expectations, problem-solving strategies, types of thinking, personality types and motivational forces (Boggs 2023; Moss 2020). Environmental factors also affect the outcomes of interactions. They are many and varied, and each has its own effect on potential outcomes. Environmental factors are similar to the aspects of the Person/s, with some being obvious and others more obscure. Some are more immediate than others – directly affecting the individual in the present – while others have shaped the individual in their past. Some can be managed by the healthcare professional within the routine of practice, while others require specific understanding and acceptance (Fitzpatrick et al 2014; Mantell & Scragg 2019; Odhayani & Khawaja 2014).

The physical environment

Physical appearance: dress and odour

The healthcare professional has immediate control over their physical appearance, specifically clothing, including a well-laundered uniform, jewellery, personal grooming, including hairstyle and hygiene. Certainly facial features and other inherited characteristics are innate and cannot be chosen, but consideration of personal codes of dress, grooming and hygiene is essential and within the control of healthcare professionals. While dress and grooming are components of body language, from the perspective of the unsure, vulnerable Person/s, the physical appearance of the healthcare professional is part of the new and unfamiliar physical environment. For example, the Person/s being able to see the face of the healthcare professional is important. It allows the Person/s to easily see facial features and expression, thereby potentially assisting them to understand the interest and intention of the healthcare professional. This therefore affects the choices of the healthcare professional during their daily grooming routine. The odours of healthcare professionals may also potentially affect the Person/s. Such odours include body odour, perfumes and aftershave. Healthcare professionals must consider the effect of their odour upon those around them and ensure they have daily showers (in hotter climates more than daily may be necessary), use deodorant with minimal fragrance and minimise the use of heavily scented sprays when grooming themselves for work. Most healthcare services have specific codes of dress for staff members, thereby eliminating the need to choose clothing and footwear every workday. However, it is important to consider the effect of personal grooming and odour upon the Person/s seen in daily practice.

- Decide why healthcare services have restrictive codes of personal appearance.
- List the reasons for and against such codes; consider healthcare interventions for individuals in various stages of the lifespan.

- Explore the identified reasons for restrictive codes of personal appearance in healthcare services – consider uniforms, hair restraint, jewellery and footwear.
  - During this exploration, consider the importance of comfort and safety for all stakeholders.
  - List the benefits and disadvantages of wearing a uniform regularly.
- Decide whether restrictive codes of personal appearance are necessary and appropriate in every healthcare setting. Provide clear, relevant and appropriate reasons for your decision.

When dressing as a healthcare professional, it is important to avoid expressions of economic status – either wealth or poverty – or personal preferences in clothing, footwear or jewellery (Holli & Beto 2023). Appearance of wealth or poverty might be intimidating, and is sometimes misinterpreted by those seeking assistance.

Familiarity with the physical environment and the usual procedures of the healthcare service

The Person/s seeking assistance

Most people feel apprehensive when entering a new environment for the first time. New environments typically produce unsure and tentative behaviours. If the new environment holds unknown procedures and perhaps pain, there might even be feelings of fear and anger. Investing time to familiarise people with a new environment can avoid any negative emotions related to the novelty of the environment and the unknown procedures associated with the environment (Beukeboom et al 2012; Chapman et al 2014; Haddad et al 2019). In such situations, it is helpful to imagine what the personal reaction of the healthcare professional might be in a similar situation; that is, when they experience unfamiliar environments with unknown procedures.

A person who had never previously been admitted to hospital, on waking from a ten-day coma asks to "get up" to go to the toilet. A helpful nurse returns a few minutes later with a commode chair on wheels. This is a standard procedure, where the person transfers onto the commode chair and the nurse wheels the person and commode to the toilet cubicle. This is appropriate for someone who is weak from lack of sustenance and exercise. Upon seeing the commode chair, the person bursts into tears and states *I don't want to go that much!*

- Can you explain this reaction? How would you react?
- Is there anything that could be done to avoid this reaction?
- If so, what? If not, why?
- Can you think of a regular procedure in your healthcare profession that might elicit a similar reaction?

Knowing where to find toilets and other necessary facilities is reassuring. However, understanding what to expect during a procedure or intervention, or as a result of a particular need, is equally important. Assisting the Person/s to become familiar with the environment – the facilities, people and procedures – is essential to ensure positive responses and outcomes.

The healthcare professional

There are times when healthcare professionals may find themselves in unfamiliar environments when assisting a Person/s. Some of these environments may feel cosy and relaxing, while others seem daunting, smelly or cluttered. (A visit to the home of a Person/s who lives adjacent to a fertiliser factory does test the ability of the healthcare professional to successfully complete their task in such an environment.) When visiting a Person/s in their home or attending to them in an unfamiliar, sometimes unexpected, environment as part of the intervention, it is important for healthcare professionals to act to minimise the anxiety resulting from the sometimes unexpected novelty of the environment (e.g. outline every procedure and expectation, always indicating the level of assistance available). In such circumstances, it is imperative that the healthcare professional continues to respond with respect and empathy, regardless of the conditions of the particular environment.

Rooms

Furniture placement and physical comfort

Various factors require consideration when choosing the type of furniture and how to place the furniture within a room. Placement of furniture can encourage or discourage interaction. Chairs side-by-side facing the same direction do not necessarily encourage communication, nor might they demonstrate interest and care. A large desk between the people communicating is not only a physical barrier; it might also be an emotional barrier. Such a desk potentially communicates a desire to maintain an emotional and physical distance. It is important to avoid using furniture as a physical barrier when providing Person/Family-centred Care. Arranging the chairs around an appropriate table, a comfortable distance apart, facing each other or adjacent to each other promotes communication that is potentially more personal and caring. This configuration facilitates eye contact, which is valued in most Western cultures, although not in some other cultures. It is important to ensure that all communicating individuals are physically comfortable before commencing the interaction. If a table is required for placement of written material, a round table allows a clear view for everyone seated at the table. If a Person is already seated, or in bed, the healthcare professional may facilitate clearer communication by placing themselves at the same level as the Person.

Waiting rooms

Waiting rooms are often crowded and noisy. Regardless of the busy nature of the room or the size of the room, there are aesthetic principles that make a waiting room more pleasant for those waiting (Beukeboom et al 2014). The colour of the room (paint and furniture), the texture and type of furniture, the lighting and ventilation create either a warm, welcoming atmosphere or a cold, clinical feeling. A room with warm features encourages a feeling of comfort, relaxation and safety, while a cold, clinical room feels impersonal and unfriendly. The first encourages people to linger, while the latter encourages people to leave as quickly as possible. The more impersonal the waiting room, the greater the likelihood of expressions of frustration and hostility (Haddad et al 2019). Such behaviour can result from personal factors or having to wait too long, but may also result from the impersonal or clinical nature of the environment.

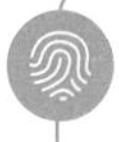

- Consider the effect of your physical comfort on your ability to concentrate, understand and remember specific details. Can you concentrate regardless of your comfort?

- Decide on the best way to establish whether a Person/s is physically comfortable. Remember the Person/s is feeling overwhelmed and vulnerable, so they may not tell you directly that they are physically uncomfortable. How will you know they are comfortable or uncomfortable? What might you do to make them physically comfortable if you establish that they are uncomfortable?

The feeling of comfort gained from sitting or lying on particular types of furniture varies from person to person according to their size, height, physical condition, age and gender. Well-equipped waiting rooms with varying types of chairs can assist to overcome these personal variations. Ventilation and natural light can contribute to the ambience of any room. However, sometimes these are not possible. In such cases, it is important to consider the colour and type of furniture to create an inviting and comfortable environment.

Treatment rooms and rooms with beds

The same principles outlined for creation of an aesthetically comfortable waiting room also apply to treatment areas. However, it is important to consider additional environmental factors when in such areas. Many treatment areas do not naturally facilitate confidential and private communication. It is important for healthcare professionals working in such environments to consider individual needs for privacy.

The need for privacy may vary according to personality type and the emotional state of the individual at any given time. Consistent consideration of these needs will promote personal disclosure when required and the development of rapport. It is important to consider the difference between visual privacy and auditory privacy. Drawing curtains around a treatment bed or a bed in a ward or emergency department does not guarantee complete privacy. A private room will facilitate personal communication, while in a public space, the depth of the interaction may be restricted to protect confidentiality, producing only superficial discussion or interactions.

Avoiding distractions and interruptions

The use of a private room for discussion of personal information is very important, but it may not achieve personal disclosure if there are constant distractions. Environmental distractions come from such things as the telephone, people, regular or loud noises, particular objects in the room and sometimes movement outside a window (Liu et al 2014; Sanderson & Grundgeiger 2015; Spooner et al 2014).

Personal and emotional communication require concentration and focus. Distractions disturb the flow of the communication, making this focus difficult. Restoring the concentration and information flow during exploration of emotion is often difficult. More importantly, responding to distractions communicates that the distraction is more important to the healthcare professional than the communicating Person/s (Liu et al 2014). Thus, avoidance of such distractions is very important. This is achieved by not answering the telephone, leaving a message indicating interruptions or disturbances are not acceptable (e.g. a sign on the door saying "Do Not Disturb"), decreasing or removing distracting noises and/or objects where possible, and organising the seating to avoid distractions seen through a window. If in a hospital ward, it is appropriate to arrange a time when there are no expectations from other healthcare professionals or visitors.

Some sounds are so much a part of the environment that the healthcare professional no longer notices them, such as sounds from equipment or machinery. These sounds are often necessary and unavoidable, but they may be distracting to a Person/s unfamiliar with the environment. In such situations, it may be necessary to recognise and explain the distraction, potentially encouraging the individual to attempt to ignore it if possible. Sometimes the simple acknowledgement and/or explanation of the distraction may assist the individual to ignore it and focus on the interaction.

Temperature

Different healthcare settings have different constraints relating to resources and type of service. This may affect the presence of temperature controls within the setting. The external climate may make temperature alterations desirable. Healthcare services in very cold climates usually have heating; however, those in hot, humid climates may not always have air-conditioning. In such situations, the behaviour of those within the healthcare service may reflect the temperature. If there is a pattern of irritability among people in those services – Person/s and staff alike – consideration of the heat in the environment may explain the "emotional temperature" (Haddad et al 2019).

Warm temperature and poor ventilation can encourage drowsiness, which will limit the quality of the communication. Feeling cold can be equally detrimental to communication, with the physical temperature of the Person/s dominating their responses. Where possible, when climate control is lacking, control the temperature using compensatory measures, as discomfort from temperature affects the mood and the achievement of effective communication. It may be important to remember that individuals respond differently to temperature. Remember the temperature should suit the Person/s not the healthcare professional.

- List possible ways of compensating for the absence of, or a failure in, a climate-control system. Use your imagination, but be realistic – although spraying the individuals with a garden hose would be very cooling, it is unlikely to be acceptable in any healthcare service!

The physical status of the Person/s in particular environments

Each individual has characteristics, abilities and skills to facilitate their movement and comfort in particular environments. Children find stairs and large chairs and tables difficult to accommodate until they grow to a particular height and develop the abilities and skills to independently negotiate such objects in the environment. Extremely tall people can find the size of chairs and tables and the height of benches equally challenging, regardless of their abilities and skills. Individuals with physical limitations restricting their ability to negotiate particular environments, may find such objects a barrier to participation and independent functioning. It is important for a healthcare professional to consider the abilities and skills of the individuals seeking their assistance in order to adjust the environment to accommodate the needs of those individuals. Ramps with rails, the heights of chairs and tables, the heights of beds and toilets – in fact, the height of anything the Person/s must negotiate within the environment of the particular healthcare profession – may be significant. Assistive devices (with appropriate explanations of their use and the reasons for their use) to facilitate independent functioning for such individuals will reduce potentially negative emotions and increase the possibility of positive outcomes of communication and interventions.

Trust, empathy, positive rapport and a therapeutic relationship can compensate for deficits in the physical environment. However, these develop over time, and an unfriendly clinical environment without acknowledgement of the reality of the environment, creates an initial impression that is potentially difficult to overcome.

The emotional environment

The emotional state and emotional response of individuals seeking assistance create a particular emotional environment, which, in many cases, requires direct attention from the healthcare professional. Direct and immediate attention to emotions can save time and effort for both the Person/s and the healthcare professional. The emotional environment within an individual may be as simple as feeling a sense of disappointment because they believe they should be able to manage their condition themselves, or a sense of inconvenience because they require assistance for something simple and relatively minor. It may be due to loss of family or future plans (Carpenter et al 2022). However, it may be more complex because of previous experiences with healthcare services. It may also originate from other social/emotional environments external to the healthcare service. If working in palliative care or oncology, the emotional environment of a Person/s who has a life-limiting illness is complex and requires management and collaboration to ensure positive outcomes for all stakeholders (Anderson et al 2021). Consideration of the emotional environments of those seeking the assistance of a healthcare professional has numerous benefits to contribute to Person/Family-centred Care and satisfying outcomes.

Formal versus informal environments

Different occasions and places demand different types of behaviour; some more formal than others. In formal situations, individuals are expected to adhere carefully to particular norms. These norms might require the use of the family name when addressing an individual; they might require only speaking when asked a question; or they might perhaps require a controlled use of language. For example, the language and behaviour used in a courtroom is very different from the language and behaviour used with friends at a sporting event. The expected formality of a situation will affect the emotional response of the individual, their comfort when communicating and their willingness to communicate about personal matters.

The various expectations and demands of the formality of the environment affect the individual. More formal situations may create a more tentative and apprehensive emotional response in an individual. Less formal situations can promote relaxation, generally encouraging willingness to discuss personal matters at a deeper level.

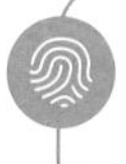

- On a separate piece of paper, list the environmental factors that facilitate your ability to talk about yourself at more than a superficial level.

- Discuss in groups the implications of the above factors for a healthcare professional.

Emotional responses to environmental demands

Emotional responses to the immediate environment

There is a continual and dynamic interaction between the individual and their immediate environment. This interaction creates a particular emotional environment. This will vary according to the dominant need at any given time. If the personal emotional needs dominate an individual and the environment does not accommodate these needs, the stress level for that individual increases as they attempt to meet the demands of both self and the environment (Levine 2013). In such circumstances, it is beneficial for the healthcare professional to note and, where possible, accommodate the emotional environment of the Person/s. Something as simple as the position of the healthcare professional (e.g. standing over someone or standing too close or too far away) may evoke a negative response in particular individuals. Unfamiliarity with the surroundings, the individuals and the associated intervention or procedure in the environment can also create a particular emotional environment for the individual. This emotional environment may affect their responses and the quality of their interactions. It is possible to alleviate these particular emotional environments with direct attention, acknowledgement and action.

Emotional responses to an external environment

Individuals often exhibit emotions because of an emotional environment established from a source external to the immediate environment of the healthcare service. Potential contributing causes of negative emotional environments include financial stress, social stress, physical discomfort or anxiety about an unknown future. It is not the role of every healthcare professional to treat the causes of the dominating emotional environment. However, validation of the associated emotions, empathic responses and referral to a relevant professional will reduce the consequences of the particular emotional environment (Beukeboom et al 2012; Lui et al 2014; Margolies et al 2015).

Mrs Gilles is a 78-year-old who lives alone with her cat. She is currently attending for weekly treatment. She generally appears happy and eagerly enters into collaborative goal-setting and relevant interventions. Her level of improvement suggests she is implementing the particular regimen suggested by you as her healthcare professional.

One particular day, you intend to introduce Mrs Gilles to a more demanding "home program" during her treatment session. You have a positive relationship with her and often talk about her past and present life when she attends. She appears to enjoy attending.

When Mrs Gilles arrives she seems a little teary, but smiles when she sees you.

You have two choices:

- to investigate her apparent tendency to tears, or
- ignore it.

The treatment environment demands a happy and willing-to-participate Mrs Gilles.

At this point, her emotional environment does not appear to be dominating her responses. She is able to respond to the demands of the treatment environment, continuing her collaborative way of interacting.

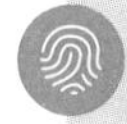

- What will you do? You decide to ignore it – you have a full day and decide you simply do not have the time to investigate.

The next time Mrs Gilles attends it is obvious she has not been implementing her home program; in fact, she seems to be back to her status of three weeks ago. She is teary and, although participating, does not smile or look at you.

The emotional environment of Mrs Gilles is now beginning to dominate. She is no longer able to meet the demands of the treatment environment, demonstrating an inability to continue her treatment regimen at home.

You are busier this week with more appointments than normal because you are going on holidays at the end of the week. You decide to ignore the emotional environment surrounding Mrs Gilles, hoping it will be better when you return from holidays. You think to yourself that most emotional things improve with time and a colleague will see her while you are away.

You return from holidays two weeks later to find that Mrs Gilles has not attended since you went on holidays. You ring her and she tells you she has been lying in bed since the last time you saw her. She says she cannot be bothered to get out of bed anymore.

What will you do? You know Mrs Gilles was improving with your intervention.

You ask her a few questions, but she is reluctant to talk to you. You finally ask her about her cat – she often talked lovingly about the cat, stating she had nothing else since the death of her husband. Mrs Gilles suddenly sobs uncontrollably – the cat had died the first week when she was teary! The interaction identifying the cause of the tears took more than 15 minutes.

- How long would it have taken to investigate the cause of the tears (the emotional environment affecting the Person) when you first noticed the tears?
- Might it potentially have created a different scenario for Mrs Gilles?

In groups of no more than four:

Have one person play Mrs Gilles and another play a healthcare professional, who validates the cause of the tendency to tears, with empathic responses and questions.

- Time how long it takes to validate the emotions and demonstrate empathy.
- Discuss the possible direction of the conversation with Mrs Gilles.
- Should the healthcare professional discuss the emotions related to grieving (see Section 4) and strategies for dealing with the death of the cat?

Failure to note and accommodate the internal or external emotional environment of the individual can have negative consequences. Responding to the emotional environment does not usually take excessive amounts of time and has benefits for all involved individuals. The ultimate benefit for the individual is improved outcomes, also saving time for the healthcare professional if explored immediately.

The cultural environment

Individuals grow and develop in specific cultural environments. Cultural environments do not necessarily originate from ethnicity; every group (including families) has unique cultural norms governing expectations and behaviour. Cultural environments determine how individuals view themselves, how they view others and how others view them (Henderson 2019; Williams 2022).

Examination and understanding of the cultural context of an individual provides information about the rules and norms governing their life, both individually and within groups. Cultural environments influence the values of societies and of individuals. These values directly affect expectations and goals within the culture and outside the particular culture (Whelan et al 2018). Shared values and expectations (i.e. the cultural worldview) are inherent in cultural groups; thus individuals from those groups are often unable to verbalise the details of these values and expectations. An appreciation and accommodation of the specific worldview of the individual seeking assistance promotes positive communication and Person/Family-centred Care.

Personal space

Different cultures have different norms determining personal space, that is, the distance individuals stand or sit from each other during a communicative interaction. Recognising variations in ideas of personal space is important when relating to people from a different culture. If the Person/s uses non-verbal cues demonstrating emotional discomfort by moving away from standing or sitting a particular distance apart, the Person/s has adjusted their emotional environment by positioning himself or herself in relation to the other people, according to their cultural expectations. It is important not to move closer in response, but to establish the cause of the movement away and to accommodate the response. The healthcare professional should try to remain in their original location, even if it feels uncomfortable, impersonal and distant. If the healthcare professional does move closer, they may "chase the Person/s around the room" or produce distress or discomfort throughout the discussion. Alternatively, if a Person/s moves closer when interacting, demonstrating emotional distress unless they remain closer, this may demonstrate a different cultural norm governing personal space. Variations in ideas of personal space when interacting, whether sitting or standing, require awareness in the healthcare professional and accommodation or explanation of the positioning needs in the particular circumstances.

Colour

Colours can communicate different emotions to different individuals. Some of this communication is culturally determined and some results from individual preferences. Different cultures assign sometimes totally opposite meanings to the same colours (Devito 2021). Colour may encourage a relaxed attitude, while others might create excitement. Consideration of the effects of colour in the environment may promote relaxation and calm.

Time

Different cultural environments have a different awareness of, and often place a different emphasis on, time and its effect on behaviour. Some cultures measure time by the movement of the Earth around the Sun, that is, *a seasonal calendar*. In these cultural environments, the seasons regulate the lives and expectations of the people. If the winter is long and cold, then that season determines the cultural expectations of interactions between people at that time. If there is little seasonal change in a particular location, then the cultural environment is unlikely to demand different ways of relating as the year progresses. Some cultures regulate their interaction by the movement of the Moon around the Earth (phases of the Moon) – the *lunar calendar*. In these cultural environments, the movement of the Moon determines the expectations and norms governing interactions between people and events at particular times. This means that a New Year celebration can sometimes occur in late February, and Easter can occur in mid-March. Other cultures regulate their interactions by the movement of the Earth on its axis – a *24-hour schedule* based on the spinning of the Earth. In these cultural environments, the 24-hour clock regulates the events and expectations of the people. In other cultures, time has a different significance and is unrelated to schedules throughout the day.

Understanding cultural differences

The regard for time and adherence or non-adherence to a schedule in different cultures delivers different messages. Some cultures value adherence to the time schedule above other cultural or social demands. In Western cultures, punctuality communicates respect, whereas being late communicates the opposite. Other cultures consider the adherence to "being on time" as less relevant than particular cultural or social demands – so much so that they may not attend a previously made appointment and don't consider it necessary to notify the healthcare professional of their inability to attend. When differences in perceptions of the significance of time cause difficulties in healthcare, it may be important to sensitively communicate to a Person/s that the reality for the healthcare professional of many appointments in one day makes it difficult to see someone after or before their allocated time.

In some cultures, inviting people to have or do something requires repeating the request three times before the individual answers in the affirmative. In other cultures, lack of an affirmative response after the first request might indicate that the individual is ambivalent about accepting the invitation. For example, in some parts of China it is sometimes polite to ask an individual three times if they would like a drink or join in a meal. If the request occurs once, the person may indicate a definite *no*, regardless of their desire for a drink. It is not until the occurrence of the third request that they might indicate their desire for a drink. In other cultures, where one request is the expected norm, the first answer indicates the desire or lack of desire for a drink.

A cultural environment influences many components of human behaviour, too many to consider in this chapter (see Chapter 16). It is the responsibility of the healthcare professional to acknowledge and accommodate the cultural variations in all interactions. Fulfilling this responsibility requires an awareness of the personal cultural expectations of the healthcare professional and their emotional responses to variations in cultural expectations (Mantell & Scragg 2019). It also requires an awareness of the cultural differences of the Person/s. Such awareness potentially prepares healthcare professionals to humbly open themselves to exploring and understanding those differences. Understanding cultural differences empowers the healthcare professional to accommodate variations in the diverse cultural environments potentially represented by both the individuals seeking their assistance and their colleagues in the particular healthcare service.

Environments affecting sexuality

Different cultures may have differing sexual and moral expectations. These differences may affect the willingness of a Person/s to discuss sexuality (Butler & Langlois 2022). They may also determine the significance of sexual experiences for particular individuals and the expectations of individuals relating to sexual intimacy (Honeycutt & Milliken 2021). A person raised in an environment that practises regular casual sexual relationships would make particular assumptions about sexual practices and may either exhibit similar practices or carefully control any sexual activity. A sexually abused person may avoid any kind of physical touch or may have a fragile self-image, limiting their ability to relate sexually or communicate about sexual matters.

It is important that healthcare professionals understand that different individuals may have different sexual habits and preferences (McAuliffe et al 2020) and often differing levels of willingness to discuss sexuality. Some individuals may practise sexual abstinence, others casual sexual relationships, and others may prefer sexual experiences with people of the same gender.

Such sexual practices and preferences may or may not be the preference of the healthcare professional. However, it is important to be aware of these various sexual environments to ensure appropriate and positive non-judgemental responses to such individuals.

In addition, healthcare services often face difficulties in developing policies for regulation of sexual activity for both staff and Person/s (Butler & Langlois 2022). There is also limited education dedicated to training healthcare professionals to manage and address the sexual needs of the Person/s (Verrastro et al 2020). This results in a limited consideration of the sexual needs and environment of the Person/s, despite the role and ability of particular healthcare professions to consider these needs (Fennell & Blair 2019; Ravenhill et al 2020; Traumer et al 2019).

The social environment

Individuals typically mature in the context of other individuals. The social environment of an individual consists of all the social relationships they experience with people and animals. Such relationships can be encouraging and supportive, discouraging and unhelpful, or a combination of both. The social environment of the Person/s seeking assistance can influence their responses and their ability to communicate effectively.

Family

A supportive family can assist the healthcare professional (Holli & Beto 2023). When desired, and if appropriate, supportive family members should be included in establishing and supporting the goals of the collaborative process between the Person/s and the healthcare professional. If the social environment of a family is a place of abuse and discouragement, or control and constraint, this will shape the communication style of the individual. The behaviour associated with this type of social environment is not always interactive or easy. Understanding this behaviour might be difficult; however, it is important in such cases that the healthcare professional relate to the individual with acceptance, consistency and definite boundaries. The creation of a safe, predictable environment for such a Person/s within the context of the healthcare service is the immediate goal of the healthcare professional.

Pets

A relationship with a pet is often of great significance to a person (e.g. a dog or guinea pig to a child, a horse to a female adolescent, or a dog, bird or cat to an ageing person). Different cultures or geographical settings may mean that the animal is different (it may even be a whale), but, if it is a pet, the animal may serve to be the most significant comforting social relationship for a particular individual. Healthcare professionals must accommodate the significance of a pet when assisting individuals who value a particular pet. Discussion about the pet can assist in developing rapport and continuing the therapeutic relationship.

Friends, neighbours, interest groups and sporting teams

The social environment, including groups outside a family, is often significant to an individual. Friends, neighbours, special purpose groups or sporting teams may provide a social environment that reinforces the value of the individual, providing affection and affirming them in a unique way. Such friends or groups may become more significant for the individual who lives alone. However, these social environments may also be the context for either unintentional or intentional abuse (e.g. a "helpful" neighbour may lock a person in a room thinking they are protecting them). Particular social environments in some circumstances may explain unreasonable behaviour by a Person/s .

Institutional social environment

A healthcare professional may assist an individual whose primary social environment is an institution. These individuals may have different styles of communication according to their experiences within the particular institution. Such institutions may have rules governing daily events and timing of those events. This may also be the first time the Person/s has either been in a shared room with a non-family member or, alternatively, in a room alone. In this situation, it is important for the healthcare professional to demonstrate behaviour to reflect both the general and specific purposes of the healthcare professions (see Chapters 2, 3 and 4).

The social environment of each healthcare service team may vary. It is important that healthcare professionals resolve any personal responses to their colleagues in their healthcare environment to avoid negatively affecting those seeking their assistance.

- Brainstorm and list possible strategies for managing an unsupportive social environment. Note these are not age-specific needs and occur throughout the lifespan.
- List strategies for managing an unsupportive family.
- List strategies for managing the loss of a special pet.
- List strategies for managing lost social environments through relocation of the family home, decrease in or loss of physical abilities, or the death of someone significant.
- List strategies for managing experiences from institutional social environments – whether pleasant or unpleasant.

The spiritual environment

Individuals adopt particular elements of spirituality, creating their own spiritual environment for many reasons. It takes many forms, but regardless of the form, spirituality is fundamental to human experience (Ronaldson 2014). It determines what is important to an individual and the beliefs governing their choices in daily life (O'Toole & Ramugondo 2018). Some individuals simply adopt the dominant spiritual environment of their native culture, while others may choose a particular spiritual environment. The spiritual environment of an individual may be more relevant to particular healthcare professions than others, thus some healthcare professionals may appropriately choose not to relate to this environment (Mir & Sheikh 2010). Regardless of the relevance of spiritual issues to the particular healthcare profession, it is important that healthcare professionals demonstrate respect and sensitivity to the way in which the spiritual environment may assist in the management of the health issue and healing of the individual seeking assistance (Haddad et al 2019). Healthcare professionals can choose to relate to or to ignore the spiritual environment of the Person/s (Egan & Reese 2019; Moss 2020). However, some indicate that spiritual care is essential to achieve Person-centred Care (O'Toole & Ramugondo 2018; Phelps et al 2012; Ronaldson 2014). Many Western healthcare professionals prefer to avoid discussing spiritual environments, finding it awkward (Ford et al 2012; Phelps et al 2012). However, growing interest in spirituality has produced an increasing body of knowledge, thereby providing guidance for the use of spiritual understanding in the practice of healthcare professionals (Miller 1999; Miller & Thorensen 2003; O'Toole & Ramugondo 2018; Richards & Bergin 2005; White 2006). Acknowledging and accommodating the spiritual environment of the Person/s can create deeper understanding of that environment, as well as encouraging the individual in the use of images, medicine and rituals typical of that environment. The use of these elements of a particular spiritual environment may promote participation, healing and increased function (Eckermann et al 2010).

- Consider the scenarios in Section 4 about the Persons/s experiencing a life-limiting illness and their family. Decide how you will accommodate each environment for these Person/s.

Chapter summary

Healthcare professionals may experience multiple environmental demands from various dynamically related environments while fulfilling their role. These demands may arise from the physical, emotional, cultural, sexual, social and spiritual environments of the healthcare professional, the particular healthcare service or those of the Person/s. It is the responsibility of healthcare professionals to overcome any personal and negative responses to the specific environmental demands experienced as part of their role. Successfully accommodating the demands of particular environments while practising as a healthcare professional will ensure positive outcomes and Person/Family-centred Care.

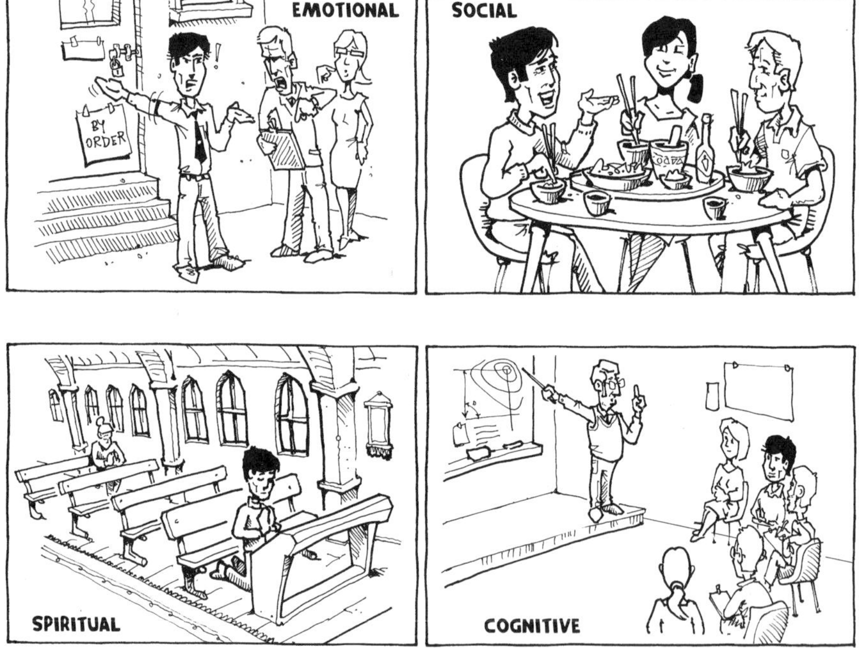

FIGURE 12.1
The cultural, spiritual, social and emotional environments can be paralysing.
Courtesy Roger Harvey © Elsevier Australia.

REVIEW QUESTIONS

1. Various environments form a dynamic system that affect each individual. These environments include:

   i. ____

   ii. ____

   iii. ____

   iv. ____

   v. ____

   vi. ____

2. List seven elements of the physical environment that affect communication with the individual seeking assistance.

   i. ____

   ii. ____

   iii. ____

   iv. ____

   v. ____

   vi. ____

   vii. ____

3. Name three ways the healthcare professional can accommodate the emotional environment.

   i. ____

   ii. ____

   iii. ____

4. Cultural environments vary and the healthcare professional must be open to differences between their own cultural environment and those of the individuals seeking assistance. Healthcare professionals must respond with willingness to understand and accommodate such differences. Name three culturally-specific elements requiring understanding.

   i. ______________________________

   ii. ______________________________

   iii. ______________________________

5. What differences can occur in sexual environments?

   i. ______________________________

   ii. ______________________________

   iii. ______________________________

6. What might social environments include?

   i. ______________________________

   ii. ______________________________

   iii. ______________________________

   iv. ______________________________

7. Why is the spiritual environment of each individual important?

____

____

____

____

References

Anderson, N.E., Robinson, J., Moeke-Maxwell, T., Gott, M., 2021. Paramedic care of dying, deceased and bereaved in Aotearoa, New Zealand. Progress in Palliative Care, 29(2), 84–90.

Beukeboom, C.J.L., Langeveld, D., Tanja-Dijkstra, K., 2012. Stress-reducing effects of real and artificial nature in a hospital waiting room. Journal of Alternative and Complementary Medicine, 18(4), 329–333.

Boggs, K., 2023. Interpersonal relationships: Professional communication skills for nurses, 9th ed. Elsevier, St Louis, MO.

Butler, J., Langlois, D., 2022. Consent, capacity and client sexuality policies in healthcare. Healthcare Management Forum, 35(3), 190–194.

Carpenter, C.R., Betz, M., Doering, M., et al., 2022. Emergency department communication in persons living with dementia and care partners: A scoping review. Journal of Medical Directors Association, 23(8), 1313.e15–1313.e46.

Chapman, R., Smith, T., Martin, C., 2014. Qualitative exploration of the perceived barriers and enablers to Aboriginal and Torres Strait Islander people accessing healthcare through one Victorian Emergency Department. Contemporary Nurse, 48(1), 48–58.

Devito, J.A., 2021. The interpersonal communication book, 16th ed. Pearson, Boston.

Eckermann, A., Dowd, T., Chong, E., et al., 2010. Binaŋ Goonj: Bridging cultures in Aboriginal health, 3rd ed. Elsevier, Sydney.

Egan, G., Reese R.J., 2019. The skilled helper: A problem management and opportunity approach to helping, 11th ed. Cengage, Boston MA.

Fennell, R., Blair, G., 2019. Discussing sexuality in health care: A systematic review. Journal of Clinical Nursing, 28(17–18), 3065–3076.

Fitzpatrick, N., Breen, D.T., Taylor, J., et al., 2014. Parental satisfaction with paediatric care, triage and waiting times. Emergency Medicine Australasia, 26(2), 177–182.

Ford, D., Downey, L., Engelberg, R., et al., 2012. Discussing religion and spirituality is an advanced communication skill: An exploratory structural equation model of physician trainee self-ratings. Journal of Palliative Medicine, 15(1), 63–70.

Haddad, A.M., Purtilo, R.B., Doherty, R.F., 2019. Health professional and patient interaction, 9th ed. Elsevier/Saunders, St Louis, MO.

Henderson, A., 2019. Communication for health care practice. Oxford University Press, Melbourne.

Holli, B.B., Beto, J.A., 2023. Nutrition counselling and education skills: A practical guide, 8th ed. Jones & Bartlett, Burlington, MA.

Honeycutt, A., Milliken, M.A., 2021. Understanding human behavior: A guide for healthcare providers, 10th ed. Cengage Learning, Boston.

Levine, J., 2013. Working with people: The helping process, 9th ed. Pearson, San Antonio.

Liu, W., Manias, E., Gerdtz, M., 2014. The effects of physical environments in medical wards on medication communication processes affecting patient safety. Health and Place, 26(1), 188–198.

Mantell, A., Scragg T., (eds) 2019. Reflective practice in social work, 5th ed. Sage, Chichester.

Margolies, R., Gurnaney, H., Egeth, M., et al., 2015. Positioning patient status monitors in a family waiting room. Health Environments Research and Design Journal, 8(2), 103–109.

McAuliffe, L., Fetherstonhaugh, D., Bauer, M., 2020. Sexuality and sexual health: Policy in Australian residential aged care. Australasian Journal of Ageing, 39(Supp 1), 59–64.

Miller, W.R. (ed.), 1999. Integrating spirituality into treatment: Resources for practitioners. American Psychological Association, Washington DC.

Miller, W.R., Thorensen, C.E., 2003. Spirituality, religion and health: an emerging research field. American Psychologist, 58(1), 24–35.

Mir, G., Sheikh, A., 2010. "Fasting and prayer don't concern the doctors ... they don't even know what it is": Communication, decision-making and perceived social relations of Pakistani Muslim patients with long-term illnesses. Ethnicity and Health, 15(4), 327–342.

Moss, B., 2020. Communication skills in health and social care, 5th ed. Sage, London.

Odhayani, A.A., Khawaja, R.A., 2014. Patient's satisfaction: Insight into access to service, interpersonal communication and quality of care issues. Middle East Journal of Family Medicine, 12(8), 24–30.

O'Toole, G., Ramugondo, E., 2018. Occupational therapy and spiritual care. In: Carey, L.B. & Mathisen, B. (eds). Spiritual care in allied health practice. Jessica Kingsley, London.

Pati, D., Harvey, T.E., Pati, S., 2014. Physical design correlates of efficiency and safety in emergency departments. Critical Care Nursing Quarterly, 37(3), 299–316.

Phelps, A., Laudervale, K., Alcorn, S., et al., 2012. Addressing spirituality within the care of patients at the end of life: Perspectives of patients with advance cancer; oncologists and oncology nurses. Journal of Clinical Oncology, 30(20), 2538–2544.

Ravenhill, J.P., Poole, J., Brown, S.D., et al 2020. Sexuality, risk, and organisational misbehaviour in a secure mental healthcare facility in England. Culture, Health and Sexuality, 22(12), 1382–1397.

Richards, P.S., Bergin, A.E., 2005. The need for a spiritual strategy for counseling and psychotherapy, 2nd ed. American Psychological Association, Washington DC.

Ronaldson, S., 2014. Spirituality in palliative care nursing. In: O'Connor, M., Lee, S., Aranda, S. (eds), Palliative care nursing: A guide to practice, 3rd ed. Ausmed, Melbourne.

Sanderson, P.M., Grundgeiger, T., 2015. How do interruptions affect clinician performance in healthcare? Negotiating fidelity, control, and potential generalizability in the search for answers. International Journal of Human-1 Studies, 79(1), 85–96.

Spooner, A.J., Corley, A., Chaboyer, W., et al., 2014. Research paper: Measurement of the frequency and source of interruptions occurring during bedside nursing handover in the intensive care unit: An observational study. Australian Critical Care, 28(1), 19–23.

Traumer, L., Jacobsen, M.H., Laursen, B.S., 2019. Patients' experiences of sexuality as a taboo subject in the Danish healthcare system: A qualitative interview study. Scandinavian Journal of Caring Sciences, 33(1), 57–66.

Verrastro, V., Saladino, V., Filipoo, P., et al., 2020. Medical and health care professionals' sexuality education: State of the art and recommendations. International Journal of Environmental Research and Public Health, 17(7), 2186.

Whelan, M., Ulrich, E., Ginty, J., et al 2018. Journeys to Jamaica: A healthy dose of culture, competence, and compassion. Journal of Christian Nursing, 35(2), E21–E 27.

White, G., 2006. Talking about spirituality in healthcare practice: A resource for the multi-professional healthcare team. Jessica Kingsley, London.

Williams R., 2022. Cultural safety frameworks: Principles into practice. In: Edmondson, W., Williams, R., (eds), Burda-Burda Balayi health professionals and Indigenous health: Working at the interface. Oxford University Press, Melbourne.

SECTION 3

Managing realities of communication as a healthcare professional

CHAPTER 13

Holistic communication contributing to holistic healthcare

Chapter objectives

Upon completing this chapter, readers should be able to:

- reflect upon the importance of holistic communication
- list some characteristics of holistic communication
- appreciate the required elements for holistic communication, specifically respect, confidentiality and empathy
- demonstrate awareness of and skills in the appropriate use of empathy, touch and silence to achieve holistic communication
- list the various meanings of the concept of holistic and/or integrative healthcare
- consider and develop strategies to overcome the difficulties associated with providing holistic and/or integrative healthcare.

Holistic communication

Holistic communication requires healthcare professionals to apply the principles of effective communication to every unique individual within the context of their practice. As stated previously, these individuals include other healthcare professionals (some in the same interprofessional team and others not), support staff and people seeking care. Holistic communication requires a willingness to communicate about contexts, life experiences, thoughts, emotions, needs and desires, because in so doing the healthcare professional will relate to all interrelated aspects of the whole Person/s (Honeycutt & Milliken 2021; Moss 2020; White 2006; Young et al 2014; see Chapter 9). It requires respectful and effective use of empathy, touch and **silence** to empower the Person/s. When communicating holistically, it is also important to understand that the individual perspectives of each Person/s, as well as previous and present events, influence the choice of topics of communication and the interpretation of events and messages during communication (Gordon & Druckman 2018; Harms & Pierce 2019). These also affect results of communication.

Holistic communication requires healthcare professionals to consider the various environments relevant to the Person/s (Duke Integrative Medicine 2019; Chapter 12). It also requires consideration of elements of the particular context of the interaction, as these will affect the quality and success of the communication (Liu et al., 2014; Chapter 12). The immediate context involves the resources associated with the service (both people and objects) and the various interrelated aspects of the individual at the time. It is necessary for healthcare professionals to consider and care for these aspects within themselves, as well as within those with whom they communicate (Devito 2021; Doherty 2021; Haddad et al 2019; Stein-Parbury 2021).

Haddad and colleagues (2019) note that it is essential to understand that the Person/s seeking assistance will attribute a different significance, most often a greater significance, to their need than the healthcare professional. They may be aware of the implications of their need from a physical perspective and this may be the reason they are seeking assistance. The Person/s will also perceive the emotions, thoughts and social experiences associated with their need. In addition, many will also experience a spiritual element relating to their background, values and beliefs. Awareness of variations in the level of significance and influence of the aspects, perspective and context of the individual will assist the healthcare professional to communicate holistically (Dudgeon et al 2022).

- As a healthcare professional, what would be your response to the following questions from a Person/s?
  - Can you tell me where I can perform my daily prayers while I am in hospital?
  - Can I talk with you about my religious beliefs?
  - Can I ask my family to bring me a copy of the writings of my faith while in hospital?
  - May I keep my placenta please?
  - I must go back to where I was born to "finish off" (die). When will I be able to go?
  - Can I use the medicine made by my Elder (Aboriginal or Torres Strait Islander) or Tohunga (Māori) or Indigenous medicine person?
  - Can I use herbal remedies as well?
  - Can you tell me where I can have an abortion? My husband and I are not ready to have children.
  - Can I also have acupuncture while having your treatment?
  - Can I also have physiotherapy while having acupuncture?
  - You won't tell my father he is dying, will you? It is not our way.
- How should healthcare professionals respond to these requests?
- Is there anything they should or should not do in response to these requests?

Holistic communication requires genuine and sincere care, acknowledging the uniqueness of each individual (Lisenbee 2022). It requires a flow of expression and interchange between people and significant beings – pets, nature, God/life force and others around them. It acknowledges the importance of individuals recognising and understanding that humans share their humanity (Keegan & Drick 2016; Moss 2020). Humans, regardless of ethnicity, culture, gender, age, status, intelligence, material possessions or any other factor, share the same needs and concerns. Recognition of this fact assists healthcare professionals to humbly accept diversity to achieve holistic communication (Booth & Kaylor 2018; Mathibe-Neke & Mondell 2018), thereby creating collaborative, therapeutic relationships in practice (Honeycutt & Milliken 2021). Holistic communication requires consideration of more than the symptoms of the Person/s (Newton 2018) or their physical aspect (White et al 2018). It requires exploration of all aspects (physical, social, cognitive, emotional and spiritual) to achieve care of the whole person (Falkenheimer 2018). It also requires understanding of their perspective to ensure both quality of care and also maintenance of health and social function (Reeve 2018; Wang et al 2018). Such communication and resultant care increases health and wellbeing, thereby improving health outcomes while decreasing workload and the cost of healthcare (Fletcher & Barrett 2018).

An essential criterion in holistic communication: respect

As mentioned in Chapter 2, respect is a foundational component in achieving Person/Family-centred Care, a trusting relationship and thus positive outcomes (Linnet Olesen & Jørgensen 2023). Respect is essential in order to achieve these aims and more (Jiménez-Herrera 2023). Respect is more than an attitude or a value about viewing people from a particular perspective (Egan & Reese 2019). It provides the basis for appropriate behaviour (Mathibe-Neke & Mondell 2018), resulting in holistic communication.

The demonstration of respectful behaviour towards the Person/s requires healthcare professionals to respect themselves (see Chapters 6–8). Respecting the self protects the health and wellbeing of the healthcare professional. It also maintains satisfaction, contributing to the fulfilment of both personal and professional goals (Haddad et al 2019).

Demonstration of respect requires commitment to competent communicative and interpersonal practice – Person-centred Care. While the behaviours demonstrating respect are often nonverbal, they are easily recognised as respectful.

Defining respect

Respect is an underlying personal value determining both attitudes and actions, making it difficult to define. The following attempt to define respect combines various definitions of this value. Respect does not entail responding to an individual positively merely because of their status, position or role in society. It is not based on liking or admiring someone. Respect is an interest in and acknowledgement of the Person/s, their viewpoint and their emotions (Stein-Parbury 2021). It assumes that everyone has innate worth and value. Respect allows everyone to be themselves and to express themselves honestly without condemnation, ridicule or criticism (Egan & Reese 2019; Mathibe-Neke & Mondell 2018). It does not impose personal values, and thus expresses no judgement (Davis & Musolino 2016). Respect believes in the potential of each individual providing the basis for actions to assist in achieving this potential. It believes that individuals are valuable, regardless of their appearance or actions, past and present (Mathibe-Neke & Mondell 2018). Respect values the Person/s regardless of age, colour, racial group, position, uniform, state, relationship, social status or other characteristics (Booth & Kaylor 2018). It gazes past the negatives and positives to the inherent worth at the core of the Person/s (Haddad et al 2019) – a worth shared by all human beings.

Demonstrating respect

The following attitudes, characteristics or behaviours demonstrate respect: interest, warmth, friendliness, approachability, active concern, humility, honesty, authenticity, responding to the needs of the Person/s and carefully considering those needs (Haddad et al 2019).

It is not always easy to demonstrate respect, even with shared values, beliefs and positive feelings towards someone. Demonstrating respect when the Person/s acts contrary to the values and beliefs of the healthcare professional can be challenging. In such situations, it can be difficult to recognise the worth of the individual – to believe in the reality of that worth and to act according to that worth.

- Discuss possible strategies that would overcome the barriers to demonstrating respect when relating to someone who you might find difficult to respect.

The Person/s seeking healthcare is vulnerable, thus responsibility lies with the healthcare professional to demonstrate respect. It is imperative for the healthcare professional to act to communicate the importance of the Person/s – worthy of the investment of time and energy. Also important is acceptance of the individual and being available for them, regardless of their role, dysfunction, disfigurement or the demands on your time. Rogers (1967) suggests it is beneficial to expect or believe that somehow the Person/s will be able to overcome the current challenges; that they will persevere and reach the established goals. In situations where the Person/s appears resistant and uncooperative, it is important that the healthcare professional demonstrates understanding of their perspective and their feelings, assisting as necessary to achieve collaboration. While challenging, it is also important to demonstrate respect when personal values and expectations are different to those of the Person/s. Respect does not mean that the Person/s can manipulate or avoid responsibility for their actions. Respect requires the healthcare professional to challenge the Person/s to act to achieve the established goals of the intervention (Egan 2014; Egan & Reese 2019). Respect is a foundational value that is essential for effective and positive communication in all healthcare professions (Hampton 2013).

Cultural expectations

Demonstrating respect can cause difficulty for healthcare professionals when relating to Person/s from particular cultural groups (see Chapters 16 and 17). Different cultures have a variety of expectations related to respectful behaviour and thus may expect particular behaviour in specific situations as a demonstration of respect. Some of these behaviours relate to non-verbal cues (e.g. eye contact; see Chapter 10) or the use of particular colours in specific circumstances (Devito 2021). Other behaviours relate to specific actions when first meeting or seeing each other after an initial introduction (e.g. some cultures allow men to embrace and kiss in public, others have particular handshakes, while others kiss twice or maybe three times on the cheek, depending on the situation and the culture). Some cultures demonstrate respect according to gender and/or age, and thus expect particular behaviours related to the gender and/or age of either the healthcare professional or the Person/s. When working with people from different cultural backgrounds it is essential to seek information about attitudes and expected behaviour governed by and relating to respect.

Using names as a sign of respect

The name of an individual has particular meaning and generally identifies them. Using the name of the Person/s indicates interest and acknowledges them as separate from other people. It indicates their value, thus demonstrating respect. Asking an individual the name they prefer is very important when first communicating. Some individuals from particular generations or cultures prefer the use of their family name (e.g. Mr Thomas or Mrs Berk), finding the use of their given name offensive. Using the preferred name during subsequent communicative interactions continues to demonstrate respect, thereby contributing to the development of a therapeutic relationship.

- If you are in an unfamiliar place, how do you feel if someone greets you by using your name?
- What does this mean for a practising healthcare professional?

Confidentiality demonstrates respect

Confidentiality refers to ensuring that information remains within a particular context (Stein-Parbury 2021; see Chapter 19). It is another way of demonstrating respect. All information about the Person/s is confidential. Confidentiality involves keeping information private. The information, whether written or verbal, is available only to those with the right to access that information. It is important that healthcare professionals avoid sharing any information about the Person/s they assist in any context, except at work. This includes both professional and/or personal networking sites (see Chapter 23). It requires healthcare professionals to restrict what information they provide, to whom they provide the information and when they provide that information. Some of this information is recorded in particular records or databases. Any such records should not leave the healthcare service setting, nor should databases be accessed anywhere but on the healthcare service premises except for legal reasons. Such records or databases should not be taken off or accessed off the premises to complete an entry, nor should they be left for easy access on a desk or screen overnight. It is important to understand that this includes sharing any information about a Person/s on networking sites. This also includes results of any assessments or procedures.

When gathering information, it is important to indicate to the Person/s whether particular information will be shared, how it will be shared, with whom it will be shared, and the reason for sharing the information. Many healthcare services require the Person/s to sign an informed consent form before commencing services. These forms generally indicate who may receive information about the Person/s.

Another essential criterion in holistic communication: empathy

Empathy has received some discussion previously in this book. However, as expressing empathy is essential in healthcare, it requires further consideration.

Empathy is a process (Rogers 1975) that requires a healthcare professional to enter:

> *... the private perceptual world of the other and becoming thoroughly at home in it ... It includes communicating your sensing of his world as you look with fresh and unfrightened eyes at elements of which the individual is fearful. It means frequently checking with him for the accuracy of your sensings, and being guided by the responses you receive ... To be with another in this way means that for the time being you lay aside the views and values you hold for yourself in order to enter another's world without prejudice ... (p. 4).*

This definition reveals the reality of the complexity of expressing empathy. Unlike many definitions of empathy, it makes the healthcare professional responsible for their emotional response to the Person/s. It demands that the healthcare professional express emotional sensitivity, demonstrating understanding of the emotions (Williams et al 2014a; Williams et al 2014b). It also requires them to separate themselves from their values and personal prejudices (Morales 2014). The definition requires the healthcare professional to "feel" with the Person/s in a non-judgemental manner. It requires the healthcare professional to patiently listen and reflect on what they hear in order to respond with empathy. It requires the healthcare professional to avoid giving advice, regardless of their experience or understanding. In addition, it requires the healthcare professional to avoid interrupting, except to either affirm the Person/s without words or to encourage further expression of the emotions. The healthcare professional verbally and non-verbally expresses empathy – through their actual words and how they express those words. Expressions of empathy require the healthcare professional to make no assumptions about the accuracy of their perceptions of the emotions in the Person/s, only that they request verification of those perceptions. It is the seeking of verification that allows the healthcare professional to remain himself or herself while focusing on the Person/s.

In contrast to empathy, *sympathy* is the expression of the experiences, feelings and perspectives of the healthcare professional, placing the focus upon their experiences, feelings and perspectives rather than those of the Person/s (Lamothe et al 2014). Experiencing events that are similar to those of the Person/s may assist the healthcare professional when communicating. However, this can also lead the healthcare professional to assume they know exactly how the Person/s is feeling. This "feeling" can assist understanding or it can create an illusion of understanding potentially limiting the expression of empathy. That is, this "feeling" may communicate either authentic understanding or a nonchalance that is inappropriate, depending on how the healthcare professional communicates the commonality of experience. While in some circumstances self-disclosure may increase satisfaction for a Person/s, it is often safest to avoid sharing a similar experience with the Person/s, to avoid placing focus on the healthcare professional instead of the Person/s and potentially inappropriate outcomes (Moss 2020). When communicating with empathy, it is important to focus only on the needs and reactions of the Person/s.

The importance and result of empathy for the seeker of assistance

Empathy has a positive effect for both the healthcare professional and the Person/s. The context of the particular healthcare service, while familiar to the healthcare professional, is unfamiliar to the Person/s seeking the assistance of that service. Each Person/s has a reason for seeking assistance, potentially creating confusion and fear in them. There may also be factors and events in the life of the Person/s, past or present, which cause confusion and fear, independent of the current reason for seeking assistance. In such circumstances, the emotional need for understanding and acceptance becomes the dominant need. The needy and fearful Person/s seeks that understanding and acceptance from anyone offering it.

Making an effort to enter the perspective of the Person/s without judgement is a sign of respect (Egan 2014). It communicates understanding and acceptance, thereby encouraging expression and exploration of sometimes debilitating emotions. It reassures the Person/s that their emotions are not "crazy", potentially facilitating management of confusion and fear in unfamiliar and sometimes unpleasant situations. Empathy can empower the Person/s to "take control" in a seemingly out-of-control situation, thereby facilitating a change in their management of the situation and how they relate to themselves. This reality indicates that empathy is a central component of holistic communication and Person/Family-centred Care (Davis & Musolino 2016).

Person-centred Care and solving the problem

Divide the entire group into pairs. If there is an odd number, have one person observe the progress of the pairs. Role-play the following roles.

Nancy: You have not been attending the healthcare service for predetermined appointments. You enjoy the healthcare professional who telephones however, you are reluctant to explain your lack of attendance at the mutually agreed time for appointments. (The student "playing" Nancy must decide the reason why you have not been attending – you may discuss your reason with the group facilitator or instructor if appropriate.) Do not initially give the reason to the person playing the part of the healthcare professional; wait until you experience feelings of safety and affirmation. Reasons for not attending might include illness; concern about someone in your family; a sick pet; nausea because of a new liquid oral medication that smells and tastes horrible, despite the existence of a more palatable flavoured variety; pain that makes showering very slow and tedious, and so forth.

Healthcare professional: You are aware of the number of people waiting to see you, but you are intent on establishing why Nancy has failed to attend over the past two weeks. You really want to assist Nancy, so you persist when she is reluctant to provide an explanation for her absence. Demonstrate how you communicate both for Nancy-centred practice (using empathic responses) and to gather the information you need to assist her.

- How successful was the healthcare professional?
- How long did it take to express empathy and identify the issue?
- Does confidentiality affect this scenario? If so, how? How will you manage it if Nancy requires referral to another healthcare professional?
- Did the person playing the healthcare professional achieve their goals?
- How did Nancy feel?
- What assisted Nancy to trust and disclose?
- What made it difficult for Nancy to trust and disclose?

Repeat the role-play, swapping roles and changing the reason for Nancy's non-attendance, discussing any differences.

Empathy is a time-saving tool for the healthcare professional. Willingness to explore the needs and issues of the Person/s promotes expression of the feelings associated with those needs and issues, thereby building a collaborative therapeutic relationship (Reeve 2018). The expression of these feelings can facilitate a sense of control for the Person/s. The healthcare professional should note and acknowledge the feelings immediately, and should encourage their expression to avoid difficulties and further problems. An immediate empathic approach allows efficient provision of appropriate interventions. It usually ensures collaboration with and effective fulfilment of the needs of the Person/s.

The use of touch with or without empathy

Touch is a powerful, non-verbal form of communication. The habit of touching to communicate reflects a personal style of communicating, and should not be forced if it is not naturally part of the communicative style of the healthcare professional. The reality that different personality types have different communication styles (Hall et al 2014; Literat & Chen 2014) means that sometimes individuals, including the Person/s, may find it difficult to communicate through touch. However, when there is a connection and resultant rapport, a gentle touch on the shoulder, a pat on the arm or a squeeze of the hand, for many, demonstrates awareness of their plight. A gentle touch typically communicates a desire to collaborate to fulfil the needs of the Person/s without causing offence (Holli & Beto 2023), regardless of the personal style of communication. It is important that the healthcare professional carefully observes responses to touching and avoids touching if there is a negative response. Asking permission to use touch before touching may avoid a negative response. If there is established rapport and the touch is intended to comfort and encourage – indicating support and empathy – the Person/s usually senses this and appreciates the touch.

Each culture has norms that govern touch conventions when communicating. Sexual harassment is a reality in many professional workplaces. Awareness of the norms governing sexual behaviour for a particular workplace is essential for all healthcare professionals in order to avoid communicating inappropriately when using touch.

- List the social norms governing touching in each culture represented in the group. (If it is a monocultural group, discuss any experience of different norms governing touching – even within families.)
- Consider greeting, handshaking, kissing on the cheek, introducing, saying goodbye, variations in touching because of age and gender, comforting an upset person who is familiar, comforting an upset person who is a stranger, and any other situations that might include communication by touching.
- Compare the differences in the social norms governing touching in different situations.
- List ways in which these differences might guide the practice of a healthcare professional.

Touching can provide feedback about the emotions of the Person/s. A gentle touch may inform the healthcare professional that the individual who appears relaxed and in control feels unsure and requires encouragement. This previously unnoticeable information encourages the healthcare professional to communicate empathy by investing time and energy in exploring these distressing emotions.

Parents and significant others communicate emotions through touch with their children. In families, touch is a powerful form of communication, expressing parental or sibling emotion. Kisses, cuddles, tickles and rumbles are fun and comforting; they communicate ease, acceptance, love and affection (Greene et al 2015). This manner of touch produces positive emotions in both the person touching and the person receiving the touch. Potentially physical expressions of anger, frustration and disapproval communicated through either touch or tone of voice produce negative emotions and responses. Various types of touch, whether producing positive or negative emotions, can acclimatise an individual to respond in a particular manner when touched by anyone. Healthcare professionals who use touch within their treatment media should consider the reaction of anyone they touch. Careful awareness of the responses and needs of children when touching is essential because this provides information about the touch experiences of that child. Accurate knowledge of the touch experiences of a child, if managed appropriately, has the potential to restore and protect the emotional growth of the child and their future ability to both give and receive touch to express concern.

When used appropriately to communicate, touch can be a powerful tool for the healthcare professional who feels comfortable touching others.

Silence to comfort

Silence can be a powerful and comforting communication device. Words are sometimes inappropriate. Saying nothing to someone – just being with them – can be more appropriate than words in particular circumstances, especially with Indigenous peoples (see Chapter 17).

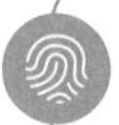

- How comfortable are you with silences in conversations?
- What is your natural tendency when there is a silence in a conversation?
- What does that mean for you as a healthcare professional?

When listening, the healthcare professional is silent; however, because the Person/s is speaking, the interaction is not silent. Refraining from speaking while listening, in combination with concentrating and focusing on the speaker, demonstrates skills in listening as well as interest and respect (Stein-Parbury 2021). There are occasions while communicating, however, when words are inappropriate or inadequate. In these cases, just being with a Person/s and saying nothing indicates interest, care, respect and even empathy. There are occasions when the Person/s does not seek words but the presence of an interested and caring healthcare professional. A carer or relative found sitting outside the room of their seriously ill or dying family member may not desire verbal communication but the non-verbal, silent presence of a previously known, concerned and interested healthcare professional. This presence communicates care and – even though the healthcare professional may be skilful in verbal expressions of empathic care – simply sitting quietly with the Person/s can fulfil the needs of the Person/s at that time.

When the Person/s has difficulty expressing themselves verbally, it is appropriate in some healthcare professions to silently perform an activity with them in an interested and observant manner to build rapport. The possible people with whom a healthcare professional might use this type of silence include children, people with mental health disorders or communication difficulties, people experiencing severe pain and people in palliative care units.

Different cultures have different uses for silence. Some cultures find that silence communicates more effectively than words. When communicating with a vulnerable Person/s from a different culture, it is important to clarify the uses and effects of silence.

Silence, when used appropriately, can powerfully communicate interest, regard and a desire to assist where possible.

Effective and holistic communication with any individuals relating to the healthcare professional requires understanding of all involved individuals; that is, both self and the Person/s. It requires an understanding of the constituent, interrelated aspects of the Person, respect and expressions of empathy, perhaps including touch and silence, along with knowledge of the roles of the various healthcare professions. While holistic communication requires an investment of time, it is essential for effective communication, and promoting positive outcomes.

Holistic care

The principle of holism always considers the Person/s to be a whole, regardless of the specific needs of or demands upon that Person/s at a particular time (Burkhardt 2015). The concept of holism is not a new idea for many healthcare professions (Dossey et al 2016; Honeycutt & Milliken 2021; White 2006). In fact, some healthcare professions have developed because of a holistic philosophy of care.

There are various ways of understanding **holistic care**. It can mean inclusive care that accommodates diverse cultural and spiritual systems (Selman et al 2014), in particular the medicine of traditional Indigenous healers and the traditional interventions of Eastern cultures (Hope & Rosa 2018). Holistic care can also mean **complementary and alternative medicine (CAM)** (Dossey et al 2016), as opposed to traditional medical care. A holistic concept of healthcare is the basis of CAM (Honeycutt & Milliken 2021), and thus some consider holistic care as synonymous with CAM. In some countries, there is a move towards the term "integrative care", combining conventional (medical) and complementary therapies (Australasian Integrative Medicine Association [AIMA] 2019; Burkhardt 2015; Poplar 2014). Some healthcare professions perceive holistic care as the consideration of the whole Person/s – every aspect of the unique individual (American Nurses Association [ANA], & American Holistic Nurses Association [AHNA], 2019; Duke Integrative Medicine 2019) – using a variety of interventions depending on the needs of the individual. In these professions, holistic care means avoidance of focusing upon one aspect of the individual over another aspect (McIlfatrick & Hasson 2014). It requires recognition that healthcare is more than a focus upon the physical needs of the individual (Johnson 2014; Wang et al 2018).

Holistic care fulfils more than the immediate needs relevant to the particular healthcare profession; it recognises there are many causes contributing to and emotions relating to those needs (Newton 2018). It recognises that the immediate needs may arise from more than the physical aspect of the Person/s, even though the need initially may appear to be physical (Reeve 2018). Holistic care understands there is more than one way to fulfil a need and to achieve healing. It considers the less obvious and often forgotten aspects of the psychological/emotional, spiritual and social/cultural functioning of the individual. It acknowledges that health is more than physical wellbeing, but includes spiritual, emotional, cognitive and social wellbeing (Dossey & Luck 2016; Patz 2014; World Health Organization [WHO] 1946, 2008).

- Consider the aspect of the Person/s (physical, emotional, cognitive, social or spiritual) to which you feel most comfortable relating. Why? Have each group member explain which aspect of a Person/s they would feel most comfortable relating to in their healthcare profession.
- As a group, decide which aspect of the Person/s is the easiest to relate to or address. Discuss why.
- As a group, decide which aspect is the most difficult to address. Discuss why. Suggest strategies that might assist in overcoming this difficulty.
- Share the group decisions with the entire class/group.

Holistic care does not merely treat symptoms, but also searches for causes, understanding there are often multiple causes arising from and relating to every aspect of the Person/s. Mutual respect is the foundation of holistic care, and it assumes equality (see Chapters 2 and 9) within the therapeutic relationship. Mutual respect seeks involvement from the Person/s in the collaborative goal-setting and decision-making associated with their care and future (Blaszko

Helming 2020; Young et al 2014). In holistic care, the responsibility for change and healing lies within the Person/s. The role of the healthcare professional is to facilitate and empower the Person/s to achieve their particular health-related goals (Honeycutt & Milliken 2021).

Unless specifically taught to provide holistic care, a developing healthcare professional may require a role model and experience in their profession to consistently provide holistic care (Mathibe-Neke & Mondell 2018). It is possible for a healthcare professional who practises within a particular specialty area to provide holistic care, despite a focus upon their specialty area. Regardless of the situation, it is always possible to consider the whole Person/s while practising as a healthcare professional (Sims-Gould et al 2010). Holistic care is fundamental in achieving Person/Family-centred Care in any healthcare service and thus should be an aim of every healthcare professional.

Holistic care includes consideration of context

To provide holistic care, it is important that healthcare professionals consider the interrelating aspects of the whole Person/s, regardless of the presence of an obviously dominating aspect at any one time (Fletcher & Barrett 2018). It is also important to remember that individuals with whom healthcare professionals communicate develop within diverse and multiple contexts. Recognition of these contexts is essential when communicating (Harms & Pierce 2019; Honeycutt & Milliken 2021; Haddad 2019; White 2006). Some consider these contexts to be physical, financial, cultural and social (family or kinship groups, friends, colleagues or acquaintances), while others consider them to also include a spiritual element (Booth & Kaylor 2018; Colbert 2003; White 2006). Regardless of their composition, these contexts provide experiences, promoting either positive or negative responses within the cognitive, psychological and spiritual functioning of the individual. Such responses ultimately affect the physical and social aspects of the individual (Colbert 2003; Golman 2007) and, therefore, all of these contexts require the understanding and recognition of healthcare professionals (Christian 2014).

The requirements of holistic care

There are currently many healthcare professions, each with their particular expertise and focus. An awareness and understanding of the various healthcare professions is important to ensure holistic care and positive outcomes (WHO 1946). Openness to the involvement of multiple healthcare professionals when assisting individuals, regardless of the presence of an inter-professional or multidisciplinary team, increases the potential for holistic care and positive outcomes (White 2006).

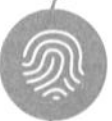

- Which aspect(s) of the Person does your particular healthcare profession focus upon?
- How can you ensure holistic care for those seeking your assistance?
- Divide a page into two, top to bottom.
  - On one side, make a list of every healthcare profession you know.
  - On the other side, list the aspect(s) upon which that healthcare profession focuses. If you are not sure, do some research and then list the aspect(s).

- Compare your list with two others and adjust it according to research relating to the contents of the other lists, requesting clarification where necessary.
- How can you use this list to ensure holistic care to empower the individual to achieve their goals and transform their functioning?

Each of the individuals below is awaiting a diagnosis relating to particular physical symptoms; however, this is what they express:

1. A 43-year-old regularly expresses anxiety about their diagnosis.
2. A 17-year-old expresses stress because of university entrance examinations and assessments.
3. A 7-year-old just wants to continue playing weekend sport.
4. A 54-year-old male with an intellectual disability wants to marry his 32-year-old girlfriend who also has an intellectual disability.
5. A 28-year-old over-eats constantly because of anxiety and fear.
6. A 45-year-old expresses disappointment that their same-gender partner of 20 years has recently been unfaithful.
7. A 76-year-old expresses distress over their lost cat.
8. A 52-year-old expresses confusion because of their dementing parent.
9. A 39-year-old expresses despair because of their dying child.
10. A 60-year-old is depressed because they cannot attend their religious group.
11. A 32-year-old has just given birth to her first (much-awaited) child. She has been told the child has Down Syndrome and she expresses devastation.
    - Decide how to best acknowledge and fulfil each of these expressed needs.
    - What would your healthcare profession do to assist each Person/s?
    - How can you ensure holistic care for these people?

Holistic care requires consideration of the whole Person/s; however, it also requires care of self. This requires reflection and self-awareness while practising as a healthcare professional. This awareness will guide and promote necessary change. Holistic care also requires healthcare professionals to assume responsibility for themselves – for their thoughts, words, actions and related outcomes. This, of course, requires healthcare professionals to balance their personal and professional needs (Dossey et al 2016). Holistic care requires healthcare professionals to acknowledge the effects of their professional encounters and seek assistance as necessary. Such care of self will develop and strengthen holistic communication (Portillo & Cowley 2011).

- Choose a scenario from Section 4. Consider both the male and female in the chosen scenario.
- Identify and list how you will achieve holistic communication and care with the Person/s in that scenario.

Chapter summary

The healthcare professional must achieve effective and holistic communication with all stakeholders in practice. Such communication requires a willingness to communicate about individual needs, different perspectives of various experiences, thoughts relating to the condition of the Person/s and

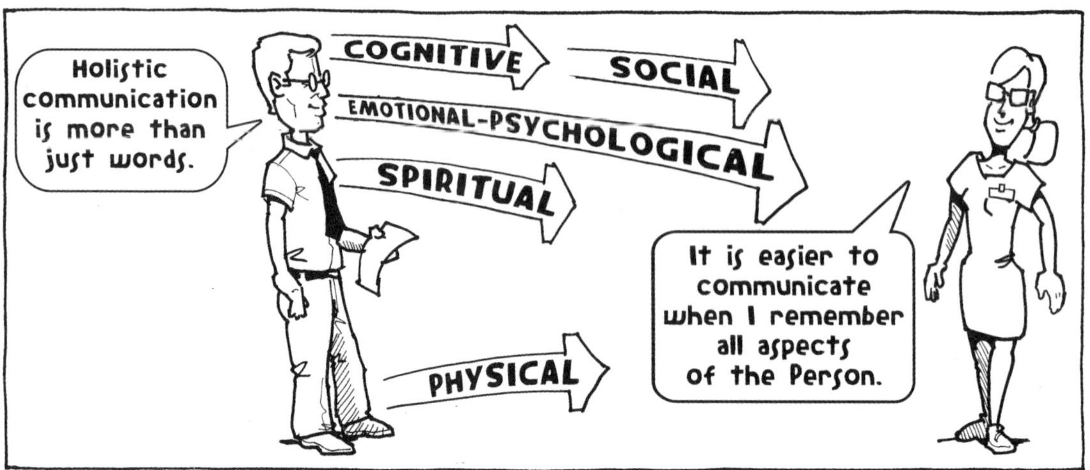

FIGURE 13.1
Holistic communication considering all aspects of the whole Person/s.
Courtesy Roger Harvey © Elsevier Australia.

their aspirations and goals for the immediate and long-term future. It acknowledges the unique nature of each individual interacting with the healthcare professional. Holistic communication is founded on respect of self and others. This respect facilitates demonstration of genuine and sincere care, based upon knowledge of all aspects of the Person/s. This knowledge promotes expressions of empathy; confidentiality; Person-centred Care; effective communication and empowerment for the Person/s and the healthcare professional. Holistic communication considers and promotes holistic care. Holistic care recognises that the needs of a Person/s seeking assistance may arise from more than the physical aspect. It considers underlying causes of the presenting symptoms and, as necessary, refers to other appropriate healthcare professionals. This requires a clear understanding of the roles of other healthcare professionals and how to contact or refer to particular services.

REVIEW QUESTIONS

1. What does holistic communication require?

   i. ______________________________

   ii. ______________________________

   iii. ______________________________

iv. ____________________

v. ____________________

2. State three important elements of holistic communication.

i. ____________________

ii. ____________________

iii. ____________________

3. What should healthcare professionals be willing to communicate about?

i. ____________________

ii. ____________________

iii. ____________________

iv. ____________________

v. ____________________

vi. ____________________

4. What are the three meanings of holistic care?

i. ____________________

ii. ____________________

iii. ____________________

5. What does holistic care require?

i. ____________________

ii. ____________________

iii. ____________________

6. Why does holistic care require knowledge of the role of other healthcare professions?

____

____

____

7. What should healthcare professionals be willing to communicate about?

   i. ____

   ii. ____

   iii. ____

   iv. ____

   v. ____

   vi. ____

References

American Nurses Association (ANA), & American Holistic Nurses Association (AHNA), 2019. Holistic nursing: Scope and standards of practice, 3rd ed. American Nurses Association Nursing Knowledge Centre, Ohio.

Australasian Integrative Medicine Association (AIMA), 2018. What is integrative medicine? Available at: www.aima.net.au./what-is-integrative-medicine

Blaszko Helming, M.A., 2020. Relationships. In: Blaszko Helming, M.A., Shields, D.A., Avino, K.M. et al., Dossey & Keegan's Holistic Nursing: A handbook for practice. Jones and Bartlett Learning, Burlington MA.

Booth, L., Kaylor, S., 2018. Teaching spiritual care within nursing education: A holistic approach. Holistic Nursing Practice, 32(4), 177–181.

Burkhardt, P., 2015. Holistic and integrative nursing understanding our roots. Beginnings (American Holistic Nurses' Association), 35(1), 5–33.

Christian, K.E., 2014. The diabetes one-stop: An off-the-road person-centered care model. Beginnings (American Holistic Nurses' Association), 34(6), 6–9.

Colbert, D., 2003. Deadly emotions: Understand the mind body spirit connection that can heal or destroy you. Thomas Nelson, Nashville, TN.

Davis, C.M., Musolino, G.M., 2016. Patient practitioner interaction: An experiential manual for developing the art of healthcare, 6th ed. Slack, Thorofare, NJ.

Devito, J.A., 2021. The interpersonal communication book, 16th ed. Pearson, Boston.

Doherty, R.F., 2021. Ethical dimensions in health professions, 7th ed. Elsevier, St Louis, MO.

Dossey, B., Luck, S., 2016. Self-assessment. In: Dossey, B., Keegan, L., Barrere, C.C., et al., (eds), Holistic nursing: A handbook for practice, 7th ed. Jones & Bartlett Learning, Burlington, MA.

Dossey, B.M., Keegan, L., Barrere, C.C., et al., (eds) 2016. Holistic nursing: A handbook for practice, 7th ed. Jones & Bartlett, Burlington, MA.

Dudgeon, P., Derry, K., Platell, M., et al., 2022. Social and emotional wellbeing and healing from trauma. In: Edmondson, W., Williams, R., (eds). Burda-Burda Balayi health professionals and Indigenous health: Working at the interface. Oxford University Press, Melbourne.

Duke Integrative Medicine, 2019. What is integrative medicine? Online. Available at: dukeintegrativemedicine.org/about-us/what-is-integrative-medicine

Egan, G., 2014. The skilled helper: A problem management and opportunity approach to helping, 10th ed. Brooks/Cole, Belmont CA.

Egan, G., Reese R.J., 2019. The skilled helper: A problem management and opportunity approach to helping, 11th ed. Cengage, Boston, MA.

Falkenheimer, S.A., 2018. Prime: Partnerships in international medical educational an oral history of the development of an international network in whole person medicine and whole person teaching. Ethics and Medicine, 34(2), 87–102.

Fletcher, J., Barrett, S., 2018. Improving holistic assessment of chronic wound: How to meet patient expectation using the new Best Practice Statement. Wound UK, 14(5), 92–95.

Golman, C., 2007. Social intelligence: The new science of human relationships. Random House, London.

Gordon, R.A., Druckman, D., 2018. Non-verbal communication as behaviour: Approaches, issues and research. In: Hargie, O. (ed.), The handbook of communication skills, 4th ed. Routledge, New York.

Greene, C.A.F., Julian, D., Ward-Zimmerman, B., et al., 2015. Please break the silence: Parents' views on communication between pediatric primary care and mental health providers. Families, Systems and Health, 33(2), 155–159.

Haddad, A.M., Purtilo, R.B., Doherty, R.F., 2019. Health professional and patient interaction, 9th ed. Elsevier/Saunders, St Louis, MO.

Hall, M.B., Guidry, J.J., McKyer, E.L.J., et al., 2014. Association analysis of reported attitudes and culturally competent behavior engagement among public health employees. Journal of Health Disparities Research and Practice, 7(3), 15–24.

Hampton, R., 2013. Communication for working with Indigenous Australian. In: Hampton, R., Toombs, M. (eds), Indigenous Australians and health: The wombat in the room. Oxford University Press, Melbourne.

Harms, L., Pierce, J., 2019. Working with people: Communication skills for reflective practice, 2nd Canadian ed. Oxford University Press, Ontario.

Holli, B.B., Beto, J.A., 2023. Nutrition counselling and education skills: A practical guide, 8th ed. Jones & Bartlett, Burlington, MA.

Honeycutt, A., Milliken, M.A., 2021. Understanding human behavior: A guide for healthcare providers, 10th ed., Cengage Learning Boston.

Hope, S., Rosa W., 2018. Holistic care of the spirit: The use of entheogens in patients with advanced serious illness. Beginnings, 38(4), 8–21.

Jiménez-Herrera, M.F., 2023. The moral compass in care: From ethics to professionalism (Editorial). Scandinavian Journal of Caring Sciences, 37, 1–2.

Johnson, B., 2014. Healing services team: A holistic interdisciplinary approach to inpatient care at the Cleveland Clinic. Beginnings (American Holistic Nurses' Association), 34(3), 12–26.

Keegan, L., Drick, C.A., 2016. Dying in peace. In: Dossey, B.M., Keegan, L., Barrere, C. et al. (eds), Holistic nursing: A handbook for practice, 7th ed. Springer, New York.

Lamothe, M.B., Boujut, E., Senasni, F., et al., 2014. To be or not to be empathic: The combined role of empathic concern and perspective taking in understanding burnout in general practice. BMC Family Practice, 15(1), 15–30.

Linnet Olesen, M., Jørgensen, R., 2023. Impact of the person-centred intervention guided self-determination across healthcare settings: An integrated review. Scandinavian Journal of Caring Sciences, 37, 37–59.

Lisenbee, M., 2022. Holistic Nursing: A way of being in the world. Beginnings, 42(6), 4–5.

Literat, I., Chen, N.-T.N., 2014. Communication infrastructure theory and entertainment-education: An integrative model for health communication. Communication Theory, 24(1), 83–103.

Liu, W., Manias, E., Gerdtz, M., 2014. The effects of physical environments in medical wards on medication communication processes affecting patient safety. Health and Place, 26(2014), 199– 98.

Mathibe-Neke, J.M., Mondell, T., 2018. Facilitate a holistic midwifery care: A teaching strategy. Africa Journal of Nursing and Midwifery, 19(1), 190–208.

McIlfatrick, S., Hasson, F., 2014. Evaluating a holistic assessment tool for palliative care practice. Journal of Clinical Nursing, 23(7/8), 1064–1075.

Morales, J.B., 2014. The relationship between physician emotional intelligence and quality of care. International Journal of Caring Sciences, 7 (3), 704–710.

Moss, B., 2020. Communication skills in health and social care, 5th ed. Sage, London.

Newton, E., 2018. Embracing a holistic approach to patient care. Radiologic Technology, 89(5), 516–517.

Patz, S., 2014. Holistic assessment in person-centered care. Beginnings (AHNA), 34(1), 10–22.

Poplar, J., 2014. Holistic care in high risk pregnancy. International Journal of Childbirth Education, 29(4), 68–71.

Portillo, M.C., Cowley, S., 2011.Working the way up in neurological rehabilitation: The holistic approach of nursing care. Journal of Clinical Nursing, 20(11/12), 1731–1743.

Reeve, J., 2018. Primary care redesign for person-centred care: delivering an international generalist revolution. Australian Journal of Primary Health, 24, 330–336.

Rogers, C., 1967. On becoming a person. Constable, London.

Rogers, C., 1975. Empathic: an unappreciated way of being. The Counselling Psychologist, 5(2), 2–10.

Selman, L., Speck, P., Barfield, R.C., et al., 2014. Holistic models for end of life care: Establishing the place of culture. Progress in Palliative Care, 22(2), 80–87.

Sims-Gould, J., Wiersma, E., Arseneau, L., et al., 2010. Care provider perspective on end-of-life care in long-term-care homes: Implications for whole-person and palliative care. Journal of Palliative Care 26(2), 122–129.

Stein-Parbury, J., 2021. Patient and person: Interpersonal skills in nursing, 7th ed. Churchill Livingstone Elsevier, Sydney.

Wang, J.J., Yang, Y.Y., Liu M.Y., 2018. Holistic healthcare for the aged: Concepts and strategies. Journal of Nursing, 65(2) 5–12.

White, C., McVeigh, C., Foster, S., et al., 2018. Evaluation of the European Certificate of Holistic Dementia Care programme. European Journal of Palliative Care, 25(2), 82–88.

White, G., 2006. Talking about spirituality in healthcare practice: A resource for the multi-professional healthcare team. Jessica Kingsley, London.

Williams, B., Brown, T., Boyle, M., et al., 2014a. Levels of empathy in undergraduate emergency health, nursing, and midwifery students: A longitudinal study. Advances in Medical Education and Practice, 5, 299–306.

Williams, B., Brown, T., McKenna, L., et al., 2014b. Empathy levels among health professional students: a cross-sectional study at two universities in Australia. Advances in Medical Education and Practice, 5, 107–113.

World Health Organization (WHO), 2008. Primary care: Putting people first. In: World Health Report. WHO, Geneva, Switzerland. Online 7 October 2019. Available at: reliefweb.int/report/world/world-health-report-2008-primary-health-care-now-more-ever

World Health Organization (WHO), 1946. Preamble to the Constitution of the World Health Organization as adopted by the International Health Conference, New York, 19–22 June, 1946; signed on 22 July 1946 by the representatives of 61 States (Official Records of the World Health Organization, no. 2, p. 100) and entered into force on 7 April 1948.

Young, J., Cund, A., Renshaw, M., et al., 2014. Improving the care of cancer patients: Holistic needs assessment. British Journal of Nursing (Oncology Supp) 24(1), 17–20.

CHAPTER 14

Effective interprofessional communication within multidisciplinary teams

Chapter objectives

Upon completing this chapter, readers should be able to:

- apply the components of the model of Person-centred Care to members of a multidisciplinary team
- identify the aspects of collaborative teamwork in the relevant code of conduct and/or standards
- demonstrate understanding of the importance of interprofessional communication for effective multidisciplinary care
- demonstrate understanding of the requirements of multidisciplinary care
- state and explain the benefits of multidisciplinary care
- outline the challenges of and their effects upon multidisciplinary communication for team members
- suggest ways to overcome the challenges of multidisciplinary communication within the team.

PLEASE NOTE: In the literature, multiple terms refer to communicating or working with practitioners from other disciplines in healthcare, including interdisciplinary care; interprofessional care, multidisciplinary care and teamwork. This chapter generally uses multidisciplinary communication, collaboration and thus care (MDC), with some use of team or teamwork.

ADDITIONAL NOTE: In the context of multidisciplinary teamwork, the concept of the Person/s is not only the individual requiring assistance, but also includes the other members of the team. Therefore, all aspects of the model discussed in Chapter 2 requires both consideration and application to other team members when working within a team, whether or not a multidisciplinary team.

Multidisciplinary care has become more common in healthcare provision in the last few decades. This more regular occurrence may result from a worldwide increase in the complexity of healthcare systems (Showstark et al 2023; Will et al 2019). In fact, one healthcare professional alone is able to provide safe Person/s care. However, the worldwide increase in the need for care of chronic conditions and palliative conditions, in combination with an ageing population and the increasing cost of healthcare, highlights the importance of and need for multidisciplinary teams (James et al 2018; Martin et al 2023). The World Health Organization (WHO), in understanding the effect of multidisciplinary teamwork to enable integrated and holistic care, also supports multidisciplinary collaboration and care to contribute to the provision of comprehensive care and to address the global health needs (WHO 2010; 2016). Additionally, this multidisciplinary collaboration increases the appropriate use of available resources relevant to the care of the Person/s, potentially contributing to achievement of Person/Family-centred Care. It also reduces the possibility of negative outcomes, due to the shared understanding of the needs of the Person/s from the perspective of each team member, thereby ensuring effective and satisfactory care. In addition, registration bodies and national boards of every healthcare discipline require effective multidisciplinary communication of all relevant Person/s information and respectful collaboration (sharing appropriate skills, knowledge and experience) to benefit the Person/s (AHPRA & National Boards 2022; Health & Care Professions Council UK 2016).

Realities of multidisciplinary communication

Multidisciplinary communication occurs multiple times every day for most healthcare professionals (Dickson & Peelo-Kilroe 2021). It typically involves communicating with people from various professions (e.g. teachers, voluntary staff, sometimes police, firefighters, organisational staff, managers) and other healthcare professionals (e.g. assistants, case managers, counsellors, dieticians, general practitioners, medical specialists, nurses, occupational therapists, paramedics, physiotherapists, psychologists, service managers, social workers, speech pathologists). Effective multidisciplinary communication and collaboration promotes effective, holistic, integrated, sustainable, safe and quality care for all Person/s (Flanagan et al 2020; James et al 2018; Martin et al 2023; McInerney et al 2022; Mulholland et al 2020), along with continuity of care (Reed et al 2021), thereby potentially increasing Person/s satisfaction (Will et al 2019), while also ensuring positive health outcomes (Filho et al 2023; Fink-Samnick 2019; Stadick 2020). This indicates the importance of multidisciplinary communication for achieving effective collaboration, thereby producing a requirement for appropriate provision of care by multidisciplinary teams (Boggs 2023; Schot et al 2020).

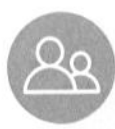

In small groups, consider the components of the model of Person-centred Care, discussed in Chapter 2.

- How might each component relate to relationships between healthcare professionals within multidisciplinary teams?
- How might each component contribute to positive relationships with individuals from other healthcare disciplines?
- Suggest how to ensure the achievement of each of these components when relating to other healthcare professionals while practising in your own discipline.

With the entire (large) group, share and discuss:

- how to ensure the achievement of each component during challenging interdisciplinary and/or multidisciplinary interactions.

The benefits of multidisciplinary communication and thus collaborative care

The discussion above mentions various benefits of multidisciplinary communication resulting in effective collaboration and thus quality care. An important benefit is the provision of effective care and thus the improvement of health outcomes (WHO 2010). It enables healthcare professionals from diverse backgrounds with different skills working together to provide holistic and safe care, thereby addressing global health needs (WHO 2016). The provision of holistic and comprehensive care that considers often complex needs is only possible with a multidisciplinary team. Such a team, consisting of practitioners with their particular "scope of practice" or focus and thus unique Person/s-related goals, enables integration of comprehensive care, thereby improving health outcomes (Williams et al 2021).

Inclusion of multiple disciplines in the care of the Person/s also encourages advocacy for the specific (often unique) needs and desires of that Person/s (Carter et al 2021; Nsiah et al 2020). A healthcare professional presenting the specific needs of the Person/s (being their voice) can increase the quality of care and thus the overall health outcomes, including relevant care before and after discharge. It also contributes to improving the quality of the therapeutic relationship, along with potentially contributing to equity in the provision of care for all Person/s. Such advocacy seeks to advance the health and wellbeing of every Person/s, regardless of their condition or background. This, then supports the decision-making and desires of the Person/s. A strong therapeutic relationship can also assist the Person/s to understand and navigate the complexity of the health and social system. This can empower them to express their own needs when experiencing the complexity of the health systems. Such advocacy contributes to achieving all components of Person/Family-centred Care.

Multidisciplinary communication increases the possibility of providing effective care, by highlighting the needs of the Person/s. Discussion of these needs occurs during case conferences. This discussion encourages all represented healthcare professionals to understand the needs of the Person/s and their possible contribution to enhance the quality of care and thus ultimate health outcomes. This contribution promotes the satisfaction of all involved in the provision of care. This satisfaction has the potential to improve the reputation of the health service and relevant healthcare professionals, thereby increasing the trust and sense of safety for the current Person/s and all future Person/s (Bashatah et al 2020; Carter et al 2021).

Multidisciplinary teams have also been shown to increase the continuity of care (Hustoft et al 2019). Continuity of care requires continuous relationships between the Person/s and the healthcare professional. This care is possible with multidisciplinary teams. They provide the opportunity for the Person/s to connect and collaborate with all team members, although often in depth with a particular team member, one of their choice. This particular therapeutic relationship, involving rapport and empowerment, provides the possibility of all team members understanding the needs and perspective of the Person/s. This can then ensure that the Person/s receives ongoing and appropriate care from all team members, resulting in achievement of the unique goals of each Person/s, over time. This achieves both continuity of care and sustainable, timely and ongoing care, along with Person/Family-centred-Care.

There are sometimes ethically challenging situations in healthcare. These situations often result from conflict between personal values, principles and interests combining to make particular decisions difficult. In such situations, there is evidence to suggest the benefit of discussing these dilemmas with other healthcare professionals (Fischer-Grönlund et al 2021). Multidisciplinary teams make such discussions with individuals from diverse backgrounds, possible. Such discussion contributes to all healthcare professionals understanding that they are not alone when experiencing ethical dilemmas. This can result in reduction of stress for the individual healthcare professional, thereby contributing to their ability to focus on achieving Person-centred Care. This can also contribute to increasing the confidence and self-efficacy of the healthcare professional when making ethically challenging decisions, thereby affecting future collaboration with other healthcare professionals and related care.

The above discussion indicates the many benefits of multidisciplinary communication, collaboration and care. However, such communication and care can have associated challenges, often resulting in avoidance of communicating with other healthcare professionals during practice. This can be challenging; however, if managed appropriately, it has the potential to increase the quality of relationships and thus the effectiveness of the multidisciplinary team. This contributes to achieving Person-centred Care for all Person/s.

Requirements of multidisciplinary communication or teamwork

Multidisciplinary communication can be complex. It requires understanding of the role of the different healthcare professionals in the team (Clark 2014; Cruz et al 2017; Olvera et al 2020); respectful and trusting relationships among team members (Lynch et al 2021); relevant technology (Slaghmuylder et al 2022); and technical staff to support the use of the particular technology; along with support from organisational leaders and policymakers (Mulholland et al 2020; Vrijmoeth et al 2022) and appropriate policy and procedural guidelines (Bashatah et al, 2020). Remember that achieving effective verbal and non-verbal communication is the focus of this book. Therefore careful consideration and application of the content of the book, including the skills and underlying self-awareness, will empower all readers to achieve the goals of effective multidisciplinary communication, regardless of the reactions of other healthcare professionals or Person/s.

As mentioned above, multidisciplinary communication, collaboration and effective teamwork require demonstration of all components of the model of Person-centred Care (see Chapter 2). Mutual respect is essential amongst team members (Hustoft et al 2018). However, demonstrating respect is not always easy when others do not respect or understand you or your role. Nevertheless, respect is essential for developing trust and positive relationships within healthcare. This trust is important in time-scarce, pressured situations, affecting levels of collaboration and thus quality of safe care (Barnard et al 2020) and creativity within the team (Liu 2021). These positive relationships contribute to the ongoing achievement of exploration and thus mutual understanding of the roles of other healthcare professionals (Flanagan et al 2020; Machin et al 2019; Preston et al 2018). This is important, to ensure clear understanding of each role and the associated focus of care (Clark 2014; Cruz et al 2017), along with understanding of how the roles of each discipline can complement each other, thereby encouraging effective collaboration.

The components of mutual understanding contribute to effective collaboration, an essential component of multidisciplinary care (Machin et al 2019). This collaboration empowers team members in ethical decision-making and in provision of appropriate and effective care. This collaboration also provides an understanding of how each discipline can complement each other in practice. This improves care, while potentially reducing the length of time in hospital, thereby reducing the pressure on hospitals (Preston et al 2018; Walton et al 2020).

Another important aspect of multidisciplinary care is easy access to records and data platforms (Bereznicki et al 2021). Such access allows all team members to read the entries of any team member, thereby contributing to their understanding of the provided care for each unique Person/s, along with details relating to the requirements of their care (Dickson & Peelo-Kilroe 2021; Foronda et al 2016). This contributes to the provision of timely, safe, appropriate and effective care for the Person/s from all relevant healthcare professionals.

An important requirement of multidisciplinary collaboration and care is consideration of the current culture of the health service. Multidisciplinary or interdisciplinary care requires an encouraging and collaborative workplace culture among all employees of the health service, including each discipline in the team (Preston et al 2018). Changes in a negative workplace culture can occur from an increase in respectful and trusting relationships among all staff. This can produce a workplace with expectations of collaborative multidisciplinary care.

In small groups, consider how to consistently achieve positive interdisciplinary relationships within multidisciplinary teams.

- Suggest how to ensure positive collaboration when relating to uncooperative colleagues.
- Suggest how to ensure positive collaboration in time-limited, pressured interactions with other health professionals.

With the entire group, share and discuss the answers to the above questions.

Multidisciplinary communication, collaboration and care require an affirming, collaborative workplace culture; one that encourages acceptance of diversity and collaboration with all employees of the health service, including every represented discipline, in the team (Preston et al 2018). A positive change in workplace culture may require consideration and adjustment of relevant procedures for each team member. Workplace culture should encourage all individuals to succeed with a strong sense of self-efficacy. Self-efficacy is a belief and confidence in the ability of an individual to provide effective care for each Person/s, relevant to their profession; that is, to succeed in the required role (Dickson & Peelo-Kilroe 2021; Williams et al. 2017). This enables effective interpersonal relationships and thus communication, thereby ensuring a sense of self-worth, resulting in effective care. In some situations, positive cultural change has the potential to reduce hospital admissions, re-admission after a short period post-discharge and thus costs of health services. A positive and encouraging workplace culture can provide safe care, increase Person/s satisfaction, while also achieving Person/Family-centred Care.

Consider times when you have worked with other people.

- List what you found challenging.
- How did **you** contribute to these challenges?

Draw a table with three columns and three headings: Challenge; My contribution; Overcome by:

1. Identify the challenge.
2. State the effect of your responses to the challenges, whether positive or negative.
3. Indicate how you overcame or how you might have overcome the challenge. Keep your table for discussion with other members of the group about overcoming challenges.

Challenges of multidisciplinary communication, collaboration and care

There are various challenges that affect teams with multiple disciplines. Some have been implied in the above discussion. Certainly time pressures, in combination with limited resources, have the potential to reduce motivation to interact in multidisciplinary communication. The challenge of limited motivation, and sometimes discomfort when relating to other healthcare professionals, requires a determined effort to integrate all team members into communicating about and developing care for the Person/s.

In small groups, from the previous individual reflection, consider the listed challenges. Choose one challenge from each group member and discuss ways to overcome each of the chosen challenges.

- Identify the strength and limitation of each suggested method for overcoming each challenge.
- Suggest alternative methods of overcoming each challenge.

Share and discuss one effective method of overcoming a difficult challenge with everyone in the session.

One important requirement mentioned above is the need for all team members to understand the role of the other people in the team (Boggs 2023; Franz et al 2020; McInerney et al 2022; Olvera et al 2020; Paxino et al 2022; Reed et al 2021; Stadick 2020). This understanding enables team members to refer the Person/s to the relevant team member for appropriate care. Limited exposure to a particular health discipline and thus to the focus, knowledge and skills of individuals from that discipline, will affect the interactions and communication with those particular individuals. While challenging, this indicates the importance of exploring the role and expertise of all represented health disciplines in the team.

A negative attitude to a particular healthcare professional may arise from limited experience of that discipline or perhaps a previous negative experience with a member of that discipline, or sometimes the reputation of another member of that discipline (Mulholland et al 2020). It may also relate to the current culture of the particular health service and possibly related policies and/or procedures (Bashatah et al 2020). In addition, limited efforts to understand particular disciplines can result in an overlapping of aspects of roles in some disciplines and therefore a waste of time for those disciplines. This requires negotiation to ensure each discipline performs their role without overlapping, to avoid duplication of assessments or interventions (Martin et al 2023).

The limited understanding of other disciplines is increased by the tendency to train healthcare professionals separately. This typically results in a limited understanding of discipline-specific roles, terminology and often associated abbreviations (Mulholland et al 2020). This discipline-specific language and associated roles contribute to the identity of each individual discipline, often being an important aspect of the identities of the discipline. However, understanding each discipline (both their language and their expertise) is essential for effective multidisciplinary communication, collaboration and resultant care (Reed et al 2021). This suggests the need for interprofessional education (Filho et al 2023), or at least regular multidisciplinary experiences during training. This training also produces different styles of communication (Foronda et al 2016). This has the potential to limit effective communication, often creating frustration and limiting trust between team members.

Sandra is a member of a multidisciplinary team dedicated to Person-centred Care and appropriate outcomes within an acute care ward of a hospital. She often does not complete all the tasks related to her particular profession. In fact, she is often seen many times a day smoking outside, rather than fulfilling the requirements of the role of her profession and her position (head of her discipline, managing two other healthcare professionals of that discipline) in the team.

Consider the different ways of responding and how to respond in a Person-centred manner to this colleague when you are a team member from the same health profession who often has to complete tasks Sandra was expected to perform.

- How would you relate to Sandra?
- How would you manage her behaviour?

List the possible ways of relating and managing her behaviour when you are team leader who has recently been assessing team members in a review process. This requires consideration of the behaviour of team members. This consideration identifies that Sandra is the only team member not fulfilling the expectations of her role and position in the team.

- How will you address this issue?
- How will you manage the effect of her behaviour on other team members?

Multidisciplinary communication and teamwork requires respectful and trusting relationships within the team. This can be difficult if some team members experience difficulties working with other people (Stadick 2020). Where there is such a difficulty, it is important to invest time into developing respectful and trusting relationships within the team. This will also positively affect the work culture and the effectiveness of multidisciplinary communication. Regular team meetings or case conferences are essential to discuss the needs and desires of the Person/s (Dickson & Peelo-Kilroe 2021). This requires a regular dedicated time and the attendance of all team members. This will also require preparation for the discussion of each Person/s during the meeting. This may be challenging in the time-pressured environment of healthcare. However, such meetings have the potential to increase team cohesion and understanding of each other and the roles. Regular informal exchange of information can also assist in the sharing of recent, relevant information. This will potentially affect the actions of team members between case conferences and therefore the resultant care.

Multidisciplinary communication, collaboration and resultant care requires access to technology and reliable staff to support the use of the technology. The increase in the use of electronic medical records and the improvement in the electronic interface, contributes to effective communication among all team members. Electronic medical records allow all team members to share information about the Person/s. They can read the entries of each team member, thereby potentially increase their understanding of the role and purpose of the interventions. This will enable a definite benefit: the provision of integrated and appropriate care by all team members

(Barnard et al 2020). However, this can be challenging if there is no technical support or if there is limited support affecting the reliability of the interface and the ability to use the interface. It also requires regular upgrades of devices and software, not always automatic without appropriate support staff. This requires willingness of the health service to fund these upgrades, which may be challenging.

Electronic records: points to remember

Many health services use electronic forms of notes, records and files (databases) for recording information about the Person/s. It is important that each healthcare professional learns and conforms to the expectations and requirements of the health service regarding electronic records (see Chapter 22). It is also important to remember the principles for recording information presented in Chapter 22. Confidentiality of information entered into an electronic database is also essential (see Chapter 19). Leaving Person/s information on the computer screen while interacting with others, regardless of your location, is inappropriate and does not conform to confidentiality requirements. Discussing Person/s-related information or assessment results with anyone, without the consent of the Person/s, is also inappropriate and potentially dangerous for the healthcare professional and the Person/s.

Another potential challenge relating to multidisciplinary care is the attitude and expectation of employers (often those funding the service) and sometimes colleagues. Limited understanding and experience of multidisciplinary teamwork in healthcare, along with the role and effect of multidisciplinary teamwork, can reduce the support and agreement to encourage such care by employers. Unfortunately, this can result in limited motivation to promote or encourage multidisciplinary care. Organisational guidelines and policy, typically created by employers, and procedures, often created by leaders of a profession, can also contribute to limited encouragement for teamwork despite the abilities and willingness of any healthcare professionals to contribute to multidisciplinary care (Mulholland et al 2020). This challenge can be increased by a limited understanding of the benefits to the health service of multidisciplinary care. The policies of a health service may affect the work culture, sometimes restricting team members and reducing ability to provide appropriate care. This indicates the possible impact of leadership upon the work culture (Paxino et al 2022).

Mistimed communication or failure to report particular information, limited preparation for team meetings or irregular team meetings, can also be challenging in a multidisciplinary team. This may produce conflict among team members. Any conflict will affect team efficiency and willingness to honestly discuss any opinions about the Person/s, while also eroding the trust amongst team members. This can be difficult to manage. However, in order to ensure effective communication it is essential to resolve any causes of miscommunication and reasons for conflict.

In groups, consider the challenges identified and discussed in the above text. Choose two from the list and discuss possible ways to overcome both of the chosen challenges.

- Consider the role of your discipline and associated pressure to ensure safe care.
- Suggest at least two methods of overcoming each of the chosen challenges.

Share and discuss your suggested method of overcoming the chosen challenges with the large group.

Overcoming challenges relating to multidisciplinary communication, collaboration and care

The previous discussion contained suggestions relating to methods of overcoming the challenges of achieving effective multidisciplinary communication, collaboration and care. However, an essential and initial method of overcoming some of the challenges is that of acknowledging, understanding, respecting and accepting the role difference and the particular focus of each healthcare professional. This will contribute to the development of respectful and trusting relationships among all team members. Development of these relationships may require activities to develop cohesion and trust within the team. These activities, while using valuable time, will develop the required trusting relationships to ensure effective communication, collaboration and appropriate care from all members of the multidisciplinary team. This can be challenging in a time-pressured environment. However, investing time to develop this trust produces positive results, encouraging acceptance of diversity, thereby affecting communication, collaboration and resultant care. Development of an understanding of the values of the team is usually required to provide appropriate and effective care and to demonstrate the required characteristics of the team. These characteristics, of a respectful, trusting, validating and collaborative team, will improve the quality of care and the relationships with the Person/s (Lynch et al 2021; Paxino et al 2022; Stadick 2020).

As mentioned above, training of all health service stakeholders about the benefits of multidisciplinary teams is often lacking. Understanding the role, expertise and thus capabilities of each team member is important for all employees of a health service. This often requires training (Machin et al 2019; Mulholland et al 2020; Preston et al 2018; Reed et al 2021) and promotion of the expertise of each discipline in the team to promote understanding among employees of and Person/s using the service. This training can increase understanding of the benefits of multidisciplinary teams. It can also begin the process of changing the culture of the service to encourage the establishment of multidisciplinary teams (James et al 2018). Such integration increases the trust among team members, while also producing an awareness of the benefits of the contribution of each member of the team. This then results in more equitable and sustainable care for each Person/s, and therefore the overall quality of their care (James et al 2018).

An essential requirement to overcome the challenges of multidisciplinary care is the creation of appropriate practices and often protocols to guide the integration of each team member into the team and the use of multidisciplinary teams (Mulholland et al 2020; Preston et al 2018). Development of such protocols; for example, how to accommodate and integrate the different roles of each team member, including the expectations relating to the contribution and requirements of each team member, will increase the possibility of each team member being both confident and able to contribute to the multidisciplinary care for any Person/s. Creating the protocols will require contributions from all represented disciplines. The development of such protocols may be complex, because of the complexity of the situation and environment. However, collaborating with relevant healthcare professionals could enhance all future interactions, thereby benefiting the quality of care for all Person/s. The process may require training to recognise and appreciate the abilities of each team member and the realities of teamwork. The creation of appropriate protocols has the potential to develop a connection, collaboration and trust between team members, producing a cohesive and effective multidisciplinary team. The resultant cohesion from this connection and collaboration potentially improves both the quality of care and the satisfaction of the Person/s (Carter et al 2021; Walton et al 2020). This collaboration encourages interdisciplinary support from colleagues in the team when experiencing challenging events in daily practice (Cameron et al 2021), a beneficial aspect for all multidisciplinary team members.

In small groups, choose and discuss one of the suggested methods of overcoming the chosen challenge.

- Consider the strengths of the suggested method.
- Consider the possible limiting factors affecting the suggested method.
- Suggest other possible methods of overcoming the chosen challenge.

Share and discuss other possible methods of overcoming one challenge with the large group.

Chapter summary

The occurrence of multidisciplinary teams is common in many health services. There is a global recognition of the importance and effectiveness in healthcare of multidisciplinary teams. This mandates consideration of aspects of multidisciplinary communication and resultant collaboration in achieving effective, safe and quality care. There has been documentation and publications about the benefits of multidisciplinary communication, collaboration and resultant care. These teams increase the provision of effective, continuous and equitable care, thereby increasing overall satisfaction with healthcare. They empower team members to provide safe and quality care and the Person/s to achieve their desires and fulfil their needs, thereby improving their health and wellbeing. Multidisciplinary teams support ethical decision-making and the development of confidence and self-efficacy in team members.

Multidisciplinary communication and collaboration requires clear understanding of the role and focus of each team member to ensure relevant and appropriate care and to avoid overlapping or repeating care. This understanding contributes to the essential development of respectful and trusting relationships within multidisciplinary teams. Multidisciplinary communication, collaboration and care also requires relevant technology and staff to support the use of technology. It also requires the support of service managers, policymakers and team leaders to ensure a healthy work culture, appropriate and collaborative team relationships and quality care. The underlying requirements of effective multidisciplinary teams are the components of the model of Person/Family-centred Care. There are various challenges related to the realities of healthcare from multidisciplinary teams. The most important of these is respectful and trusting relationships between team members. Overcoming the challenges related to multidisciplinary teams requires particular attitudes and behaviour, based upon commitment and understanding from all employees of every health service in order to manage the complexity of the realities of healthcare in the twenty-first century.

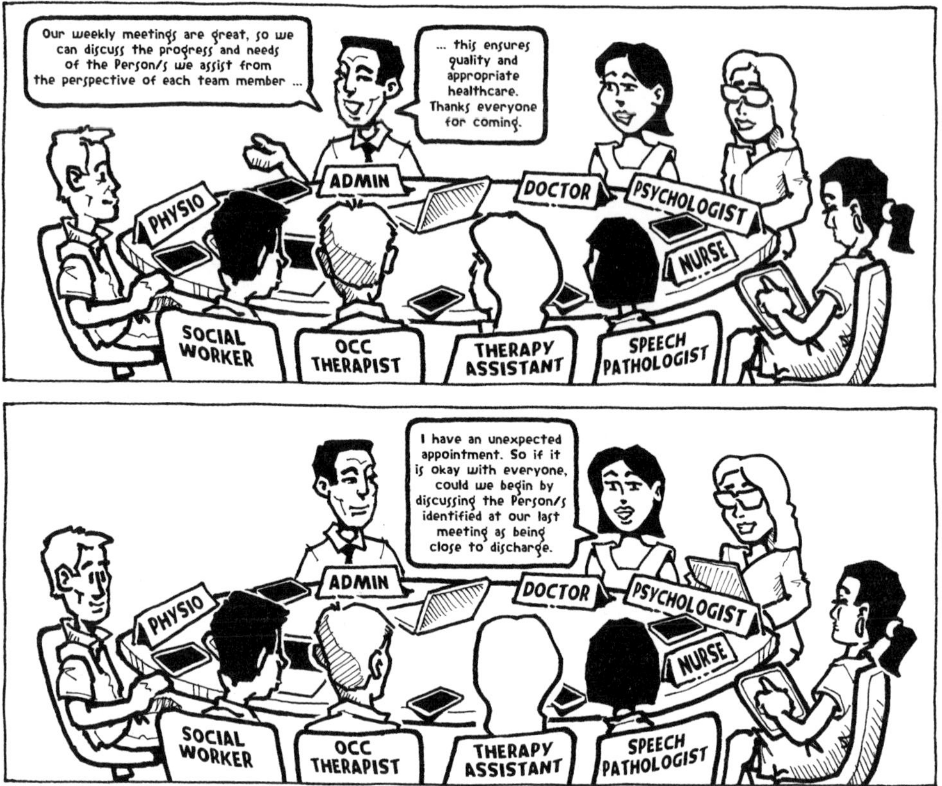

Figure 14.1
Multidisciplinary communication ensures quality care and appropriate outcomes.
Courtesy Roger Harvey © Elsevier Australia.

REVIEW QUESTIONS

1. Define a multidisciplinary team.

2. Locate (provide the relevant link) and summarise the registration requirements relating to multidisciplinary team communication and collaboration for your discipline.

____

____

____

Link – http:// ______________________________

3. List four realities of multidisciplinary teams.

   i. ______________________________

   ii. ______________________________

   iii. ______________________________

   iv. ______________________________

4. State four benefits of multidisciplinary teams in healthcare.

   i. ______________________________

   ii. ______________________________

   iii. ______________________________

   iv. ______________________________

5. Identify and explain three requirements of multidisciplinary teams.

   i. ______________________________

   ii. ______________________________

   iii. ______________________________

6. Outline three major challenges relating to communication in multidisciplinary teams.

   i. ______________________________

   ii. ______________________________

   iii. ______________________________

7. Outline how to overcome the three chosen challenges for multidisciplinary teams.

   i. ______________________________

   ii. ______________________________

   iii. ______________________________

References

Australian Health Practitioners Regulation Authority (AHPRA) & National Boards, 2022. Code of conduct. AHPRA & National Boards, Sydney.

Barnard, R., Jones, J., Cruice, M., 2020. Communication between therapists and nurses working in inpatient interprofessional teams: Systematic review and meta-ethnography. Disability and Rehabilitation, 42(10), 1339–1349.

Bashatah, A.S., Al-Ahmary, K.A., Arifi, M.A., et al., 2020. Interprofessional cooperation: An interventional study among Saudi healthcare teaching staff at Kind Saud university. Journal of Multidisciplinary Healthcare, 13, 1537–1544.

Bereznicki, B.J., Caruso, V., Errey, J.A., et al., 2021. Interprofessional education for pre-clinical medicine, paramedicine and pharmacy students. Medical Education, 55(5), 643.

Boggs, K., 2023. Interpersonal relationships: Professional communication skills for nurses, 9th ed. Elsevier, St Louis, MO.

Cameron, C., Lunn, T.M., Lanos, C., et al., 2021. Dealing with dying – progressing paramedics' role in grief support. Progress in Palliative Care, 29(2), 91–97.

Carter, A.J.E., Arab, M., Cameron, C., et al., 2021. A national collaborative to spread and scale paramedics providing palliative care in Canada: Breaking down silos is essential to success. Progress in Palliative Care, 29(2), 59–65.

Clark, P.G., 2014. Narrative in interprofessional education and practice: Implications for professional identity, provider-patient communication and teamwork. Journal of Interprofessional Care, 28(1), 34e39.

Cruz, L.C., Fine, J.S., Nori, S., 2017. Barriers to discharge from inpatient rehabilitation: A teamwork approach. International Journal of Health Care Quality Assurance, 30(2), 137–147.

Dickson, C., Peelo-Kilroe, L., 2021. Being person-centred in community and ambulatory services. In: McCormack, B., McCance, T., Bulley, C. et al., (eds). Fundamentals of Person-centred health practice. Wiley-Blackwell, London.

Filho, J.R.F., Fernandes, M.N.F., Gilbert, J.H.V., 2023. The development of interprofessional education and collaborative practice in Latin America and the Caribbean: Preliminary observations. Journal of Interprofessional Care, 37(1), 168– 72.

Fink-Samnick, E., 2019. Leveraging interprofessional team-based care toward case management excellence: Part 1, history, fundamentals, evidence. Professional Case Management, 24(3), 130–141.

Fischer-Grönlund, C., Brännström, M., Zingmark, K., 2021. The "one to five" method – A tool for ethical communication in groups among healthcare professionals. Nurse Education in Practice, 51(2021), 102998.

Flanagan, E., Chadwick, R., Goodrich, J., et al., 2020. Reflection for all healthcare staff: A national evaluation of Schwartz Rounds. Journal of Interprofessional Care, 31(1), 140–142.

Foronda, C., MacWilliams, B., McArthur, E., 2016. Interprofessional communication in healthcare: An integrative review. Nurse Education in Practice, 19, 36–40.

Franz, S., Muser, J., Thielhorn, U., et al., 2020. Inter-professional communication and interaction in the neurological rehabilitation team: A literature review. Disability and Rehabilitation, 42(11), 1607–1615.

Health and Care Professions Council, 2016. Standards of conduct, performance and ethics UK, Health and Care Professions Council, London.

Hustoft, M., Biringer, E., Gjesdal, S., et al., 2018. Relational coordination in interprofessional teams and its effect on patient-reported benefit and continuity of care: A prospective cohort study from rehabilitation centres in Western Norway. BMC Health Services Research, 18(1), 719.

Hustoft, M., Biringer, E., Gjesdal, S., et al., 2019. The effect of team collaboration and continuity of care on health and disability among rehabilitation patients: A longitudinal survey-based study from western Norway. Quality of Life Research, 28(10), 2773–2785.

James, K., Jones, D., Kempenaar, L., et al., 2018. Occupational therapists in emergency departments: A qualitative study. British Journal of Occupational Therapy, 81(3), 154–161.

Liu, H-Y., 2021. The relationship between swift trust and interaction behaviors on interdisciplinary and non-interdisciplinary teams in nursing education. Nurse Education in Practice, 51, 102977.

Lynch, B., Barron, D., McKinlay, L., 2021. Connecting with others. In: McCormack, B., McCance, T., Bulley, C. et al., (eds). Fundamentals of Person-centred health practice. Wiley-Blackwell, London.

Machin, L.L., Bellis, K.M. Dixon, C., et al., 2019. Interprofessional education and practice guide: Designing ethics-oriented interprofessional education for health and social care students. Journal of Interprofessional Care, 33(6), 608–618.

Martin, A.K., Green, T.L., McCarthy, A.L., et al., 2023. Allied health transdisciplinary models of care in hospital settings: A scoping review. Journal of Interprofessional Care, 37(1), 118–130.

McInerney, J., Seedhouse, D., Pettit, M., et al., 2022. Interdisciplinary interprofessional education using an online learning environment called values exchange: A qualitative investigation. Journal of Medical Radiation Sciences, 69, 309–317.

Mulholland, P., Barnett, T., Woodroffe, J., 2020. A grounded theory of interprofessional learning and paramedic care. Journal of Interprofessional Care, 34(1), 66–75.

Nsiah, C., Siakwa, M., Ninnoni, J.P.K., 2020. Barriers to practicing patient advocacy in healthcare setting. Nursing Open, 7(2), 650–659.

Olvera, L., Smith, J.S., Prater, L., et al., 2020. Interprofessional communication and collaboration during emergent birth center transfers: A Quality Improvement Project. Journal of Midwifery and Women's Health, 65(3), 555–561.

Paxino, J., Denniston, C., Woodward-Kron, R., et al., 2022. Communication in interprofessional rehabilitation teams: A scoping review. Disability and Rehabilitation, 44(13), 3253–3269.

Preston, J., Galloway, M., Wilson, R., et al., 2018. Occupational therapists and paramedics form a mutually beneficial alliance to reduce the pressure on hospitals: A practice analysis. British Journal of Occupational Therapy, 81(6), 358–362.

Reed, K., Reed, B., Bailey, J., et al., 2021. Interprofessional education in the rural environment to enhance multidisciplinary care in future practice: Breaking down silos in tertiary health education. Australian Journal of Rural Health, 29, 127–136.

Schot, E., Tummers, L., Noordegraaf, M., 2020. Working on working together. A systematic review on how healthcare professionals contribute to interprofessional collaboration. Journal of Interprofessional Care, 34(3), 332–342.

Showstark, M., Joostem-Hagye, D., Wiss, A., et al., 2023. Results and lessons learned from a virtual multi-institutional problem-based interprofessional learning approach: The VIPE program. Journal of Interprofessional Care, 37(1), 164–167.

Slaghmuylder, Y., Pype, P., Van Hecke, A., et al., 2022. Exploring healthcare providers' perceptions of the prevention and treatment of chronic pain in breast cancer survivors: A qualitative analysis among different disciplines. PLos ONE, 17(8), e0273576.

Stadick, J.L. 2020. Understanding health care professionals' attitudes towards working in teams and interprofessional collaborative competencies: A mixed methods analysis. Journal of Interprofessional Education and Practice, 21, 100370.

Vrijmoeth, T., Wassenaar, A., Koopmans, R.T.C.M., et al., 2022. Generalist-specialist collaboration in primary care for frail older persons: A promising model for the future. Journal of the American Medical Directors Association, 23(2), 288–296.

Walton, V., Hogden, A., Long, J.C. et al., 2020. Clinicians' perceptions of rounding processes and effectiveness of clinical communication. Journal of Evaluation in Clinical Practice, 26(3), 801–811.

Will, K.K., Johnson, M.L., & Lamb, G., 2019. Team-based care and patient satisfaction in the hospital setting: a systematic review. Journal of Patient-Centered Research and Reviews, 6(2), 158–171.

Williams, A., Martin, S., Coates, V., 2021. Being person-centred when working with people living with long-term conditions. In: McCormack, B., McCance, T., Bulley, C. et al. (eds). Fundamentals of Person-centred Health Practice. Wiley-Blackwell, London.

Williams, B., Beovich, B., Ross, L., et al., 2017. Self-efficacy perceptions of interprofessional education and practice in undergraduate healthcare students. Journal of Interprofessional Care, 31(3), 335–341.

World Health Organization (WHO), 2010. Framework for action on interprofessional education and collaborative practice. WHO, Geneva. Online. Available at: iris.who.int/handle/10665/70185

World Health Organization (WHO), 2016. Framework on integrated, people-centred health services. Report by the World Health Assembly A69/35. WHO, Geneva. Online. Available at: iris.who.int/handle/10665/252698

CHAPTER 15

Managing conflict when communicating as a healthcare professional

Chapter objectives

Upon completing this chapter, readers should be able to:

- recognise the mutual benefits of communicating calmly and appropriately during conflict
- identify the usual causes of conflict
- understand the importance of identifying emotions during conflict
- discuss the different responses to conflict
- reflect upon the management of bullying
- outline the characteristics of assertive communication
- demonstrate ways of communicating assertively in difficult situations.

Most communicative interactions are relatively straightforward and, although they may require concentration and energy, do not present major challenges or difficulties. However, wherever people interact, difficulties in communication are inevitable. These difficulties can include **conflict** (Bowe et al 2014; Devito 2021; Levine 2012). Conflict involves a disagreement or clash between people. Such disagreements can be common in healthcare (Moss 2020). Such communicative interactions are not only difficult, but are also potentially unpleasant. It is beneficial for healthcare professionals to develop understanding of and skills in managing conflict – both to achieve effective communication and to develop skills and confidence when communicating (Almost et al 2010; Moss 2020). It is advantageous if healthcare professionals feel confident and skilled at calmly and appropriately resolving conflict for the mutual benefit of themselves and the vulnerable Person/s.

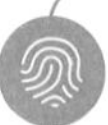

How do you feel about:

- disagreeing with someone?
- presenting a point of view that is different to a popular view?
- saying *no* to a request?
- discussing an emotionally charged topic?

Consider your answers to these questions. Your answers indicate the reality of how you face potentially difficult situations involving conflict.

Conflict during communication

Causes of conflict

Conflict while communicating can involve:

- disagreement about provision and understanding of information, reasons for decisions, supervisory feedback (Weissman et al 2010)
- differences in ideas, principles or even in people (Weissman et al 2010)
- differences in ideas about the way to organise things (Stein-Parbury 2021)
- different understanding of the same words (Purtilo et al 2014)
- different perceptions of the relative value of certain procedures (Holli & Beto 2023; Weissman et al 2010)
- the importance or order of priority of particular tasks (Weissman et al 2010)
- not understanding expectations (Eckermann et al 2010)
- differences in opinions about procedures or individuals (Henderson 2019).

These are some of the differences that potentially result in conflict and thus a difficult communicative interaction. Conflict may occur between the healthcare professional and the Person/s, but it may also occur between the healthcare professional and their colleagues (Almost et al 2010). Conflict in itself does not cause difficulty; it may facilitate positive change (Moss 2020). The management of conflict produces negative or positive results (Rakos 2018). This includes identifying the emotions contributing to the responses causing the conflict (Honeycutt & Milliken 2021). Gaining positive results from conflict situations requires self-control, typically resulting from self-awareness (Devito 2021; Thompson 2012). Such control increases the potential for validation of the emotions (Egan & Reese 2019), along with appropriate responses rather than irrational and often negative reactions (Fedoruk 2014).

Identify possible causes of conflict by discussing how the following affect communication during conflict:

- How could an understanding of your blocks to listening and barriers to emotions (see Chapter 11) assist communication during conflict? How could this understanding contribute to changing the way you communicate during conflict?
- Consider the following reasons:
  - The need to always be right.
  - The need to appear knowledgeable and/or competent.
  - The need to have control or the power in the situation

  - Being judgemental.
  - Feelings of insecurity.
- Will explicitly noting these tendencies in yourself or in others assist you to respond appropriately when communicating in difficult situations in the future? If you have these tendencies, will you need to do more than recognise them? That is, as a healthcare professional will you need to act to overcome these tendencies when communicating?

Identifying emotions during conflict

It is essential to understand how to communicate appropriately during conflict. It is therefore important to identify the severity of the emotions in all communicating parties during the conflict. This recognition will assist in deciding how to control or resolve the conflict. The severity of the emotions associated with the conflict may also indicate the effort and action required to resolve the conflict (Kassing 2011). If the emotion is simply one of uneasiness or awkwardness, it may not be too serious. The uneasiness may result from the unknown. The healthcare professional can alleviate this cause of uneasiness by providing clear and appropriate information, providing time for questions while providing the required information (Mathibe-Neke & Mondell 2018). The uneasiness may also originate from unrelated causes (e.g. tiredness, hunger or lateness). The healthcare professional asking a simple question to clarify the reason for the lack of ease may quickly resolve the awkwardness (e.g. *Are you feeling all right today?*). Alternatively, a statement to recognise (e.g. *You don't seem to be yourself today*), or to explain the discomfort (e.g. *I am sorry, I had to rush my son to emergency this morning!*) will assist in clarifying and potentially reducing the conflict in the situation.

Another emotion associated with conflict when communicating is irritation. Irritation or annoyance can occur before an interaction from waiting a long time to see the healthcare professional or during an interaction when the potential outcome of the interaction appears unsatisfactory to at least one of the people communicating. In this situation, the use of questions (e.g. *You seem irritated today – is there something upsetting you?*) or an "I" statement or question (e.g. *I feel irritated because you said you would be on time today and you were half an hour late again* or *Are you upset because of something I have done?*) can be powerful in highlighting and potentially resolving a difficult communicative event. Despite the use of "I", these responses focus on the problem. They can clarify the cause of the emotion and potentially resolve the irritation in the Person/s.

Another result of difficult communicative interactions can be misunderstandings (see Chapter 18). A misunderstanding occurs when there is a failure to understand or correctly interpret the meaning of words, ideas, intentions, associated feelings, non-verbal behaviours or actions. This may occur because of different ways of understanding and resolving conflict in different cultures (Eckermann et al 2010; Paternotte et al 2015). Such situations can cause confusion, dissatisfaction and discouragement in all communicating parties. The failure in understanding is not always easy to resolve if there were associated emotional responses. However, if one party feels misunderstood, it is possible the other communicating individuals will also feel misunderstood. Honestly acknowledging the misunderstanding, admitting any mistake and apologising is a powerful course of action with potential to resolve the conflict. This action often allows the other Person/s, if they choose, to apologise and say it is all right. Remembering that the healthcare professional is in control of their emotional responses, and can choose what they will feel and how to respond, is important in such circumstances (Drick 2012; Moss 2020).

Choosing to ignore

Expressions of negative emotions may cause discomfort for those present in the room. This reality means it is important to identify the cause and purpose of such emotional expression. Recognising the reason for the passionate expression of any negative emotion may assist the healthcare professional to determine and perhaps adjust their response. In these situations it is important to assess whether ignoring the emotional expression is the appropriate response. Sometimes an individual simply needs to express their emotions with a minimal response from another individual. It is important to attempt to assess the situation, remembering that it may be difficult to evaluate and calmly *respond* rather than reacting emotionally. One response might be to unobtrusively leave the room closing the door to promote privacy. Alternatively, the healthcare professional might remain quietly in the room until the Person/s has finished expressing the emotion. Whether or not the healthcare professional chooses to ignore the negative emotions in situations similar to these, it is best for healthcare professionals to remain calm, while avoiding a negative emotional reaction (Tregoning 2015) In addition, the healthcare professional should not absorb blame if they are *not* responsible. In contrast, however, taking responsibility if they are the cause of the emotional expression is appropriate and will potentially assist in resolving the conflict. Regardless of the cause, responding calmly and appropriately to expressions of emotion will assist the Person/s, thereby potentially achieving resolution of the situation.

Resolving negative attitudes and emotions towards another

Sometimes negative attitudes, emotions and related prejudice towards another can cause constant stress when thinking about or communicating with that individual. Such responses may occur between the healthcare professional and the Person/s, but they can also occur among colleagues. The opinion creating this stress may seem justified because of the attitudes or actions of the Person/s. However, for the healthcare professional it will be a source of constant strain. This strain could negatively affect every working relationship connected with that Person/s, and would certainly affect the thoughts and ultimately attitudes of the stressed healthcare professional (Brinkert 2010). In order to avoid habitual unproductive ways of relating to that Person/s, it is important to quickly resolve such emotions (see Chapters 6 and 7).

Unresolved stress in a relationship can result in a breakdown in both communication and the relationship. Thus changing the attitude and resolving associated negative emotions creating the stress is important. Recognition of the source of the attitude of the healthcare professional can assist in resolving the negative emotions associated with the other Person/s (see Chapters 6, 7 and 8). Investment of time to understand the Person/s and the factors producing a negative response in the healthcare professional can promote a positive attitude, assisting the healthcare professional to relate in a positive manner (Thompson 2012). It is important to remember to connect with and attend to the Person, not the emotions of the healthcare professional (Drick 2012). A focus on the positive attributes of the Person/s, as well as similarities shared in experiences or values, can also assist in changing a negative attitude. Appropriate management of conflict situations is essential in the healthcare professions, requiring self-awareness, self-control, preparation and commitment to resolution of unresolved negative emotions on the part of the healthcare professional (Henderson 2019; Tregoning 2015).

What is your natural tendency or usual way of responding?

- Do you avoid conflict at all costs by remaining silent and saying nothing?
- Do you remove yourself from conflict as quickly as you can?
- Do you do anything to appease the person and stop the conflict?
- Do you retaliate and fight to win?
- Do you defend the attacked opinion, idea or person?
- Do you become involved in the expressed emotion?
- Do you think negatively about a person and avoid that person wherever possible?
- Do you find a way of compromising to resolve the conflict?

Which of these reactions promotes feelings of satisfaction for everyone? If your natural tendency promotes a feeling of "losing" or "winning" in an interaction, how might you change this tendency to protect your rights and the rights of the Person/s?

Patterns of relating during conflict

There are always underlying requirements guiding communicative interactions in the healthcare professions, whether or not the interactions involve conflict. During any type of communication, but particularly during conflict, it is important to focus on the needs of the Person/s. Remember that they have a right to feel and to express their differences of opinion or their emotions (Thompson 2021). However, they do not have a right to "abuse" another person, regardless of the strength of their emotions. Respect for and protection of the rights of self and the Person/s, as well as the need for Person/Family-centred Care and goals must guide all communicative responses during conflict (Delaney 2018; Haddad et al 2018; Harms & Pierce 2019; see Chapter 2). Understanding the difference between aggressive, passive and assertive responses assists healthcare professionals to protect their own rights and the rights of others while achieving positive results during conflict. Awareness of these differences empowers healthcare professionals to develop the skill of responding appropriately using assertiveness, rather than reacting with a fight or flight reaction. Skills in assertiveness assist in the confident and constructive management of conflict situations.

Passive

The individual who relates passively during conflict does not express their perceptions, ideas or opinions. The belief that they do not have the right to express or feel anything can be the basis of this response. A belief, often because of past experiences, that there is no point in expressing their thoughts as no-one will listen, might also contribute to a **passive** reaction. Limited confidence, self-esteem and self-respect produce passive responses. It is interesting to note that encountering regular and repeated passive responses from an individual may negatively affect the confidence, self-esteem or self-respect of the receiver or communicative partner. As a result, this communicative partner may eventually relate passively in many communicative events due to decreased confidence, self-esteem and self-respect.

Aggressive

The individual with an aggressive pattern of relating during conflict expresses their perceptions, opinions and feelings in a manner that intimidates or attacks other communicating individuals.

Their **aggressive communication** manner expresses the desire to be right and make everyone else agree with them, thus indicating they are right; or it expresses a desire to achieve what they want regardless of the feelings of others. Aggression expresses the desire to "win". This manner precipitates various reactions in listeners: fight (aggression – *I will win this*) or flight (escape from the uncomfortable situation and emotions) or fear/freeze (afraid to move for fear of consequences).

Passive-aggressive

It is possible for individuals to express a combination of passivity and aggression. This typically involves the individual fluctuating between these two ways of relating. Their manner of relating will depend upon the context and the events preceding a particular interaction. Individuals expressing a **passive-aggressive** response may avoid relating to specific people (people they perceive are responsible for the conflict they experience because of negative emotion). However, if their responsibilities require interactions with that specific person, they may express aggression and/or passivity depending on the previous events. In such cases, the person expressing passive aggression rarely discusses the reason for their responses with the responsible individual. For example, say student A is *not* allocated to a placement site, which they state they listed as a preference. However, another student (B), who did not list that placement site as a preference receives that site. Student A does not discuss their perception of the allocation process with the appropriate individual. They instead exhibit passive-aggressive responses whenever in class, by disengaging from class activities and consistently using their computer or mobile phone. If asked a question about the content of the class, they either ignore the question (pretending not to hear) or respond using aggressive body language and tone of voice. A focused, caring discussion, attempting to identify the cause of these unusual responses, reveals their anger and frustration and the related cause. Discussing and identifying the cause may contribute to resolving the emotions. If action is required to assist in resolving the cause, perhaps an apology or, where possible, a change in a system, may contribute to a permanent resolution of the contributing emotions. If there is limited possibility of addressing the cause, the discussion and awareness of "genuinely being heard" may assist the individual to manage the emotions causing the passive-aggressive responses.

Assertive

The *assertive* individual expresses their perceptions, ideas or opinions in a manner that respects the worth and rights of others to have and express perceptions, ideas or opinions, while controlling any negative emotions (Beesley et al 2018). **Assertive communication** affirms the interests and rights of the self and the other (Craig & Banja 2010). It facilitates positive collaborative communication outcomes, strengthening relationships (Devito 2021; Moisoglou et al 2014; Rakos 2018). It is therefore the preferred manner of responding during difficult communicative interactions (Alberti & Emmons 2017). An assertive healthcare professional ensures they have heard without dominating or withdrawing. They seek to resolve the conflict in order to improve relationships, interactions and ultimately healthcare (Rosenstein et al 2014).

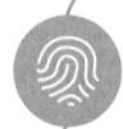

Create assertive ways of responding to the following:

- You are angry because a colleague promised to assist you with something (e.g. cleaning the storeroom) and instead they read research articles all day.
- You are struggling with a task and a colleague is watching you struggle without attempting to assist you.

- You have one day of leave promised, and now, without explanation, the decision has been reversed and you have heard that someone else has leave that day instead of you.
- A person is yelling and swearing at you and you have no idea of the cause of their emotional expression.
- A Person seeking your assistance appears preoccupied and is not listening to you.

In groups of no more than four:

- Discuss possible assertive responses to three of the above situations. Decide if there might be any other ways of managing the situation.
- Share the ideas of the group with the large group.

Bullying

When practising as a healthcare professional it is possible to experience or observe bullying (Henderson 2019). Bullying is a particular pattern of relating, otherwise known as harassment. An individual who bullies consciously seeks to demean or devalue another individual (Stein-Parbury 2021).

Healthcare professionals may bully each other or bully the Person/s. In addition, family members may bully the Person/s receiving the intervention. It is uncomfortable to experience or to observe bullying. It is one form of conflict within the workplace that creates feelings of intimidation. It usually begins because of differences or ineffective communication, typically establishing an uncomfortable environment or atmosphere (Crossman et al 2011). It can negatively affect the motivation, health and wellbeing of particular individuals (Losey 2011; Rosenstein et al 2014; Ttofi 2011), as well as potentially affecting intervention outcomes. It can originate from insecurity in particular individuals, who may find communicative interactions difficult, compensating for these feelings by intimidating or threatening people who create uncomfortable feelings in them (Hayes 2011; Healey 2011).

Bullying typically includes negative verbal and non-verbal messages, which are difficult for everyone observing those messages. Bullying may take the form of repeatedly stating negative or threatening things to a person or about a person. These statements are usually designed to create a negative view of the person in an attempt to intimidate them or to destroy their reputation (Crossman et al 2011). Bullying may also include passive responses, including failure to respond ("the silent treatment"), ignoring requests or failing to follow instructions or communicate information. Bullying definitely includes attempts to threaten or intimidate, belittle, inappropriately question the abilities or skills of another and question the ability of an individual to perform a task (Hutchinson et al 2010). All of these patterns of relating produce conflict potentially between individuals, and definitely within the "victim". A healthcare service experiencing bullying can be depressing and very negative for everyone in the service.

This book is unable to explore the wide range of possible bullying scenarios or the many ways of managing these scenarios because of the many variations. However, most healthcare services have policies and procedures to manage bullying within the workplace. Some have a designated person to contact if there is bullying in the workplace. If experiencing bullying, it is important to avoid "gossiping" about the "bully" and instead seek the assistance of an experienced healthcare professional. Such assistance should encourage development of strategies to respond assertively and to manage the resultant feelings of injustice and misunderstanding. If observing bullying, it is equally important to discuss the situation with an appropriate, experienced person in order to avoid acceleration of the bullying and assist the relevant individuals to resolve the issues and cease the bullying behaviour. It is important that the person prone to bullying is given assistance to resolve the feelings that produce their bullying behaviour. Consideration and application of how to communicate assertively when experiencing bullying may assist; however, resolution of the resultant negative emotions is essential to ensure a positive atmosphere in the particular health-care service. See Chapter 23 for an exploration of cyberbullying (the use of electronic communication to harass a person, typically by sending messages of an intimidating or threatening nature).

Communicating assertively

The following points are suggestions of how to be assertive when communicating.

- Establish the cause/problem and focus on it, not the emotions.
- Remain calm and avoid responding in an emotional manner (Harms & Pierce 2019; Tregoning 2015).
- Avoid placating with *What's your problem? Calm down, you're OK.*
- State the facts about the situation; do not evaluate or judge (Devito 2021).
- Listen carefully, allowing the person to finish each sentence (McLean 2011).
- Use "I" statements (Archee & Gurney 2024).
- Take responsibility for your feelings and actions (Holli & Beto 2023).
- Be aware of your non-verbal behaviours; use a relaxed body position (McLean 2011).
- Use normal speed and tone of voice (Devito 2021).
- Avoid talking slowly because this may appear patronising.
- Observe carefully the non-verbal behaviours of the upset Person.
- State how the problem affects you, not how you feel about the situation.
- If appropriate, gently and calmly repeat a question or statement until the person hears and responds (e.g. *Shall we talk about how to solve this now?*). The timing of such questions is significant and may negatively or positively affect the situation (Rakos 2018).
- Emphasise collaboration, asking the Person/s to contribute their thoughts throughout the discussion (Palanisamy & Verville 2015; Rosenstein et al 2014).
- Be mindful of the perspective of the upset individual and characteristics of effective communication (Swain & Gale 2014).
- Seek achievable solutions requiring specific action within a particular specified timeframe.

Use the above points on communicating assertively while role-playing the following cases. It may assist if the players choose names for their roles.

During each role-play, have observers classify every statement or question according to whether the behaviour constitutes communicating assertively.

Role-play 1

Person 1: You are the supervisor of Person 2. You feel angry because Person 2 is always late in completing their work and it reflects badly on you.

Person 2: You do your best every day with limited assistance and do not really understand the problem. The work will be done, just maybe not on time.

Role-play 2

Person 1: You are a young healthcare professional seeing Person 2 for the first time. They have previously received assistance from your healthcare service, but the healthcare professional who saw them is no longer available. You sense they are disappointed and do not really want to see you.

Person 2: You are disappointed that you have to see the healthcare professional, Person 1, because you had a good relationship with the previous healthcare professional. You really do not want to see Person 1 because they seem too young and you are not sure you have the energy to develop a relationship with another healthcare professional; however, you do not want to hurt their feelings.

Role-play 3

Person 1: You are the supervisor of Person 2, a student who has been discussing confidential matters with students from other healthcare professions, in the dining hall. During their orientation you outlined confidentiality, ethical practice and legislation. You indicated what these meant in practice and asked questions to clarify their meaning.

Person 2: The needs of some of the people assigned to you are overwhelming and there has been no time to talk about this, except during lunch or after work.

Role-play 4

Person 1: You are a healthcare professional who feels Mrs Stathos can continue living in her home. You have consulted all the healthcare professionals assisting Mrs Stathos and intend to organise various supports (weekly home care and shopping, daily nurses for showering, meals on wheels) and attendance at a weekly program to maintain her in her home. Person 2 has requested an appointment with you, and you feel he disagrees with you. You intend to show him how Mrs Stathos can stay safely and independently at home.

Person 2: You are married to Mrs Stathos's daughter. You know how forgetful and dependent Mrs Stathos has become because your wife has been caring for her, often staying with her overnight. You are really angry that this young healthcare professional (Person 1) thinks they know what is best for ***your*** family; you think they have no idea. You intend to make sure Mrs Stathos is placed in residential care – not in a nursing home, but in a "village" with her own serviced unit.

Role-play 5

Person 1: You are a healthcare professional who has been assisting Terry, a young man with paraplegia. You have been working consistently with him and his motivation to walk again is maintaining his mood. You are furious with a new colleague (Person 2) because they have just told him it is unlikely he will walk again. You have experience with people like Terry, and in the past you have seen young men with worse damage than Terry walk (with assistive equipment, but walking independently of another person) against all medical odds. You feel this colleague is ignorant and should not have spoken to Terry about him walking in the future.

Person 2: You are new to the Spinal Injuries Department and heard the doctor say that Terry would probably not walk again. You feel it is important to be honest, so you tell Terry he will probably not walk again. You cannot understand why Person 1 is upset.

Chapter summary

It is important that the healthcare professional develops strategies and skills to manage conflict situations in a calm, effective and resolute manner. Recognition of the emotions causing the conflict begins the process of resolution. Perceptions of the emotions behind the conflict require validation through honest statements or questions relating to these perceptions. Validation of perceptions promotes a clearer understanding of the cause of the conflict in the individual expressing the emotion. It allows disengagement from the argument and a focus on possible resolution of the emotions and the problem. Questions asked with an appropriate tone of voice can diffuse the expression of strong emotions, for example, *You are obviously upset. Can you tell me about the problem?* Or *Do you want to tell me why you are shouting?* Such questions allow focus on solving the problem rather than on the emotions that are creating the argument or emotional behaviour.

Resolution of conflict in difficult situations is facilitated by acceptance of differences, compromise and assertive collaboration with a calm focus on problem-solving. It is important for the healthcare professional to develop confidence in managing interactions involving conflict. Such confidence develops with self-awareness, self-control, appropriate supervision and mentoring, specific instruction in conflict management, understanding of possible management strategies and, ultimately, experience.

In groups of no more than four:

- choose a scenario from Chapter 24, “Person/s experiencing strong negative emotions”.
- consider the provided information relevant to the chosen scenario.
- discuss appropriate strategies for managing these emotions for both the male and female scenario.
- suggest how to achieve a positive response while responding to the Person/s in the scenarios.
- assign a role (Person/s or healthcare professional) to two of the group members and role-play each scenario. The observing members of the group note the responses of the members role-playing and identify their type (aggressive, passive, passive-aggressive, assertive) and reaction (positive or negative).
- list appropriate and relevant responses to manage the conflict.

Running a little behind.
Be with you soon.
HELP ME!!

THIS
Wonder why he is so upset?
OR THIS
I can see you are angry.
What do you need?
!!

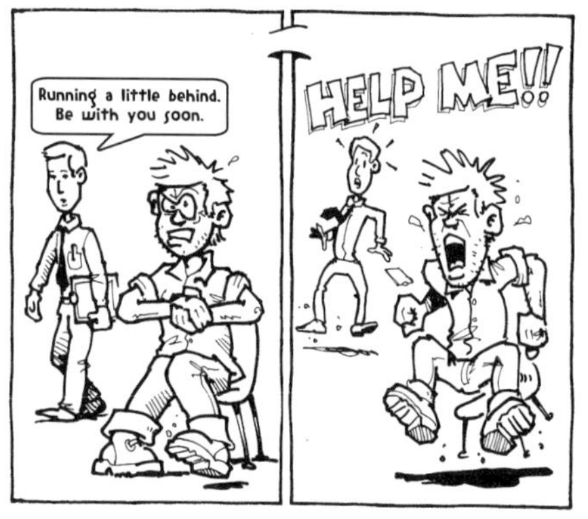

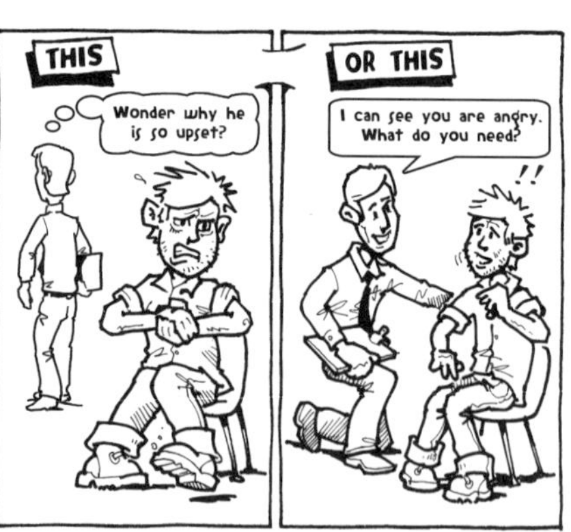

FIGURE 15.1
The conflict environment can be paralysing.
Courtesy Roger Harvey © Elsevier Australia.

REVIEW QUESTIONS

1. Define conflict.

2. State the major cause of conflict.

3. What is your natural tendency when communicating during conflict? Suggest at least two ways of overcoming this tendency if it is unproductive.

   i.

   ii.

4. Describe ways of resolving each emotion during conflict.

5. Describe ways of resolving your negative attitudes towards particular people.

6. In your own words, describe one of the ways of responding during conflict.

____

____

____

7. In your owns words, list five ways of communicating assertively. Provide examples of each.

   i. ____

   ii. ____

   iii. ____

   iv. ____

   v. ____

References

Alberti, R., Emmons, M., 2017. Your perfect right: Assertiveness and equality in your life and relationships, 10th ed. Impact, Oakland, CA.

Almost, J., Doran, D.M., Hall, L.M., et al., 2010. Antecedents and consequences of intra-group conflict among nurses. Journal of Nursing Management, 18 (8), 981–992.

Archee, R., Gurney, M., 2024. Communicating as professionals, 4th ed. Cengage Learning, Melbourne.

Beesley, P., Watts, M., Harrison, M., 2018. Developing your communication skills in social work. Sage, London.

Bowe, H., Martin, K., Manns, H., 2014. Communication across cultures: Mutual understanding in a global world, 2nd ed. Cambridge University Press, Melbourne.

Brinkert, R., 2010. A literature review of conflict communication causes, costs, benefits and interventions in nursing. Journal of Nursing Management, 18(2), 145–156.

Craig, K., Banja, J.D., 2010. Speaking up in case management, part I: Ethical and professional considerations. Professional Case Management, 15(4), 179–187.

Crossman, J., Bordia, S., Mills, C., 2011. Business communication for the global age. McGraw-Hill, Sydney.

Delaney, L.J., 2018. Patient-centred care as an approach to improve health care in Australia. Collegian, 25(1), 119–128.

Devito, J.A., 2021. The interpersonal communication book, 16th ed. Pearson, Boston.

Drick, C.A., 2012. In good times and bad: Holistic communication. Beginnings (AHNA), 32(1), 10–11.

Eckermann, A., Dowd, T., Chong, E., et al., 2010. Binaŋ Goonj: Bridging cultures in Aboriginal health, 3rd ed. Elsevier, Sydney.

Egan, G., Reese R.J., 2019. The skilled helper: A problem management and opportunity approach to helping, 11th ed. Cengage, Boston MA.

Fedoruk, M., 2014. Essential competencies for the registered nurse. In: Fedoruk, M., Hofmeyer, A. (eds), Becoming a nurse: An evidence-based approach, 2nd ed. Oxford University Press, South Melbourne.

Haddad, A.M., Purtilo, R.B., Doherty, R.F., 2018. Health professional and patient interaction, 9th ed. Elsevier/Saunders, St Louis, MO.

Harms, L., Pierce, J., 2019. Working with people: Communication skills for reflective practice, 2nd Canadian ed. Oxford University Press, Ontario.

Hayes, R., 2011. Rising above bullying: From despair to recovery [electronic resource]. Jessica Kingsley, London.

Healey, J., 2011. Dealing with bullying. Spinney Press, Thirroul.

Henderson, A., 2019. Communication for health care practice. Oxford University Press, Melbourne.

Holli, B.B., Beto, J.A., 2023. Nutrition counselling and education skills for dietetics professionals, 8th ed. Jones & Bartlett, Burlington, MA.

Honeycutt, A., Milliken, M.A., 2021. Understanding human behavior: A guide for healthcare providers, 10th ed. Cengage Learning, Boston.

Hutchinson, M., Jackson, D., Wilkes, L., et al., 2010. A new model of bullying in the nursing workplace. Advances in Nursing Science, 32(2), E60–E71.

Kassing, J.W., 2011. Stressing out about dissent: Examining the relationship between coping strategies and dissent expression. Communication Research Reports, 28(3), 225–234.

Levine, J., 2013. Working with people: The helping process, 9th ed. Pearson, San Antonio.

Losey, B., 2011. Bullying, suicide, and homicide: Understanding, assessing, and preventing threats to self and others for victims of bullying [electronic resource]. Taylor & Francis, Hoboken.

Mathibe-Neke, J.M., Mondell, T., 2018. Facilitate a holistic midwifery care: A teaching strategy. Africa Journal of Nursing and Midwifery, 19(1), 190–208.

McLean, S., 2011. The basics of interpersonal communication, 2nd ed. Allyn & Bacon, Boston.

Moisoglou, I., Panagiotis, P., Galanis, P., et al., 2014. Conflict management in a Greek public hospital: Collaboration or avoidance. International Journal of Caring Sciences, 7(1), 75–82.

Moss, B., 2020. Communication skills in health and social care, 5th ed. Sage, London.

Palanisamy, R., Verville, J., 2015. Factors enabling communication- based collaboration in interprofessional healthcare practice: A case study. International Journal of e-Collaboration, 11(2), 8–27.

Paternotte, E., van Dulmen, S., van der Lee, N., et al., 2015. Factors influencing intercultural doctor–patient communication: A realist review. Patient Education and Counseling, 98(4), 420–445.

Rakos, R.F., 2018. Asserting and confronting. In: Hargie, O. (ed.), The handbook of communication skills, 4th ed. Routledge, New York.

Rosenstein, A.H., Dinklin, S., Munro, J., 2014. Conflict resolution: Unlocking the key to success. Nursing Management, 45(10), 34–39.

Stein-Parbury, J., 2021. Patient and person: Interpersonal skills in nursing, 7th ed. Churchill Livingstone Elsevier, Sydney.

Swain, N., Gale, C., 2014. A communication skills intervention for community healthcare workers reduces perceived patient aggression: A pretest–postest study. International Journal of Nursing Studies, 51(9), 1241–1245.

Thompson, N., 2021. People skills, 5th ed. Red Globe Press, London.

Thompson, N., 2012. The people solutions sourcebook, 2nd ed. Palgrave Macmillan, Basingstoke.

Tregoning, C., 2015. Communication skills and enhancing clinical practice through reflective learning: A case study. British Journal of Healthcare Assistants, 9(2), 66–69.

Ttofi, M.M., 2011. Health consequences of school bullying [electronic resource]. Emerald, Bradford.

Weissman, D.E., Quill, T.E., Arnold, R.M., 2010. The family meeting: Causes of conflict. Journal of Palliative Medicine, 13(3), 328–329.

CHAPTER 16

Culturally responsive communication to accommodate cultural diversity in healthcare

Chapter objectives

Upon completing this chapter, readers should be able to:

- define culture and culturally responsive communication
- clarify the importance of culturally responsive communication
- reflect upon the notion of cultural safety in practice
- describe factors affecting culturally responsive communication
- develop useful strategies to achieve culturally responsive communication
- list the necessary steps required for the use of an interpreter.

The use of the word "responsive" to describe **responsive cross-cultural communication** reflects the reality that unless born into or "growing up" in a specific culture, developing competence – an expectation of proficient communication and functioning within that culture (Dwyer et al 2018) – is a complex and challenging task. "Responsive" suggests the need for **open**, receptive and empathic communication, or effectively communicating despite differences in cultural expectations of communication. This can seem overwhelming, and, for some, impossible. The word responsive was chosen in order to encourage readers to begin the journey of becoming confident and open cross-cultural communicators whenever and wherever they experience cultural diversity.

Introduction

Effective communication requires the healthcare professional to understand that there are *different ways of "doing and being"* (Wilcock & Hocking 2015). These ways of "doing and being" result in many different patterns of daily life. To become a culturally responsive healthcare professional, it is essential to explore being and doing aspects of other cultures (Delaney et al 2018). The values and beliefs of groups generate these everyday patterns, **customs** or traditions (Haddad et al 2019). Some consider it difficult to define *culture* (Bahreman & Swoboda 2016; Truong et al 2017a). However, for this discussion culture is seen as the word commonly used to describe the learnt patterns of perceiving, interpreting, adapting and relating to the world. These patterns develop from within the context of a group or community (Paternotte et al 2015). Culture is not innate; it is learnt from the relevant group (Liu et al 2023). It influences every person and every activity, every day (Devito 2021). Despite this influence, culture is often quite invisible to the members of the original group (Ramsden 2002). It typically consists of unconscious patterns encouraging individuals to expect everyone to "do and be" in similar patterns or customs (Liu et al 2023).

This chapter may begin the process of exploring culturally responsive communication; however, it is important to note that becoming a culturally responsive communicator can be an experiential process requiring a lifetime of learning about other cultures. As such, the chapter cannot provide an exhaustive understanding of appropriate communication or work practices with people from all cultural groups, but it can provide awareness of the cultural diversity in the world and ways to embrace, accept and begin to understand and accommodate this diversity. This growing diversity, recognised by governments, mandates the need for culturally responsive communication in healthcare services (Australian Commission on Safety and Quality in Health Care (ACSQHC) 2011; Darnell & Hickson 2015; Paternotte et al 2015). Responsive cross-cultural communication has been identified as improving both quality of care and health outcomes (Indigenous Allied Health Australia; 2015; Jennings et al 2018; Minnican & O'Toole 2020; Mollah et al; 2018; Olaussen & Renzaho 2016; Smith et al 2017; Truong et al 2017b; Ward et al 2018).

Before beginning this journey, it is important to remember that no culture ranks more highly than any other culture; cultures are merely different (Johnson & Withers 2018; Wells et al 2016). In addition, this chapter presents a model in order to assist healthcare professionals experiencing diversity. Exploring aspects of the model can assist healthcare professionals to develop culturally responsive communication and to explore and accommodate some of these aspects with the Person/s.

During daily practice, healthcare professionals will relate to individuals from both "large" and "small" cultures (Holliday et al 2021). A **"large" culture** is one that has extensive membership and considerable impact upon its members in all aspects of life. The culture of a nation is an example of a "large" culture. A **"small" culture** is one that has a smaller membership, usually affecting the lives of the members only when fulfilling roles expected by that small group culture. Thus, "small" cultures may have a restricted impact on the everyday lives of the members. An example of a "small" culture is a particular healthcare profession, healthcare service or sports group. Typically, healthcare professionals will experience cultural differences with the Person/s (including colleagues), whether they are from other countries, other socioeconomic groups or other "small" cultures. They will also experience cultural differences with other healthcare professionals. These differences develop within particular group settings, potentially affecting the outcomes of communication and thus, services.

Defining culture

It is important to examine and thereby achieve some understanding of the notion of culture to assist the healthcare professional to achieve culturally responsive communication. The concept of culture is complex, with considerable depth (Jacobson 2022). Culture varies over time and there are currently many ways of explaining this notion. This may explain why some consider culture difficult to define! Haddad and colleagues (2019) and Gilligan and colleagues (2019) present culture as a broad concept embracing all aspects of life, including customs, beliefs, technological achievements, language and the history of that particular group and similar groups. Thus culture has material and non-material aspects affecting daily life (Beltram 2011). Liu and colleagues (2023) suggest that culture produces a shared identity and unity within a group. Devito (2021) states that culture relates to the specific life habits within a particular group of people. This suggests that culture is the shared and systematic ways of living within a particular society or group. Similarly, culture can be described as a system of beliefs, values and behaviours characterising a particular group (Egan & Reese 2019; Haddad et al 2019; Holland 2018a; Stein-Parbury 2021; Verderber & MacGeorge 2015). However, the influence of life experiences, personal perceptions and current emotions, results in the expression of culture being unique to each individual at any point in time (Johnson & Withers 2018; Passi 2018).

None of these descriptions of culture are contradictory. They all suggest the relationship of culture to group membership as an unconscious expression of similarities (congruence) or shared meaning or identity within that group. Groups might express their culture through their particular beliefs, spirituality, language, family roles, ways of living and working, expectations, dress, artefacts, artistic expression, attitudes, food, remedies, identity and non-verbal behaviours, as well as through the value they place on their land (Dade-Smith 2016; Kinébanian & Stomph 2010; Parbury & Lamberton 2006; UNESCO 2002). Each generation shares these patterns of behaviours and understanding with each new generation. However, it is important to note that culture evolves and changes with time. This typically occurs when members of the cultural group experience different ways of "being and doing". Such changes can also occur with advances in technology and availability of previously unknown or unavailable commodities or services.

Cultural identity affecting culturally responsive communication

Cultural identity is unique to each individual, typically developing from group membership. However, cultural identity, is complex for every individual. Every individual has membership within various groups. Each group has a distinctive cultural identity, thereby contributing to a unique cultural identity for every individual (Holliday et al 2021). Group members develop particular identities relating to the values, traditions, beliefs and expectations associated with membership of that group. Examples of such groups include families, sporting teams, special interest groups, religious groups, school groups, class groups and activity groups. Membership of many groups affects the overall identity of every individual because of the unique common experiences and expectations of each group. Thus each individual has a unique identity reflecting his or her cultural and/or ethnic origins. However, cultural identities are complex and rarely static. Biles (2018) indicates that for many Indigenous groups, sharing their stories strengthens cultural identity. However, changes in cultural practices, beliefs and values affect these identities, as individuals adapt to the changes around them. This complexity indicates that healthcare professionals should abandon any stereotypical idea of other cultures or of individuals from those cultures (Olivares & Pena 2014). An awareness of the complex nature of cultural identity (both of the healthcare professional and the Person/s) is essential when communicating with people from diverse backgrounds (McClimens et al 2014). This awareness facilitates acceptance of the uniqueness of every individual and their differing perceptions of the world (Alvarez et al 2014; Passi 2018). For a deeper exploration of cultural identity, please see Chapter 17.

Defining culturally responsive communication

The worldwide increase in cultural diversity (Ceo-DiFrancesco et al 2020; Ward et al 2018) mandates consideration of communication with culturally diverse individuals to achieve effective communication and appropriate services. Understanding the cultural backgrounds of these diverse populations will also inform relevant interventions (Balkozar 2019). In order to achieve culturally responsible communication and appropriate services, it is important for healthcare professionals to understand that cultures differ (Mollah et al 2018; Noe et al 2014). It is also important for healthcare professionals to understand that each person has diverse experiences, worldviews, beliefs, attitudes and values affecting their understanding of power and privilege (Eckermann et al 2010; Likupe 2014; McClimens et al 2014). This understanding allows consideration of this diversity during healthcare interactions (Indigenous Allied Health Australia 2015). Such understanding is especially important for healthcare professionals because the relationship between the healthcare professional and the Person/s can be seen to have an inbuilt power imbalance, potentially affecting communication. This reality is especially relevant in communicative interactions with individuals from various Indigenous cultures because many have histories or experiences that potentially negatively affect their expectations of the relationship with any healthcare professional (Jennings et al 2018; Noe et al 2014).

Cultural safety

Perceptions of power and privilege, in combination with any previous experiences of a relationship with a healthcare professional (with its inbuilt power imbalance), may suggest to many Indigenous People that they should not trust a healthcare professional (Eckermann et al 2010; Jennings et al 2018). It is this reality, evident wherever there are Indigenous People relating to healthcare services, which led to the development of the notion of **cultural safety**. This concept developed because of the power imbalance in healthcare services in Aotearoa New Zealand during the mid-1990s (Papps & Ramsden 1996). However, it is relevant to every healthcare professional providing care in any healthcare service. It often relates to systems, typically disempowering the Person/s or groups. The notion of cultural safety embraces all diverse groupings, regardless of age, gender, sexual preferences and disability. The discussion around this notion indicates that the power, prejudice and attitude in the healthcare professional can negatively affect healthcare service outcomes. It is not merely about creating safety for the Person/s in healthcare services. It highlights the importance of respecting and accepting the Person/s, of embracing differences and valuing their opinions (Barnett & Kendall 2011; Holland 2018b; Noe et al 2014).

Cultural safety considers everyone unique, potentially empowering each individual (Eckermann et al 2010). It provides opportunities for the Person/s to contribute and exercise some power over the healthcare intervention process (Levoy 2014a; Ramsden 2001, 2002). The model of Person/Family-centred Care (see Chapter 2) – a foundation for all interactions in healthcare – allows every individual to retain their identity, in this instance their cultural identity, throughout the healthcare process. It mandates acceptance of the Person/s and their chosen lifestyle and a willingness to collaborate in a therapeutic relationship to promote equality (Chan et al 2015; Levoy 2014b; National Health and Medical Research Council (NHMRC) 2006; Nursing Council of New Zealand 2011).

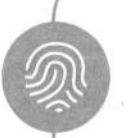

- Define safety.
- What generally creates feelings of safety for you?
- What might create the feeling of safety in healthcare practice?
- What might limit experiencing feelings of safety in healthcare practice?
- How might you avoid these limitations when practising as a healthcare professional?

The notion of cultural safety highlights the importance of tactful and compassionate acceptance of the different cultures represented by the individuals relating to the healthcare professional. It identifies the need to involve the Person/s in any healthcare process (Darnell & Hickson 2015).

Dean (2001) states that it is impossible to be "completely culturally competent" in every culture, perhaps unless born into that culture. Even then, individual interpretation and expression of the culture produces both material and non-material changes to expressions of their culture. In the healthcare professions, the concept of **cultural competence** relates to making ethical, sound and culturally appropriate decisions during daily healthcare (Wells et al 2016). Regardless of their level of competence, the healthcare professional must be open to and accepting of the different cultures encountered during practice, to achieve culturally responsive communication. Culturally responsive communication involves being aware of, sensitive to and appreciative of the cultural variations common among individuals and groups, mandating respect for these variations (Eckermann et al 2010; Egan & Reese 2019; Holland 2018b; Likupe 2014; Minnican & O'Toole 2020). It invites the healthcare professional to acknowledge the validity of the other culture (Bowe et al 2014), rather than ridiculing or trivialising it. Culturally responsive communication requires an effective and sensitive healthcare professional who is willing to explore, accept and embrace cultural differences. It requires knowledge, mutual respect and negotiation (Haddad et al 2019) to achieve effective communication. Such communication can achieve satisfying outcomes specific to the skills of the healthcare professional and the needs of the Person/s.

Why consider cultural differences?

Every individual has a culturally determined perspective affecting his or her understanding, expectations and styles of communication, and of healthcare (Minnican & O'Toole 2020). This reality mandates consideration of cultural differences. These differences produce a diversity of behaviours, but they also produce the health beliefs and behaviours of individuals. These health beliefs and behaviours can profoundly affect expectations and the ultimate outcomes of any healthcare service (Balkozar, 2019; Haddad et al 2019).

Individuals vary in their responses to physical and psychological distress; these variations affect the responses of both the healthcare professional and the Person/s. Particular health beliefs often regulate these responses. It is initially surprising to realise that different people have different beliefs and behaviours associated with their health. Therefore, it is important to resist applying personal health beliefs to those seeking healthcare to avoid negatively affecting communication.

A model of culturally responsive communication

There are many closely related factors contributing to achieving culturally responsive communication. These factors exist in a dynamic system, subject to regular change. They are intimately connected and constantly affect each other. This model highlights some of these factors in order to remind the healthcare professional of the importance of these factors and the need to accommodate them, or, if affecting them personally, to control and/or resolve these factors while providing healthcare (Fig. 16.1).

The central and pivotal component of the model is the healthcare professional who is responsible for achieving culturally responsive communication. The healthcare professional must demonstrate particular characteristics to achieve effective communication. Awareness of these characteristics allows the healthcare professional to demonstrate them consistently, thereby communicating more effectively when experiencing cultural diversity. The first characteristic – *motivation* to learn both about other cultures (Ziaian & Xiao 2015) and display the other characteristics – is foundational to achieving responsive, and thus effective, cross-cultural communication. Secondly, critical *self-awareness* is essential in all communicative events, providing a foundation for culturally responsive communication (Darnell & Hickson 2015; Hall et al 2014; Indigenous Allied Health Australia 2015; Likupe 2014; McClimens et al 2014; Mir et al 2015; Paternotte et al 2015; Queensland Health 2010; Taylor 2017; World Health Organization (WHO) 2018).

This self-awareness contributes to being *other-aware*, or aware of the Person/s encountered in practice, potentially liberating the healthcare professional to communicate effectively with

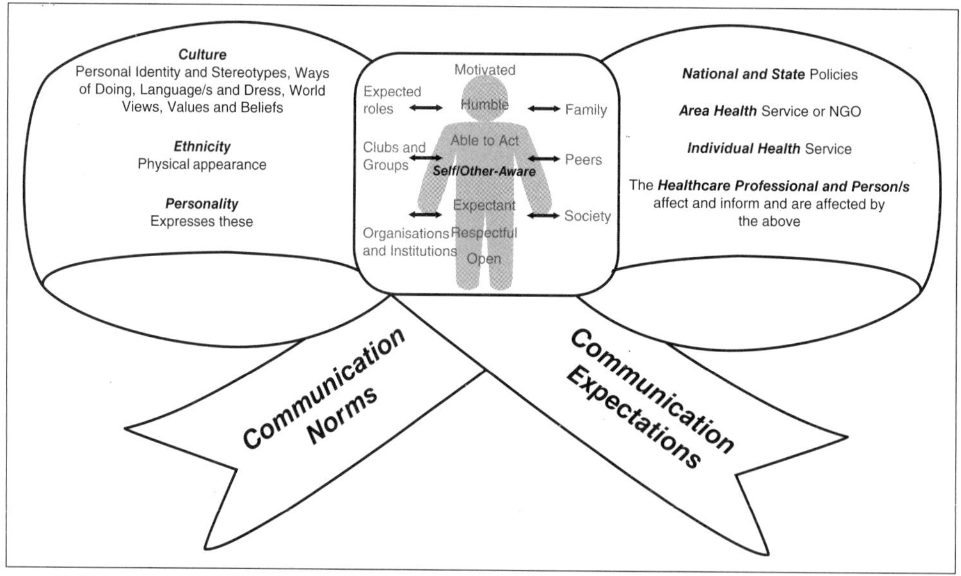

FIGURE 16.1
A model of culturally responsive communication.

cultural sensitivity. In addition, critical self-awareness promotes humble understanding that no-one is better than another person, but merely different (Xiao et al 2018). Such *humility* promotes an open willingness to learn about and embrace differences without judgement, an essential requirement for a healthcare professional (Hampton 2013). It also promotes an understanding that individual cultures implicitly guide judgements and interpretation of others, thereby empowering the healthcare professional to restrict the effect of their personal culture when relating to others. Humility also empowers the healthcare professional to take responsibility for any mistakes they make while relating, thereby promoting an appropriate apology for any such errors.

Critical self-awareness and humility can also encourage the healthcare professional to accommodate these differences and therefore be able to be *expectant* of positive communication outcomes while interacting with the culturally diverse Person/s. This expectation will non-verbally communicate hope to the vulnerable and possibly fearful Person/s, therefore promoting development of the features of Person-centred Care. Indigenous Allied Health Australia (2015) states that culturally effective care extends and consolidates Person-centred Care. The abovementioned characteristics contribute to another mandatory characteristic in healthcare professionals: to demonstrate *respectful* attitudes and behaviours (Likupe 2014; McClimens et al 2014; Noe et al 2014). These characteristics ensure an open healthcare professional committed to culturally responsive communication. However, such communication is rarely possible when the healthcare professional is *unable to act*, either because of **cultural norms** or an inability to communicate because of cognitive or physical causes or differences in language. There are strategies that can overcome the last few causes of an inability to act; however, it is more challenging to overcome the cultural reasons limiting the actions of the particular healthcare professional. The abovementioned characteristics are key for any healthcare professional when communicating with a culturally diverse Person/s.

Also central to this model are group contexts surrounding and influencing the individual healthcare professional. This indicates that each healthcare professional and Person/s develops and exists within the context of various social groups. These groups influence the ability to achieve culturally responsive communication. Membership of these groups produces particular *roles* that may contribute to the development of skills relating to communication, and can influence effectiveness while communicating. The *family* group has a lasting effect on communication styles, typically preparing, or perhaps not preparing, the healthcare professional and Person/s for competence in settings with differences. In addition, the family often defines the expected roles of individual family members. Other groups that affect the healthcare professional and Person/s include the wider *society,* which has norms and expectations influencing the family and thus their members. The related norms and experiences of interacting with *peer* groups, such as sports *groups,* single-purpose *clubs,* such as chess or quilting clubs, or licensed clubs, also influence expectations of communication. The *organisation* or *institution* has a considerable effect on the expectations and behaviours of the healthcare professional (Alvarez et al 2014). These contexts are not limited to the employing organisation or institution, but relate to any group with whom the healthcare professional or Person/s must relate to successfully perform their roles and fulfil their responsibilities. They often mandate culturally responsive communication and may provide support to produce such communication. All of the above contribute to the development of skills in communication.

The intrinsic factors influencing the healthcare professional and Person/s are another component of the model. They influence communication in diverse situations. The *culture* of an individual, as mentioned above, is often invisible or assumed, and consequently the healthcare professional or Person/s may not be able to articulate actual expectations of their personal culture. However, it does affect their *personal* and *cultural identity*, and may contribute to particular assumptions or *stereotypes* influencing their communicative ability. It will determine their particular *"ways of doing"* or living their everyday life, whether private or professional. It will initially determine their *values and beliefs*, the *rules* governing their life and their *worldview*. The ethnicity of an individual is often obvious and although not always conclusive, it can determine their *physical appearance*, the *languages* they speak, along with their style and type of *clothing*. These factors are both material and non-material aspects of culture (Beltram 2011) and, while some are less obvious, they affect the healthcare professional and the Person/s. However, the healthcare professional and the Person/s will interpret and *express* these factors according to their individual *personality*. These factors combine to affect the healthcare professional, the Person/s and their expectations of and skills in culturally responsive communication.

Language

Words, non-verbal behaviours and intention can have different meanings among people from the same culture and can cause difficulties in communication. For example, asking someone for dinner for some means a meal at midday, for others a meal around 5.30 p.m., and still others, a formal meal after 8.00 p.m. It is not surprising then that individuals from different cultures experience communication difficulties because of variations in meanings of words and non-verbal behaviours (Beesley et al 2018; Boggs 2023). For example, directional nods and shakes of the head have different meanings in different cultures, so this can cause miscommunication (see Chapter 18).

The external factors influencing the healthcare professional, their practice and the Person/s are another component of the model. While these factors do guide healthcare professional behaviour, the healthcare professional can also influence these external realities.

The *national and state policies* guide and support each area healthcare service, relevant non-government organisations (NGO) and private practices. These policies determine expectations for communication and behaviour among all healthcare professions, whether in the private or public sector. In turn, the *area healthcare service* and/or *NGO* supports particular healthcare services, implementing relevant policies. This support can include such things as recruiting, training and networking. The *individual healthcare service* supports and directs the healthcare professional, implementing and monitoring norms and expectations for communication and behaviours. It also supports the Person/s, indicating their rights and expressions of satisfaction or complaint. The healthcare professional and the Person/s interact and communicate within the context of the above factors. They can, however, through collaborative agreement, affect and inform all of the above, even at the level of policy. The healthcare professional can achieve this through active involvement with their national professional body.

The norms and expectations of communication are an underlying component of culturally responsive communication. These are important and in the context of the healthcare professions affect all elements or features of this model.

Understanding context

Understanding a particular context can promote effective communication (Bowe et al 2014). The context of the Person/s can affect communication and mutual understanding. Similarly, the context of a healthcare service is confusing and unfamiliar for many individuals, even if it is within their own culture (Victorson et al 2014), but for someone from a different culture it is often frightening (Hasnain et al 2011). It is important to understand that the particular contexts affect the expectations and emotions of each communicating individual – both the Person/s and the healthcare professional – and thus the effectiveness of communication.

Ethnocentricity

When an individual believes their particular method or way of approaching a situation is superior and indeed the best way, they are **ethnocentric**. Haddad and colleagues (2019) state that ethnocentricity is a common phenomenon in healthcare professionals and can negatively affect communication. Olaussen and Renzaho (2016) discuss the situation of healthcare professionals using the same style of communication for everyone, regardless of differences. This could suggest a tendency towards ethnocentricity.

A man from a different culture was admitted to hospital with a stroke. His family was absent. The healthcare professionals were curious as they settled the man into the ward. His language skills seemed adequate because he asked appropriate questions and responded appropriately when asked to do something. However, he sat by the bed quietly and passively; he did not look around or relate to anyone.

Around 4.30 p.m. people of varying ages from the same culture arrived and the healthcare professionals assumed they were family. The man suddenly seemed happy and took an interest in what was happening. These people brought woven mats, food, plates and utensils with them. In an out-of-the-way corner of the ward they placed the mats on the floor and served the food onto plates. One person – an older lady – sat by the man and assisted him to eat his meal. The rest of the family sat on the mats on the floor, eating together, including the man in all the interactions while talking quietly in their own language. They were obviously all enjoying themselves.

- What are the possible explanations for the behaviour of this man? Do you think it strange?
- What are the possible explanations for the behaviour of this family? Do you think it strange?
- How would you respond to this behaviour?
- One response is to ask to join them on the floor – suggest other appropriate responses.

- List the possible ways of responding.
  - What are the possible consequences of these responses?
  - What is a culturally responsive response?

The behaviour in the scenario above is regarded as "strange" in a Western culture, and there were negative responses from various healthcare professionals. Some were direct expressions of personal biases and attitudes, while others were personal attitudes expressed through healthcare service regulations. In most situations it is important – and in situations such as the one described above, it is essential – to consider more than the behaviours, by exploring in depth the multifaceted and complex reasons for the behaviours (Haddad et al 2019). Different situations and countries have different services available. The family in the above scenario came from a country where hospitals do not provide many services, thus the family was expecting to do everything for the person in hospital, including supplying meals, providing clothes and assisting with showering and toileting. In addition, their culture values mealtimes as social occasions and therefore they could not imagine their relative having a meal without all family members present. In their culture, a person is alone when they are among strangers. Understanding cultural differences in this situation provided explanations for the "strange" behaviour and facilitated a compromise that met the needs of all involved in the care of this culturally different man and his family.

- Consider the previous scenario and outline the:
  - needs and expectations of the Person/Family
  - needs and expectations of the healthcare professionals
  - expectations of the healthcare service.
- Brainstorm ways of compromising to be culturally accommodating while still completing the required routines of healthcare professionals and meeting the work, health and safety requirements of the healthcare service.

In situations presenting cultural differences, it is important to accept, appreciate and accommodate diversity (Egan & Reese 2019). If the healthcare professional merely recognises the differences, this may separate and create distance. However, perception and appreciation of the similarities will promote connection and development of rapport (Likupe 2014). In such situations, it is important that culturally different individuals experience acceptance and understanding, not judgement, defensiveness and misunderstanding, possibly from fear of differences.

Managing personal cultural assumptions and expectations

It is relevant to remember that cultural differences do not only occur between people from different countries, but also between people from different socioeconomic backgrounds, contexts, states or provinces, Indigenous groups, religious groups, occupations, societies and families. Cultural variations can also occur between different healthcare professionals. In fact, there is a limitless number of variations.

Cultural differences occur in everyday life in material and non-material ways (Beltram 2011), including practices relating to handshakes, greetings, what to talk about, what to avoid talking about, the meaning and use of colours, personal space, eye contact, humour, music and songs, ways to wash and dry clothing, food (including its value, ways to prepare it, timing of meals and how to arrange the place of eating), habits of personal hygiene/personal cleaning rituals, bed linen and ways of arranging a bed, spirituality and religious practices, expression of beliefs and values, understanding and meaning of the land, artistic expression, to name a few.

The list is extensive and could fill many pages. In the healthcare professions it is important to understand that for particular individuals there are differences that might affect the outcome of the healthcare service (Darnell & Hickson 2015; El Amouri & O'Neill 2014; Likupe 2014). Consideration of cultural difference is essential when planning outcomes for individuals and groups. When establishing goals, it is easy to apply the cultural values, assumptions and expectations of the healthcare professional, thereby limiting Person/Family-centred Care.

A southern European family lives with several generations in four adjacent houses. The retired father, Giuseppe, is recovering from surgery that established he has inoperable brain tumours. He currently requires assistance to complete simple self-care tasks. The healthcare professionals involved are reluctant to suggest how long he might live.

Each healthcare professional (HcP) has different thoughts about what should happen.

HcP1 suggests he should go to a hospice to die.

HcP2 suggests he needs more time to recover from surgery.

HcP3 suggests placing him in a high-dependency unit.

HcP4 says that his daughter cannot see her mother managing if Giuseppe goes home.

HcP5 suggests that with the right assistance he could die at home.

HcP6 suggests that talking to the family is important.

HcP7 suggests that asking Giuseppe might be a good idea.

HcP8 says that Giuseppe should not be told that he will die soon (his prognosis).

- Consider each response and decide what the HcP assumes, values and fears.
- Which of the responses do you consider is the one that suits the family?

The family conference includes HcP 1, 4 and 5, as well as several members of the family, including his wife Roma, his eldest son, his youngest daughter and the wife of his youngest son.

The aim of the conference is to establish where Giuseppe will go upon discharge. Each healthcare professional explains the options. The first discusses hospice care and states that they feel it would suit everyone. The second indicates that they understand certain members of the family are concerned about managing if Giuseppe goes home, and supports this view. While both these healthcare professionals are explaining the options, Giuseppe's wife cries uncontrollably. The third healthcare professional outlines the possible assistance that is available if Giuseppe goes home, carefully explaining the possible difficulties, but stating that Giuseppe may be more independent when he recovers from the surgery. As the third healthcare professional (HcP5) explains, Roma begins to listen and stares at this healthcare professional. When this healthcare professional finishes, Roma stands and says in broken English *That is what we want – Giuseppe to come home*. She states this emphatically and says it will mean that he can die at home. A family argument ensues, with some family members supporting Roma and others supporting the idea of Giuseppe being told what is happening and going where he can receive expert Care.

- Suggest ways to manage this situation so that Giuseppe and his family receive Person/Family-centred Care.

- What do you feel you would want if Giuseppe was your husband? Or father?
- What does this feeling indicate about your personal values?

In order to provide Person/Family-centred Care, healthcare professionals must avoid applying particular **cultural assumptions** and expectations to those seeking their assistance.

Strategies for achieving culturally responsive communication

It is important for healthcare professionals to expand their understanding of and accept cultural differences across the myriad cultures they experience every day (Harms & Pierce 2019), including the cultures within different healthcare professions. There is evidence that many healthcare professionals, despite their willingness to learn, are unsure of how to achieve culturally responsive communication (Hughson et al 2018; Mollah et al 2018; Truong et al 2017a; Watt et al 2016; Watts et al 2018; Xiao et al 2018). Many strategies contribute to positive experiences in cross-cultural communication. At this point it seems appropriate to mention that culturally effective communication also requires all the components of the model of Person/Family-centred Care (see Chapter 2).

Critical self-awareness

The first step in achieving culturally responsive communication is to critically evaluate personal and individual cultural values, beliefs, traditions and worldviews (Curtis et al 2019; Hall et al 2014; Haddad et al 2019; Holli & Beto 2023; Queensland Health 2010). It is difficult to be a culturally responsive healthcare professional if unaware of personal biases (Darnell & Hickson 2015; Likupe 2014). If unaware of personal cultural biases, it is impossible to confront any tendency to stereotype (McClimens et al 2014) (see Chapter 8), as this limits the potential to understand and accept different cultures; in fact, any kind of difference or diversity.

Personal commitment to understanding and accommodating differences

The requirements of effective communication (see Chapters 1 and 2) are the basis of culturally responsive communication (Haddad et al 2019). Commitment and willingness to implement these foundational requirements will assist healthcare professionals to adopt appropriate strategies when communicating with people from cultures that are different from their own. Such commitment will assist the healthcare professional to predict the needs when communicating with individuals from different cultures, thereby improving the possibility of a collaborative therapeutic relationship and positive outcomes.

Exposure and learning

An effective way to communicate across cultures is to become familiar with the relevant culture(s) (Devito 2021). There are many ways to achieve this familiarity, including reading books and articles written by individuals from the culture about the culture, watching relevant movies (beware of bias), reading information on the internet and socialising with friends from the particular culture. Another way to achieve familiarity with a culture is to approach the culturally different Person/s with an open, accepting attitude and express interest within the context of the practice. Asking questions about traditions, values, life meaning and expectations (Chan et al 2015), as well as asking about styles of communication, can increase understanding. This understanding provides the knowledge of the culture, thereby contributing to developing appropriate and sufficient skills for culturally responsive communication. Discussion about the cultural differences as the healthcare professional conducts their interventions, can be reassuring for both the individual and the healthcare professional. Such discussion might also highlight similarities, providing an interface for connection (Gilligan et al 2019; Stein-Parbury 2021. Haddad and colleagues (2019) suggest that the healthcare professional should embrace the differences and consider the interaction an opportunity to learn about the other culture. It is important when considering cultural differences to also consider the unique individual, because often there are individual variations limiting the application of a general understanding of any cultural norm.

Investment of time to negotiate meaning and ensure understanding

There is a certain amount of insecurity about communicating with someone who is from a different culture, speaks a different language, or has differing values, beliefs and traditions, even when it is only a different healthcare language and belief. Investment of time and energy to understand the individual is imperative. There is no reason to be afraid because, while it is important for the healthcare professional to restructure their worldview to accommodate and understand the differences, they do not necessarily need to profess, internalise or assimilate these differences in their everyday life. Cultural understanding simply allows the healthcare professional to demonstrate respect of the worldview, which will assist in developing rapport and fulfilling the needs of the Person/s (Darnell & Hickson 2015).

Anticipation of difficulties

There are a variety of possible difficulties within any communicative interaction. Anticipation of these difficulties may assist the healthcare professional to develop appropriate responses (Verderber & MacGeorge 2015). The healthcare professional can overcome some of the difficulties associated with achieving culturally responsive communication by being aware of their personal cultural attitudes, the aspects of that culture, along with the factors affecting culturally effective communication (Henderson 2019; Queensland Health 2010).

A common difficulty in intercultural communication can be the lack of a common language. This creates apprehension for both the healthcare professional and the Person/s, potentially reducing positive outcomes (Ramos et al 2014; Rorie 2015). An open and relaxed demeanour will assist any attempt to connect with the individual, despite the lack of a shared language. When communicating without a common language, anticipating the need for an interpreter is paramount.

Using an interpreter

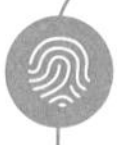

- What difficulties might arise when using an interpreter?
- When using an interpreter, who do you predict will most easily develop rapport with the Person/s?
- How could the healthcare professional use the interaction to build rapport?

Discuss your answers with other members of the large group.

When considering the use of an interpreter to achieve culturally responsive communication, it is important to first note that there are different types of interpretation (Bowe et al 2014). The **interpreter** translates information while it is being presented during **simultaneous interpretation**. This type of interpretation does not usually occur when translating for one person, but often occurs when there is a group of listeners. Simultaneous interpretation is common when interpreting for groups of people who have a hearing impairment. This type of interpretation is demanding because the interpreter "speaks" at the same time as the speaker, and must concentrate and listen carefully in order to accurately interpret the meaning.

Alternatively, **sequential interpretation** allows the speaker to present a small portion of the information, then the interpreter translates this portion. During this type of interpretation, only one person speaks at any one time. Sequential or consecutive interpretation is the usual form of interpretation for interactions in the healthcare professions.

There are also two styles of interpretation. **Transliteration** is the exact translation of each word or sound spoken, regardless of meaning; such utterances often have limited meaning. **Interpretation** is the translation of the meaning of the utterance, regardless of the spoken sound or word. Each style of interpretation has limitations potentially affecting comprehension of all parties. In either style it is important to ensure the interpreter understands the meaning of the message.

There are particular steps required to use an interpreter effectively. This process requires skill, focused concentration and careful planning, just as the act of interpreting itself requires skill, concentration and specific knowledge of both languages. Many interpreters, unless particularly trained in the use of medical terminology (Stein-Parbury 2021), may find medical or technical words unfamiliar, so it is best to avoid using professional jargon and, where possible, untrained interpreters (Amery 2017; Finset 2018; Zendedel et al 2018).

It is important to understand that professionally trained interpreters are not always available. In remote areas, interpreters may not be available at all, while in other areas, there are interpreters for only a limited number of languages. In some areas, telephone interpreters are available; they usually require an appointment made in advance. It is possible to use colleagues as interpreters if available, but remember that colleagues are rarely trained for interpreting and thus may require additional consideration while interpreting. In some situations, healthcare professionals might use family members to interpret. This practice is not always recommended and can cause family tension. The use of an *adult* family or community member might be appropriate for information about progress or the need for the toilet, for example, but it can be inappropriate to use such an individual to give complicated information relating to a diagnosis, prognosis or the future.

When using an interpreter, it is important to prepare the interpreter. The healthcare professional should advise the interpreter of the purpose of the interview, and if possible introduce them to the Person/s prior to the discussion, especially if discussing sensitive topics; in some cases, the discussion may require the interpreter to be the same gender as the Person/s (Stein-Parbury 2021).

Essential steps when using an interpreter

1. Establish the purpose of the interaction requiring an interpreter – for both the interpreter and the Person/s.
2. Schedule and book an appropriate time for everyone required for the interaction. It is important to organise an interpreter in advance. Allow time to brief the interpreter concerning the purpose of the interaction before the commencement of the interaction with the Person/s. Interpreters can be late for good reason, so briefing them by telephone may be necessary.
3. If appropriate, prepare the questions and information for discussion using an interpreter. When using an interpreter it is easy to forget a point or to deviate from the original plan. It is therefore important to organise the points carefully to ensure coverage of all necessary information.
4. Clarify any areas of uncertainty in the mind of the interpreter. It is important to establish a signal to indicate when an item of information is too long. All people involved in the interaction should know the meaning of this signal.

5. Introduce everyone. Remember the healthcare professional and the Person/s are the focus of the interaction. Take care to concentrate on maintaining or developing rapport with the Person/s, not the interpreter. Introduce the purpose of the interaction to the Person/s.
6. Speak to and look at the Person/s, not the interpreter. It is important that the interpreter connects with the Person/s; however, development of a relationship between them is unnecessary and may detract from the purpose of the interaction. They may have an immediate rapport because they share a common language and this will assist the Person/s to relax, but it is important to focus on the purpose of the interaction because the interpreter is available for a limited time. Maintain control of the interaction; the interpreter is there to assist not to conduct the interaction.
7. Use small "chunks" of information, not long sentences. Make the points clear and minimise jargon or colloquialisms to avoid misinterpretation or reinterpretation of the content. It is important to keep a mental note of what has been covered and what is yet to be covered as the interaction progresses.
8. Carefully observe the non-verbal reactions of the Person/s.
9. Ask questions in response to these non-verbal reactions, for example, *You appear unhappy about that – am I right? What do you need to know or how can we help you to feel happier?* Because it is often difficult to know exactly what has been communicated, asking questions to clarify and verify understanding throughout the interaction is essential when using an interpreter (Harms & Pierce 2019).
10. If appropriate, ask the Person/s to summarise the information to demonstrate their understanding. Include time to answer any unrelated questions or address any concerns. Remember the importance of disengagement or concluding the interaction in the development of a therapeutic relationship with the Person/s.

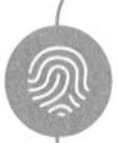

- Consider the reasons for and against using a family member as an interpreter.
- When might it be appropriate to use a family member? (e.g. when asking about matters such as improvement in symptoms, or the habits of the Person within the family)
- When might it be **in**appropriate to use a family member? (e.g. when giving bad news or asking intimate personal questions).

Share your ideas with members of the large group.

The culture of each healthcare profession

Individual healthcare professions have underlying philosophies, values, assumptions, beliefs, expectations and habits specific to that profession. These generate particular knowledge and behaviours in the everyday activities of each healthcare profession. Therefore, each healthcare profession has a "culture" specific to that profession. These cultures generate differences between healthcare professions. Each profession has a particular concept of the Person/s, and the role of the Person/s and the profession in the healing process (Honeycutt & Milliken 2021). Each profession has a particular understanding of various concepts (e.g. pain, disability, illness, health, wellbeing) and each has a particular role when relating to these concepts relevant to that particular profession. While there are variations in values and beliefs, many professions value Person/Family-centred Care and all share the common value of mutual respect and developing rapport.

The culture of disease or ill-health

The culture that may be the most difficult to understand, unless experienced personally, is the **culture of disease or ill-health**, whether chronic or acute, sudden or gradual. During their working week, healthcare professionals consistently relate to people who live in this culture of disability. Achieving effective communication to accommodate this culture is challenging, but as rewarding as communicating effectively with individuals from different backgrounds.

Chapter summary

Culture refers to the material and non-materials aspects of a group. These aspects represent the values and beliefs of a particular group generating patterns of behaviour. While a healthcare professional can never understand a culture completely unless they are part of it, it is important that they are open to and accepting of the different cultures encountered while providing healthcare. The model presented in this chapter highlights factors affecting communication for each healthcare professional as they consider how to be culturally responsive communicators in their daily workplace. It highlights particular characteristics to enhance communication in culturally diverse situations. It also identifies inherent and external factors affecting the healthcare professional and the Person/s. These require consideration when communicating with Person/s from different cultures. Culturally responsive communication can be achieved through consideration and application of this model, along with investment of time to negotiate meaning and achieve mutual understanding. Where this requires the use of an interpreter, there are necessary steps to ensure effective communication. The above discussion outlines aspects of culturally responsive communication contributing to Person/Family-centred Care.

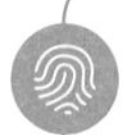

Consider all the information in Chapter 28 relevant to Scenario 5, "A Person/s who speaks a different language to the healthcare professional".

- List what you would do to ensure culturally responsive communication.
- Consider questions you might ask to ensure achievement of all aspects of Person/Family-centred Care
- Outline how your use of an interpreter will contribute to achieving effective communication with the Person/s from this scenario.

People, like bow ties, come in all colours, shapes and sizes.

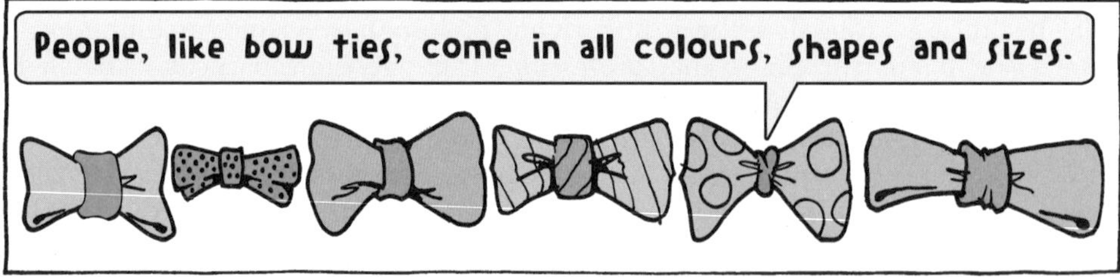

FIGURE 16.2
Accommodating and embracing diversity facilitates effective communication.
Courtesy Roger Harvey © Elsevier Australia.

REVIEW QUESTIONS

1. What must healthcare professionals understand about themselves to be committed to culturally responsive or effective cross-cultural communication?

2. Create your definition of "culture".

3. What are some of the differences affecting culturally responsive communication?

4. How might members of a culture express the cultural characteristics of the culture?

5. List three factors affecting culturally responsive communication and give examples of each factor.

   i.

   ii.

   iii.

6. What promotes openness to cultural diversity in a healthcare professional?

7. List some strategies to assist healthcare professionals to avoid applying their personal cultural biases when communicating with culturally diverse people.

____

____

____

8. In your own words, outline the ten steps for effective communication while using an interpreter.

   i. ____

   ii. ____

   iii. ____

   iv. ____

   v. ____

   vi. ____

   vii. ____

   viii. ____

   ix. ____

   x. ____

References

Alvarez, K., Marroquin, Y.A., Sandoval, L., et al., 2014. Integrated health care best practices and culturally and linguistically competent care: Practitioner perspectives. Journal of Mental Health Counseling, 36(2), 99–114.

Amery, R., 2017. Recognising the communication gap in Indigenous health care. Medical Journal of Australia, 207(1), 13–15.

Australian Commission on Safety and Quality in Health Care (ACSQHC), 2011. Patient-centred care: Improving quality and safety though partnerships with patients and consumers. Australian Government, Sydney Australia. Online. Available at: www.safetyandquality.gov.au/sites/default/files/migrated/PCC_Paper_August.pdf

Bahreman, N.T., Swoboda, S.M., 2016. Healthcare diversity: Developing culturally competent communication skills through simulation. Journal of Nursing Education, 55(2), 105–108.

Balkozar, A., 2019. Culture, compassion and competency: When culture is more than a backdrop. Journal of the American Academy of Child and Adolescent Psychiatry, 58(10), S125–S126.

Barnett, L., Kendall, E., 2011. Culturally appropriate methods for enhancing the participation of Aboriginal Australians in health-promoting programs. Health Promotion Journal of Australia, 22(1), 27–32.

Beesley, P., Watts, M., Harrison, M., 2018. Developing your communication skills in social work. Sage, London.

Beltram, R., 2011. Cultural dimensions of occupation analysis. In: Mackenzie, L., O'Toole, G. (eds), Occupation analysis in practice. Wiley-Blackwell, London.

Biles, K., 2018. Strengthening relationships: We all need a place to call home. Emergency Medicine Australasia, 30, 857–858.

Boggs, K.U., 2023. Interpersonal relationships: Professional communication skills for nurses, 9th ed. Elsevier, St Louis, MO.

Bowe, H., Martin, K., Manns, H., 2014. Communication across cultures: Mutual understanding in a global world, 2nd ed. Cambridge University Press, Melbourne.

Ceo-DiFrancesco, D., Dunn, L.S., Solorio, N. 2020. Transforming through reflection: Use of student-led reflections in the development of intercultural competence during a short-term international immersion experience. Internet Journal of Allied Health Sciences and Practice, 18(2), Article 8.

Chan, F., Berven, N.L., Thomas, K.R. (eds), 2015. Counselling theories and techniques for rehabilitation and mental health professionals, 2nd ed. Springer, New York.

Curtis, E., Jones, R., Tipene-Leach, D., et al., 2019. Why cultural safety rather than cultural competency is required to achieve health equity: A literature review and recommended definition. International Journal for Equity in Health,18(1), 174.

Dade-Smith, J.D., 2016. Australia's rural, remote and Indigenous health, 3rd ed. Elsevier, Sydney.

Darnell, L.K., Hickson, S.V., 2015. Cultural competent patient-centered nursing care. The Nursing Clinics of North America, 50(1), 99–108.

Dean, R., 2001. The myth of cross-cultural competence: Families in society. Journal of Contemporary Human Services, 86, 623–630.

Delaney, C., Doughney, L., Bandler, L., et al., 2018. Exploring learning goals and assessment approaches for Indigenous health education: A qualitative study in Australia and New Zealand. Higher Education, 75(2), 255–270.

Devito, J.A., 2021. The interpersonal communication book, 16th ed. Pearson, Boston.

Dwyer, J., O'Donnell, K., Willis, E., et al., 2018. Equitable care for Indigenous people: Every health service can do it. Asia Pacific Journal of Health Management, 11(3),11–17.

Eckermann, A., Dowd, T., Chong, E., et al., 2010. Binaŋ Goonj: Bridging cultures in Aboriginal health, 3rd ed. Elsevier, Sydney.

Egan, G., Reese R.J., 2019. The skilled helper: A problem management and opportunity approach to helping, 11th ed. Cengage, Boston MA.

El Amouri, A., O'Neill, S., 2014. Leadership style and culturally competent care: Nurse leaders' views of their practice in the multicultural care settings of the United Arab Emirates. Contemporary Nurse, 48(2), 135–149.

Finset, A., 2018. Among the topics of this issue: Health literacy and interpreter-mediated communication. Patient Education and Counseling, 101(1), 1.

Gilligan, C., Outram, S., Buchanan, H., 2019. Communicating with people from culturally and linguistically diverse backgrounds. In: Levett-Jones, T. (ed.), Critical conversations for patient safety, 2nd ed. Pearson, Sydney.

Haddad, A.M., Purtilo, R.B., Doherty, R.F., 2019. Health professional and patient interaction, 9th ed. Elsevier/Saunders, St Louis, MO.

Hall, M.B., Guidry, J.J., McKyer, E.L.J., et al., 2014. Association analysis of reported attitudes and culturally competent behavior engagement among public health employees. Journal of Health Disparities Research and Practice, 7(3), 15–24.

Hampton, R., 2013. Communication for working with Indigenous Australian. In: Hampton, R., Toombs, M. (eds), Indigenous Australians and health: The wombat in the room. Oxford University Press, Melbourne.

Harms, L., Pierce, J., 2019. Working with people: Communication skills for reflective practice, 2nd Canadian ed. Oxford University Press, Ontario.

Hasnain, M., Connell, K.J., Menon, U., et al., 2011. Patient-centered care for Muslim women: Provider and patient perspectives. Journal of Women's Health, 20 (1), 73–82.

Henderson, A., 2019. Communication for health care practice. Oxford University Press, Melbourne.

Holland, K., 2018a. Culture, race and ethnicity: Exploring the concepts. In: Holland, K. (ed.), Cultural awareness in nursing and health care: An introductory text, 3rd ed. Routledge, New York.

Holland, K., 2018b. Cultural care: Knowledge and skills for implementation in practice. In: Holland, K. (ed.), Cultural awareness in nursing and health care: An introductory text, 3rd ed. Routledge, New York.

Holli, B.B., Beto, J.A., 2023. Nutrition counselling and education skills: A practical guide, 8th ed. Jones & Bartlett, Burlington, MA.

Holliday, A., Kullman, J., Hyde, M., 2021. Intercultural communication: An advanced resource book for students, 4th ed. Routledge, New York.

Honeycutt, A., Milliken, M.A., 2021. Understanding human behavior: A guide for healthcare providers, 10th ed. Cengage Learning, Boston.

Hughson, J-A., Marshall, F., Daly, J.O., et al., 2018. Health professionals' views on health literacy issues for culturally and linguistically diverse women in maternity care: Barriers, enablers and the need for an integrated approach. Australian Health Review, 42(1),10–20.

Indigenous Allied Health Australia, 2015. Cultural Effectiveness in action: An IAHA framework. Indigenous Allied Health Australia, Canberra.

Jacobson, J., 2022. Wisdom on the 3 Cs – Compassion, culture and Courage. American Journal of Tropical Medicine and Hygiene, 106(1), 10–11.

Jennings, W., Bond, C., Hill, P.S., 2018. The power of talk and power in talk: A systematic review of Indigenous narratives of culturally safe healthcare communication. Australian Journal of Primary Health, 24(2), 109–115.

Johnson, R., & Withers, M., 2018. Cultural competence in the emergency department: Clinicians as cultural learners. Emergency Medicine Australasia, 30, 845–856.

Kinébanian, A., Stomph, M., 2010. Diversity matters: Guiding principles on diversity and culture. World Federation of Occupational Therapists (WFOT), Amsterdam.

Levoy, B., 2014a. Culturally competent care. Chiropractic Economics 60(19), 25–27.

Levoy, B., 2014b. Does your practice provide culturally competent care? Podiatry Management, 33(3), 45–46.

Likupe, G., 2014. Communicating with older ethnic minority patients. Nursing Standard, 28(40), 37–43.

Liu, S., Volcic, Z., Gallois, C., 2023. Introducing intercultural communication: Global cultures and contexts, 4th ed. Sage, London.

McClimens, A., Brewster, J., Lewis, R., 2014. Recognising and respecting patients' cultural diversity. Nursing Standard, 28(28), 45–52.

Minnican, C., O'Toole, G., 2020. Exploring the incidence of culturally responsive communication in Australian healthcare: The first rapid review on this concept. BMC Health Services Research, 20(1), 1–14.

Mir, G., Meer, S., Cottrell, D., et al., 2015. Adapted behavioural activation for the treatment of depression in Muslims. Journal of Affective Disorders, 180, 190–199.

Mollah, T.N., Antoniades, J., Lafeer, F.I., et al., 2018. How do mental health practitioners operationalise cultural competency in everyday practice? A qualitative analysis. BMC Health Services Research, 18(1), 480.

National Health and Medical Research Council (NHMRC), 2006. Cultural competency in health: A guide for policy, partnerships and participation. Commonwealth of Australia, Canberra.

Noe, T.D., Kaufman, K.E., Kaufman, L.J., et al., 2014. Providing culturally competent services for American Indian and Alaska Native veterans to reduce health care disparities. American Journal of Public Health, 104(S4), S548–S554.

Nursing Council of New Zealand, 2011. Guidelines for cultural safety, the Treaty of Waitangi and Māori health in nursing education and practice. Nursing Council of New Zealand, Wellington.

Olaussen, S.J., Renzaho, A.M.N., 2016. Establishing components of cultural competence healthcare models to better cater for the needs of migrants with disability: A systematic review. Australian Journal of Primary Health, 22(2),100–112.

Olivares, M., Pena, C., 2014. Teaching health sciences students about culturally sensitive communication between health professionals and patients from diverse cultures. International Journal of Bilingual Education and Bilingualism, 18(1), 115–126.

Papps, E., Ramsden, I., 1996. Cultural safety in nursing: The NZ experience. International Journal of Quality Health Care 8, 491–497.

Parbury, N., Lamberton, K., 2006. Survival: A history of Aboriginal life in NSW, 2nd ed. Ministry of Aboriginal Affairs, Sydney.

Passi, N., 2018. Looking forward, looking back: An Indigenous trainee perspective. Emergency Medicine Australasia 30, 862–863.

Paternotte, E., van Dulmen, S., van der Lee, N., et al., 2015. Review: Factors influencing intercultural doctor–patient communication: A realist review. Patient Education and Counseling, 98 (4), 420–445.

Queensland Health, 2010. Five cross cultural capabilities for clinical staff. Division of the Chief Health Officer, Brisbane, Queensland.

Ramos, R., Davis, J.L., Antolino, P., et al., 2014. Language and communication services: A cancer centre perspective. Diversity and Equality in Health and Care, 11(1), 71–80.

Ramsden, I., 2002. Cultural safety and nursing education in Aotearoa and Te Waipounamu. New Zealand Council of Nursing, Auckland.

Ramsden, I., 2001. Defining cultural safety and transcultural nursing. Nursing New Zealand, 7(1), 21–26.

Rorie, S., 2015. Using medical interpreters to provide culturally competent care. AORN Journal, 101(2), 7–9.

Smith, K., Fatima, Y., Knight, S., 2017. Are primary healthcare services culturally appropriate for Aboriginal people? Findings from a remote community. Australian Journal of Primary Health, 23(3), 236–242.

Stein-Parbury, J., 2021. Patient and person: Interpersonal skills in nursing, 7th ed. Churchill Livingstone Elsevier, Sydney.

Taylor, A., 2017. Getting it right: Culturally safe approaches to health partnership work in low to middle income countries. Nurse Education in Practice, 24, 49–54.

Truong, M., Gibbs, L., Paradies, Y., et al., 2017a. "Just treat everybody with respect": Health service providers' perspectives on the role of cultural competence in community health service provision. ABNF (Association of Black Nursing Faculty) Journal, 28(2) 34–43.

Truong, M., Gibbs, L., Paradies, Y., et al., 2017b. Cultural competence in the community health context: "We don't have to reinvent the wheel". Australian Journal of Primary Health, 23(4), 342.

UNESCO, 2002. Universal declaration on cultural diversity. UNESCO, Paris.

Verderber, K.S., MacGeorge, E.L., 2015. Inter-Act. Interpersonal communication: Concepts, skills and contexts, 14th ed. Oxford University Press, New York.

Victorson, D., Banas, J., Smith, J., et al., 2014. eSalud: Designing and implementing culturally competent ehealth research with Latino patient populations. American Journal of Public Health, 104(12), 2259–2265.

Ward, A., Mandrusiak, A., Levett-Jones, T., 2018. Cultural empathy in physiotherapy students: A pre-test post-test study utilising virtual simulation. Physiotherapy, 104(2018), 453–461.

Watt, K., Abbott, P., Reath, J., 2016. Cross-cultural training of general practitioner registrars: How does it happen? Australian Journal of Primary Health, 22(4), 349–353.

Watts, K.J., Meiser, B., Zilliacus, E., et al., 2018. Perspectives of oncology nurses and oncologists regarding barriers to working with patients from a minority background: Systemic issues and working with interpreters. European Journal of Cancer Care, 27(2), 1–8.

Wells, S.A., Black, R.M, Gupta, J., 2016. Culture and occupation: Effectiveness for occupational therapy practice, education and research, 3rd ed. AOTA Press, Bethesda, MD.

Wilcock, A.A., Hocking, C., 2015. An occupational perspective of health, 3rd ed. Slack, Thorofare, NJ.

World Health Organization (WHO), 2018. Human Rights. Online. Available at: www.who.int/news-room/fact-sheets/detail/human-rights-and-health

Xiao, L.D., Willis, E., Harrington, A., et al., 2018. Improving socially constructed cross-cultural communication in aged care homes: A critical perspective. Nursing Inquiry, 25(1), 11.

Zendedel, R., Schouten, B.C., van Weert, J.C.M., et al., 2018. Informal interpreting in general practice: Are interpreters' roles related to perceived control, trust and satisfaction? Patient Education and Counselling, 101(2018), 1058–1065.

Ziaian, T., Xiao, L.D., 2015. Cultural diversity health care. In: Fedoruk, M., Hofmeyer, A. (eds), Becoming a nurse: An evidence-based approach, 2nd ed. Oxford, Melbourne.

CHAPTER 17

Healthcare professionals communicating with Indigenous Peoples

Chapter objectives

Upon completing this chapter, readers should be able to:

- employ the four Rs – Remember, Reflect, Recognise and Respond – to achieve reconciliation and respect for empowering all interactions with Indigenous Peoples
- appreciate the importance of using terms appropriately when communicating with Indigenous Peoples
- apply the general principles of effective communication when communicating with Indigenous Peoples
- analyse and recognise the importance of cultural identity in communication
- reflect upon the relevance of pre-contact and post-contact history for Indigenous Peoples
- appreciate and synthesise the factors affecting the establishment of cultural safety when working with Indigenous Peoples
- apply specific communication principles relevant to Indigenous Peoples
- recognise potential barriers to effective communication when communicating with Indigenous Peoples.

NOTE: The use of Indigenous Peoples throughout this chapter is not intended to offend, but rather to be inclusive of all original inhabitants of lands.

ADDITIONAL NOTE: It is not possible to be an expert in all cultural ways of living. The author as a non-Indigenous Person is far from being an expert, nor is this chapter able to make experts of all readers, whether or not they have an Indigenous background. However, it can begin the exploration of communicating with and empowering Indigenous communities who may have "ways of doing and being" that differ from those of the healthcare professional.

This chapter will potentially begin the journey for some and continue it for others in understanding and embracing the communication needs of Person/s who were the original inhabitants of a region or country, that is, **First Nations** or **Indigenous Peoples**.

Indigenous communities are typically community-based, with the community rather than the individual forming the basis of their society. Therefore, for this chapter the overarching goal of communication will be to achieve Family/Community-centred goals and Care. This means that the model underpinning effective communication in this chapter is a Community-centred model rather than a Person-centred model.

Correct use of terms

History and inappropriate attitudes dominate relationships with Indigenous groups around the world (Edmondson 2022). This often means that non-Indigenous colonists and their descendants demonstrate attitudes and use discriminatory and offensive terms to refer to Indigenous Peoples. Therefore, it is important for healthcare professionals to avoid causing offence by ensuring they understand and use the appropriate, current terms when relating to Indigenous Peoples. While this is not always true in many countries, in Australia the terms used evolve continually when describing Aboriginal and Torres Strait Islander Peoples (Cultural Capability Enablers' Network [CCEN] 2016; NSW Ministry of Health 2019; Queensland Health 2010). This provides a challenge for every Australian healthcare professional to know the most current terms, as the appropriate use of terms is essential for the development of trust, therapeutic relationships and Family/Community-centred goals and Care. Using the current terms also contributes to positive experiences contributing to Indigenous Peoples continuing to seek care from health services.

Suggest ways a healthcare professional might ensure appropriate use of terms to avoid offending Indigenous Person/s when communicating with them.

The 4 Rs for reconciliation: Remember, Reflect, Recognise, Respond

Indigenous Allied Health Australia (IAHA) has suggested four relevant words and related actions beginning with "R" to assist anyone relating to Indigenous Peoples. These words suggest considered thought and, in some instances, actions, to assist healthcare professionals in any country interacting with Indigenous Peoples. R*emember*, R*eflect*, R*ecognise* and R*espond* challenges any healthcare professional when communicating with any individual; however, they are particularly important concepts when assisting Indigenous Peoples.

Remember

As mentioned above, the events of history around the world when Indigenous Peoples were assumed to be inferior (often based upon stereotypical attitudes) meant that they experienced removal from their language, culture and land; disempowerment and death (Biles 2018; Tomas 2018). In many countries, including Australia, children were forcibly removed from their families, in order to teach them the ways of the settlers and to deconstruct their cultural identity. These events were justified by thoughts that it was in the best interest of the Indigenous Peoples.

These events are not only regrettable, but also in many cases have created challenging and often continuing unacceptable situations for Indigenous Peoples (Hampton & Toombs 2013; Passi 2018; Schramm & Walter 2022). The reality of these events has resulted in substandard conditions and major health disparities for many Indigenous peoples throughout the world (Bainbridge et al 2015; Edmondson 2022; Sherwood 2018). It is important to remember and reflect upon these events, not to create a sense of guilt, but rather a sense of understanding and awareness of the historical realities (Dudgeon et al 2014; Saggers et al 2011). These events continue to affect many Indigenous Peoples in the present as they attempt to relate to health services (Eckermann et al 2012; Ewan & McCoy 2011; Jennings et al 2018; Lovett 2018).

Reflect

Remembering is vital; however, without critical reflection (producing change in attitude and behaviour) it can be futile (Gerlach 2015). Reflection about these events produces understanding and the ability to demonstrate respect and empathy in order to develop trust and a collaborative therapeutic relationship. Respect (unconditional positive regard for all) is an essential underlying element of healthcare (Minnican & O'Toole 2020) and it is mandatory when assisting Aboriginal and Torres Strait Islander Peoples (CCEN 2016; Crowden 2013). It ensures satisfying, culturally appropriate and safe care, producing positive outcomes. This can take time when assisting Indigenous Peoples (Crowden 2013; Eckermann et al 2012). As these characteristics of care (respect, empathy and trust) affect the final outcomes of the health service, it is vital that healthcare professionals reflect upon these historical events. It is sobering to note that there are still people alive in some countries who remember the violence/death experienced by Indigenous Peoples (Australia being one such country). It is equally sobering to realise some Indigenous Peoples in some communities continue to experience this disparity, prejudice and violence today. In Australia, the continuing health statistics are a constant reminder of this reality (Abbott et al 2014; Australian Institute of Health and Welfare (AIHW) 2015; 2023, Chapman et al 2014; Durey et al 2011; Hornosty et al 2017; Hunt et al 2015; Walker et al 2014).

- Remember the events of history (typically including violence and death, separation from land, family and lifestyle, discrimination and so forth) relating to the Indigenous Peoples in your country.
- How do you think you and your family would have responded if you had been in their place?

Given that you would have had limited methods of resisting:

- How would you feel if you had been separated from your family and sent away?
- How would you feel if you were forced to do menial labour with minimal rewards or pay?
- How do you think the Indigenous Peoples in your country felt?

It is also essential to reflect about personal worldviews, biases and values to ensure demonstration of genuine respect and empathy (Paul & McKivett 2022; see Chapters 7 and 8).

Recognise

The events of history in many countries have radically reduced the number of Indigenous Peoples. However, for the generations who remain, it is important to recognise the resilience of

Indigenous Peoples. This characteristic produced people who were originally well adapted to and thrived in their often-severe environments. In the present, it produces people who attempt various ways not only to survive but also to thrive in their current situations.

Respond

An appropriate response requires constant **collaborative** and culturally safe care reflecting equality and true reconciliation (Ramsden 2001). This care requires time and perseverance to establish mutual understanding, beginning with consistently demonstrating respect, and a therapeutic relationship (Eckermann et al 2012; Hampton 2013). It requires humility (understanding personal and system biases to develop and maintain respectful processes to develop mutual trust) and a willingness to learn about both language (effective cross-cultural communication) and "ways of doing" (see Chapter 16). Remembering, reflecting and recognising potentially promote responses to enable and enhance the characteristics discussed in Section 1 of this book. These characteristics are essential in healthcare professionals committed to Person/Family-centred Care and often in the case of Indigenous Peoples, Community-centred care.

There is no definitive formula for relating to Indigenous Peoples; however, the four Rs provide a foundation for any healthcare professional relating to Indigenous communities. Recognition, reflection, respect and application of the overarching purpose of healthcare professionals when communicating will "build upon" these Rs and assist in achieving effective communication and positive outcomes (Alford et al 2014).

There are also specific principles that are useful in all communicative circumstances and will therefore be beneficial when communicating with Indigenous Peoples. Before exploring these principles, it is important to consider the reality of cultural identity.

The complexity of cultural identity

Cultural identity is complex because each individual is a member of many different groups with a unique culture affecting their cultural identity. In each of these groups, every individual has a particular identity that is unique to that group (Anngela-Cole et al 2010; Hampton & Toombs 2013; Holliday et al 2021; see Chapter 16). The **nationality** of the individual provides a particular cultural identity, including values, traditions, beliefs (including health beliefs) and expectations (of self and others) specific to that **nation**. Membership of other groups – families, clans (in New Zealand *iwi* = tribe and *hapū* = subtribe), communities, sporting groups, religious groups, educational groups, employment groups and political groups – creates additional aspects of cultural identities that relate to and affect the national and/or cultural identity of each person. Membership of each group provides a connection through common experiences and expectations unique to the group. However, each member has a different, unique identity (see Chapter 16).

List the groups of which you are a member. Choose two of these groups:

- How has membership of each group shaped how you view yourself?
- How has membership of these groups affected how others view you?
- How has membership of these groups affected what you expect of others?

People with Indigenous descent also have unique identities reflecting their original ethnicity, group or nation. Their connection to the values, beliefs, traditions and expectations of that group influences their cultural identity and their appreciation of that identity. Levels of identity and connection vary for many Indigenous People. If an individual has lived their entire life with their **kinship group** at a traditional birthplace, their cultural identity will strongly reflect their particular group. Traditional knowledge and customs will guide their daily life. If an individual was separated from their birthplace and kinship group at some point, their cultural identity may reflect other influences in combination with the influence of their ethnic or national origin. An Indigenous Person/s who lives in a large metropolis may or may not take pride in their cultural identity. They may have only vague expectations of adhering to cultural traditions and customs, although they may acknowledge particular spiritual and relational values and beliefs.

In Australia, there are over 250 Aboriginal and Torres Strait Islander nations with differing cultures and languages. However, common core values are shared throughout the country. These values include family and kinship (a collective identity), caring and sharing (maintaining harmony), and a spiritual connection with and love of the land (Country). While **Māori** have less variation in their distinctive groups, they share a sense of connection to space and belonging. This is reflected in *Tūrangawaewae* – a place to stand, a place to belong to, a seat or location of identity.

In most countries there is a broad range of connection with and adherence to traditions among Indigenous Peoples. In Australia, for example, many rural Aboriginal and Torres Strait Islander Peoples have replaced walking with horses or motorised forms of transport. However, the same people continue to value the land (Country), along with their traditional ceremonies and singing (Smith 2016). In New Zealand, many Māori have absorbed "ways" from the dominating culture of the colonists. However, they still believe in and use traditional remedies to augment or replace the healthcare practices of the dominant culture. In the Pacific, various Indigenous Peoples may use modern equipment to fulfil the traditional occupation of fishing. However, the same people continue to make traditional mats for use in their houses and for particular ceremonies. In many places in Asia, Indigenous Peoples use mobile phones to communicate, but still plough their fields using buffalo. In many places in Northern Canada, the skidoo has replaced the traditional use of the dog sled for transport and sometimes even hunting. However, the same people still create unique clothing, reflecting membership of their particular kinship group (Christian 2014). It is important to remember that the culture of all Indigenous Peoples is neither static nor uniform. Each culture and individual within that culture is continually changing and adapting to the influences upon themselves or upon their community (Crowden 2013; Johnson & Withers 2018; see Chapter 16).

The complexity of cultural identity indicates that it is important for healthcare professionals to recognise the factors affecting that identity. It is also essential for healthcare professionals to acknowledge the variations within Indigenous Peoples, thereby prohibiting the stereotypical labelling of any individual because of their ethnicity or nationality. Aboriginal and Torres Strait Islander Peoples clearly exemplify this fact, as they are two distinct groupings, with multiple subgroups. The Torres Strait Islander Peoples have an origin, culture and identity distinct from the many Aboriginal nations originating on the mainland and Tasmania. These many Aboriginal groups also have languages, cultures and identities that are distinct from each other and from those of the various groups of Torres Strait Islander Peoples.

There is a long history of stereotyping many Indigenous Peoples, dating from the arrival of Europeans in most colonised countries. Indigenous Peoples may also stereotype non-Indigenous people and sometimes even other Indigenous individuals or groups. It is the responsibility of the healthcare professional to consider their own tendency to stereotype and adjust their knowledge and attitudes to avoid stereotyping any Indigenous Person/s. It is also important that the healthcare professional behaves to reduce the tendency of some Indigenous Peoples to negatively stereotype non-Indigenous healthcare professionals (Chapman et al 2014; CCEN 2016; Eckermann et al 2012; Hunt et al 2015). Healthcare professionals must base their care on respect, empathy and trust, in order to achieve satisfying and positive outcomes when delivering healthcare. This is essential when working with Indigenous Peoples.

Principles of care for healthcare professionals when working with Indigenous Peoples

Creating culturally responsive interactions and cultural safely for Indigenous Peoples

Understanding the concept of cultural safety is essential when relating to Indigenous Peoples from any country. Healthcare respecting, supporting and empowering the cultural identity and wellbeing of an individual produces cultural safety (Kaunihera Manapou Paramedic Council 2020; Nursing Council of New Zealand 2011). Such care is more than mere awareness or sensitivity; it mandates attitudes of equality and collaboration with the **Indigenous community** (Lowell 2013; Tomas 2018). It allows the Indigenous community to have power when receiving healthcare interventions – it is Community-centred care. It values their opinion (Barnett & Kendall 2011). It recognises their unique endocrinology, along with their unique biological functioning and their ideas of health and wellbeing (Podham et al 2019). It also requires action resulting from critical reflection about the personal values of the healthcare professional (DiGiacomo et al 2010; Gerlach 2015; Stein-Parbury 2021) and evaluation of their personal attitudes and beliefs (Australian Health Practitioner Regulatory Agency (Ahpra) & National Boards 2022; Kaunihera Manapou Paramedic Council 2020; Paramedicine Board of Australia (Ahpra) 2021; see Chapters 6, 7 and 8). It requires the healthcare professional to **acknowledge** and **accept** that their own values and beliefs may be different to those of the Indigenous Person/s they assist in their daily care (Eckermann et al 2012; Supreme Court of Queensland 2016).

This acknowledgement and acceptance should assist the healthcare professional to avoid discriminating and imposing their own values onto the Indigenous Person/s. Culturally safe healthcare also requires awareness of and reflection about the culture and values of the particular health service (Alvarez et al 2014; Noe et al 2014; Walker et al 2014). It is important that the healthcare professional evaluates how their values, attitudes and beliefs and those of the relevant health service affect the Indigenous Person/s they assist in their daily practice.

It is equally important for healthcare professionals to evaluate the quality and outcomes of the assistance Indigenous Person/s receive from their health service. Such evaluation requires awareness and appreciation of the perceptions and lives of Indigenous Person/s, their kinship groups and communities. These perceptions develop while receiving assistance, whether past or present, and should contribute to any evaluation of a health service. The histories of the relationship of Indigenous Person/s with the Europeans who have colonised their country also affect these perceptions. The result of such reflection and evaluation should result in the achievement of cultural safety (equal sharing and collaboration in the healthcare process) for Indigenous Person/s because of adjustments and improvements in the health service and the care of the healthcare professional.

In contrast, lack of cultural safety exists when any individual behaves in a manner that challenges, denies, diminishes, demeans or disempowers the cultural identity and wellbeing of any individual within a health service (Nursing Council of New Zealand 2011).

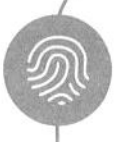

- What actions or words demean or deny your identity?
- How do you feel when this happens?
- What might you do to avoid doing this to an Indigenous Person/s?

Emilia is a 5-year-old Australian girl with blonde hair and blue eyes who has come to you for assistance. You have developed a good relationship, based on respect, trust and rapport, with her mother, Jill. Your assessment of Emilia indicates that choice of school will be significant and could affect her learning and therefore her future.

Her mother feels safe and comfortable with you and discusses the pros and cons of the local schools with you. She indicates that one school, a distance away, has extra funding for children with an Indigenous background. You are unsure of the meaning of this comment – you have not noticed any indication of heritage on Emilia's record or file and the appearance of Jill and her three children suggest there is no Indigenous background. You assume Jill is concerned that if Emilia attends that school she will not have the assistance she requires because of the presence of an Indigenous cohort. You say it would not be good for Emilia to experience reverse discrimination because of her ethnicity (i.e. to miss out because she does not have an Indigenous background).

Jill bristles and coldly explains that her mother was taken from her family post-contact with Europeans (one of the stolen generation) and thus Jill did not know until recently she had an Aboriginal heritage. She states a family that was discriminatory against people with her background raised her mother, and so she now has to adjust to the fact that she is one of the people about whom she previously thought negatively. While her husband, who she married before she discovered this fact, says it makes no difference to him, she struggles to establish her cultural identity, often avoiding disclosing her heritage. This makes her reticent to place Emilia, despite her eligibility, at the school that has specific funding for children with an Aboriginal background.

You are generally an accepting person and have good friends with Indigenous backgrounds. You regret your assumptions and offensive comment. You are aware that you could have been assisting Jill to resolve her struggle, experience acceptance and establish her cultural identity.

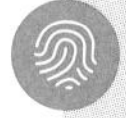

- What could you have done to ensure cultural safety for Jill and her three children?
- What will you do now to retrieve the relationship and encourage her to continue bringing Emilia for assistance?

Note: When treating children it is essential that the healthcare professional assist the *family*, not just the individual child, because it is the context of the family that typically dominates the development of the child. In addition, it is the parents who know the child better than anyone and are invaluable in providing a true picture of the child and their abilities. When working with Indigenous Peoples, it is important to involve the *community* in the interventions, to assist the *community* in managing the illness or disease.

There are several factors contributing to the creation of equality in collaborative healthcare relationships. These result in cultural safety and thus positive and satisfying outcomes for Indigenous Peoples. These require examination.

The importance of history

As mentioned above, the awareness and understanding of pre- and post-contact history is a factor contributing to the creation of cultural safety and thus positive outcomes (Jennings et al 2018; Smith et al 2017). For many Indigenous Peoples (particularly those who are older), it is highly significant because historical factors have created negative perceptions and mistrust of non-Indigenous or **mainstream** healthcare systems (Australian Government Department of Health 2022). Thus, pre- and post-contact history requires close consideration.

Pre-contact history

Before contact with Europeans, many Indigenous groups in various places around the world existed in harmony with their spiritual and physical environments, and in varying levels of harmony with each other for generations upon generations. Each group had its own traditional languages; culture; specific identity, including dress, artefacts, spiritual explanation of their existence; rules of behaviour, including expectations of the individual and the group, kinship rules, remedies, methods of artistic expression, methods of providing food and water, and laws governing their daily lives. The groups (although rarely hierarchical in Australia) had designated leaders or groups of members who understood and protected their values, traditions and laws. As protectors of these values, traditions and laws, these leaders had particular levels of wisdom and understanding and thus were often the decision-makers for the group and the individuals within the group.

In Australia pre-contact, there were around 300 distinct groups of Aboriginal and Torres Strait Islander Peoples with their own language, culture, identity, kinship rules, boundaries and laws for relating to other groups (Australian Government Department of Health 2022). Aboriginal groups had inhabited Australia for approximately 60 000 years pre-contact. These groups did not always relate well to each other and some still experience tension today.

In New Zealand pre-contact, there was one Māori language. However, more than one group existed and these groups did not always experience harmonious relations. The Māori inhabited New Zealand for approximately 300 years before the arrival of Europeans. While there was a treaty (*te Tiriti O Waitangi: The Treaty of Waitangi*) in 1840 between the Māori and particular non-Indigenous People, that treaty was not ratified by the non-Indigenous colonial government of the time. This meant that the rights of the Māori were not recognised, although it became impossible to ignore their organised existence. This resulted in post-contact stress, leading to inequality today.

Post-contact history

In many cases, when European contact occurred with the Indigenous Peoples of a region or country, the Indigenous groups were not structured or organised in ways recognisable to the non-Indigenous People. In many places in Australia, "contact" resulted in violence and devastation through loss of access to their traditional food sources (Eckermann et al 2012), while introducing diseases or from deliberate attempts to kill and/or control these groups. This control often placed members of "non-compatible" groups together in reserves or missions. Lack of understanding, multiple incorrect assumptions and misplaced social theories by non-Indigenous People post-contact often resulted in histories establishing negative expectations in the minds of the affected Indigenous Peoples. For example, in Australia there was deliberate segregation in society that also occurred in hospitals. Hospital staff often placed Aboriginal and Torres Strait Islander Peoples on the verandah or in unneeded areas of the hospital to keep them separate from non-Indigenous People. Many older Aboriginal and Torres Strait Islander Peoples still remember such actions, thereby contributing to current negative expectations of health services. These expectations continue in many places today because of continued discriminatory attitudes and behaviour by many non-Indigenous People within health services. In some sectors of Australian society, however, there has been a slow awakening and recognition of the social, emotional, spiritual and cultural damage caused post-contact to Aboriginal and Torres Strait Islander Peoples. In New Zealand, there has been a similar awakening reflected in the *Treaty of Waitangi Act* 1975, which recognises the effects of colonisation on the Māori.

Knowledge and understanding of pre-contact and post-contact history is important in the creation of culturally appropriate healthcare. However, genuine Remembering and Reflection creating synthesis of the history, Recognising and producing an appropriate Response (including awareness of the personal bias and stereotypes of the healthcare professional) to this history are all essential when communicating with Indigenous Peoples.

Other factors

Many factors affect feelings of safety; some of these factors relate to cultural differences. Some have greater impact on healthcare than others, but all are significant in the creation of culturally appropriate and effective care.

- It is important to understand that communication styles vary (regardless of ethnic background!) For example, the use of eye contact for some Aboriginal and Torres Strait Islander Peoples and for Māori (Metge & Kinloch 1978) can be a sign of disrespect rather than a sign of attentive listening. Others may avoid eye contact if they feel uncomfortable from being made conspicuous or embarrassed or ashamed or if they feel they are being patronised. Some will not look at an individual of the opposite gender. Some Indigenous Peoples may feel it is unnecessary to answer a question when the answer is obvious. Some may also consider it impolite to answer a question immediately, and thus they will pause before answering a question. The use of direct questions in some cultures (not just Indigenous cultures) is rude and thus when requesting personal information it is best to ask open or indirect questions (see Chapter 4). For some, direct questioning creates fear and discomfort from feelings of interrogation (Hampton 2013; Lowell et al 2012). In many cases, telling a story of someone with a particular difficulty (similar to that of the particular individual) may elicit information about the needs of the Person/s. It is important to accept and accommodate differences in communication style wherever possible.

In groups, choose a condition relevant to your health profession.

- Together construct a story of a Person with symptoms and difficulties typical of the chosen condition.
- Have one person read the story to the group – adjust the details as necessary.
- Consider how this story might encourage someone to identify their symptoms and difficulties.

- It is important to understand that many Indigenous Peoples define the *notion of family* differently to non-Indigenous People. For example, in an Indigenous context Aboriginal and Torres Strait Islander Peoples, Māori and many Pacific Islanders may call and consider someone a brother, sister, uncle or auntie when, if related, there is only a distant relationship, or if they are from the same birth location. In some Indigenous groups, a community Elder may have an important place within a family group, regardless of biological connection.
- Equally important is understanding that there are differences in *concepts of spirituality* among Indigenous Peoples. They may consider their spiritual needs more important than their physical status (Waran et al 2016). For many, spirituality includes a special relationship with the land or with nature. It may relate to a responsibility to ensure harmony/balance between physical and spiritual realms (Crowden 2013). It is possible for each Indigenous Person to have unique spiritual requirements that are integral to the provision of healthcare, whether the requirements are related to a special custom or the expectation of particular behaviour when someone is ill. For example, a particular person in the "family" is expected and expects to care for a relative with a life-limiting illness. This person may consider caring for this relative to be more important than employment, and thus if they are unable to continue working while caring for this ill person they will resign from their employment without a second thought.
- It is important to understand that *kinship obligations* (for Māori reflected in the concept of *whanaungatanga*, an obligation of giving and receiving) may result in large numbers of people either visiting or accompanying the Person/s. Accommodating this factor may mean provision of a particular area or room for the Indigenous Peoples accompanying the Person/s. Expectations of particular behaviour may also relate to kinship obligations and mutual reciprocity (Crowden 2013). For example, when a mother is ill among the Aboriginal and Torres Strait Islander Peoples, most often the eldest daughter expects to fulfil the role of carer.
- Also important is the reality that Indigenous Peoples experience *differences in life circumstances*, family histories, community and social determinants of health. Many Indigenous Peoples live in imposed poverty with living conditions that a non-Indigenous Person would not tolerate. Therefore, many Indigenous Peoples experience diseases related to poverty. Life expectancy may be shortened in many Indigenous communities, with general levels of health below the average for the non-Indigenous population (Abbott et al 2014; Australian Institute of Health and Welfare [AIHW] 2023; Hunt et al 2015; Nielsen et al 2014). For example, in Australia, the Yawuru people of the West Kimberley country (Western Australia) commonly experience a premature death of one of the members of the community, often on a weekly basis (ANTaR 2007). Aboriginal and Torres Strait Islander Peoples typically have life expectancies that are 20 years less than those of the total Australian population, while Indigenous Peoples in Canada typically have life expectancies that are between 5 and 14 years less than those of the Canadian population (Hornosty et al 2017). In Australia, the death rates in the 35–54-year age group are five to six times higher than in the general population (AIHW 2015). Such health-related facts exist for many Indigenous Peoples (see ANTar.org.au). Māori also experience differences in health-related statistics (Durie 2007; Ministry of Health (NZ) 2018). (For facts relating to Māori, see Ministry of Health (NZ) 2018; Durie 2007). These facts often result in unresolved grief and a sense of loss, for both the past and present, in Indigenous communities. Recognition of this reality is important for the creation of equality to empower collaboration in therapeutic relationships.
- It is important to remember that Indigenous Peoples will *react differently to people and the healthcare environment*. Some Indigenous Peoples find it difficult to seek assistance, or to continue to

seek assistance, because of factors, such as separation from the people in their communal group; arrangement of the environment and rooms in health services and thus restrictions on particular types of behaviour; and unfamiliar people who apparently do not understand or want to understand their customs and often their previous experiences with health services. These realities can affect the creation of culturally appropriate and effective healthcare.

- Any person with a different cultural background will be affected by differences in *education and language*. For many rural and remote Indigenous Peoples, English is a second, third or sometimes fourth language, and thus they may require an interpreter (see Chapter 16), preferably from an organisation dedicated to that particular Indigenous group. If there is no known organisation dedicated to the appropriate Indigenous group, it is essential to remember that the Indigenous Person/s will have their own sociolinguistic and sociocultural expectations affecting the interaction (Bowe et al 2014; Eckermann et al 2012; Hampton 2013). It is also important to note that many Indigenous Peoples have their own dialect of the language of the non-Indigenous colonists. In Australia, many Aboriginal and Torres Strait Islander Peoples have a particular dialect of English that is in many cases a significant part of their cultural identity. The use of their own dialect without an interpreter may contribute to pauses of varying lengths as the Person/s silently translates the message into their dialect to facilitate their understanding, thereby attempting to avoid misunderstandings. Acceptance of variations in the dialects of English may be important for creating cultural safety.
- Understanding that Indigenous Peoples may have *different attitudes, understanding and approaches to illness*, health, death and disability contributes to establishing culturally appropriate and effective care. Some Indigenous groups in Asia believe particular disabilities are a punishment for wrong behaviour, thus disability brings shame. Generally, in such cultures it is unacceptable for individuals with disabilities to relate in public. Some Indigenous groups in the Pacific and Australia attribute disease and death to sorcery or curses rather than biomedical causes. It is interesting to note that the word "health" may not always have a direct equivalent in some languages of Indigenous Peoples. For Aboriginal and Torres Strait Islander Peoples, "health" is often about **wellbeing**. Wellbeing is not related to illness, but rather to connection with and harmony within kinship groups and, for many, connection with traditions and the land.
- For many Indigenous Peoples, having a *same-gender healthcare professional* to assist them contributes to their sense of safety and wellbeing. In many cases, the Indigenous Person/s may not attend repeat appointments if they have a healthcare professional of the opposite gender assisting them.
- Establishing cultural safety for Indigenous Peoples requires an understanding that *different values*, and *"ways of doing and caring"* in rural and remote areas may result in behaviours that seem foreign and sometimes unacceptable to the values and ways of the non-Indigenous healthcare professional. These ways of caring have been practised for thousands of years, and, if accepted and creatively accommodated, can produce culturally effective care and safety, thereby removing reluctance to access non-Indigenous health services.
- Another cultural difference affecting equal collaboration and cultural safety is *traditional methods of managing illness and death* (Healing Forum UNSW 2014). Such methods are often foreign to non-Indigenous healthcare professionals. However, inclusion of such practice in the care of Indigenous Peoples (e.g. the use of traditional healers and foods) can contribute to their spiritual, emotional, psychological, social and often physical comfort.
- The impact of the *imbalance of power* in the relationship between the healthcare professional and the Indigenous Person/s is a crucial factor affecting the creation of culturally responsive

communication and effective healthcare. This imbalance occurs even when there is no cultural difference, because of the greater familiarity of the healthcare professional with the health system and the particular health profession. When assisting Indigenous Peoples, however, this imbalance is heightened in some cases because of the social, economic and educational advantage of the healthcare professional. In many countries, previous government policies relating to Indigenous Peoples have influenced the expectation of a power imbalance from the perspective of Indigenous Peoples. This, in turn, influences (often limiting) the potential development of equality, collaboration and empowerment within therapeutic relationships and thus the creation of cultural safety. It is important that the healthcare professional behaves in a manner that respects and accommodates, thereby earning respect in return. In some instances the healthcare professional may need to advocate for cultural differences in order to create a collaborative balance of power rather than a dominating one.

- Appropriate *training* in understanding cultural differences for all staff in a health service may contribute to achieving culturally relevant and appropriate healthcare. However, it is the application of this training that produces both safety and competence.
- *Investing* time to learn about cultural differences and discovering ways to accommodate these differences and include them in practice will contribute to culturally responsive communication, healthcare and therefore positive outcomes.
- Avoid making assumptions about the community and the people within the community, as every individual is unique with particular ways of expressing their culture (Johnson & Withers 2018; Strobel et al 2019). Critical self-awareness is essential to avoid such assumptions (see Chapters 7 and 8).

All of the above factors affect the creation of cultural safety for Indigenous Peoples. They require consideration and accommodation when providing health services for Indigenous Peoples from both the Southern and Northern Hemispheres. These factors provide a foundation for the principles guiding the care of a healthcare professional when assisting Person/s with Indigenous backgrounds.

Identify which of the above factors affecting feelings of cultural safety you feel are most important to you.

In groups of four, divide the **factors** affecting feelings of cultural safety among the large group to ensure consideration of all the listed factors.

- Suggest ways that an individual healthcare professional might accommodate each factor.
- Suggest ways that your health profession or health service might accommodate each factor.
- Suggest ways that you or your health profession might advocate for accommodating each factor in healthcare.

Factors contributing to culturally responsive communication with Indigenous Peoples

Many of the factors contributing to the creation of cultural safety also influence the achievement of effective communication with Indigenous Peoples. However, the following factors relate *specifically* to communication with Indigenous Peoples.

- The direct and confident "professional" manner encouraged in non-Indigenous healthcare professionals may be offensive to some Indigenous Peoples, especially when discussing sensitive information. In such situations, *a softly spoken, informal manner* is more appropriate. An established relationship (this may take time) based on respect, trust and rapport encourages effective communication with Indigenous Peoples.

- When receiving a referral to see a Person/s with an Indigenous background, it is important to consider the *correct people to approach or to include* if providing important information about the future of the Person/s. Include all appropriate people in discussions about the intervention plan and where appropriate the discharge plan. As mentioned, when a mother is ill it is often the eldest daughter who needs to know the medication or intervention regimen, not the Person herself. It may be important to approach a **local Elder** (*Kaumātua* [male] or *Kuia* [female] Māori Elder) before initiating contact, or have an Elder present when discussing future intervention or discharge (Renhard et al 2015).
- Establish how to *contact the local community Elder or relevant organisation* connected specifically with the cultural background of the Person/s. Establish communication links with the specialist organisation, either at an institutional level or a personal level, depending on the situation. Seek the advice or direct involvement of an Indigenous Health Worker as they are trained specifically to liaise between the Person/s and the healthcare professional to ensure understanding and to accommodate the communication and cultural needs of the Person/s to promote quality healthcare. The Indigenous Health Worker, while trained in health, is typically a member of the community in which they work and thus has "first-hand" experience and understanding of the cultural expectations of the Person/s. They also know who should be involved and how to engage the Person/s and relevant services.
- *Avoid making assumptions* based on appearance, living conditions, people present, and commitment to traditional beliefs and customs.
- Remember the person who is entitled to give *consent* may not be present despite the presence of a close relative.
- Use an Indigenous Health Worker or Medical Liaison Officer from the *particular Indigenous group* if communicating complex information or bad news (Crowden 2013). Isaacs and colleagues (2010) and Millis and colleagues (2010) state that collaboration is a key factor of successful communication opportunities with Indigenous Peoples. Clarify with the interpreter before the discussion the appropriate terms for particular concepts. For example, "death" and "dying" are words that may not be used in some Indigenous communities.
- Using *Open communication* to embrace differing communication styles contributes to culturally safe and effective communication. It is important to avoid imposing any particular values, expectations or ways of performing tasks onto the Indigenous Person/s. It is also important to avoid correcting the spoken expression of Indigenous Peoples, including children, because this indicates lack of acceptance of their particular dialect and a desire to impose the use of the dialect of the healthcare professional.
- *Explore the cultural background* of the Person/s or family and community. Ask the Indigenous Health Worker for information about specific *communication behaviours* and relevant *cultural needs*. Accommodate these differences where possible. Explain the requirements of the health service and remain open to possible ways of complying with these requirements while accommodating the cultural needs of the Person/s or community.
- Sometimes the *questions* asked by healthcare professionals are *offensive* to an Indigenous Person/s because of the nature of the questions or the gender of the person asking the questions. If direct questions are not a feature of their communication style, they may find them intimidating (Hampton 2013). In addition, questions may appear *silly* if the answers seem obvious. It is important for healthcare professionals to state the need to ask many questions

in an apologetic, concerned manner. *Explain* that everyone seeking assistance from this health service usually answers these questions and the information will not affect their access to services. Reassure them of *privacy* and *confidentiality* of the collected information.

- *LISTEN.* Skills in listening are essential when communicating; however, many Indigenous Peoples feel that non-Indigenous People do not take the time to listen (Harms & Pierce 2019; Renhard et al 2015). This reality may originate in the different uses of silence and questions/answers in some Indigenous cultures.
- Consider using a method of providing information that will maximise understanding. Many Indigenous cultures use *storytelling* as a means of sharing information. Storytelling is part of the cultural identity of many Indigenous Peoples (Biles 2018). Using a story about a person with a particular condition or difficulty may allow the Indigenous Person/s to understand the requirements of the healthcare professional or to recognise their own condition and related needs. For example, telling a story about someone with diabetes and their experience of the relevant intervention may allow the Indigenous Person/s to see they too have diabetes and to understand how to control that condition.
- Allow sufficient *time for processing of information.* **Verify** understanding of the given information and seek clarification where required about that information from an Indigenous member of staff or individual from the relevant Indigenous organisation (Australian Government Department of Health 2014). Remember some Indigenous Peoples may be translating the information into their own dialect or language and thus may require longer to process information.
- *Invest time to establish trust* and a therapeutic relationship with the Person/s and the members of the community who care for them. This may take longer than expected depending on the previous experience of the Person/s with healthcare professionals. Many Indigenous Peoples are accustomed to non-Indigenous people talking and filling the silences (Harms & Pierce 2019; Metge & Kinloch 1978). Therefore, establishing a relationship may require investment of time to sit quietly and listen, or simply sit. Learning some of their language or particular, relevant terms can assist in developing trust (Hampton 2013).
- Provide *time for discussion* and explanation during all stages of the healthcare process. Where possible, include an Indigenous Health Worker or Medical Liaison Officer of the same cultural background for any discussion.
- *Observe* and *validate non-verbal cues.* Where direct questions are not the cultural norm, express a possible interpretation of the non-verbal cues and wait for a response. For example, if an Indigenous Person/s has their eyes averted or head turned away, the healthcare professional might ask a specific question in a non-confronting, non-patronising manner. For example, *I can see you are not happy (frightened, etc); Are you feeling pain?* This manner of questioning validates their feelings and allows them to feel and agree or disagree with the assumption. For some Indigenous Peoples, however, if the healthcare professional has made the correct assumption about the cause of the non-verbal cues they will not answer because the answer seems obvious. Remember non-verbal cues may have particular meanings that are different from the understanding of the healthcare professional.
- *Silence* has a particular role in many Indigenous communities. It is a positive element of communication facilitating learning about a person through thought and observation. Silence is an acceptable part of communicating. It allows time for a person to process information, "feeling" those around them and understanding the environment.
- Indigenous Peoples may *communicate discomfort through silence* and this has particular implications for a healthcare professional. The silence may indicate physical pain. However, it

may also indicate that it is inappropriate to respond to particular questions or comments from an individual of the opposite gender. As mentioned, silence may also represent translation time.

- *Lack of response* may possibly indicate an inability to physically hear the message and this requires particular action on the part of the healthcare professional.
- Some may respond with a nod, which while indicating they hear you, may not indicate understanding. They may feel it is impolite to ask questions and thus they do not pursue mutual understanding (Hampton 2013).
- Some may respond with "yes" for every question. If this occurs it is important to explore the understanding of the Person/s. Whether or not they are understanding, they may feel "yes" is the expected answer to all questions. Skilful use of a trained Indigenous Health Worker or Medical Liaison Officer may assist in gathering reliable information.

In a group:

- decide which of the above factors affecting communication are least familiar to you.
- choose the five least familiar factors to the group and decide how a healthcare professional might accommodate each factor.

Barriers to culturally responsive and effective communication

Many Indigenous Peoples have experiences suggesting most non-Indigenous healthcare professionals have limited knowledge of or lack of interest in Indigenous cultures, and are generally not interested in accommodating Indigenous cultures (Bailie et al 2010). These experiences often result in Indigenous Peoples avoiding seeking healthcare from non-Indigenous healthcare professionals and health services. They may also result in the Indigenous Person/s not returning for repeat visits.

The following are causes of **culturally unsafe communication** by healthcare professionals. They were identified by Indigenous Peoples as providing barriers to effective communication.

- The presence of *stereotypes* and preconceptions may govern the behaviour of both the healthcare professional and the Indigenous Person/s. These occur when the healthcare professional fails to identify and change their often unconscious personal biases, prejudices and stereotypes (Strobel et al 2019). For example, assuming an Indigenous Person presenting to the emergency department with slurred speech is drunk – is not appropriate – they may be experiencing potentially life-threatening symptoms of specific undiagnosed disorders, including but not limited to diabetes.
- Failure to establish a *sense of equality and collaboration* within the healthcare process, making cultural safety impossible.
- Failure to explore the *actual meaning of words or behaviours*, because words may have a different meaning for the Indigenous Person/s. For a non-Indigenous Person, "home" may mean a house, but for an Indigenous Person/s they are at home when they are with their kinship group, whether or not that group is in a house. Failure to explore the meaning of words can limit communication in the same way that failure to explore the meaning of particular behaviour can limit communication. For example, exploration of the meaning of silence, averted

head and/or eyes, non-attendance, repeated attendance after discharge, or failure to complete the required at-home tasks may assist the healthcare professional to provide appropriate assistance and develop rapport. This could be done using a "story" presenting the reactions of a similar Person/s to explore meaning of reactions. If unsure, consult the Indigenous Health Worker.
- Failure to *understand* that some Indigenous Peoples provide the answer they think the healthcare professional desires. Indigenous Peoples may do this because they do not understand the request or because of multiple repeats of the same question by different healthcare professionals.
- Failure to *develop trust* and overcome any previous negative experiences with health services.
- Failure to *listen* patiently and quietly.
- Failure to *observe and explore non-verbal behaviours* in a culturally appropriate, sensitive and effective manner.
- Failure to *clarify understanding.*
- Responses that are **clichés** or automatic and therefore do not acknowledge the language and/or cultural needs and differences between the Indigenous Person/s and the non-Indigenous healthcare professional.
- Use of *inappropriate pamphlets or written information.* Using written information with visual images and no jargon or technical terms is important when communicating with most people seeking assistance, and especially with Indigenous Peoples. The use of pictures related to Indigenous Peoples can be reassuring and clarifying. It is important to seek the advice of Indigenous Health Workers or Medical Liaison Officers when preparing any written information for Indigenous Peoples.

Chapter summary

Many factors affect communication with Indigenous Peoples. These factors arise from history and prejudice, in combination with separate and shared experiences of Indigenous Peoples and often non-Indigenous People. It is important that healthcare professionals consider the relevant factors when communicating with Indigenous Peoples to ensure effective communication, culturally responsive and effective healthcare, along with Family/Community-centred Care.

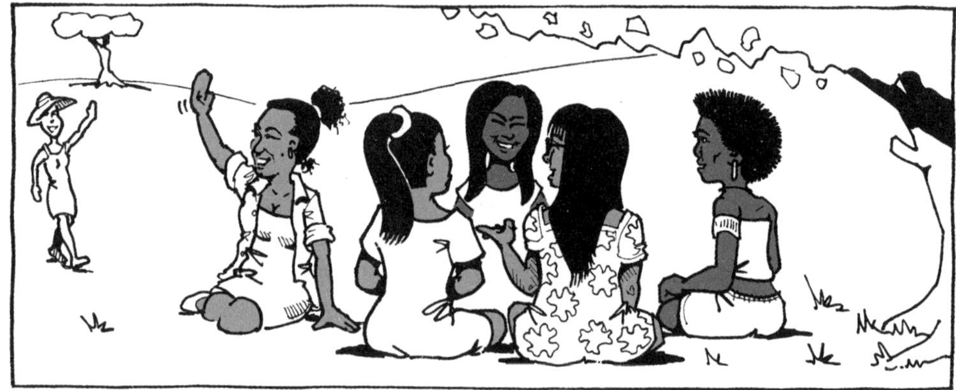

FIGURE 17.1
Equality produces positive results.
Courtesy Roger Harvey © Elsevier Australia.

REVIEW QUESTIONS

1. What is the purpose of using appropriate terms to describe their groups when relating to Indigenous Peoples?

____

____

____

2. Explain why each individual has a unique cultural identity.

____

____

____

3. How can I achieve cultural safety with Indigenous Peoples?

____

____

____

4. List the five main steps creating culturally safe care when working with Indigenous Peoples.

   i. ______________________________

   ii. ______________________________

   iii. ______________________________

   iv. ______________________________

   v. ______________________________

5. Identify eight factors affecting the creation of culturally responsive and effective communication for Indigenous Peoples. Give original examples of how a healthcare professional might *accommodate each of these factors* while delivering healthcare.

   i. ______________________________

   ii. ______________________________

   iii. ______________________________

iv. ____

v. ____

vi. ____

vii. ____

viii. ____

6. Choose and explain 10 factors contributing to the creation of culturally responsive and effective communication for Indigenous Peoples. Give examples of ways of communicating that will create effective communication with Indigenous Peoples.

i. ____

____

ii. ____

____

iii. ____

____

iv. ____

____

v. ____

____

vi. ____

____

vii. ____

____

viii. ____

____

ix. ____

x. ____

7. List seven barriers to the creation of culturally responsive and effective communication.

   i. ____

   ii. ____

   iii. ____

   iv. ____

   v. ____

   vi. ____

   vii. ____

8. Describe how a healthcare professional might overcome at least four of the barriers to culturally responsive and effective communication.

   i. ____

   ii. ____

   iii. ____

   iv. ____

References

Abbott, P., Dave, D., Gordon, E., et al., 2014. What do GPs need to work more effectively with Aboriginal patients? Views of Aboriginal cultural mentors and health workers. Australian Family Physician, 43(1/2), 58–63.

Alford, V., Remedios, L., Ewen, S., et al., 2014. Communication in Indigenous healthcare: Extending the discourse into the physiotherapy domain. Journal of Physiotherapy, 60, 63–65.

Alvarez, K., Marroquin, Y.A., Sandoval, L., et al., 2014. Integrated health care best practices and culturally and linguistically competent care: Practitioner perspectives. Journal of Mental Health Counseling, 36(2), 99–114.

Anngela-Cole, L., Ka'Opua, L., Busch, M., 2010. Issues confronting social workers in the provision of palliative care services in the Pacific Basin (Hawai'i and the US-affiliated Pacific Island nations and territories). Journal of Social Work in End-of-Life and Palliative Care, 6(3/4), 150–163.

ANTaR: Australians for Native Title and Reconciliation, 2007. Liyarn Ngarn (feature film with Patrick Dodson, Peter Postlethwaite, Archie Roach and Shane Howard). ANTaR, Australia.

Australian Government Department of Health 2022. National Aboriginal and Torres Strait Islander health workforce strategic framework and implementation plan 2021–2031. Commonwealth of Australia Department of Health, Canberra, Australia.

Australian Health Practitioner Regulatory Agency (Ahpra) & National Boards, 2022. Code of Conduct. Author, Melbourne, Australia.

Australian Institute of Health and Welfare (AIHW), 2015. The health and welfare of Australia's Aboriginal and Torres Strait Islander Peoples. Commonwealth of Australia, Canberra.

Australian Institute of Health and Welfare (AIHW), 2023. Aboriginal and Torres Strait Islander health performance framework (HPF) report. Commonwealth of Australia, Canberra. www.indigenoushpf.gov.au.

Bailie, R., Si, D., Shannon, C., et al., 2010. Study protocol: National research partnership to improve primary health care performance and outcomes for Indigenous peoples. BMC Health Services Research, 10(1), 129–141.

Bainbridge, R., McCalman, J., Clifford, A., et al., 2015. Cultural competency in the delivery of health services for Indigenous people. AIHW, Canberra, Australia.

Barnett, L., Kendall, E., 2011. Culturally appropriate methods for enhancing the participation of Aboriginal Australians in health-promoting programs. Health Promotion Journal of Australia 22(1), 27–32.

Biles, K., 2018. Strengthening relationships: We all need a place to call home. Emergency Medicine Australasia, 30, 857–858.

Bowe, H., Martin, K., Manns, H., 2014. Communication across cultures: Mutual understanding in a global world, 2nd ed. Cambridge University Press, Melbourne.

Chapman, R., Smith, T., Martin, C., 2014. Qualitative exploration of the perceived barriers and enablers to Aboriginal and Torres Strait Islander people accessing healthcare through one Victorian Emergency Department. Contemporary Nurse: A Journal for the Australian Nursing Profession, 48(1), 48–58.

Christian, K.E., 2014. The Diabetes One-Stop: An Off-the-Road Person-Centered Care Model. Beginnings (American Holistic Nurses' Association), 34(6), 6–9.

Crowden, A., 2013. Ethics and indigenous health care: Cultural competencies, protocols and integrity. In: Hampton, R., Toombs, M. (eds), Indigenous Australians and health: The wombat in the room. Oxford University Press, Melbourne.

Cultural Capability Enablers' Network (CCEN), 2016. Aboriginal and Torres Strait Islander cultural capability: Respectful language guide. CCEN, Brisbane, Australia

DiGiacomo, M., Davidson, P.M., Taylor, K.P., et al., 2010. Health information system linkage and coordination are critical for increasing access to secondary prevention in Aboriginal health: A qualitative study. Quality in Primary Care, 18(1), 17–26.

Dudgeon, P., Wright, M., Paradies, Y., et al., 2014. Aboriginal social, cultural and historical context. In: Dudgeon, P., Milroy, H., Walker, R. (eds), Working together: Aboriginal and Torres Strait Islander Mental Health and wellbeing principles and practice, second ed. Australian Government Department of Health and Ageing, Canberra.

Durey, A., Thompson, S.C., Wood, M., 2011. Time to bring down the twin towers in poor Aboriginal hospital care: Addressing institutional racism and misunderstandings in communication. Internal Medicine Journal, 42, 17–22.

Durie, M., 2007. Hauora Tangata: Māori health status. In: Broom, D., Reed, B., Dew, K., et al. (ed.), Health in the Context of Aotearoa New Zealand. Oxford University Press, Melbourne.

Eckermann, A., Dowd, T., Chong, E., et al., 2012. Binaŋ Goonj: Bridging cultures in Aboriginal health, 3rd ed. Elsevier, Sydney.

Edmondson, W., 2022. Settler colonialism: black armband or white blindfold? In: Edmondson, W., Williams, R., (eds). Burda-burda balayi: Health professionals and Indigenous health. Oxford University Press, Melbourne.

Ewan, S., McCoy, B., 2011. The national apology: A new pathway forward? In: Thackrah, R., Scott, K. (eds), Indigenous Australian health and cultures: An introduction for health professionals. Pearson, Frenchs Forest.

Gerlach, A.J., 2015. Sharpening our critical edge: Occupational oherapy in the context of marginalised populations. Canadian Journal of Occupational Therapy, 82(4), 245–253.

Hampton, R., 2013. Communication for working with Indigenous Australian. In: Hampton, R., Toombs, M. (eds), Indigenous Australians and health: The wombat in the room. Oxford University Press, Melbourne.

Hampton, R., Toombs, M., 2013. Culture, identity and Indigenous Australian Peoples. In: Hampton, R., Toombs, M. (eds), Indigenous Australians and health: The wombat in the room. Oxford University Press, Melbourne.

Harms, L., Pierce, J., 2019. Working with people: Communication skills for reflective practice, 2nd Canadian ed. Oxford University Press, Ontario.

Healing Forum, UNSW., 2014. Mapu Yaan Gurri, Mapu Marrunggirr: Healing our way. Aboriginal Affairs NSW Government, Sydney.

Holliday, A., Kullman, J., Hyde, M., 2021. Intercultural communication: An advanced resource book for students, 4th ed. Routledge, New York.

Hornosty, J., Gray, D., & Saggers, S. 2017. Canada's Aboriginal Peoples and Health: The Perpetuation of Inequalities. In Germov, J. & Hornosty, J. (eds), Second Opinion: An Introduction to Health Sociology, 2nd Canadian ed. Oxford University Press, Canada.

Hunt, L., Ramjan, L., McDonald, G., et al., 2015. Nursing students' perspectives of the health and healthcare issues of Australian Indigenous people. Nurse Education Today, 35(3), 461–467.

Isaacs, A.N., Pyett, P., Oakley-Browne, M.A., et al., 2010. Barriers and facilitators to the utilisation of adult mental health services by Australia's Indigenous people: Seeking a way forward. International Journal of Mental Health Nursing, 19(2), 75–82.

Jennings, W., Bond, C., Hill, P.S., 2018. The power of talk and power in talk: A systematic review of Indigenous narratives of culturally safe healthcare communication. Australian Journal of Primary Health, 24(2), 109–115.

Johnson, R., & Withers, M., 2018. Cultural competence in the emergency department: Clinicians as cultural learners. Emergency Medicine Australasia, 30, 845–856.

Kaunihera Manapou Paramedic Council, 2020. Standards of cultural safety and clinical competence for paramedics. Kaunihera Manapou Paramedic Council, Wellington.

Lovett, R., 2018. A history of health services for Aboriginal and Torres Strait Islander people. In: Best, O., Fredericks, B. (eds), Yatdjuligin: Aboriginal and Torres Strait Islander nursing and midwifery care. Cambridge University Press, Melbourne.

Lowell, A., 2013. "From your own thinking you can't help us": Intercultural collaboration to address inequities in services for Indigenous Australians in response to the World Report on Disability. International Journal of Speech-Language Pathology, 15(1), 101–105.

Lowell, A., Maypilama, E., Yikaniwuy, S., et al., 2012. Hiding the story: Indigenous consumer concerns about communication related to chronic disease in one remote region of Australia. International Journal of Speech-Language Pathology, 14, 200–208.

Metge, J., Kinloch, P., 1978. Talking past each other: Problems of cross-cultural communication. Victoria University Press, Wellington.

Millis, J.E., Francis, K., Birks, M., et al., 2010. Registered nurses as members of interprofessional primary health care teams in remote or isolated areas of Queensland: Collaboration, communication and partnerships in practice. Journal of Interprofessional Care, 24(5), 587–596.

Ministry of Health (NZ), 2018. Position Paper on Māori Health Analytics – Age standardisation. Ministry of Health, Wellington.

Minnican, C., O'Toole, G., 2020. Exploring the incidence of culturally responsive communication in Australian healthcare: The first rapid review on this concept. BMC Health Services Research, 20(1), 1–14.

Nielsen, A.-M., Stuart, L.A., Gorman, D., 2014. Confronting the cultural challenge of the whiteness of nursing: Aboriginal registered nurses' perspectives. Contemporary Nurse: A Journal for the Australian Nursing Profession, 48(2), 190–196.

Noe, T.D., Kaufman, K.E., Kaufman, L.J., et al., 2014. Providing culturally competent services for American Indian and Alaska Native veterans to reduce health care disparities. American Journal of Public Health, 104(S4), S548–S554.

NSW Ministry of Health, 2019. Communicating positively: A guide to appropriate Aboriginal terminology. NSW Ministry of Health, Sydney.

Nursing Council of New Zealand, 2011. Guidelines to cultural safety, the treaty of Waitangi, and Māori health in nursing and midwifery education and practice. Nursing Council of New Zealand.

Paramedicine Board of Australia, (Ahpra), 2021. Professional capabilities for registered paramedics. Ahpra, Melbourne.

Passi, N., 2018. Looking forward, looking back: An Indigenous trainee perspective. Emergency Medicine Australasia, 30, 862–863.

Paul, D., McKivett, A., 2022. Becoming culturally capable: From student to practitioner and beyond. In: Edmondson, W., Williams, R., (eds). Burda-burda balayi: Health professionals and Indigenous health. Oxford University Press, Melbourne.

Podham, M., Charles, J., & Moses A., 2019. Aboriginal and Torres Strait Islander Peoples' endocrinology health and wellness. In: Biles B., Biles J., (eds), Aboriginal and Torres Strait Islander Peoples' health and wellbeing. Oxford University Press ANZ, Melbourne.

Queensland Health, 2010. Aboriginal and Torres Strait Islander cultural capability framework 2010–2033. Queensland Government, Brisbane.

Ramsden, I., 2001. Defining cultural safety and transcultural nursing. Nursing New Zealand 7(1), 21–26.

Renhard, R., Chong, A., Willis, J., et al., 2015. Aboriginal and Torres Strait Islander Quality Improvement Framework and Toolkit for Hospital Staff (AQIFTHS), St Vincent's Hospital, Melbourne.

Saggers, S., Walter, M., Gray, D., 2011. Culture, history and health. In: Thackrah, R., Scott, K. (eds), Indigenous Australian health and cultures. Pearson, Frenchs Forest.

Schramm, T., Walter, M., 2022. Understanding Indigenous health and well-being: Policy and data sovereignty. In Edmondson, W., Williams, R., (eds). Burda-burda balayi: Health professionals and Indigenous health. Oxford University Press, Melbourne.

Sherwood, J., 2018. Historical and current perspectives of the health of Aboriginal and Torres Strait Islander people. In: Best, O., Fredericks, B. (eds), Yatdjuligin: Aboriginal and Torres Strait Islander nursing and midwifery care. Cambridge University Press, Melbourne.

Smith, J.D., 2016. Australia's rural, remote and indigenous health, 3rd ed. Elsevier, Sydney.

Smith, K., Fatima, Y., Knight, S., 2017. Are primary healthcare services culturally appropriate for Aboriginal people? Findings from a remote community. Australian Journal of Primary Health, 23(3), 236–242.

Stein-Parbury, J., 2021. Patient and person: Interpersonal skills in nursing, 7th ed. Churchill Livingstone Elsevier, Sydney.

Strobel, N., McAully, D., Sim, M., et al., 2019. Communicating with Aboriginal and Torres Strait Islander Peoples. In: Levett-Jones, T. (ed.), Critical conversations for patient safety: An essential guide for healthcare students, 2nd ed. Pearson Education, Sydney.

Supreme Court of Queensland, 2016. Equal treatment bench book, 2nd ed. Supreme Court of Queensland, Brisbane.

Tomas, I., 2018. Equity for Indigenous peoples in the emergency department: A Māori perspective. Emergency Medicine Australasia 20, 859–861.

Walker, B.F., Stomski, N.J., Price, A., et al., 2014. Perspectives of Indigenous people in the Pilbara about the delivery of healthcare services. Australian Health Review, 38(1), 93–98.

Waran, E., O'Connor, N., Zubair, M.Y. et al., 2016. "Finishing up" on country: Challenges and compromises. Internal Medicine Journal, 46(9), 1108–1111.

Further reading

Best, O., Fredericks, B. (eds), 2021.Yatdjuligin: Aboriginal and Torres Strait Islander nursing and midwifery care, 3rd ed. Cambridge University Press, Melbourne.

Ellis, R., Simms, S. (eds), 2009. The Indigenous health promotion resources guide: A national information guide for Aboriginal and Torres Strait Islander health workers, 6th ed. Aboriginal and Islander Health Worker Journal, Matraville.

Hazlehurst, K.M., 1996. A healing place: Indigenous visions for personal empowerment and community recovery. Central Queensland University Press, Rockhampton.

Mawson, S., 2021. The deep past of pre-colonial Australia. The Historical Journal, 64(5), 1477–1499.

Milroy, H., Dudgeon, P., Walker, R. (eds), 2014. Working together: Aboriginal and Torres Strait Islander mental health and wellbeing principles and practice. Australian Government Department of Prime Minister and Cabinet, Canberra.

National Public Health Partnership, 2005. Healthy children – strengthening promotions and prevention across Australia: national public health strategic framework for children 2005–2008. Australian Government Department of Health and Aged Care, Canberra.

NSW Department of Community Services, 2009. Working with Aboriginal people and communities: A practical resource. Sydney. Online. Available: www.community.nsw.gov.au.

Social Health Reference Group for National Aboriginal and Torres Strait Islanders, 2004. Social and emotional wellbeing framework for Aboriginal and Torres Strait Islander Peoples' mental health and social emotional wellbeing: 2004–2009. Australian Government Department of Health and Ageing, Canberra.

Thackrah, R., Scott, K. (eds), 2011. Indigenous Australian health and cultures: An introduction for health professionals. Pearson Education, Melbourne.

Websites and organisations

NOTE: These largely Australian websites have been found to be useful and reliable. Many of these associations or organisations also represent the equivalent health profession in New Zealand, as there is currently no related association there.

Australian Indigenous Doctors Association (AIDA). www.aida.org.au

Australian Indigenous Psychologists Association (AIPA). www.indigenouspsychology.com.au

Australian Institute of Aboriginal and Torres Strait Islander Studies. www.aiatsis.gov.au

Congress of Aboriginal and Torres Strait Islander Nurses and Midwives (CATSINaM). catsinam.org.au/

Indigenous Allied Health Australia (IAHA). https://iaha.com.au

Indigenous Dentists Association of Australia (IDAA). www.atns.net.au/reference.asp?RefID=2879

National Aboriginal and Torres Strait Islander Health Worker Association (NATSIHWA): www.natsihwa.org.au/

Useful and reliable information relevant to health professionals in various countries

New Zealand www.atns.net.au/glossary.asp: An Agreement in Principle or Heads of Agreement (AIP/HA) is an agreement entered into between the Crown and a claimant group that is part of the process for the historical settlement of grievances under the Treaty of Waitangi (1840) (extended definition).

A site relevant to communication and the health law in New Zealand can be found on the Health and Disability Commissioner website: www.hdc.org.nz/

A relevant New Zealand site relating to privacy and confidentiality can be found on the Privacy Commissioner website – www.privacy.org.nz. See: Your responsibilties/Your privacy responsibilties.

National Centre for Truth and Reconciliation (Canada) – nctr.ca/

National Collaborating Centre for Indigenous Health (Canada) – www.nccih.ca/en/

First Nations and Inuit Health and Wellness Indicators – health-infobase.canada.ca/fnih

CHAPTER 18

Misunderstandings and communication for the healthcare professional

Chapter objectives

Upon completing this chapter, readers should be able to:

- define and explain a misunderstanding
- explain the factors contributing to understanding
- describe some possible causes of misunderstandings
- develop useful strategies to reduce misunderstandings
- explain the steps for effectively resolving misunderstandings.

Communication that produces misunderstandings

All healthcare professionals must learn to manage communicative interactions when there is a failure to achieve mutual understanding about words or events (Henderson 2019; Morgan 2013). In such cases they must respond in a reasonable and calm manner (Holli & Beto 2023), even though interactions involving misunderstandings can cause discomfort and frustration (Greenberg & Weingarten 2015; Wachterman et al 2015). Both the healthcare professional and the Person/s may experience negative emotions because of misunderstandings. Misunderstandings may produce feelings of anxiety and regret, and, if serious enough, feelings of guilt or unfair judgement. Guilt, while a self-defeating emotion, is a typical reaction if lack of care on the part of the healthcare professional causes a miscommunication. However, the healthcare professional may feel misjudged if incorrectly blamed for a misunderstanding. Collaboration can avoid and resolve misunderstandings (Greenberg & Weingarten 2015). When experiencing misunderstandings, it is essential to remember the characteristics of effective communication and Person-centred Care.

It is interesting to note that communicating with care and the best intentions does not guarantee understanding (Bowe et al 2014). This indicates that the healthcare professional should avoid assuming the Person/s comprehends the message (Griffey et al 2015). The perspective of the Person/s may affect the interpretation of a message. For example, assisting someone after observing them struggling to complete a task may produce anger rather than expressions of thanks if the Person/s was intent on proving they could independently complete the task. Conversely, not assisting a struggling Person/s may also elicit anger. A means of avoiding such situations is to use a question or gesture designed to establish the desire or lack of desire for assistance. Similarly, if the Person/s expects a particular intervention that is outside the role of the health professional, this may cause miscommunication, indicating the needs for immediate clarification. Misunderstandings decrease levels of trust, therefore potentially severely affecting the therapeutic relationship. This has implications for the healthcare professional, the Person/s and the ultimate outcome of their healthcare (Greenberg & Weingarten 2015; Morgan 2013; Moss 2020; Wachterman et al 2015).

Consider a time when you experienced a misunderstanding.

- What was the cause of the misunderstanding?
- Were you the person who failed to communicate clearly or were you the person who failed to clarify the meaning?
- What were the consequences?
- How did you feel?
- Did you feel tempted to blame the other person?
- What could you have done to avoid the misunderstanding?
- What did you learn from this experience?
- What will you do next time to avoid a misunderstanding?

It is clear that a misunderstanding might generate negative emotions, but the various factors contributing to misunderstandings are not always clear. However, it is important to explore and understand the various factors potentially affecting mutual understanding in an attempt to prevent misunderstandings.

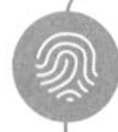

Consider your health profession and its role in various settings.

- How might you ensure the Person/s understand the role of your health profession in the different settings?

In groups of people from your health profession, discuss the ideas of group members relating to explaining the role of your profession in various settings. Agree on how to avoid misunderstandings relating to your role in that setting.

- How might you ensure the public understands the general role of your profession?
- How might you ensure the public understands its specific role in particular settings?

Factors affecting mutual understanding

Many factors affect the ability of communicating individuals to achieve mutual understanding. Some of these factors include language, word usage, making assumptions about meaning, the context, differing expectations and desires, the presence of strong emotions and/or pain, along with the time invested in or available to negotiate meaning. The possibility of misunderstanding increases if communicating individuals come from different cultural backgrounds. However, misunderstandings may also occur between individuals from the same cultural groupings (Rosen 2014).

Mutual understanding increases, although it is not guaranteed, if the interacting individuals can communicate competently in a common language. Understanding is enhanced when individuals share the same meanings for particular words. In many languages, sounds, intonation and/or words can carry multiple meanings (Harms & Pierce 2019; Nunan 2012). Difficulties can arise if one person does not know the various meanings of a particular word (see Chapter 1) and thus does not recognise the meaning of that word in a particular context. Lack of word recognition prevents understanding. This limited recognition can make it difficult to understand the sound or word in an unfamiliar context. This may occur with the use of professional jargon, commonly used healthcare abbreviations (For example OT can have different meanings to different people in particular contexts: operating theatre; occupational therapy; occupational therapist; off topic; overtime; out of town or old testament), technical words or very long monologues. This may also occur when communicating with a person for whom the language of the interaction is their second, third or fourth language (Bensing et al 2010).

Mutual understanding is also influenced by assumptions individuals make about meaning. Assumptions can develop because of experience, knowledge and understanding of the situation and context. The probability of achieving mutual understanding may be decreased if some of the individuals communicating are unfamiliar with the context of the communication, or they communicate outside the expectations of the context (Davies et al 2014; Nunan 2012).

Mutual understanding can also be influenced by differing expectations and desires. In the modern world of accessible health information and increasing health literacy using technology (see Chapter 22), the Person/s may have particular expectations or desires that differ from those of the healthcare professional (Greenberg & Weingarten 2015). Strong emotions may accompany these expectations. Unless managed appropriately, they may become negative emotions. This can produce both frustration and conflict, sometimes requiring expert assistance or particular communication strategies to achieve mutual understanding. These strategies include taking time to listen and explore the expectations without judgement. They also require calm explanation of the expectations of the healthcare professional with a willingness, where appropriate, to implement the expectations of the Person/s or to establish a compromise to ensure safety and quality of life.

Give examples of each of these seven factors that could produce miscommunication: culture, language, word usage, assumptions about meaning, expectations of the Person/s, strong emotions /pain, and the context of the health profession and/or of the words.

Of the factors limiting the achievement of mutual understanding, it is necessary to consider which of these are relevant to the health professions. Healthcare professionals relate regularly to individuals from different cultures (see Chapter 16). Misunderstandings between people from different cultures may occur because of strong emotions and expectations, as well as the meaning of particular behaviours and words (Strobel et al 2019). Openness, willingness to learn about variations in communication styles, understanding and acceptance of the variations, will assist those communicating to achieve mutual understanding. It is the responsibility of the healthcare professional to demonstrate openness and acceptance because of the vulnerability of the Person/s. This will therefore enhance the therapeutic relationship and ultimate outcome of the care (Rosen 2014).

Among healthcare professionals there is not always a common language. A healthcare professional from a particular profession may use jargon that a healthcare professional from a different profession might struggle to understand. For example, someone working in medical radiation science may not understand the terminology used by someone working in occupational rehabilitation. Or someone working in palliative care may not understand the terminology used by someone from the same profession working in the area of workplace health and safety. Individuals seeking assistance relating to their health, even when they speak the local language, may not understand any health-specific jargon or abbreviations. In such cases, if they are unable to recognise a particular word in the healthcare context, they may misinterpret the meaning. The individual struggling to understand a word will often assume the meaning if they feel uncomfortable about asking for clarification. Similarly, some Aboriginal and Torres Strait Islander Peoples will not express an inability to understand because experience tells them the healthcare professional will not listen (Eckermann et al 2010; Lowell et al 2015; Passi 2018). In all situations the healthcare professional has responsibility to negotiate mutual understanding. However, if misunderstandings do occur it is important that the healthcare professional takes responsibility to repair the misunderstanding, regardless of the cause. Misunderstandings occur wherever people interact (Henderson 2019; Morgan 2013), thus the healthcare professional will benefit from carefully considering such events and their causes to understand the causes and how to avoid them in the future.

Causes of misunderstandings

The factors affecting mutual understanding – culture, language, word meanings, assumed meanings and context – can also contribute to misunderstandings. There are additional factors potentially causing misunderstandings, however, and these are examined in this section.

Attitudes

Misunderstandings can occur because of the negative attitudes or assumptions of the interacting individuals. Non-verbal communication of judgemental attitudes may assume greater strength from the perspective of the Person/s than is actually intended by the healthcare professional (Levine & Ambady 2013). The negative emotions associated with these attitudes can create barriers resulting in misunderstandings. It is important that the healthcare professional, through reflection and critical self-awareness, fosters an attitude of openness and acceptance towards individuals who might not meet their criteria of what is acceptable. For example, vulnerable individuals from a different culture must experience an accepting, open attitude from the healthcare professional, regardless of the language they speak and their potentially differing values and/or habits. It is important that an attitude of respect, empathy and inclusion (Mendes 2020; NSW Ministry of Health 2019), as well as an attitude that focuses on the goals of the vulnerable individual saturates every encounter between the healthcare professional and the Person/s. Healthcare professionals with such underlying attitudes will automatically communicate to explore meaning and avoid misunderstandings.

It is difficult to control the attitudes of those around the healthcare professional. However, maintaining a positive and accepting attitude can influence the attitudes of others. A healthcare professional with an appropriate attitude will positively affect the Person/s, contributing to avoidance of misunderstandings and achievement of mutual understanding and satisfying outcomes (Greenberg & Weingarten 2015; Morgan 2013; Wachterman et al 2015).

Emotions

Emotions can both positively and negatively influence the outcome of communication. Emotions may be expressed non-verbally (Li & Mao 2015). It is usually possible to perceive feelings of frustration, intolerance, impatience and anger in another person, and such emotions can significantly compromise communication (Allen 2021). Unresolved emotions – whether in the healthcare professional or the Person/s – can negatively affect any communicative interaction. Failure to give adequate attention to emotions both before and during interactions can cause misunderstandings. When attempting to repair or resolve a misunderstanding, it is important for the healthcare professional to dedicate time for appropriate consideration of the emotions causing the misunderstanding.

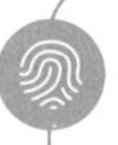

Consider an interaction in which your negative emotions and/or pain limited your ability to concentrate or understand. Perhaps you reacted emotionally to something that was said and were unable to hear the rest of the conversation, resulting in misunderstanding.

- How might you control any negative emotional responses when communicating while providing healthcare?

Relevance of context to determine the content of the message and meaning

The use of context to determine meaning varies from culture to culture, and this cultural variation can cause misunderstandings. Some cultures use verbal and non-verbal messages to construct meaning, while other cultures construct meaning using a combination of these messages as well as context. In such cultures, the circumstances (including the unique cultural and familial circumstances of the interacting people) or events that form the various environments (see Chapter 12) within which the communication occurs is the context. In these cultures the context may have greater weight than the verbal or non-verbal messages. In cultures that use context to affect meaning, the speaker, their role, their manner of communicating and their relationship to the listener(s) combine to influence the meaning; the actual words spoken may contribute only a small amount to the meaning of the message. Context is always a component of meaning – with it sometimes changing the meaning of particular words. In circumstances where the type of context changes, it is essential to focus on those aspects of the message that affect the meaning of the message and either repeat the message or ask for clarification of the meaning of the message to avoid misunderstandings. Communicating in an emergency requires explicit messages with the receivers often repeating them to ensure understanding and appropriate actions. This context requires particular message content and a particular style of communication to avoid misunderstandings. Effective communication in this context is essential, affecting intervention outcomes and potentially life or death. In contrast, communication within other less urgent healthcare settings often focuses on the needs of the Person/s – thereby affecting the therapeutic relationship. Time to consider and fulfil these needs ultimately affects quality of life, not merely life or death. In these settings there is often time to respond to various messages and/or information.

- What is important when relating to a Person/s who uses context (assumed information from their culture and family) to affect meaning?
- Should the healthcare professional adjust their manner of communicating when interacting with these Person/s? Explain why or why not.

Expectations of styles of communication

Styles of communication vary across cultures, families and situations. This reality rarely requires consideration unless communicating with individuals who expect a different style (Li & Mao 2015). Some cultures expect information to be organised in particular ways, with the major points clearly expressed first (more direct). Others seem to avoid the major point initially, only reaching it after extensive circular discussion (indirect) (Bowe et al 2014). Thus confusion may result between individuals from cultures that organise information in different ways.

Another style of communicating relates to the tolerance of **ambiguity** (Bowe et al 2014). This tolerance is higher in people who have a tendency towards an indirect style of communication. Some cultures, societies and families communicate through implied meaning – one person suggests an implied perception of a concept or idea and another then implies similar or alternative perceptions. This style of communicating is difficult to grasp if it is not the style of the culture of the healthcare professional. However, while to a novice this style appears circular and difficult to follow, the communicators are typically able to achieve mutual understanding. In contrast, a less ambiguous style of communicating involves explicit statement of points and exploration of these points. The words used to communicate directly reflect the meaning. In this style, unless there is an unconscious agenda, the communicators say exactly what they think, feel and desire. Some cultures and families use both implicit and explicit (some call them ambiguous and clear) styles of communicating, depending on the circumstances. The healthcare professional does not necessarily need to adjust their style to that of their communication partner. However, it is important to understand that the Person/s may experience more comfort, being more able to comprehend, if the language style of the healthcare professional is similar to their style (Li & Mao 2015). It may be beneficial to explain the style of the healthcare professional and to be aware of the style of the Person/s, acknowledge their style and explicitly explore the differences between the styles, using examples. This may reduce the possibility of misunderstandings.

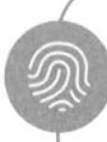

- How could direct and indirect communication styles influence understanding in the practice of the healthcare professional?
- How could the healthcare professional compensate for either style?

- Decide what style of communication your culture uses – an implicit style, explicit style or combination of both.
- Give examples of each style. State the conditions and the type of subject regulating the use of each style.
- Suggest how the healthcare professional might accommodate a different style, without insisting upon using their preferred style while interacting.

Expectations of the event or procedure

The expectations an individual might have of a health service will influence their understanding within that service. For example, if a Person/s expects to receive something that will immediately remove their symptoms, it may be distressing to learn they must have further investigations. It is important that healthcare professionals clearly explain their service and the expected steps in, results of, and reasons for particular procedures and events (see Chapters 3, 16 and 17). In particular situations, it may be important to explore the possible outcomes, if any, of not administering a particular procedure. The vulnerable Person/s may not understand the situation or the procedures well enough to know which questions to ask. Therefore, it is the responsibility of the healthcare professional to explain rather than assume the Person/s knows how, why/why not or when something might occur along with what will happen during any event. For example, everyone involved in a family conference should understand the purpose of and the usual process employed during a family conference. This allows the Person/s to clarify their expectations and/or to demonstrate their understanding of the procedure. Clear explanations will assist in avoiding misunderstandings due to particular expectations.

- List the characteristics of a clear explanation.
- Choose one of the following health service contexts: emergency, acute, rehabilitation, community, palliative care, health promotion, occupational rehabilitation or private practice.
- Write a clear explanation of the context and the kinds of "events" typically occurring in that context.

Expectations governed by cultural norms

Every culture and society, and most families, have norms affecting communicative behaviours. Such norms govern what is said, when and how (non-verbal and verbal messages) it is said according to particular situations. Lack of understanding of or familiarity with cultural norms can cause miscommunication (Buettgen & Gorman 2019; Latif 2020). It is not possible for any health professional to learn every norm for every culture, society or family (Boggs 2023; Dean 2001). However, it is important that healthcare professionals are aware of the existence of cultural norms related to communication. This awareness and resultant understanding can explain variations in communicative events, thereby empowering the healthcare professional to learn about and make allowances for these variations. Particular cultures, social groups and families have norms governing the topic of social conversation in particular situations. Some freely discuss politics, salaries and sex, and openly ask the age of a person, while others avoid these topics. Some freely discuss spiritual beliefs and values, while others avoid discussing spiritual or religious topics. Some freely express emotions, while others avoid both verbal and non-verbal expression of emotions.

Some cultures use specific combinations of words to fulfil a social function. For example, in English, *How are you?* fulfils the function of acknowledging and greeting a person. In most cases it is not a request for information about the health of a person, but simply says hello. In Chinese, *Where are you going?* or *Have you eaten?* may fulfil the same function. Understanding that different combinations of words may fulfil different functions in different cultures is important, thereby assisting the healthcare professional to avoid misunderstandings.

Strategies to avoid misunderstandings

Specific communicative behaviours can assist in avoiding misunderstandings. Most individuals have a desire to share meaning with those communicating (Bowe et al 2014) and will usually concentrate and struggle, if necessary, to understand. This is both an encouragement and a warning to the healthcare professional. It is encouraging because it indicates that those seeking assistance will want to understand and in many cases will try to understand. The warning is that in a service with limited resources, the healthcare professional may not invest the time required to achieve adequate understanding. The temptation to provide information quickly, either assuming comprehension or allowing the Person/s to assume the meaning, especially when they are struggling to understand this meaning, is dangerous. This action does not guarantee mutual understanding (Greenberg & Weingarten 2015).

Reducing the incidence of misunderstandings

The following are suggestions that can reduce the incidence of misunderstandings (Bowe et al 2014).

- Plan and prepare for the interaction. Read reports, records and relevant research related to the condition and needs of the Person/s. It is important when referring to reports, records or referrals to avoid the creation of assumptions and opinions about the needs of the Person/s, before seeing them. Remember the overarching aim of the healthcare professional is fulfilment of Person/Family-centred goals and Care.
- Understand the communication expectations of the Person/s involved in the interaction – what do they understand to be the purpose of the interaction?
- If communicating with a Person/s from another culture, become familiar with the needs, cultural expectations (Davies et al 2014) and language level of the Person/s. If necessary, schedule an interpreter or use a community member (see Chapter 16) who speaks the appropriate language of the Person/s – not someone who has the same nationality or ethnicity, but someone who speaks their language.
- Know and understand the information for discussion and organise it clearly and carefully.
- Speak clearly and avoid speaking too quickly.
- Use simple, commonly used words.
- Be specific: avoid words that do not communicate specific information (e.g. "this", "that", "then", "things", "some", "many", "over there").
- Choose the words carefully, giving consideration to other possible meanings and anticipating potential assumptions and conclusions.
- Avoid using health jargon, abbreviations or technical terms without a clear explanation of such words.
- Avoid using colloquialisms or everyday sayings specific to a local dialect or language (e.g. *He's on the road, Go with the flow, A lot, Take it easy*).
- Employ all components of effective listening.

- Observe the effect of the information on all communicators, including the personal reactions of the healthcare professional, throughout the interaction (Jegatheesan et al 2010).
- Ask for confirmation of understanding throughout the interaction (Griffey et al 2015).
- Ask for a summary of the information to determine the level of understanding (Griffey et al 2015; Morgan 2013). Calmly ask for or provide explanations if misunderstandings are apparent.
- Remember the components of effectively concluding either the interaction or the service (see Chapter 5).
- Provide clear visual summaries of the verbal discussion, using either images or simple words or verified translations into the relevant language (Morgan 2013).
- Reflect upon the interaction after completion. Reflection can assist healthcare professionals to understand themselves, the Person/s and the components and outcomes of the interaction. This can assist the healthcare professional to prepare for future communicative interactions, potentially avoiding future misunderstandings.
- When communicating within the many health professions, fostering teamwork, improving interdepartmental communication and encouraging positive interdisciplinary relationships may also minimise misunderstandings (Dickson 2021; Olvera et al 2020).

Misunderstandings are inevitable wherever individuals interact. It is important that the healthcare professional understands the causes of misunderstandings and develops confidence to manage misunderstandings. Such confidence will develop with experience, reflection, discussion and understanding of possible management strategies.

Resolving misunderstandings

The experience of misunderstanding affects individuals in different ways. As a healthcare professional, the major concern is the effect of misunderstandings on the emotions of the Person/s and on the outcomes of the service. It is also important for healthcare professionals to take care of themselves; however, resolution of the emotions of the health professional must occur separately to the resolution of the emotions of the vulnerable Person/s. The control of any frustration, impatience or intolerance on the part of the healthcare professional is essential when there is a misunderstanding. Vulnerable individuals quickly receive and interpret such negative emotions, which may contribute to further misunderstanding. Clarification of information may resolve the negative emotions associated with the misunderstanding. Resolution of the emotions resulting from the misunderstanding may accelerate the ability of the vulnerable Person/s to understand the previously misunderstood information. It is important that the healthcare professional decides which to consider first – the resolution of the emotions or the understanding of the information. The existence of a therapeutic relationship will facilitate this decision; however, resolving the emotions may facilitate understanding. The major aim of the healthcare professional at this point is to resolve the misunderstanding. Exploring and resolving any negative emotions may expediently achieve this aim. Sometimes careful explanation of the procedure and all other relevant information may also achieve mutual understanding, potentially reducing the strength of the negative emotions.

It is important in every communicative interaction to remember the components of effective communication. If the healthcare professional communicates according to these components, their action will achieve mutual understanding, resolving any misunderstandings. Restoring communication is essential for achieving the ultimate purpose of the health professions – fulfilment of Person/Family-centred goals and Care.

Refer to the activity at the beginning of this chapter.

- Was that misunderstanding resolved?
- How did you resolve any negative emotions?
- Was it resolved satisfactorily? If so, outline or list the steps used to resolve it.
- How did you ensure understanding of necessary information?
- Could you use these steps in every situation? How could they be adapted for use in any situation?

Steps to resolving misunderstandings

These steps will assist the healthcare professional in resolving misunderstandings.

1. Be aware that there is a misunderstanding. This is not always immediately obvious. However, as soon as it becomes obvious the healthcare professional has a responsibility to act to overcome the cause of the misunderstanding and thus achieve effective communication.
2. Control any negative emotions associated with the misunderstanding. If possible, resolving negative emotions before restoring communication is the most appropriate option. Time constraints may make this difficult or impossible, thus learning to control negative emotions is beneficial. The major emotions for the healthcare professional to communicate are: regret that the communication failed and a desire to achieve effective communication.
3. Take responsibility for the misunderstanding regardless of the cause or problem. It is more probable that the vulnerable Person/s will accept the actions of the healthcare professional if the health professional willingly assumes responsibility for the misunderstanding. Indicate willingness to learn from the miscommunication, implementing strategies and/or steps to avoid them in similar situations in future.
4. Understand what caused the misunderstanding. Understanding the cause will assist the healthcare professional to compensate and avoid further misunderstandings due to that cause. It may also assist the healthcare professional to consider and predict other possible causes. Preparation and planning should assist the health professional to avoid further misunderstandings.
5. It is essential to understand that isolating the cause of the misunderstanding is not a substitute for action to resolve the misunderstanding (Levine 2012).
6. Make a conscious decision to restore communication to achieve mutual understanding. This will assist the healthcare professional to persevere to overcome the barriers to understanding. It will potentially resolve the misunderstanding, thereby restoring trust and effective communication.
7. Focus on restoring understanding with clear explanation and humble validation of understanding (Wachterman et al 2015), not on the cause of the misunderstanding. If the healthcare professional focuses on restoring communication it will assist in resolving the negative emotions associated with the misunderstanding.

Chapter summary

Misunderstandings may occur for many reasons, potentially affecting the outcomes of health services. They are the opposite of mutual understanding. The factors affecting achievement of mutual understanding include language; use and meaning of non-verbal cues; word choice and recognition of the meaning of particular words in particular contexts, whether high or low contexts; assumptions about the meaning of words; strong emotions; expectations/desires and the level of understanding of the Person/s. The healthcare professional must recognise that their personal attitudes and emotions may adversely affect communication, as the Person/s will perceive any judgemental attitudes or negative emotions. Thus the healthcare professional must invest time to reflect to achieve self-awareness of any judgemental attitudes or negative emotions. They must also invest time to acknowledge and resolve the emotions of the Person/s to avoid misunderstandings. Healthcare professionals must acknowledge that the expectations of the Person/s and the limitations of the role of the healthcare professional may also cause misunderstandings. This acknowledgement will empower them to ensure mutual understanding in every interaction. Commitment to the components of effective communication and Person/Family/Community-centred Care will empower the healthcare professional to successfully manage misunderstandings and restore effective communication.

What runs in your family?
Mainly the dog. However, my husband sometimes goes for a jog.
Sorry. I did not express that clearly. Do any of your family have any particular medical conditions?

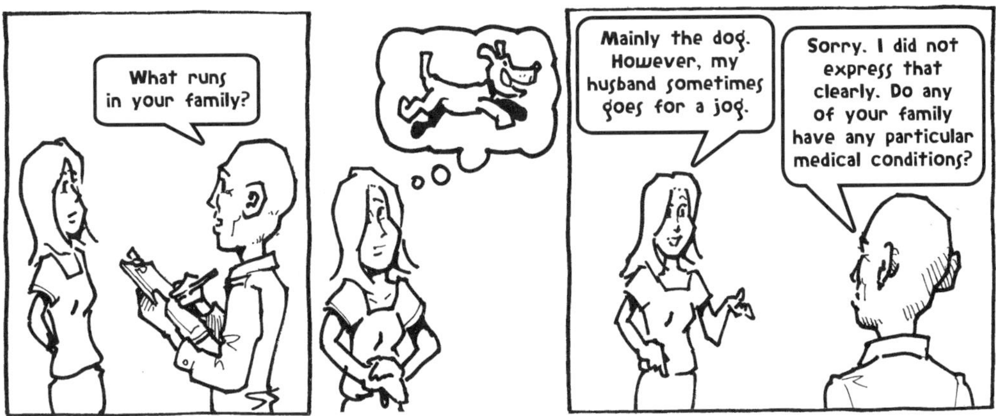

FIGURE 18.1
Clear expression gathers required information.
Courtesy Roger Harvey © Elsevier Australia.

REVIEW QUESTIONS

1. Define "misunderstanding".

____

____

____

2. List the factors that affect achievement of mutual understanding.

____

____

____

3. Give examples of how two of these factors can affect communication.

   i. ____

   ii. ____

4. Give original examples of each cause of misunderstandings.

____

____

____

5. In your own words, list four ways to reduce the incidence of misunderstandings.

   i. ____

   ii. ____

   iii. ____

   iv. ____

6. List the six steps that will assist the healthcare professional to resolve misunderstandings.

   i. ____

   ii. ____

   iii. ____

iv. ______________________________

v. ______________________________

vi. ______________________________

7. Suggest reasons for the importance of each step listed in Question 6.

i. ______________________________

____

ii. ______________________________

____

iii. ______________________________

____

iv. ______________________________

____

v. ______________________________

____

vi. ______________________________

____

References

Allen, D., 2021. Communication: The steps to take to support nervous or anxious patients, Nursing Standard, 36(2), 35 – 37.

Bensing, J.M., Verheul, W., Jansen, J., et al., 2010. Looking for trouble: The added value of sequence analysis in finding evidence for the role of physicians in patients' disclosure of cues and concerns. Medical Care, 48(7), 583–588.

Boggs, K.U., 2023. Interpersonal relationships: Professional communication skills for nurses, 9th ed. Elsevier, St Louis, MO.

Bowe, H., Martin, K., Manns, H., 2014. Communication across cultures: Mutual understanding in a global world, 2nd ed. Cambridge University Press, Melbourne.

Buettgen, A., Gorman, R., 2019. Disability culture. In: Zangeneh, M., Al-Krenawi, A., (eds). Culture, diversity and mental health – Enhancing clinical practice. Springer Nature, Switzerland.

Davies, J., Bukulatjpi, S., Sharma, S., et al., 2014. "Only your blood can tell the story" – a qualitative research study using semi-structured interviews to explore the hepatitis B related knowledge, perceptions and experiences of remote dwelling Indigenous Australians and their health care providers in northern Australia. BMC Public Health, 14, 1–23.

Dean, R., 2001. The myth of cross-cultural competence: Families in society. Journal of Contemporary Human Services, 86, 623–630.

Dickson, C., Peelo-Kilroe, L., 2021. Being person-centred in community and ambulatory services. In: McCormack, B., McCance, T., Bulley, C. et al., (eds) 2021. Fundamentals of Person-centred health practice. Wiley-Blackwell, London.

Eckermann, A., Dowd, T., Chong, E., et al., 2010. Binaŋ Goonj: Bridging cultures in Aboriginal health, 3rd ed. Elsevier, Sydney.

Greenberg, R.A., Weingarten, K., 2015. When health care professionals say "more" and parents say "enough". Paediatrics and Child Health (Commentaries), 20(3), 131–134.

Griffey, R.T., Shin, N., Jones, S., et al., 2015. The impact of teach-back on comprehension of discharge instructions and satisfaction among emergency patients with limited health literacy: A randomized, controlled study. Journal of Communication in Healthcare, 8 (1), 10–21.

Harms, L., Pierce, J., 2019. Working with people: Communication skills for reflective practice, 2nd Canadian ed. Oxford University Press, Ontario.

Henderson, A., 2019. Communication for health care practice. Oxford University Press, Melbourne.

Holli, B.B., Beto, J.A., 2023. Nutrition counselling and education skills: A practical guide, 8th ed. Jones & Bartlett, Burlington, MA.

Jegatheesan, B., Fowler, S., Miller, P.J., 2010. From symptom recognition to services: How South Asian Muslim immigrant families navigate autism. Disability and Society 25(7), 797–811.

Latif, A.S., 2020. The importance of understanding social and cultural norms in delivering quality health care – a personal experience commentary. Tropical Medicine and Infectious Disease, 5(1), 1–8.

Levine, C.S., Ambady, N., 2013. The role of non-verbal behaviour in racial disparities in health care: Implications and solutions. Medical Education, 47(9), 867–876.

Levine, J., 2012. Working with people: The helping process, 9th ed. Pearson, San Antonio.

Li, M., Mao, J., 2015. Hedonic or utilitarian? Exploring the impact of communication style alignment on user's perception of virtual health advisory services. International Journal of Information Management, 35(2), 229–243.

Lowell, A., Maypilama, E., Yikaniwuy, S., et al., 2015. Hiding the story: Indigenous consumer concerns about communication related to chronic disease in one remote region of Australia. International Journal of Speech–Language Pathology 14, 200–208.

Mendes, A., 2020. Communication in care: The importance of "soft skills". Nursing and Residential Care, 22(9), 10.12968/nrec.2020.22.9.4.

Morgan, S., 2013. Miscommunication between patients and general practitioners: Implications for clinical practice. Journal of Primary Health Care, 5(2), 123–128.

Moss, B., 2020. Communication skills in nursing, health and social care, 5th ed. Sage, London.

NSW Ministry of Health, 2019. Communicating positively: A guide to appropriate Aboriginal terminology. NSW Ministry of Health, North Sydney, Australia.

Nunan, D., 2012. What is this thing called language? 2nd ed. Macmillan International Red Globe Press, New York.

Olvera, L., Smith, J.S., Prater, L., et al., 2020. Interprofessional communication and collaboration during emergent birth center transfers: A Quality Improvement Project. Journal of Midwifery and Women's Health, 65(3), 555–561.

Passi, N., 2018. Looking forward, looking back: An Indigenous trainee perspective. Emergency Medicine Australasia 30, 862–863.

Rosen, D., 2014. Vital conversations: Improving communication between doctors and patients. Columbia University Press, New York.

Strobel, N., McAully, D., Sim, M., et al., 2019. Communicating with Aboriginal and Torres Strait Islander Peoples. In: Levett-Jones, T. (ed.), Critical conversations for patient safety, 2nd ed. Pearson, Sydney.

Wachterman, M.W., McCarthy, E.P., Marcantonio, E.R., et al., 2015. Mistrust, misperceptions, and miscommunication: A qualitative study of preferences about kidney transplantation among African Americans. Transplantation Proceedings, 47(2), 240–246.

CHAPTER 19

Ethical communication in healthcare

Chapter objectives

Upon completing this chapter, readers should be able to:

- explain the importance of ethical communication
- list and understand the characteristics of ethical communication
- appreciate the ethical responsibility of healthcare professionals when communicating about their professional life
- consider and develop strategies that ensure ethical communication and practice.

Ethical communication is essential in any healthcare profession, and typically a characteristic of everyday practice (Boggs 2023). It assists in demonstrating respect and consideration of the rights of the Person/s (Brown et al 2014; Vaz & Srinivasan 2014), while ensuring safe and appropriate care. It requires some moral sensitivity in order to avoid possible moral distress affecting the therapeutic relationship (Jiménez-Herrera 2023). Moss (2020) indicates that communication skills are not used in a "moral vacuum". Each healthcare profession has its own code with legal and ethical responsibilities (Australian Health Practitioners Regulation Agency (Ahpra) & National Boards 2022; Australian Medical Association 2016; Medical Board, Ahpra 2020; New Zealand Nurses Organisation 2019; Nursing and Midwifery Board, Ahpra 2022). These codes refer to standards of practice for the relevant healthcare profession. They are mandatory, with every relevant healthcare professional required to adhere to their relevant code (Gibson et al 2021). Therefore, it is essential to examine ethical communication in the context of particular healthcare professions.

So what constitutes ethical communication? Ethical communication relates to appropriate actions when communicating, regardless of the challenges in particular situations (Fischer-Grönlund et al 2021). It requires awareness of how to communicate to avoid harming the Person/s, to ensure safe and morally correct communication and thus healthcare (Johnstone 2019). It is necessary for the maintenance of harmonious, productive, satisfying and beneficial therapeutic relationships (Brown et al 2014; Crowden 2016; Donkor & Andrews 2011), including interprofessional relationships (Fischer-Grönlund et al 2021). Ethical communication acknowledges that the Person/s has an interest in and the right to comprehend everything they experience or hear and everything written about them, when receiving healthcare (Byrd & Winkelstein 2014; Nairn 2014).

Therefore, ethical behaviour for a healthcare professional is governed by the relevant rules for conduct related to their particular profession (Warren et al 2014). These rules typically provide guidance on how to relate and communicate while practising as a healthcare professional. However, the ability to communicate ethically also requires motivation, a caring other-focused character and critical self-awareness (Blaszko Helming et al 2020). Awareness of, and commitment to, ethical communication may depend on the familial, social and cultural background of the healthcare professional (Egan & Reese 2019; Harms & Pierce 2019; Molloy et al 2015). That is, the values and beliefs of healthcare professionals typically arise from their background and the related belief systems (Fedoruk 2015). Regardless of their origin, violation of ethical responsibilities when communicating has serious consequences for both the Person/s and the healthcare professional (Brown et al 2014; Egan & Reese 2019). Therefore, it is important for the healthcare professional to know the rules or codes of behaviour expected by their government, their profession and their particular health service (Haddad et al 2019; Warren et al 2014). This chapter examines some of these expectations and rules.

Many professionals, although aware of ethical requirements at a theoretical level, rarely consider them during everyday practice. However, it is not awareness of ethical requirements alone that produces ethical communication. It is the knowledge of, commitment to and application of these requirements into communicative behaviours that creates an ethical communicator. Devito (2021) considers every communicative act to have the potential to be constructive or destructive. This reality indicates that every communicative interaction in the healthcare professions, if ethically sound, has the potential to create and sustain constructive and satisfying therapeutic relationships and thus positive healthcare outcomes.

The main purpose of this chapter is to outline the characteristics of, and strategies to achieve, ethical communication.

Respect regardless of differences

A foundational characteristic and value of the healthcare professions is respect for *all* people, whether seeking healthcare or working alongside other healthcare professionals (see Chapter 2). This respect identifies the worth and dignity of all human beings. Crowden (2016, p. 125) states that such respect is essential for an appropriately functioning moral society. Every healthcare professional must respect the rights of all individuals. These rights include equal opportunities, equal consideration and equal treatment, regardless of status or condition (Crowden 2016; Fedoruk 2015; Harms & Pierce 2019; Staunton & Chiarella 2020). Ethical communication requires health professionals to express unconditional positive regard for all human beings (Crowden 2016; Haddad et al 2019; Rogers 1967; see Chapter 8), to effectively collaborate and empower within the therapeutic relationship. These are fundamental requirements for achieving the ultimate purpose of the health professions – Person/Family-centred Care. Expression of unconditional positive regard for all human beings is ethical and is in accordance with the Universal Declaration of Human Rights (United Nations 1948), the Human Rights Council (United Nations 2006) and the Convention on the Rights of Persons with Disabilities (United Nations 2017) and the *World Health Organisation Resource Book on Mental Health, Human Rights and Legislation* (World Health Organisation (WHO) 2005). The challenge for the healthcare professional is not usually in respecting rights, however, but in respecting the actual Person/s.

Demonstration of respect for others requires healthcare professionals first to respect themselves. Respecting and valuing self begins with an awareness of the thoughts about self, affecting self-image and self-esteem; some of these thoughts may have their origin in comments made by others. Regardless of their origin, these thoughts require reflective consideration and adjustment (Backus & Chapian 2014). If healthcare professionals find it difficult to value and respect themselves, it is imperative they seek expert assistance to maximise their potential to be effective communicators and ethical healthcare professionals.

Healthcare professionals demonstrate respect through verbal and non-verbal communicative behaviours. Such behaviours automatically reflect the underlying values and beliefs of an individual (Levine 2012). Thus critical awareness of personal values and beliefs is essential for establishing and practising ethical communication (Harms 2015; Salladay 2010, 2011; Smudde 2011).

Honesty

The truthful statement of thoughts, feelings and desires is the common understanding of honesty. The *New Shorter Oxford English Dictionary on Historical Principles* (1993) suggests that honesty is a characteristic, not merely a linguistic or social occurrence. Words such as "honourable character" and "uprightness of disposition and conduct" imply that honesty is about more than truthful statements; it is an underlying characteristic of an individual. The dictionary presents the opposites of honesty as cheating, stealing and lying. These definitions stimulate thought in order to assist the healthcare professional when considering honesty. They suggest that honesty is a characteristic generating honest statements, while also considering the needs of all interacting individuals despite the possible challenges of the situation (e.g. discussing the diagnosis of a life-limiting illness with a Person and their family).

In groups, consider this scenario.

You are very busy today, with more than the usual number of appointments. The young Person you are assisting is the same age as you and has similar interests. They are usually optimistic and relaxed when they attend, but today they suddenly begin to tell you about their feelings of depression and all the things that are going wrong in their life.

A holistic communicative approach alone, without consideration of the therapeutic relationship that is essential for positive outcomes, dictates that you should stop, actively listen, empathise and, if appropriate, seek permission to refer the Person to another relevant healthcare professional.

However, you are extremely busy and not interested in hearing anything else, because you have problems in your life, too! You do not want a reminder of these things while at work, nor do you want to fall behind today because you have a personal appointment immediately after work. Besides, there are other people waiting to see you.

- Consider the possible ways of responding. Discuss the potential outcomes of each response.
- What is the appropriate balance between the needs of the Person or those of the healthcare professional in this situation?
- What is an ethically appropriate response?

Honest responses from healthcare professionals are important. Many people seeking assistance are able to recognise a verbal or non-verbal response that is not reflecting honesty. Such responses affect the level of trust in the relationship and, if detected, potentially create anxiety in the Person/s concerning reasons for the lack of honesty (Wenger & Vespa 2010). It is important to consider particular situations and questions that may cause difficulty for the health professional in order to prepare possible responses, both spoken and emotional (Loftus & Mackey 2012). This consideration will assist in the development of a therapeutic relationship and contribute to satisfying Person/Family-centred Care. If the healthcare professional genuinely seeks the wellbeing of those with whom they interact, sensitive (non-dismissive) honest responses will develop trust and safety for all communicating individuals.

Clarification of expectations

When entering a new situation or environment, most individuals strive to understand that situation or environment. As well as feeling vulnerable, they may feel tentative or insecure and thus appreciate a friendly healthcare professional demonstrating genuine interest and concern. In such situations, it is reassuring for the Person/s to know what to expect and how to gain answers or assistance through either verbal or written information (Bladt et al 2020). Asking the Person/s to voice their expectations of the service allows clarification of any uncertainties. It is also important to ensure that the Person/s understand what to expect and the process of any procedures. Similarly, it is important to ensure the Person/s understands that they can contribute to the final decisions relating to their care (Beauchamp & Childress 2019). This can also reassure the Person/s, thereby contributing to the development of a positive relationship.

There are various ways of communicating about the available services and the rights of the Person/s. Verbal and written explanations of rights and details of procedures, with opportunity for clarification, are usually successful, potentially improving the outcomes of both the interactions and interventions. It is important to remember that written and verbal instructions in English may not always be appropriate. The Person/s may require verbal or written instruction in their preferred language, or if not possible, other forms of communication, such as picture-based communication (see Chapter 10). Provision of the required information in an appropriate manner can assist in establishing clear understanding and expectations of the interaction and or procedure.

Consent

Agreement about providing care and gathering information

Duty of care for every health professional includes introducing themselves and their service. This should be followed by asking for consent to assist the Person/s with explanations about any procedure or need to touch or move parts of their body (Malherbe 2021). In addition, in order to achieve ethical behaviour from staff, particular health services use signed agreements outlining rights, privacy and related issues for the Person/s. All Person/s are asked to sign such agreements. These agreements are explicit statements of the usually implied codes guiding the relationship between the healthcare professional and the Person/s. Such codes assume that healthcare professionals will never seek to harm the Person/s, but always seek to assist and fulfil appropriate goals for that Person/s (Haddad et al 2019). Signed agreements may provide information about the service, what to expect when receiving assistance, the responsibilities of all stakeholders and guidelines for lodging a complaint. They usually make statements about responsible use of gathered information based upon the assumption that every individual has a right to privacy (Brown et al 2014; Byrd & Winkelstein 2014; Malherbe 2021). For more information relating to privacy, see relevant government websites. In Australia, see Australian Government policies and Acts such as the *Privacy Act* 2014, *Privacy Amendment Act* 2018, *Disability Services Act* 1986 (see particular

Disability Acts for specific states in Australia) and Commonwealth Disability Strategy 2010–2020. For a similar policy in New Zealand, see the New Zealand Government (Ministry of Justice) *Privacy Act* 2019. These Acts often state that the health service agrees to protect privacy. They may indicate that healthcare professionals might share provided information with other healthcare professionals, but only for the benefit of the Person/s, never for illegal or inappropriate reasons.

Imagine you are requiring healthcare.

- If you sign an agreement to protect your privacy, what would you expect that signed agreement would mean in relation to the information you provide to different healthcare professionals about your condition and/or needs?
- Would you feel it was appropriate for a particular healthcare professional to discuss your information with another person? If so, with whom and why?
- Would you like to have access to and explanation of any notes or reports the healthcare professional(s) wrote about you?

In groups, discuss the following questions.

- What are the implications of the above answers for your role as a healthcare professional?
- How can healthcare professionals manage the implications to ensure safe and effective care?

It is important to remember that the Person/s may be more willing to provide information if the healthcare professional has explained how the information will be used and why it is necessary for them to have this information (Harms 2015; Harms & Pierce 2019; Stein-Parbury 2021). To encourage sharing of information, healthcare professionals must act to indicate they are worthy of trust (Levine 2012).

Informed consent

Although an "informed consent" agreement often refers to research involving humans (Malone 2003), within the healthcare professions it usually refers to procedures associated with a particular healthcare profession. This type of agreement requires the healthcare professional to provide clear information about the procedure, the associated risks and the expected outcome of the procedure in the appropriate languages (Doherty 2021; Haddad et al 2019). Informed consent is an attempt to give the vulnerable individual a sense of control in a situation where they often feel they have little power, control or autonomy, thereby contributing to the therapeutic relationship (Carpiniello & Wasserman 2020). In many places there are legal requirements to provide such information at an appropriate level of complexity for all Person/s. It is important to remember that the vulnerable Person/s may sign a consent form regardless of their level of understanding in order to expedite the healthcare process.

Confidentiality

Protecting shared information

The Person/s seeking assistance requires a safe "space" in which to express their feelings, thoughts and concerns. The foundation for this is a trusting therapeutic relationship (Levine

2012; Stein-Parbury 2021). It requires the healthcare professional to state explicitly what they intend to do with the shared information. It also requires indication of how the information will remain protected and confidential (Avraam et al 2022; Doherty 2021).

- Why is confidentiality important for everyone in a healthcare setting?
- Decide if all contexts require the same level of confidentiality. List possible contexts that might be more sensitive than others and require greater confidentiality. Suggest why.
- Is a healthcare professional obliged to share everything they hear from the Person/s? How should you decide what to share?
- A Person shares with you that they feel suicidal and asks you to tell no-one. What should you do?
- List ways that guarantee confidentiality for the Person/s. Consider:
  1. reports and records
  2. meeting a good friend who asks about a Person/s you are assisting
  3. a difficult encounter that leaves you drained emotionally at the end of the day
  4. frustration with other healthcare professionals.

Some of the information given by the Person/s is required for the development of appropriate interventions and should be available for all involved healthcare professionals. However, there will also be information shared that does not contribute to their overall treatment. It is often quite personal, but not always essential to share this information. Sometimes it is not obvious whether the information is necessary for the success of the overall goals. Awareness of the necessity of information increases with experience. A relatively inexperienced healthcare professional who is unsure about why someone is sharing particular information might be advised to ask the Person/s two questions. First, *Do you want me to do something about this?* Meaning: Is there any action required because of this disclosure or do you simply trust me? Second, the healthcare professional might ask whether it is acceptable to discuss the information with a more senior healthcare professional, for example, *Do you mind if I tell X what you have told me to ensure you have relevant help with this?* These questions will promote awareness in the Person/s about the type of information they are sharing and perhaps their reason for sharing it. This may be particularly important when a young person shares information with a young healthcare professional of the opposite gender. The possibility for attachment, whether romantic or not, is real and is best avoided because it can be destructive for both the Person/s and the healthcare professional. A guiding principle for deciding what information to share with other healthcare professionals should be whether the information affects the health and wellbeing of and interventions for the Person/s seeking assistance.

Mandatory communications

Mandatory communications are legal requirements relating to either abuse or neglect of individuals in society, in Australia known as mandatory **reporting** (Australian Institute of Family Studies (AIFS) 2017; Mathews & Walsh 2014) and New Zealand (Ministry of Health 2019) or inappropriate healthcare practice, which in Australia is typically known as mandatory **notification** (Ahpra 2014), and in New Zealand is known as conduct concerns (Medical Council of New

Zealand 2019). While there are variations relating to these requirements across states and countries, generally healthcare professionals are obliged to report abuse, including physical and/or sexual abuse, in some cases emotional abuse and neglect along with exposure to domestic violence (AIFS 2017; New Zealand Ministry of Health 2018).

When making notifications, the healthcare professional informs their employer, colleagues or educational providers to the relevant government authority. Mandatory communications require a belief "on reasonable grounds" that an individual is experiencing the aforementioned type of abuse (reporting) or that a healthcare professional is unfit to practice because of practising while intoxicated, or engages in sexual misconduct related to their practice, or places the public at risk because of an impairment or practising contrary to the professional standards of their profession (notification). It is important for each healthcare professional to be aware of the requirements for mandatory communications relevant to their location of practice. These can be found either through appropriate government healthcare websites or registration bodies for healthcare professionals.

Protecting information as an ethical responsibility

Health professionals have an **ethical responsibility** to protect information about the Person/s. This refers to information both read and heard. It also refers to *not* discussing assessment results on social networking sites, whether or not seeking expert advice. Such information belongs exclusively in the professional context – records, files, experiences, feelings and memories of shared information all belong at work. It is also important to remember that failing to protect confidentiality can destroy any trust between the healthcare professional and any Person/s, including colleagues, as well as potentially having legal ramifications, possibly including the risk of deregistration.

Discuss the following scenario.

You meet an ex-classmate after work. You naturally talk about your experiences at work. They ask about a Person/s you are assisting by name – a close relative of theirs. How will you respond? This is a "small" city, but you want them to value you, and you also want to be respected and successful in your profession.

Protecting the healthcare professional

There are many times when healthcare professionals simply need to "unload" the experiences, thoughts and feelings associated with the information gathered from a particular Person/s or from an entire day. The emotions and thoughts associated with a particular interaction or several interactions over a day require some form of resolution. Accumulation of these emotions, without resolution, can produce cynicism and burnout (Rupert & Morgan 2005). Discussing the emotions and ethical dilemmas with someone (preferably an appropriate healthcare professional) provides an opportunity for resolution and dissipation of the intensity of the emotions. It can also assist when experiencing ethical dilemmas in practice (Doherty 2021). Sometimes a particular Person/s makes a deep impression in the mind of the healthcare professional, and thus the healthcare professional may require time and discussion to process the depth of and the implications of this impression. Self-care for the healthcare professionals, including emotional and mental care, is as important as care for the Person/s (Skovholt & Trotter-Mathison 2016).

- Is it appropriate for the health professional to talk to a close and trusted family member if they need to "offload"? What are the ethical issues here?
- Who is an appropriate person for the health professional to "offload" to? Should the health professional ever use names?
- What are the implications when working in a small city or town?

Protecting the Person/s from breaches of confidentiality and/or gossip

Words once said are very difficult to retract, whether spoken or entered onto **social media**, regardless of their intended meaning. Words cause an immediate emotional or cognitive reaction, and it is often impossible to change those emotions, even with an explanation of the intended meaning. This means that the healthcare professional must take care when they say anything about any of the people with whom they are working – colleagues or otherwise. This includes on all social media sites (see Chapter 23).

Consider this incident alone initially.

A friend contacts you on Facebook, asking you how your knee is now, after your surgery.

You are surprised as you had not had time to tell any of your friends about the surgery – it all happened too quickly. You ask her how she knew about the surgery.

She said there was discussion of an unusual case needing knee surgery and your x-ray with your name on it was on one of her medical Facebook pages.

While you understand the benefits of discussing unusual cases on Facebook to allow extensive gathering of effective surgical methods and care, you have various responses, some negative and some positive, to being identified in this way.

- List your possible responses if this was you.

As a group, discuss the effects and possible ramifications for both the Person and the healthcare professional who allows the name of a Person they assisted to appear on social media.

- Suggest possible responses that different people (including employers and professional associations) might have to this situation.
- What would group members do to respond to this situation?
- What are the implications for the health professionals who shared identifiable information about a particular service user? Consider the Human Rights guidelines and the Code of Ethics or Conduct for your profession.
- What are the implications for all healthcare professionals?

Boundaries

Roles

Ethical communication requires definite understanding of the limits of the role of each healthcare profession and the relationship between the Person/s and the healthcare professional. Each healthcare profession has a distinct role defined by their profession. Regardless of the level of knowledge of the healthcare professional about the interventions of other healthcare professions (Honeycutt & Milliken 2021), it is important that healthcare professionals practise within the limitations of their particular profession-related knowledge and skills. This is important for ethical, legal, safety and insurance reasons.

Relationships

The limitations of the therapeutic relationship relate to the whole Person/s. There are physical, emotional, social, cognitive and spiritual reasons for healthcare professionals to practise within particular boundaries or limits. These limits include time, friendship and dependency boundaries (Haddad et al 2019; Harms 2015; Harms & Pierce 2019; Levine 2012). Each encounter with a Person/s seeking assistance should have time limits. These limits allow a change for the Person/s and for the healthcare professional to assist others and complete the requirements of their role.

Practising within the boundaries of a particular healthcare professional role means understanding the role to be that of a "therapist" not an intimate friend. If the healthcare professional needs to have a real "friendship" with a Person/s they assist, this is an abuse of the role and can potentially damage the vulnerable individual (Heron 2012). That healthcare professional must ask themself whether the relationship is fulfilling their needs rather than those of the Person/s. Being friendly within the role is essential, but is different to connecting in a personal and intimate manner.

Many of the people that healthcare professionals encounter will share personal and intimate information. This **self-disclosure** from the Person/s seeking assistance assists them and assumes a particular understanding of confidentiality (Brown et al 2104; Doherty 2021; Levett-Jones & Reid-Searl 2022). If self-disclosure occurs between people of varying genders, the healthcare professional may misinterpret the meaning of this disclosure. They may assume it is simply an expression of emotions at the time and not understand that there are expectations of a deeper relationship that the healthcare professional is unable to reciprocate. Dependence may develop along with an expectation of exclusion of all others from the relationship, removing any therapeutic benefits (Egan & Reese 2019; Haddad et al 2019).

Self-disclosure

Maintaining professional boundaries by avoiding self-disclosure is an ethical requirement of practice (Levett-Jones & Reid-Searl 2022; Warren et al 2014). However, it is sometimes appropriate for healthcare professionals to share their own experiences, although only in particular circumstances. It has been shown to enhance a therapeutic relationship with older adults (Corbett & Williams 2014), however, compromises this relationship with other age groups (Griffith & Tengnah 2013; Malone 2012). Self-disclosure on the part of the healthcare professional should only occur to promote a connection with a Person/s or to demonstrate particular strategies (Harms 2015; Harms & Pierce 2019). Self-disclosure should never occur to move the focus to the healthcare professional or to make the healthcare professional appear connected and knowledgeable. It should only take place to encourage and maintain the relationship (Devito 2021) – in this case, the therapeutic relationship.

- If someone asks you some personal questions, what should you do? For example, *Do you do drugs? Do you have children? Do you have a girlfriend/boyfriend?*
- How do you decide whether or not to answer? What criteria should you use?

Sharing information about self can develop rapport. In New Zealand, a normal process that develops rapport for Māori is disclosure about their *iwi* (tribe). In other cultures, disclosure about birthplace or immediate family is the norm. People from certain cultures may benefit from the healthcare professional disclosing particular kinds of personal information. This information might be about family, country or town of origin, events or experiences, but is not usually about deep emotional experiences or emotional reasons for their demeanour. Some individuals are more comfortable than others with sharing personal details and thus the comfort level of the healthcare professional may assist in deciding the appropriate level of self-disclosure.

Over-identification

Over-identification can cause difficulties in the therapeutic nature of a relationship (Haddad et al 2019). Over-identification may occur when a healthcare professional has experienced a very similar situation to the Person/s, for example, when assisting someone who has a child, sibling or parent with a disorder the same as those of the healthcare professional. When a healthcare professional over-identifies they can be anxious to share their experiences to indicate a connection, thereby focusing on themself rather than the Person/s. Emotional competence (Heron 2012) becomes important when the healthcare professional experiences over-identification. Emotional competence means that the healthcare professional will not allow their own experiences or emotions to affect their assistance for the vulnerable Person/s. If the healthcare professional is not able to function with emotional competence, the resultant self-focus is detrimental to the therapeutic relationship. They will fulfil the needs of the healthcare professional rather than the needs of the Person/s (Haddad et al 2019; Heron 2012).

Ethical codes of behaviour and conduct

There are principles, and, in some cases, legislation that guide and direct the behaviour of all healthcare professionals (Warren et al 2014). These principles are usually the basis for the specific code of conduct or ethics adopted by individual healthcare professions. If a particular healthcare profession does not have a code specific to their practice, government policy exists to guide their practice in ethical conduct. For example, in Australia, see the Queensland Government *Public Sector Ethics Act* 1994, the National Code of Conduct for Healthcare Workers (Queensland) 2015, the National Code of Conduct for Health Care Workers (Victoria)(2015), Queensland Health, Workplace Conduct and Ethics (2015), the Queensland Health Code of Conduct 2011 and the NSW Health Department Code of Conduct 2012. In New Zealand, see *The Health and Disability Commissioner Review of the Act & Code* 2014 and the New Zealand *Health Practitioners Competence Assurance Amendment Bill* 2019 (see Parliamentary Counsel Office 2019).

The legislation, principles and ethical codes do not define the word "ethical", nor do they necessarily provide exact answers to all ethical dilemmas experienced during practice (Banks 2020). They do, however, provide guidelines to assist a practising healthcare professional. It is important to understand that a code of ethics can produce rigid attitudes insensitive to the rights of others (Taylor 2010). This is never the intention of such a code, and healthcare professionals should use their code of conduct or ethics to encourage and empower individuals, not to paralyse them.

In small groups:

- Using the code of conduct or ethics specific to your profession, list behaviours reflecting this code.
- List characteristics of communication that conform to this code.
- What do you think this means for everyday healthcare?

Chapter summary

Ethical considerations are important when communicating within the healthcare professions and they relate to specific and correct behaviour, often mandated by a specific health profession or a government legislation. Such behaviour requires respect of self and the Person/s, regardless of similarities or differences, which is communicated both verbally and non-verbally during any interaction. Honesty is also important as the Person/s can generally detect lack of honesty, which may create anxiety about the reasons for the lack of honesty.

A Person/s who is new to a health service requires information about their rights, the service and any procedures or expectations (in some cases including consent forms), along with details about how any disclosed information will be managed to maintain confidentiality. There are also ethical boundaries in both the roles and relationships of healthcare professionals limiting self-disclosure and over-identification on the part of the healthcare professional. Ethical considerations in communication ensure satisfying and positive outcomes for all people involved in a health service.

PROTECTING EVERYONE
BOUNDARIES
MANDATORY COMMUNICATION
CODES OF CONDUCT
EXPLAINING PROCESSES
CONSENT
CONFIDENTIALITY
CLARIFYING EXPECTATIONS
RESPECT
HONESTY
ETHICAL COMMUNICATION CONSISTS OF...

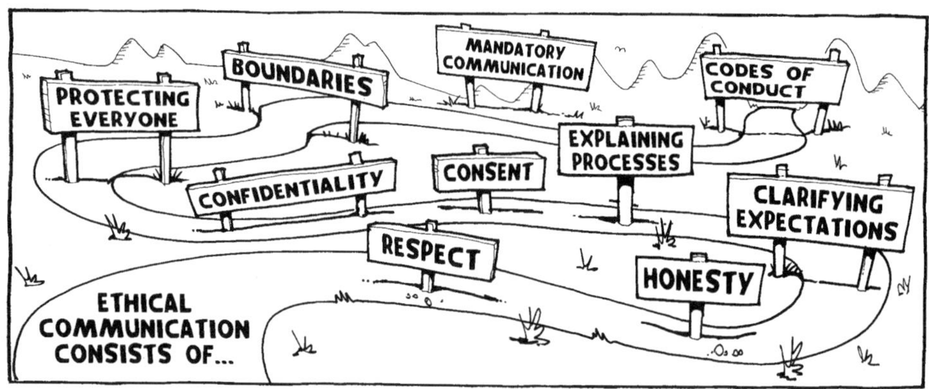

FIGURE 19.1
The components of ethical communication.
Courtesy Roger Harvey © Elsevier Australia.

REVIEW QUESTIONS

1. What does ethical communication achieve in a healthcare service?

2. Why must a healthcare professional fulfil ethical requirements?

3. A health professional must provide certain information to fulfil ethical requirements.

   i. What information must a healthcare professional provide?

   ii. What forms can this information take?

   iii. What characteristics must this information have?

4. List five things a healthcare professional must remember to ensure ethical communication.

   i.

   ii.

iii. ______________________________

iv. ______________________________

v. ______________________________

5. Define emotional competence and explain how it assists a healthcare professional to achieve ethical communication.

____

____

____

6. What are the requirements of the code of conduct relating to ethical practice relevant to your health profession?

____

____

____

References

Australian Health Practitioner Regulation Agency (Ahpra) 2014. Mandatory notifications guidelines for registered health practitioners. Ahpra, Sydney.

Australian Health Practitioners Regulation Agency (Ahpra) & National Boards, 2022. Code of Conduct. Ahpra, Sydney.

Australian Institute of Family Studies (AIFS) 2017. Mandatory reporting of child abuse and neglect. Child Family Community Australia. Online. Available at: aifs.gov.au/cfca/publications/mandatory-reporting-child-abuse-and-neglect

Australian Medical Association (AMA) 2016. Code of Ethics, AMA, Canberra.

Avraam, D., Jones, E, Burton, P., 2022. A deterministic approach for protecting privacy in sensitive personal data. BMC Medical Informatics and Decision Making, 22, 24. doi.org/10.1186/s12911-022-01754-4.

Backus, W., Chapian, M., 2014. Telling yourself the truth, 20th ed. Bethany, Minneapolis, MN.

Banks, S., 2020. Ethics and values in social work, 5th ed. Palgrave Macmillan, Basingstoke, UK.

Beauchamp, T.L., Childress, J.F., 2019. Principles of biomedical ethics, 8th ed. Oxford University Press, New York.

Bladt, T., Vorup-Jensen, T. Saedder, E., et al, 2020. Empirical investigation of ethical challenges related to the use of biological therapies. Journal of Law, Medicine and Ethics, 48, (2020) 567.

Blaszko Helming, M.A., Shields, D. A., Avino, K.M., et al., 2020. Dossey & Keegan's holistic nursing: A handbook for practice, 8th ed. Jones & Bartlett, Burlington, MA.

Boggs, K.U., 2023. Interpersonal relationships: Professional communication skills for nurses, 9th edition. Elsevier, St Louis, MI.

Brown, B., Davtyan, M., Fisher, C.B., 2014. Peruvian female sex workers' ethical perspectives on their participation in an HPV Vaccine Clinical Trial. Ethics and Behavior, 25(2), 115–128.

Byrd, G.D., Winkelstein, P., 2014. A comparative analysis of moral principles and behavioral norms in eight ethical codes relevant to health sciences librarianship, medical informatics, and the health professions. Journal of the Medical Library Association 102(4), 247–256.

Carpiniello, B., & Wasserman, D., 2020. European Psychiatric Association policy paper on ethical aspects in communication with patients and their families. European Psychiatry, 63(1), e36, 1–7.

Corbett, S., Williams, F., 2014. Striking a professional balance: Interactions between nurses and their older rural patients. British Journal of Community Nursing 19(4), 162–167.

Crowden, A., 2016. Ethics and indigenous health care: Cultural competencies, protocols and integrity. In: Hampton, R., Toombs, M. (eds), Indigenous Australians and health: The wombat in the room. Oxford University Press, Melbourne.

Devito, J.A., 2021 The interpersonal communication book, 16th ed. Pearson, Boston.

Doherty, R.F., 2021. Ethical dimensions in health professions, 7th ed. Elsevier, St Louis, MO.

Donkor, N.T., Andrews, L.D., 2011. Ethics, culture and nursing practice in Ghana. International Nursing Review 58(1), 109–114.

Egan, G., Reese R.J., 2019. The skilled helper: A problem management and opportunity approach to helping, 11th ed. Cengage, Boston MA.

Fedoruk, M., 2015. Legal responsibilities and ethics. In: Fedoruk, M., Hofmeyer, A. (eds), Becoming a nurse: an evidence-based approach. Oxford University Press, Melbourne.

Fischer-Grönlund, C., Brännström, M., Zingmark, K., 2021. The "one to five" method – a tool for ethical communication in groups among healthcare professionals. Nurse Education in Practice, 51(2021), 102998.

Gibson, C., MacDonald, K., O'Donnell, D., 2021. Professionalism and practising professionally. In: McCormack, B., McCance, T., Bulley, C., et al (eds), Fundamentals of Person-centred healthcare practice. Wiley Blackwell, Chichester.

Griffith, R., Tengnah, C., 2013. Maintaining professional boundaries: Keep your distance. British Journal of Community Nursing 18(1), 43–46.

Haddad, A.M., Purtilo, R.B., Doherty, R.F., 2019. Health professional and patient interaction, 9th ed. Elsevier/Saunders, St Louis, MO.

Harms, L., 2015. Working with people: Communication skills for reflective practice, 2nd ed. Oxford University Press, Melbourne.

Harms, L., Pierce, J., 2019. Working with people: Communication skills for reflective practice, 2nd Canadian ed. Oxford University Press, Ontario.

Heron, J., 2012. Helping the client: A creative, practical guide, 5th ed. Sage, London.

Honeycutt, A., Milliken, M.A., 2021. Understanding human behavior: A guide for healthcare providers, 10th ed. Cengage Learning, Boston, MA.

Jiménez-Herrera, M.F. 2023. The moral compass in care: From ethics to professionalism. Scandinavian Journal of Caring Science, 37, 1–2.

Johnstone, M.J., 2019. Bioethics: A nursing perspective, 7th ed. Elsevier, Sydney.

Levett-Jones, T., Reid-Searl, K., 2022. The clinical placement, 5th ed. Elsevier, Sydney.

Levine, J., 2012. Working with people: The helping process, 9th ed. Pearson, San Antonio.

Loftus, S., Mackey, S., 2012. Interviewing patients and clients. In: Higgs, J., Ajjawi, R., McAllister, L., et al. (eds), Communicating in the health sciences, 3rd ed. Oxford University Press, Melbourne.

Malherbe, J., 2021. The Protection of Personal Information Act: Its effect on clinical practice and health research. South African Journal of Occupational Therapy, 51(2), 2–3.

Malone, J.L., 2012. Ethical professional practice: Exploring the issues for health services to rural Aboriginal communities. Rural and Remote Health, 12, 1891.

Malone, S., 2003. Ethics at home: Informed consent in your own backyard. International Journal of Qualitative Studies in Education, 16, 797–815.

Mathews, B., Walsh, K., 2014. Mandatory reporting laws. In: Hayes, A., Higgins, D., (eds), Families, policy and the law. Australian Institute of Family Studies, Sydney.

Medical Board, Ahpra, 2020. Good medical practice: A code of conduct for doctors in Australia. Ahpra, Melbourne.

Medical Council of New Zealand, 2019. Conduct and competence concerns. Online. Available at: www.mcnz.org.nz/our-standards/fitness-to-practise/conduct-and-competence-concerns/

Molloy, J., Evans, M., Coughlin, K., 2015. Moral distress in the resuscitation of extremely premature infants. Nursing Ethics, 22(1), 52–63.

Moss, B., 2020. Communication skills in health and social care, 5th ed. Sage, London.

Nairn, T.A., 2014. What we have here is a failure to communicate: The ethical dimension of health literacy. Health Progress, 95(4), 61–63.

New Zealand Ministry of Health, 2019. Health Practitioners Competence Assurance Amendment Bill. Online. Available: www.health.govt.nz/our-work/regulation-health-and-disability-system/health-practitioners-competence-assurance-act.

New Zealand Ministry of Health, 2018. Family Violence and sexual violence. Online. Available at: www.tewhatuora.govt.nz/our-health-system/preventative-healthwellness/family-violence-and-sexual-violence.

New Zealand Nurses Organisation, 2019. Guideline – Code of ethics, 2019. NZNO, Wellington.

Nursing and Midwifery Board Ahpra, 2022. Code of conduct for midwives. Ahpra, Melbourne.

Nursing and Midwifery Board Ahpra, 2022. Code of conduct for nurses. Ahpra, Melbourne.

Rogers, C., 1967. On becoming a person. Constable, London.

Rupert, P.A., Morgan, D.J., 2005. Work setting and burnout among professional psychologists. Professional Psychology, Research and Practice, 36, 544–550.

Salladay, S.A., 2011. Ethical problems: Communication under surveillance. Nursing, 41(4), 12–13.

Salladay, S.A., 2010. Ethical problems: Communication, getting the nod. Nursing, 40(4), 18–19.

Skovholt T.M., & Trotter-Mathison, M., 2016. The resilient practitioner: Burnout and compassion fatigue prevention and self-care strategies for the helping professions, 3rd ed. Routledge, New York.

Smudde, P.M., 2011. Focus on ethics and public relations practice in a university classroom. Communication Teacher, 25(3), 154–158.

Staunton, P., Chiarella, M., 2020. Law for nurses and midwives, 8th ed. Churchill Livingstone Elsevier, Sydney.

Stein-Parbury, J., 2021. Patient and person: Interpersonal skills in nursing, 7th ed. Elsevier, Sydney.

Taylor, B.J., 2010. Reflective practice for healthcare professionals. Open University Press, Maidenhead, England.

The new shorter Oxford English dictionary on historical principles, 1993. Oxford University Press, Oxford.

United Nations, 2017. Convention on the rights of persons with disabilities. Online. Available at: www.un.org/development/desa/disabilities/convention-on-the-rights-of-persons-with-disabilities/convention-on-the-rights-of-persons-with-disabilities-2.html

United Nations, 2006. Human Rights Council. Online. Available at: www.ohchr.org/en/hr-bodies/hrc/about-council

United Nations, 1948. Universal declaration of human rights. Online. Available at: www.un.org/en/about-us/universal-declaration-of-human-rights

Vaz, M., Srinivasan, K., 2014. Ethical challenges and dilemmas for medical health professionals doing psychiatric research. Indian Journal of Medical Research, 139(2), 191–193.

Warren, J., Ahls, C., Asfaw, A.H., et al., 2014. Ethics issues and training needs of mental health practitioners in a rural setting. Journal of Social Work Values and Ethics, 11(2), 61–75.

Wenger, N.S., Vespa, P.M., 2010. Ethical issues in patient–physician communication about therapy for cancer: Professional responsibilities of the oncologist. The Oncologist, 15, 43–48.

World Health Organization (WHO), 2005. WHO resource book on mental health, human rights and legislation. WHO, Geneva Switzerland.

Further reading

Australian Government, Department of Social Services, 2023. Disability Services Act Commonwealth of Australia, Canberra.

Australian Government, Department of Social Services, 2021. Australia's Disability Strategy 2021–2031. Available at Australia's Disability Strategy Hub through the Disability Gateway: disabilitygateway.gov.au

Australian Government, 2018. National statement on ethical conduct in human research (2007). Updated 2018. National Health and Medical Research Council. Available at: nhmrc.gov.au

Australian Human Rights Commission, 2011. Disability standards and guidelines. Available at: www.humanrights.gov.au/disability_rights/standards/standards.html

Health and Disability Commissioner (New Zealand). The Health and Disability Commissioner Review of the Act and Code 2014. Review website. Available at: www.hdc.org.nz/your-rights/about-the-code/review-of-the-act-and-code-2014/

Minister of Health, 2023. Rural health strategy, New Zealand Ministry of Health, Wellington. Available at: health.govt.nz

New South Wales Department of Ageing, Disability and Home Care, 2014. Disability Inclusion Act, No 41. Available at: legislation.nsw.gov.au

New South Wales Government Ministry of Health, 2015. NSW Health Code of Conduct. Available at: www1.health.nsw.gov.au/pds/Pages/doc.aspx?dn5PD2015_049

New Zealand Government, 1993. Privacy Act. Available at: www.legislation.govt.nz/act/public/1993/0028/latest/DLM296639.html

New Zealand Health and Disability Commissioner, 2023. The Health and Disability Commissioner Review of the Act and Code 2023. Review website. Available at: www.hdc.org.nz/your-rights/about-the-code/review-of-the-act-and-code-2024/

Office of the Australian Information Commissioner (OAIC), 2014. Australian Privacy Principles, Australian Government. Available at: www.oaic.gov.au/privacy/australian-privacy-principles

Queensland Department of Health, 2015. Workplace Conduct and Ethics (Policy Number E1(QH-POL-113). Available at: www.health.qld.gov.au/__data/assets/pdf_file/0034/395980/qh-pol-113.pdf

Queensland Government, 1994. Public Sector Ethics Act. Current as March 2023. Available at: legislation.qld.gov.au

Queensland Health, 2022. The national code of conduct for healthcare workers (Queensland). Available at: www.health.qld.gov.au/__data/assets/pdf_file/0034/395980/qh-pol-113.pdf

United Nations Enable, 2007. About us: Secretariat for the convention on the rights of persons with disabilities. Available at: www.un.org/esa/socdev/enable/disabout.htm#:,:text5Themajor.ojectives.persons.with.disability

United Nations Department of Economic and Social Affairs, n.d. Standard rules on the equalization of opportunities for persons with disabilities. Available at: www.un.org/development/desa/disabilities/standard-rules-on-the-equalization-of-opportunities-for-persons-with-disabilities.html

Useful websites

Codes of conduct (mainly Australian) and codes of ethics for some healthcare professions

Ambulance: Ambulance Service of NSW, 2012. Code of conduct. Available at: www.ambulance.nsw.gov.au

Dental Hygiene: Dental Hygienists Association of Australia, 2023. Code of practice. Available at: www.dhaa.info In Search enter: Code of Practice – this will take you to Code of Ethics

Dietetics: Dieticians Association of Australia, 2023. Code of Conduct for Dieticians and Nutritionists. Available at: www.daa.asn.au Enter: Code of Conduct

National Code of Conduct for Healthcare Workers: Queensland. Queensland Health, 2015. The national code of conduct for healthcare workers (Queensland). Available at: www.health.qld.gov.au

National Code of Conduct for Healthcare Workers: Victoria. Department of Health. Available at: www.health.vic.gov.au/health-workforce-regulation/national-code-of-conduct-for-healthcare-workers

Nursing and Midwifery: Australian Nursing and Midwifery Council, 2018. Code of professional conduct for nurses in Australia. Available at: www.Nursingmidwiferyboard.gov.au

Occupational Therapy: Occupational Therapy Australia, 2022. National code of conduct. Available at: www.occupationaltherapyboard.gov.au/Codes-Guidelines/Code-of-conduct.aspx

Osteopathy: New South Wales Osteopaths Registration Board, 2014. Code of conduct for board members. Available at: www.osteopathyboard.gov.au/codes-guidelines.aspx

Physiotherapy: Australian Physiotherapy Association, 2022. A revised Code of conduct. Available at: australian.physio/inmotion/revised-code-conduct

Podiatry: Australian Podiatry Association, 2022. Code of conduct. Available at: www.podiatry.org.au/natabout/code-of-conduct

Radiography/Radiation Therapy: Australian Society of Medical Imaging and Radiation Therapy, 2017. Guidelines for professional conduct for medical radiation professionals. Available: www.asmirt.org/asmirt_core/wp-content/uploads/125.pdf

Social Work: Australian Association of Social Workers, 2020. Code of ethics. Available at: www.aasw.asn.au

Speech Pathology: Speech Pathology Australia, 2020. Code of ethics. Available at: speechpathologyaustralia.org.au

Traditional Medicine: Australian Traditional-Medicine Society, 2019. Code of conduct. Available at: www.atms.com.au/ Enter: Code of conduct

Work Health and Safety: Safe Work Australia Code of practice. Available at: www.safeworkaustralia.gov.au/law-and-regulation/codes-practice

Workplace Conduct and Ethics (Policy Number E1(QH-POL-113). Queensland Health, 2015. Available at: www.health.qld.gov.au

CHAPTER 20

Remote or long-distance healthcare communication:
1 The typically unseen healthcare professional

Chapter objectives

Upon completing this chapter, readers should be able to:

- define and discuss long-distance communication
- list types of long-distance communication typically used in healthcare: written reports, electronic records, mobile devices, video/teleconferences, and the internet
- describe the characteristics of long-distance communication
- explain the advantages of long-distance communication
- justify the principles for use of long-distance communication
- explain and discuss the limitations of remote, online collaboration tools
- develop strategies for appropriate use of remote communication, including written information, mobile devices, biomedical wearable devices, video/teleconferences, email, SMS, search engines and professional chat rooms.

NOTE: While the use of the word "you" does not reflect appropriate professional style and has been avoided in previous chapters, it has been used in the text (not merely in the activities) in Chapters 20, 21, 22 and 23 in an attempt to reinforce the importance of the information.

Long-distance professional communication involves communication over large distances. Wherever individuals and families live in rural and remote locations, long-distance communication is a reality. This typically means that healthcare may require technological and written forms of communication. For more than 50 years, healthcare professionals have consistently used written reports and telephones to communicate information remotely about appointments, expectations, interventions, test results, needs, future plans and various other issues related to the Person/s. Today, however, worldwide technological developments allow healthcare professionals to communicate electronically using mobile devices and the internet (video/teleconferences for telehealth)

(Anstey Watkins et al 2018; Boggs 2023; Davies et al 2014; Fouad 2014; Gagnon & Sabus 2015; Haddad et al 2019; see Chapter 21). Such electronic forms of communication include computer-mediated communication (CMC) and eMobile devices with related apps (Wilson et al 2021). They are typically forms of communication over distances and increasingly forms of communication when not attending for face-to-face care. They are used to provide and monitor healthcare for relevant Person/s, as well as to guide and support the healthcare providers (Boggs 2023; Davies et al 2014; Luz et al 2015). The increasing use of biomedical sensors to monitor and treat some diseases has further enabled remote forms of communication and thus care. These devices communicate information about the status and activity levels of the Person/s. Some also monitor vital signs remotely, providing information for the relevant healthcare professional about abnormalities. This information results in increased immediacy and efficiency of care, regardless of location and distance.

While there are advantages and disadvantages of new and old forms of long-distance communication, they are a necessary feature of healthcare for individuals and families living in remote locations, and increasingly for those living with chronic debilitating conditions.

In groups, discuss the following.

- Consider the amount of time you spend communicating every day and how you communicate.
- What forms of communication might people living in remote locations use in the twenty-first century?
- What might be the reasons for using these particular forms of remote communication?
- Suggest possible causes of disruption to communication in remote locations that are out of the control of the user.
- Do you think most people living in remote locations will typically have access to communications technology?

Societies, professions, families and individuals respond differently to remote forms of communication. Remote forms of communication potentially increase the convenience and speed of communication and receiving assistance when requiring care (De Ville 2001; Fouad 2014; Hamida et al 2015; Surantha et al 2021). However, these are not the only factors determining responses to remote communication. Each form has specific characteristics influencing responses. These characteristics include convenience, control, speed of delivery, preparation time, level of formality and thought required, reusability, sometimes the absence of non-verbal cues to complement meaning, irreversibility, legal implications, security, and access to appropriate technology (Armfield et al 2010; Boggs 2023; Klammer & Pöchhacker 2021). Many of these characteristics are desirable for healthcare professionals; however; some have implications worthy of consideration.

Characteristics of remote forms of communication for the health professional

There are a number of characteristics of long-distance forms of communication for the healthcare professional that require consideration (see Table 20.1).

TABLE 20.1
Characteristics of remote forms of communication for the health professional.

Characteristic	Telephone	Video/ teleconference	Email or SMS	Written report	Networking sites
Convenience	Y	Y	Y	D	Y
Control for caller/sender	Y	Y	Y	Y	Y
Immediate delivery time	Y	Y & N	D	D	Y
Quick preparation time	Y	N	Y	N	Y
Formality required	D	D	Y	Y	D
Thought required	Y	Y	Y	Y	Y
Repeated use	Y	Y	Y	Y	Y
Permanent record	D	D	Y	Y	Y
Non-verbal cues present	Y	Y	N	N	D
Legally binding	D	D	Y	Y	Y
Availability	Y	D	D	Y	D
Reliability	Y	D	D	Y	D
Security	D	D	N	D	N
Privacy	D	D	N	Y	N

Key: Y = definitely a characteristic; D = depending on the situation; N = not usually a characteristic.

It is interesting to consider the characteristics of each form of remote communication typically used in the healthcare professions. The often-popular electronic forms are not always as available or as reliable as many suggest (Devito 2021). Many countries and rural areas do not have technological resources available, or they have unreliable access to such resources. Therefore, it can be difficult for healthcare professionals to achieve effective communication when relying only on electronic forms of remote communication in the healthcare professions.

- List the remote forms of communication typically used in the healthcare professions.
- List the advantages and disadvantages of each of the remote forms of communication.
- Suggest ways to overcome the disadvantages.
- Explain why the following statement is or is not true and explain your answer:

Direct (speaking on the telephone or Skype) personal contact is a necessary component of long-distance communication.

Convenience, immediacy and cost are factors that are increasingly important in healthcare services, due to rising demand for and, in many places decreases in, resources and funding.

Most healthcare services adopt practices to increase efficiency and improve outcomes. Thus, many are adopting electronic methods for storing and accessing records, sharing techniques, and communicating within and beyond the health service (e.g. internal and external email) (Boggs 2023; Levine 2012; see Chapters 21 and 22). Many healthcare services and professions promote electronic forms of networking for support and professional development of employees in remote settings (Ashar et al 2010; Maeder et al 2010). However, the nature of the healthcare professions suggests that direct personal contact will always be a necessary component of long-distance communication.

There is discussion about the "paperless" modes of communicating because some healthcare professionals still prefer hard copies of information (Haddad et al 2019; Levine 2012). It is interesting but difficult to predict the preferred form of long-distance communication for healthcare professionals in the future. There is an increase in the use of electronic forms of communication, both for gathering information and providing information. Person/s portals allow the Person/s to provide relevant information and the healthcare professional to access and then gather any additional information to prepare appropriate care (Boggs 2023).

Principles governing professional remote communication

There are important principles governing remote communication among healthcare professionals (see Table 20.2). These principles relate directly to the characteristics of an effective healthcare professional (see Chapter 7), but are sometimes forgotten in remote (especially email) forms of communication (Bevan et al 2011; Boucher 2010; Devito 2021; Yao et al 2010). One essential component of professional remote communication is demonstrating effective listening and appropriate non-verbal skills. This may be challenging if you are unseen. However, awareness of the effect of the voice and ensuring mutual understanding of all messages will contribute to effective remote communication.

The principles governing remote communication are especially important in healthcare services without support personnel to assist with preparation of documents. When composing and preparing written forms of remote communication for healthcare, it is beneficial to ask a

TABLE 20.2
Principles governing professional remote communication

Use:	Avoid:
• Polite forms of words and constructions • Formal language and expression Clear explanations of any jargon or technical terms* • Correct spelling and grammar – always check before sending • Concise, accurate and clear statements – one idea to one sentence	• Abrupt, impolite messages • Colloquial or everyday expressions • Unexplained use of jargon • Spelling and grammatical errors • Long and rambling sentences

*Technical terms are words that may have one meaning in everyday use but assume a different meaning in the context of professional communication.

colleague to proofread the document (for spelling and grammatical errors, appropriate levels of civility and formality along with clarity and accuracy) before sending it.

These principles or "points to remember" govern all types of remote communication. In combination with these principles, the following strategies guide the use of types of long-distance communication within the healthcare professions.

Electronic records

Many health services now use electronic forms of notes, records and files (databases) for recording information about the Person/s and any interactions with the healthcare professional (Doherty 2021). It is important that the healthcare professional learns and conforms to the expectations and requirements of the healthcare service regarding electronic records (see Chapter 22). It is also important for the healthcare professional to remember the principles for recording information presented in Chapter 22. Confidentiality of information entered into an electronic database is essential (see Chapter 19). All Person/s information MUST be managed to ensure the confidentiality/privacy and thus the dignity of the Person/s (Doherty 2021). Leaving Person/s information on the computer screen while interacting with others either in the room or out of the room is inappropriate and does not conform to confidentiality requirements. Taking information or assessment results for a Person/s off-site on a USB stick (even when encrypted) without consent is inappropriate and potentially dangerous for the healthcare professional and the Person/s.

- Discuss how taking personal information off-site on a USB stick might be dangerous.

Telephones

A telephone conversation allows the use of suprasegmentals – the non-verbal features of the voice – for negotiation of meaning. It is best to avoid using the telephone to deliver bad news, to explain a complicated procedure or solve a complicated problem (Haddad et al 2019). There are important strategies to assist in the achievement of effective verbal telephone communication.

Strategies for verbally using a telephone

Answering a call

Many healthcare services have a method of recording information about callers, and it is important to use the designated system. However, there are some principles to guide the actions of the healthcare professional when answering a telephone call.

- When answering a call, it is important to clearly and slowly state your name and the name of the health service.
- If possible, find the person and connect them with the caller.
- If the healthcare service employee is unavailable, record the name of the caller, the time they rang, their number and the purpose of their call in the designated system. Ask them to spell

their name if necessary and read their telephone number back to them to check the accuracy of the number before terminating the call.

- Reassure the caller that you will pass the information to the relevant healthcare service employee. Explain that this individual is busy and encourage the caller to call again if they have not heard from the healthcare service employee within a particular time frame. If possible, suggest a time when the healthcare service employee might be available to have a telephone conversation.
- Thank the caller for calling, if possible, using their name.

In groups, discuss the following:

- Decide if there is any other consideration that will make answering a call during a working day either more professional or clearer for the caller than the points listed above.
- Consider the perspective of the caller and list reasons for each of the above points.

Making a call

- Prepare for the call – gather all appropriate documents, a pen and a piece of paper or diary before making the call.
- It may be beneficial to compile a list of points for coverage during the call to avoid wasting time or forgetting important points.
- State your name and place of work, the purpose of the call and the name of the particular individual to whom you wish to speak.
- Exercise patience if there is a delay in locating the required individual; it may be helpful to do something that is not demanding while waiting. When connected, ensure the delay does NOT affect your attitude or tone of voice. (If receiving a call, apologise for any delay caused and maintain pleasant responses if the caller is a little impatient.)
- If the Person/s is unknown to you, it is advisable to begin with a formal tone and reducing the degree of formality to coincide with the development of rapport.
- Articulate carefully to ensure production of clear speech (remember non-verbal features of the voice – the suprasegmental features – see Chapter 10).
- Avoid talking when the other Person/s is talking.
- Clarify all points and confirm understanding of important points.
- Listen carefully and if necessary, take notes.
- Give feedback to indicate understanding, whether of agreement or otherwise.
- Remember that there is only the voice to influence meaning and therefore the conversation may require explicit verbalisation of any non-verbal behaviour or emotions.
- Allow time for clarification and discussion of additional points if required by the other Person/s.
- Remember to thank the Person/s when finished and say goodbye.
- It may be important to provide written confirmation of the conversation.

If teleconferencing facilities are unavailable, a mobile phone using the speaker function may be used for a long-distance meeting. When teleconferencing, it is important when the remote individuals (those not present) are speaking that those present in the room listen carefully before beginning to speak, thereby allowing the remote individuals to finish their point. The remote people will be unable to notice the non-verbal cues of those present and thus may not realise when someone wishes to speak.

Strategies for using short messaging service (SMS)

Healthcare services are increasingly using the short messaging service (SMS) on mobile phones (i.e. texts) to confirm information or appointment times (Fedoruk 2014). Thus, it is important to consider the content of such messaging. When communicating using an SMS as part of a healthcare service, it is important to:

- use the name of the receiver of the message
- avoid using abbreviations typical of an SMS
- state each point clearly and succinctly, where necessary using punctuation to indicate each point
- use a name (either your name or the name of the healthcare service) at the end of the SMS to ensure the receiver knows who sent the message.

In groups:

- List the possible points for inclusion in an SMS to a Person/s to confirm their appointment.
- Together, write and agree upon the content of such an SMS.

Strategies for using an answering service or voicemail

When recording a message to advise there is no-one from the service available to answer the call, it is important to:

- clearly state the name of the service for the caller and state there is currently no-one available to answer the call
- provide instructions for how to leave a message, for example, *After the tone, state your name and number and the date and time of your call*
- state that someone will respond to the call as soon as possible
- thank them for calling (this could also be stated at the beginning of the message).

When leaving a telephone message, it is important to:

- clearly state your name and place of work, the purpose of the call and the name of the individual who should receive the message. State the return phone number carefully, perhaps twice, to allow easy transcription of the message.
- articulate carefully to produce clear speech
- avoid speaking rapidly or running words together
- as a reminder, record details of the date and time of the call in your diary or another relevant place.

When receiving a recorded telephone message, it is important to:

- write the message in a particular place, recording the date and time of receipt of the message (e.g. diary or phone message book). Avoid pieces of paper because they are easily lost.
- phone the individual to indicate receipt of the message and the relevant response (Haddad et a 2019). Indicate action taken by marking the received message in some manner or record the date and time of your response.

Using video/teleconferencing or Skype/Zoom/Teams for professional development and meetings

(For information relating to provision of remote healthcare see Chapter 21.)
Video/teleconferencing using Skype, Zoom or Teams involves the use of technical devices allowing either a simultaneous visual, telephone or computer connection with multiple people from multiple sites. These connections allow communication without individuals leaving their workplace or home (Dixon 2010). A tele-, Skype, Zoom or Teams conference is not particularly anxiety-provoking because it simply requires people to sit and either listen or talk. Some people at a remote site during such a connection may need to do something to assist their concentration or focus, as they may be unable to see the people at the other sites. Taking notes about the details of the conversation or required action as a result of the conversation may assist this potential for boredom or limited concentration. A videoconference uses a camera, and this can produce consternation for some individuals. Such consternation usually reduces with exposure to the videoconferencing process. If you are at a remote site and there is a camera, it is important to engage in the interaction. Completion of an obviously unrelated task (reading or writing) may appear rude, regardless of the relevance of the activity. It would be courteous to indicate that you will be taking notes throughout the meeting, to indicate the reason for not always looking at the interacting group.

Benefits

Communicating in this form is beneficial for:

- networking
- health professionals in remote settings
- saving time
- reducing travel costs
- allowing non-verbal behaviours to establish meaning
- sharing ideas with previously inaccessible individuals
- receiving assistance for problem-solving
- sharing new procedures with remote sites
- professional development.

Strategies for using video/teleconferencing, Skype, Zoom or Teams connection

- When conducting a video/teleconference, Skype, Zoom or Teams meeting it is important to "book" the facilities and schedule a mutually convenient time or regular meeting time with all relevant sites. It is essential to notify everyone expected to be in the meeting of the meeting details.
- When conducting a video/teleconference, Skype, Zoom or Teams meeting, it is important that every member of the meeting uses their camera to indicate their presence in the meeting.
- When conducting a video/teleconference, Skype, Zoom or Teams meeting, introduce each site. If the interacting individuals are unknown to each other, allow time for the individuals to introduce themselves and their roles. If the individuals are known, name those present and restrict introductory details to new people.
- When conducting a video/teleconference, Skype, Zoom or Teams meeting, remember to have the individuals identify themselves each time they speak, unless their name appears under their image.

- When conducting a videoconference, Skype, Zoom or Teams, it is essential to include all the connected sites in the discussion and the presentation of ideas or procedures.
  - Ask for confirmation of visual, auditory and cognitive understanding.
  - Ask for comments or questions from all sites.
- When conducting such a remote visual conference, it is important to repeat anything that is not in range of the microphone. This is especially important during question time.
- When finishing a video/teleconference, Skype, Zoom or Teams meeting, say goodbye to each site separately.
- Encourage people leaving the tele/videoconference to indicate they are leaving before terminating the connection. If they know they must leave earlier than the scheduled time, they should indicate this at the beginning of the meeting, and before they terminate the connection. This is important, as it advises those remaining in the conversation whether there were technical complications or a deliberate termination of the connection.

The internet

Email

People often forget that email is neither private nor secure (Boggs 2023; Levine 2012; Snyder 2010; Snyder & Cistulli 2011). It is possible to forward any email anywhere. As an email passes through a server, a copy appears on that server and is held there, whether deleted from or remaining in an inbox. There are also issues of consistent access to the technology relating to email. Not all sites or individuals have reliable access, and some may simply not have reliable access to this technology (Rennie et al 2010).

Despite these drawbacks, people often prefer email because it allows the sender and receiver control of their time and ideas. There are important strategies to assist in the achievement of effective email communication.

- Decide on the purpose of the email.
- Include a title in the subject box. The title indicates the content of the email to capture the attention of the recipient.
- Use a salutation (e.g. *Dear …*). The use of a given name will depend upon the purpose of the email and the relationship with the recipient. Use *Hi …* thoughtfully in professional emails.
- Remember that every email is a legal document.
- Decide if you need to copy (cc) someone else into the email and in some cases, it may be essential to copy yourself into the email.
- Use the appropriate tone for the audience; the tone (polite and friendly with an appropriate level of formality) and content of professional emails should be different to that of personal emails.
- Use well-constructed sentences to assist the individual reading the email.
- Explain critical comments carefully and politely.
- Use careful constructions to avoid appearing abrupt and even rude (Devito 2021).
- Use careful constructions to avoid ambiguity and misinterpretation.
- Describe any emotions carefully because they are unseen.
- Describe any relevant non-verbal cues because they are also unseen.
- Avoid capital letters because they are considered equivalent to SHOUTING!
- Compose requests for clarification politely, giving reasons for the need for clarification.
- Avoid abbreviations (see Chapter 22) or emoticons (Devito 2021) in professional emails.
- Write what you mean and read and edit before sending.

- Use a final salutation or signature appropriate to the tone and purpose of the email. A computer-generated signature is beneficial for professional emails because it ensures that role, position and contact details accompany every sent email.
- Ensure the email is going to the right person before sending!
- Use an explanatory sentence when including an attachment to confirm the contents of the attachment.
- Reduce the size of large attachments by saving them in a compressed format. When creating or saving an attachment in a particular format, remember that the recipient may not have the software required to access the attachment.
- Check for the correct address if an email is undeliverable. Undeliverable emails may also mean that the inbox of the recipient is full.
- Reply to every email that is not a mass "company" email; acknowledgement of receipt is polite and reassuring for the sender.

Email is convenient and, in many cases, immediate. It allows control and is beneficial in augmenting face-to-face contact with those who interact with the healthcare professional (De Ville 2001). However, there are disadvantages requiring careful consideration when communicating remotely using email.

- Using the above bullet points, compile a list of advantages and disadvantages of using email.
- Suggest realistic ways of overcoming the disadvantages.

Search engines

The use of search engines to locate information and practice-related research is common in the healthcare professions where there is appropriate technology. The value of a search engine lies in connection to multiple websites. Locating the required websites can be frustrating until an appropriate search word or combination of search words provides satisfactory results. It is important to consider the reliability of a website when sourcing information from individual sites. It is relatively simple to construct a website, so there are multitudinous websites with particular agendas and biases. When seeking evidence for practice or assessment tasks, it is possible to access websites that are less than reliable and not always reputable. Thus, it is important for healthcare professionals and students to exercise care when using any information obtained from a website.

Online collaboration tools

Professional chat rooms and wiki spaces

There are particular protocols governing all internet-based chat rooms; the basis of these protocols is a desire for and commitment to respectful communication (see Chapter 23). Professional chat rooms and wiki spaces allow worldwide exploration of alternative protocols, procedures and management strategies (Meenan et al 2010; Mills et al 2010). When relating to healthcare professionals or Person/s from other cultures through chat rooms, it is important to remember the factors affecting culturally appropriate communication (Woolley et al 2013; see Chapters 16 and 17).

Chapter summary

Long-distance communication is a permanent fixture in healthcare professions and has legal implications. It can take the form of reporting in hard copy and digital format or the use of the internet to communicate relevant information. There is also increasing use of video/teleconferencing, Skype, Zoom or Teams to physically separated sites. Long-distance communication, while convenient and immediate, can have particular disadvantages requiring the consideration of any healthcare professional communicating remotely. It is important for healthcare professionals to use remote forms of communication appropriately and politely to benefit from the advantages of this form of communication. Long-distance communication can save time, connect people who might otherwise be isolated, and provide the latest relevant information and procedures for relevant Person/s and interested healthcare professionals.

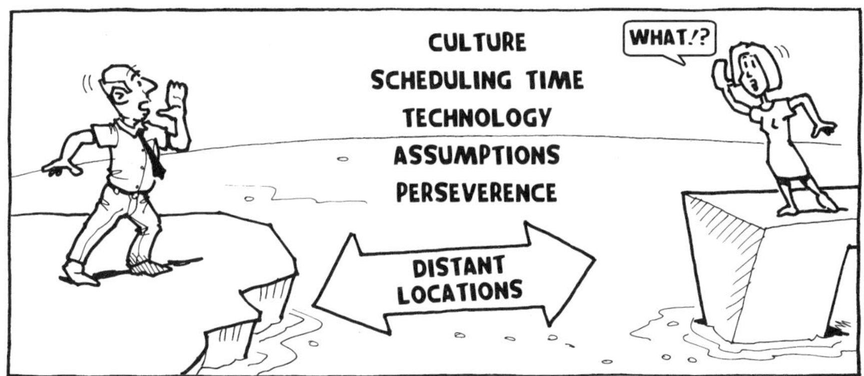

FIGURE 20.1
Long-distance communication has particular components.
Courtesy Roger Harvey © Elsevier Australia.

REVIEW QUESTIONS

1. Using your own words, define long-distance communication.

2. List the types of long-distance communication typically used among healthcare professionals.

3. State the advantages of long-distance communication.

4. Suggest ways of overcoming the disadvantages of long-distance communication.

5. Using a telephone:

    i. What is it important to do when answering a telephone call for a healthcare service?

    ii. What is important when preparing to communicate professionally over the telephone?

iii. Briefly describe an effective telephone conversation.

____

____

____

iv. List the things to remember when using an SMS to confirm information or appointments.

____

____

____

v. List the things to remember when using an answering service.

____

____

____

6. Video/teleconferencing, Skype, Zoom or Teams:

i. Outline the benefits of video/teleconferencing, Skype, Zoom or Teams.

____

____

____

ii. Briefly, describe an effective videoconference, Skype, Zoom or Teams call.

____

____

____

7. Categorise each point listed in the "Email" section of this chapter into one of three categories:

Civility	Practicality	Reality

References

Anstey Watkins, J.O.T., Goudge, J., Gómez-Olivé, F.X., et al., 2018. Mobile phone use among patients and health workers to enhance primary healthcare: A qualitative study in rural South Africa. Social Science and Medicine, 198(2018), 139–147.

Armfield, N.R., White, M.M., Williams, M.L., et al., 2010. Clinical services and professional support: A review of mobile telepaediatric services in Queensland. Studies in Health Technology and Informatics, 161, 149–158.

Ashar, R., Lewis, S., Blazes, D.L., et al., 2010. Applying information and communications technologies to collect health data from remote settings: A systematic assessment of current technologies. Journal of Biomedical Informatics, 43(2), 332–341.

Bevan, J.I., Jupin, A.M., Sparks, L., 2011. Information quality, uncertainty, and quality of care in long-distance caregiving. Communication Research Reports, 28(2), 190–195.

Boggs, K., 2023. Interpersonal relationships: Professional communication skills for nurses, 9th ed. Elsevier, St Louis, MO.

Boucher, J.L., 2010. Technology and patient–provider interactions: Improving quality of care, but is it improving communication and collaboration? Editorial. Diabetes Spectrum 23(3), 142–144.

Davies, J., Bukulatjpi, S., Sharma, S., et al., 2014. "Only your blood can tell the story" – a qualitative research study using semi-structured interviews to explore the hepatitis B related knowledge, perceptions and experiences of remote dwelling Indigenous Australians and their health care providers in northern Australia. BMC Public Health, 14, 1–23.

De Ville, K.A., 2001. Ethical and legal implications of e-mail correspondence between physicians and patients. Ethics Health Care, 4 (1), 1–3.

Devito, J.A., 2021. The interpersonal communication book, 16th ed. Pearson, Boston.

Dixon, R.F., 2010. Enhancing primary care through online communication. Health Affairs, 29(7), 1364–1369.

Doherty, R.F., 2021. Ethical dimensions in health professions, 7th ed. Elsevier, St Louis, MO.

Fedoruk, M., 2014. Legal responsibilities and ethics. In: Fedoruk, M., Hofmeyer, A. (eds), Becoming a nurse: An evidence-based approach. Oxford University Press, Melbourne.

Fouad, H., 2014. Implementation of remote health monitoring in medical rural clinics for web telemedicine system. International Journal of Advanced Networking and Applications 6(3), 2300–2307.

Gagnon, K., Sabus, C., 2015. Professionalism in a Digital Age: Opportunities and considerations for using social media in health care. Physical Therapy, 95(3), 406–414.

Haddad, A.M., Purtilo, R.B., Doherty, R.F., 2019. Health professional and patient interaction, 9th ed. Elsevier/Saunders, Philadelphia.

Hamida, S.T.-B., Hamida, E.B., Ahmed, B., 2015. A new mHealth communication framework for use in wearable WBANs and mobile technologies. Sensors, 15(2), 3379–3408.

Klammer, M., Pöchhacker, F. 2021. Video remote interpreting in clinical communication: A multimodal analysis. Patient Education and Counseling, 104(2021), 2867–2876.

Levine, J., 2012. Working with people: The helping process, 9th ed. Pearson, San Antonio.

Luz, S., Masoodian, M., Cesario, M., 2015. Disease surveillance and patient care in remote regions: An exploratory study of collaboration among health-care professionals in Amazonia. Behaviour and Information Technology, 34(6), 548–565.

Maeder, A., Hovenga, E.J.S., Kidd, M.R., et al., 2010. Telehealth and remote access. Studies in Health Technology and Information, 151, 239–254.

Meenan, C., King, A., Toland, C., et al., 2010. Use of a Wiki as a radiology departmental knowledge management system. Journal of Digital Imaging, 23(2), 142–151.

Mills, J.E., Francis, K., Birks, M., et al., 2010. Registered nurses as members of interprofessional primary healthcare teams in remote or isolated areas of Queensland: Collaboration, communication and partnerships in practice. Journal of Interprofessional Care, 24(5), 587–596.

Rennie, E., Crouch, A., Thomas, J., et al., 2010. Beyond public access? Reconsidering broadband for remote Indigenous communities [online]. Communication, Politics and Culture, 43(1), 48–69.

Snyder, J.L., 2010. Email privacy in the workplace: A boundary regulation perspective. Journal of Business Communication, 47, 266–294.

Snyder, J.L., Cistulli, M.D., 2011. The relationship between workplace e-mail privacy and psychological contract violation, and their influence on trust in top management and affective commitment. Communication Research Reports 28(2), 121–129.

Surantha, N., Atmaja, P., Wicaksono, M., 2021. A review of wearable Internet of Things device for healthcare. Procedia Computer Science, 179, 936–943.

Wilson, M.A., Fouts, B.L., Brown, K.N., 2021.Development of mobile application for acute pain management in US military healthcare. Applied Nursing Research, 58, 151393.

Woolley, T., Sivamalai, S., Ross, S., et al., 2013. Indigenous perspectives on the desired attributes of medical graduates practising in remote communities: A Northwest Queensland pilot study. Australian Journal of Rural Health, 21 (2), 90–96.

Yao, J., Wan, Y., Givens, G.D., 2010. Using web services to realize remote hearing assessment. Journal of Clinical Monitoring and Computing, 24(1), 41–50.

CHAPTER 21

Telehealth or telecommunication:
2 The seen but not-in-the-room healthcare professional

Chapter objectives

Upon completing this chapter, readers should be able to:

- demonstrate understanding of the current realities of healthcare services
- state the meaning of telehealth in healthcare
- list and define the various terms used to describe the use of technology to deliver remote healthcare
- identify the positive outcomes of using telehealth
- list and explain the challenges associated with using telehealth
- demonstrate understanding of the requirements of telehealth
- explain and demonstrate the requirements of effective communication using telehealth.

Healthcare throughout the world is experiencing increasing demands and financial strain. The sustainability of the current in-the-room model of healthcare is threatened by these realities (Carati & Margelis 2013). This is especially true when experiencing a global pandemic, COVID-19 (Sibson 2021). Another reality is that many rural and remote locations are some distance away from required healthcare resources. This creates additional demands on and cost of healthcare services, in many cases reducing the accessibility of healthcare for individuals in rural and remote areas (Reese et al 2015). The difficulty of recruiting healthcare professionals to work in these rural and remote locations is an additional reality affecting the equitable provision of healthcare to all individuals requiring such care (Parsons et al 2017). The families requiring healthcare while living in rural areas also experience difficulties accessing healthcare services. They often have to travel long distances and perhaps be away from home for extended periods of time depending on the health condition and the required interventions. This, of course, has financial implications, especially if the Person is unable to work during those times.

Returning to these rural locations after receiving healthcare typically creates further difficulties relating to maintaining the status achieved while receiving healthcare interventions. For some individuals, decreased mobility or chronic illnesses impact on the ability to access healthcare, regardless of location. These realities typically produce stress for the Person/s experiencing such circumstances, thereby contributing to the challenges of managing their health needs in rural locations. Telehealth or telecommunication allowing remote healthcare provides an appropriate alternative for these individuals, in their place of residence, while also contributing to Person-centred-Care (Dyb et al 2021). This facilitates provision of effective healthcare using face-to-face, but not-in-person interactions, improving both communication and care (Fong et al 2020; Henderson 2019). In addition, telehealth appointments replacing in-person appointments, have been shown to increase equity of healthcare for individuals in rural and remote communities (Batt et al 2021). This is changing the delivery of healthcare throughout the world (Boggs 2023).

The use of technology (telehealth or telecommunication) to address some of the above-mentioned realities has been increasing for several decades (Binks 2017; Boggs 2023; Li et al 2018; Rogante et al 2010; Sibson 2021). This use of technology to deliver and monitor healthcare is becoming more necessary with the increase in disease; a worldwide ageing population and a decrease in the number and availability, within many health professions, of appropriate specialist healthcare professionals (Speyer et al 2018; Stavas et al 2018; van Houwelingen et al 2015). Telehealth increases the ability to provide quickened responses to health emergencies (Jaffe et al 2021; New Zealand Ministry of Health 2017). It is also proving to be an appropriate form of healthcare for conditions requiring long-term management, allowing daily interaction and early identification of changes in status, thereby encouraging immediate and appropriate care (Bernocchi et al 2016; Kamei et al 2018). It is important to note that telehealth is different to the videoconferencing used among healthcare professionals for professional development and meetings – it refers to providing actual Person/s-focused healthcare, regardless of location. Telehealth facilitates delivery of healthcare for the Person/s and carers in their particular environment or context (Campbell et al 2019; Czaja, 2016).

Telehealth or telecommunication (as with in-person interactions) allows all communicating individuals to see each other and interact within their surroundings while not in the same room. It also allows the healthcare professional to see the effects of injuries or changes in function, despite not being in the same room. The improvement in technology and increasing access to internet services in remote areas have increased the use of telehealth for remote healthcare (Dudley 2018).

In Australia, these improvements have led to the planning of a national strategy for the use of telehealth by The Australasian TeleHealth Society. They suggest creation of particular key groups with the most to gain from the use of telehealth: aged care, those lacking mobility and those in rural and remote locations (Carati & Margelis 2013). Telehealth has also been successfully used within the prison system for more than a decade, thereby improving care and safety for all in that context (Binks 2017). Telehealth provides a "tele-presence" of the healthcare professional for the Person/s, to provide appropriate healthcare in their "home", potentially producing feelings of safety and acceptance of the care in the Person and carers. It allows provision of important aspects of the healthcare process, including consultations, assessments, diagnosing, establishing relevant goals and interventions of various kinds, along with information provision and ongoing monitoring of the needs of the Person/s and their carer. This contributes to the achievement of effective communication while enhancing healthcare, regardless of the diagnosis, limited mobility or distance. These visual, technology-driven consultations also support personal interactions with the Person/s, including relevant family members, resulting in the development of mutual understanding and a therapeutic relationship, while promoting awareness of non-verbal messages. Telehealth also allows the presence of several healthcare professionals simultaneously throughout a session, thereby providing appropriate alternatives to in-person healthcare for all individuals.

There are various terms used to describe the use of technology while providing healthcare. These are some of those terms: telehealth, telepractice, teleconsultation, telemonitoring, telecare, telehome-monitoring or telehomecare, telesurveillance, telemedicine, telenursing and telerehabilitation. Some are used interchangeably, depending on the understanding of the individual using the term, while others are used with a particular meaning. These different meanings appear to depend on the purpose of the remote telecommunication. However, regardless of the particular terms, they all refer to using technology and remote methods of information gathering and provision, along with other aspects of the healthcare process, to fulfil the unique healthcare needs of particular individuals. In this chapter see Table 21.1 for the meanings of these terms.

TABLE 21.1
Terms use to describe communication using technology in healthcare

Term	Definition and potential effect
Telehealth / Telepractice	Relates to immediate access to a relevant healthcare professional to provide healthcare, including assessing symptoms, providing interventions and education relating to the health needs of various and sometimes chronic health conditions. It contributes to achieving effective communication, with the potential to improve the health and quality of life of both the Person and their carers, without them leaving their home or the healthcare professional leaving their location.
Teleconsultation	Relates to accessing expert or specialist medical or relevant practitioner advice to guide on-site or out-of-hospital assessment and relevant interventions.
Telemonitoring / Telecare / Telehomecare or Telehome-monitoring / Telesurveillance	Relates to the use of devices in the place of residence/home or sometimes worn by the Person, to monitor the condition and functioning of the Person. These devices gather information, sending it to a monitoring device or service to provide alerts about the status and needs of the Person (Surantha et al 2021), promoting effective communication, immediate responses and appropriate care.
Telemedicine / Telenursing	Relates to remote provision of medical services, including nursing care for the Person/s in their place of residence to enable remote provision of clinical reviews to monitor and manage health conditions, thereby assisting in avoiding potential deterioration in the condition.
Telerehabilitation	Relates to the remote provision of rehabilitation from relevant healthcare professionals. This may include education, exercise regimes, activity programmes, and other relevant interventions (sometimes virtual) for both the Person and their carers.

Adapted from Binks, 2017, p. 478.

There are a variety of outcomes discussed in the literature relating to the use of telehealth. Some are obvious benefits, while others are challenges requiring further consideration and guidelines for the ongoing use of telehealth for any healthcare professional when providing healthcare.

The positive outcomes from using telecommunication

The requirement of Person-centred Care in health care is discussed throughout the world and mandated in healthcare policies in many countries (Dyb et al 2021). Such care is considered possible during in-person healthcare; however, Person-centred Care (P-cC) is also considered a foundational aspect of telehealth (Dudley 2018; Hines et al 2017). It is understood to be possible to build a positive therapeutic relationship, regardless of distances between the Person/s and the healthcare professional, using telehealth (Hines et al 2017; Kruse et al 2018). This relationship development is made possible by everyone being able to see each other and observe the non-verbal messages of each communicating individual, allowing demonstration of respect, expressions of empathy, development of trust and thereby rapport. This facilitates effective listening and active collaboration. In addition, it also facilitates equitable access to healthcare, regardless of location (Parsons et al 2017; Wilkes-Gillan & Lincoln 2018). It also provides access to and implementation of recent evidenced-based interventions, regardless of location (Vismara et al 2012).

Together, identify how to achieve demonstrations of respect, expressions of empathy, development of trust and thereby rapport when interacting using video interactions. Consider what the technical interface might require of the healthcare professional to achieve all aspects of P-cC.

Telehealth is reported to reduce the cost of healthcare (Binks 2017; Dudley 2018; Sitton-Kent et al 2018), after meeting the initial cost of the required technology. The removal of the need to travel to provide care, the need for the associated ownership, insurance and maintenance of vehicles, possibly accommodation and meals for the healthcare professional, definitely contributes to the reduction in cost. The time spent travelling, to provide in-person care reduces available time for other healthcare-related tasks, thereby affecting cost and efficiency of care. Telehealth potentially reduces all these costs, while also reducing the fatigue associated with travelling (O'Brien Cherry et al 2017).

Telehealth provides immediate off-site safe care in any location (Fong et al 2020; Kruse et al 2018). It also potentially provides access to specific diagnostic equipment through consultation with relevant clinicians (Armour & Helmer 2021). This not only reduces attendance at the emergency department, it also reduces admissions, re-admissions and thus hospital costs (Binks 2017; Giordano et al 2009; Gruber-Baldini et al 2022; Kamei et al 2018; Voerman & Nickel 2017), along with reducing waiting lists for in-home healthcare (Vismara et al 2012).

While decreasing these, telehealth also potentially increases both early implementation of care for identified needs (Choi & Oakley 2021; Kruse et al 2018) and the number of possible consultations within a day (Rogante et al 2010). It allows ongoing assessment and care, including ongoing rehabilitation using individually designed programs for use at home. There is evidence of this improving recovery and maintaining achievements from inpatient care related to stroke (Bernocchi et al 2016), while also reducing carer fatigue and burden post stroke (Chen et al 2017). This is often achieved by providing opportunities for remote discussion to assist in problem-solving relating to the particular condition (Brokmann et al 2016; Campbell et al 2019; Choi & Oakley 2021; Fisk et al 2020) and the challenges of their environment, thereby providing unique P-cC.

The involvement of the carer in telehealth interactions has benefits for both the carer and the Person, thereby improving outcomes. There is also evidence relating to improvement in aspects of the condition or in functioning in daily life for individuals experiencing other conditions, including: asthma (van der Meer et al 2009), autism (Pickard et al 2016), cardiology (Dalleck et al 2011), chronic obstructive pulmonary disease (COPD) (Liu et al 2013), fragile X syndrome (McDuffie et al 2016), diabetes (Chow et al 2014), paediatrics (Campbell et al 2019), palliative care (James et al 2021) and post-traumatic stress disorder (PTSD) (Kruse et al 2018), to name a few. Telehealth also facilitates ongoing monitoring of progress after discharge in order to adjust interventions as necessary, thereby potentially maintaining previously achieved improvements, while also identifying any decline in the condition. In addition, telehealth has positive results when providing education relating to the associated needs of the health condition (Rush et al 2018). This telehealth education has been repeatedly identified as effectively increasing the knowledge and understanding of the Person/s regarding their condition and the management of their condition (Kamei et al 2018; Parsons et al 2017; Rush et al 2018). Telehealth also increases the knowledge and awareness of the healthcare professional about the particular context and the associated supports and challenges of the Person/s in their current situation or place of residence (O'Brien Cherry et al 2017).

Therefore, regular use of telehealth facilitates implementation of relevant in-home healthcare interventions. This also facilitates improvement in functioning and quality of life, empowering safety in daily life (Binks 2017; Rush et al 2018; Sitton-Kent et al 2018) and often the development of skills (Victorson et al 2014). The timely achievement of this can depend on the reliability of the network technology in the particular location (Hüzmeli et al 2017). It certainly promotes the sharing of new procedures with remote services, thereby potentially contributing to improved outcomes. Telehealth does not disadvantage the particular Person/s, with there being no difference in improvement between home or in-person care at the healthcare service (Bradford et al 2015; Henderson et al 2013; Lin et al 2014). Telehealth, by providing ongoing care regardless of location, increases the convenience and efficiency of the care (Fong et al 2020; Sitton-Kent et al 2018). It is also a quality and effective form of managing care for individuals experiencing long-term chronic conditions, without them having to leave their place of residence (Chen et al 2017). All of the above points increase the satisfaction of the Person and their carer, along with the healthcare professional and their employer.

Together, choose a typical assessment used in your healthcare profession and plan how you would conduct this assessment using telehealth.

Challenges relating to using telecommunication

Achieving effective communication is essential, although not always straightforward when delivering healthcare, regardless of the mode of delivery. However, regardless of its importance in healthcare, effective communication can be potentially more challenging when using telehealth. Firstly, remember that at the foundation of all healthcare interactions are the elements of Person-centred Care (P-cC). However, when using telehealth, they are vital to ensure relevant, meaningful and quality healthcare. Allowing the distance, not-in-person interaction or events in the immediate environment, to negatively affect the quality of the interaction with the Person/s does not reflect P-cC nor achieve satisfactory health outcomes. This indicates the need for those healthcare professionals using telehealth to be skilled and experienced in their particular profession (Binks 2017; Dudley 2018; Hines et al 2017; Sitton-Kent al 2018). In addition, it is essential for the healthcare professional to identify the needs relevant to their particular profession and to be proficient in the use of the required technology for telehealth (van Houwelingen et al 2020), in order to achieve effective communication and therefore develop appropriate goals and interventions. The referral should assist you; however if not, a quick phone call to establish the relevant needs may be necessary.

As touch is not possible during telehealth interventions, for effective healthcare provision, this gathered information would assist you to establish whether or not there is a need for an in-person interaction requiring physical interaction between the Person/s and the healthcare professional (Henry et al 2018). This will then determine your next step of either making an in-person appointment in a particular location or scheduling a telehealth session. In addition, considering the personal details, including the age and gender of the Person/s, may indicate their possible response to the use of telehealth. Individuals of particular ages and sometimes genders may find the use of the required technology challenging, due to lack of knowledge about the systems, therefore requiring more training, support and possible assistance when using the technology (Campbell et al 2019; Speyer et al 2018). Some may simply have personal preferences for in-person healthcare, therefore demonstrating resistance to or scepticism about remote healthcare (Kruse et al 2018).

Regardless of the individual responses to the use of telehealth, as with any healthcare interaction, it is essential to explain the process and what to expect from the overall telehealth process (including establishing relevant goals from gathered information and assessments) and the expected process throughout each telehealth session (The Royal Australian College of General Practitioners [RACGP] 2014). In addition, it may be necessary to explain how to use the equipment, adjust sound settings and, if appropriate, where to position the camera/microphone, along with what to do if the system freezes or "drops out" during the session. Explanations relating to interruptions in the system may be more appropriate when they occur rather than when first connecting through telehealth. If possible, it may also encourage relevant actions in such circumstance if the Person and carer have written instructions relating to interruptions.

It is important when beginning any interaction to introduce yourself and your role (see Chapter 3). It is equally important to establish the identity of the Person/s, to ensure that you are interacting with the right Person/s. In the initial telehealth interaction, this requires a short discussion confirming their name, contact details and the details of their condition and symptoms. In order to establish interpersonal trust, this **may** also include discussion of the realities of their condition and how it affects their life, along with discussion of their family members, pets, interests and so forth, to achieve mutual understanding of their needs. Investing time to develop the therapeutic relationship and to maintain that relationship is an important requirement of using telehealth (Henry et al 2018). It is also essential to ensure consistent focus on the remote interaction, for both the Person and the healthcare professional. When communicating remotely, it is possible to become distracted by occurrences in the immediate environment (McDuffie et al 2016). Thus it is important to prepare the environment to avoid distractions or interruptions during any telehealth interactions. It may be appropriate to mention this to the Person/s, to avoid inappropriate interruptions from pets, phones or family members. It certainly requires thought to assist the healthcare professional to avoid any such distractions or interruptions (e.g. a sign on the relevant door or notifying relevant colleagues to avoid interruptions or turning the phone to silent!).

Devices, trained personnel and secure internet connection

Telehealth communication requires particular equipment (device), software and staffing. These include a computer or tablet/iPad or mobile phone, and an external camera, if there is not one inbuilt in the computer/tablet. Each device must have the relevant software for the interface, whether Skype, Zoom, Teams, or other relevant systems. If the healthcare professional has informed and signed consent to record the remote interaction, they will require particular additional software. Of course, these devices will require connection to the internet with either a cable or wireless (Wi-Fi) connection to conduct a telehealth interaction. There are various challenges associated with these needs. Despite many individuals owning these devices now, the cost and continued maintenance of such equipment can limit the use of telehealth, for both the healthcare professional and the Person/s. Health employers/services committed to the use of telehealth must provide both the devices; the software; technical support to maintain them and troubleshoot; a secure encrypted internet connection, staff to organise the appointments and training for all relevant staff in both using the interface and in troubleshooting when experiencing difficulties (van Houwelingen, Moerman et al 2016; van Houwelingen, Ettema et al 2020). In some cases, it may be important to provide training for the Person and their carers in the use of both the devices and the software.

These requirements can create barriers relating to using telehealth, regardless of the need and benefits (Speyer et al 2018). However, they are necessary when using telehealth to ensure provision of efficient and effective healthcare. Of course, they all require ongoing financial investment after the initial investment of purchasing the relevant equipment and software, and investing in training the employees. This may be challenging for some services, and for some Person/s.

It is also important for healthcare professionals using telehealth to be able to provide assistance to troubleshoot for the Person/s if they experience difficulty. This will require training in and familiarity with the process and the use of the telehealth interface along with effective troubleshooting behaviour. Each individual using telehealth will also require knowledge and understanding of the guidelines or protocols of their particular employer for telehealth interactions, to ensure they adhere to these guidelines whenever using telehealth (Moss 2020). In some locations, with the increasing need for telehealth, these guidelines are in the development stage (Binks 2017). Regardless of the existence of these local guidelines, it would also be beneficial to become familiar with and regularly review the national guidelines, either from the government or the relevant healthcare profession (Australian Government Department of Health and Aged Care 2019; NSW Agency for Clinical Innovation 2015). This should avoid any negative consequences of using technology when delivering healthcare.

An additional challenge when using telehealth is the reliability and speed of the connection to the internet, despite the presence of all the necessary requirements. This can vary in particular rural, remote or high-rise locations, depending on infrastructure, accessibility and usage of others in the area, along with particular weather in some locations. Some health services have tele-hubs with dedicated trained staff, several internet servers and back-up hardware to reduce service interruptions (Giodano et al 2009). However, in areas without these hubs, telehealth accessibility to rural and remote areas can vary, depending on the reliability of the infrastructure and in some cases the quality of the equipment in the place of residence and the workplace. It can be useful for a technology expert associated with the workplace to provide advice relating to equipment and ways of maintaining a connection despite challenges. An additional concern relating to internet connections is confidentiality and security (Kruse et al 2018). Some individuals have negative perceptions of using telehealth for various reasons; however, one reason may relate to the **security** and privacy of the interface (Kamei et al 2018). This concern can often be the reason for reluctance or resistance from some healthcare professionals, the Person and carer to use telehealth, making it essential to secure telehealth connections, thereby encouraging trust in this type of healthcare (Australian College of Rural and Remote Medicine [ACRRM] 2011).

It is an ethical requirement of using telehealth to have secure connections. It is therefore important to ensure security of all relevant networks (with encryption or a firewall) and to assure the Person and carer of the security of your telehealth connection. Encryption secures internet connections, ensuring access from only those authorised to participate in the telehealth session. A firewall limits use of the particular connection to only authorised individuals.

These security measures can be implemented in either hardware or software, indicating the importance of a technology expert in telehealth services. It is also important to inform the Person, the carer and any other relevant organisations of the privacy and security of the connection and each telehealth session (Sitton-Kent 2018). This may overcome their reluctance and encourage them to engage with telehealth. They also need to understand that the healthcare professional will be entering the details of the session into the relevant secure medical record, as they would for an in-person session (NSW Agency for Clinical Innovation 2015).

Suggest ways to overcome the challenges associated with using telehealth to achieve Person-centred Care. Remember your previous discussion in this chapter.

Requirements for effective communication

Healthcare professionals require particular understanding and communication skills when using telehealth. One consideration is to understand the variations in the login time of particular systems (Li et al 2018). This consideration will facilitate effective use of time and timely connection with the Person/s to maintain the appointment time. If possible, it is important to telephone the Person/s if the connection requires more time than usual or if events prevent you from connecting for their telehealth session. Also important is preparing for each session, including gathering all necessary documents and equipment, and considering the purpose of and planning for each session, as you would for an in-person session. This will contribute to protecting the therapeutic relationship and future collaborative interactions, thereby establishing a "tele-presence" to empower the Person. As with any interaction in healthcare, it is important to consider your choice of words to achieve mutual understanding and effective communication. Therefore, telehealth interactions require respectful attitudes, especially as the connection occurs in the place of residence. It is therefore important to be non-judgemental in verbal and non-verbal messages.

Considering the effect of your non-verbal skills and the associated messages is essential for telehealth delivery. Perhaps even more than in-person interactions, the tone of voice and speed of speaking are essential considerations to ensure effective communication. It may be possible to fail to observe non-verbal responses to your messages; therefore, greater awareness of your own non-verbal messages will promote development of the therapeutic relationship and, again, effective communication. In order to combat this possibility it is important to maintain eye contact and visual focus – and if unsure of the meaning, asking for clarification and perhaps the cause of any facial expressions. If you are not looking at the Person/s, perhaps completing a related task, it is important to explain your actions, indicating that you are still engaged in the remote interaction. This will encourage the Person and carer to also engage. Demonstrating empathy without touch may require stronger and more specific verbal messages and perhaps exaggerated movement in non-verbal messages (Henry et al 2018).

The presence of these elements of effective communication and Person/Family-centred Care will allow the Person/s to understand you are a "real" person, not an actor on television or artificial intelligence (AI). They also have the potential to encourage the Person/s to implement the interventions between each session in the place of residence, thereby improving outcomes and satisfaction for everyone.

As mentioned above, it is also important to be aware of aspects of the environment to enhance the interactions. These aspects include consideration of lighting and noise to ensure optimal interactions during the telehealth session. All of these elements of a telehealth session contribute to achieving Person/Family-centred Care and effective communication in a potentially challenging method of delivering healthcare.

Choose a scenario from Section 4 relevant to your profession. Identify a context of practice typical of your healthcare profession that is applicable to the chosen scenario. Outline an intervention typical of that context, considering the length of each session and the number and content of each session. Specify how you would implement that intervention using telehealth.

Chapter summary

The global challenges associated with provision of healthcare have resulted in the increased use of telehealth or telecommunication. This form of communication requires the use of technology and relevant software to communicate effectively with individuals not-in-the-room or on-site. The reasons for using this form of communication have produced variations in the meaning of each term. In healthcare, telehealth can be used to connect virtually with the Person/s and their carers to identify their current needs (telehealth or telepractice) or with specialist physicians for expert guidance or, if relevant, with other practitioners (teleconsultation). The use of telehealth has seen a decrease in the cost of providing healthcare, along with a decrease in remote residents attending hospital and, in some circumstances, avoidance of deterioration of a condition or even prevention of a condition developing. It is also useful for monitoring functioning and needs for Person/s and carers experiencing a life-limiting illness (telemonitoring or telehomecare).

However, there are challenges associated with the use of telehealth. These include the cost and maintenance of the equipment and software; having the required skills and confidence to use telehealth and both the healthcare professional and the Person/s acknowledging and believing in the effectiveness of telehealth for effective care in comparison with in-the-room or in-Person care. Certainly, telehealth requires a secure and operational internet or wi-fi connection. This may vary according to location, time of day and sometimes weather conditions. In these circumstances an appropriate staff member with the relevant training or a family member with understanding of the technology and system to manage the technology and software, is essential. Training in the use of the technology and software is important. This training can be provided by appropriate healthcare staff. A specific service regularly using telehealth makes the provision of a trained technology expert crucial. The ability to troubleshoot when experiencing difficulties is also necessary. When preparing to use telehealth the healthcare professional must consider lighting, external noise and how to reduce interruptions. All the above requirements contribute to the achievement of Person/Family-centred Care, effective communication and thus provision of effective healthcare using telecommunication or telehealth.

Today I want to check your right shoulder movement. Can you lift your arm over your head yet?

Quite an improvement. You must have been doing those exercises I demonstrated three weeks ago.

It's so good to be able to use my arm again. Being able to see you like this has been great for me. I could see how to do these exercises.
I agree. It helps us both.

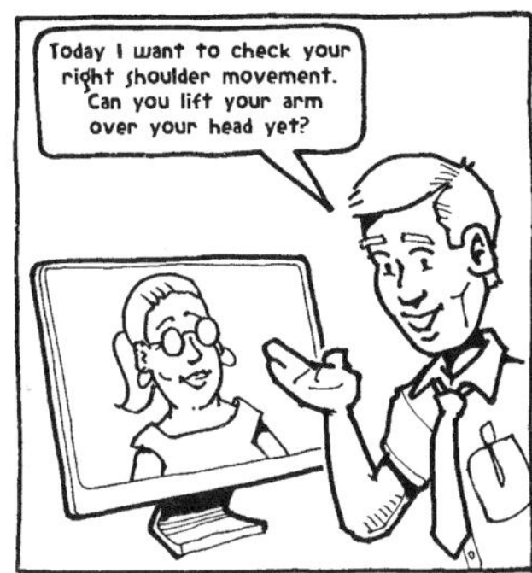

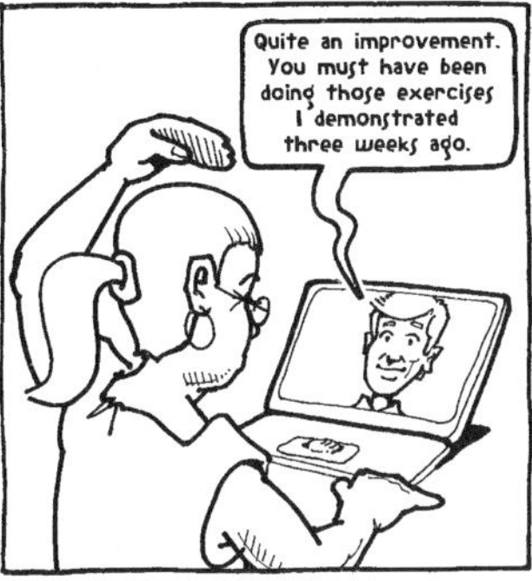

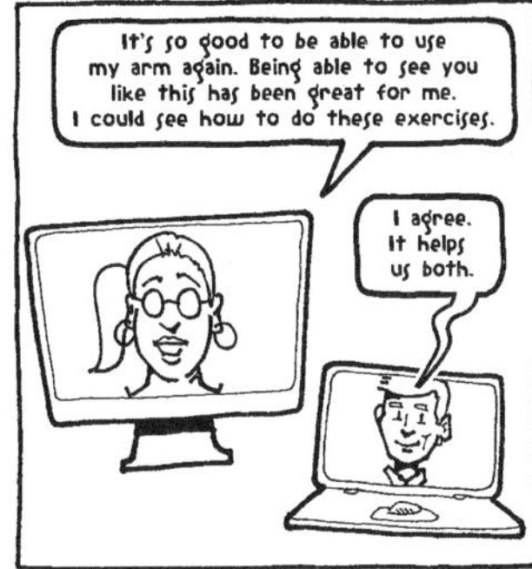

FIGURE 21.1
Telehealth allows remote but face-to-face healthcare.
Courtesy Roger Harvey © Elsevier Australia.

REVIEW QUESTIONS

1 Using your own words, define telehealth /telecommunication.

___

___

___

2 List the terms used when discussing telehealth. Using your own words define each term.

___

___

___

3 State, in your own words, the advantages of visual communication using relevant technology.

4 Create a table outlining each of the outcomes of using telehealth. Identify who benefits: the Person/s, the healthcare professional and/or the healthcare service.

Outcome	Person/s	Healthcare professional	Healthcare service

5 List the challenges associated with telehealth while delivering healthcare.

6 Explore and record guidelines relating to telehealth for your particular health profession.

7 Consider the communication requirements of a telehealth session and suggest how to ensure they are present in every telehealth intervention.

8 Create a checklist to ensure effective and secure use of telehealth or remote communication.

____

____

____

____

____

References

Armour, R., Helmer, J., 2021. Paramedic-delivered teleconsultations: A scoping review. Australasian Journal of Paramedicine, 18, 1–7.

Australian College of Rural and Remote Medicine (ACRRM), 2011. Connecting health services with the future: Guidance on security and privacy issues for clinicians. Australian College of Rural and Remote Medicine, Brisbane.

Australian Government Department of Health and Aged Care, 2019. Better Access Telehealth Guidelines. Australian Government, Canberra. Online. Available at: www.health.gov.au

Batt, A., Hultink, A., Lanos, C., et al., 2021. Advances in community paramedicine in response to COVID-19. Canadian Standards Association, Toronto, Ontario.

Bernocchi, P., Vanoglio, F., Baratti, D., et al., 2016. Home-based surveillance and rehabilitation after stroke: A real-life study. Topics in Stroke Rehabilitation, 22(2), 106–115.

Binks, R., 2017. District nursing in the digital era. British Journal of Community Nursing, 22(10), 478–483.

Boggs, K., 2023. Interpersonal relationships: Professional communication skills for nurses, 9th ed. Elsevier, St Louis, MO.

Bradford, N.K., Caffery, L.J., Smith, A.C., 2015. Awareness, experiences and perceptions of telehealth in a rural Queensland community. BMC Health Services Research, 15, 427–437.

Brokmann, J.C., Conrad, C., Roissaint, R., et al., 2016. Treatment of acute coronary syndrome by telemedical supported paramedics compared with physician-based treatment: A prospective, interventional multicenter trial. Journal of Medical Internet Research, 18(12), e314.

Campbell, J., Theodoros, D., Russell, T., et al., 2019. Client, provider and community referrer perceptions of telehealth for the delivery of rural paediatric allied health services. Australian Journal of Rural Health, 27(5), 419–426.

Carati, C., Margelis, G., 2013. Towards a national strategy for telehealth in Australia 2013–2018. Australasian Telehealth Society. Online. Available at: www.aths.org.au

Chen, J., Jin, W., Dong, W.S., 2017. Effects of home-based telesupervising rehabilitation on physical function for stroke survivors with hemiplegia: A randomised control trial. American Journal of Physical Medicine and Rehabilitation, 96(3), 152–160.

Choi, A., Oakley, A., 2021. A retrospective review of cutaneous vascular lesions referred to a teledermatology clinic. Journal of Primary Health Care, 13(1), 70–74.

Chow, W.L., Jiang, J., Cho, L.W., 2014. Telehealth for improved glycaemic control in patients with poorly controlled diabetes after acute hospitalization – a preliminary study in Singapore. Journal of Telemedicine and Telecare, 20(6), 317–323.

Czaja, S., 2016. Long-term care services and support systems for older adults: The role of technology. American Psychologist, 71(4), 294–301.

Dalleck, L.C., Schmidt, L.K., Lueker, R., 2011. Cardiac rehabilitation outcomes in a conventional versus telemedicine-based programme. Journal of Telemedicine and Telecare, 17, 217–222.

Dudley, S., 2018. The benefits of using tele-practice to support rural families. Connections, 15(2), 12.

Dyb, K., Berntsen, G.R., Kvam, L., 2021. Adopt, adapt, or abandon technology-supported person-centred care initiatives: Healthcare providers' beliefs matter. BMC Health Services Research, 21, 240.

Fisk, M., Livingstone, A., Pit, S.W., 2020. Telehealth in the context of COVID-19 changing perspectives in Australia, the United Kingdom and the United States. Journal of Medical Internet Research, 22(6), e19264.

Fong, B., Fong, A.C.M., Li, C.K., et al., 2020. Telemedicine technologies: Information technology in medicine and telehealth, 2nd ed. John Wiley, Chichester, UK.

Giordano, A., Scalvini, S., Zanelli, E., et al., 2009. Multicenter randomised trial on home-based telemanagement to prevent hospital readmission of patients with chronic heart failure. International Journal of Cardiology, 131(2009), 192–199.

Gruber-Baldini, A.L., Quinn, C.C., Roggio, A.X., et al., 2022. Telemedicine for older adult nursing home residents to avoid emergency department visits: The experience of the NHTeleED Project in Maryland. Journal of American Medical Directors Association (JAMDA), 23(8), 1311–1312.

Henderson, A., 2019. Communication for health care practice. Oxford University Press, Melbourne.

Henderson, C., Knapp, M., Fernández, J-L., et al., 2013. Cost effectiveness of telehealth for patients with long term conditions (Whole Systems Demonstrator telehealth questionnaire study): Nested economic evaluation in a pragmatic, cluster randomised controlled trial. BMJ, 2013, 346, f1035.

Henry, B.V., Ames, L.J., Block, D.E., et al., 2018. Experienced practitioners' views on interpersonal skills in telehealth delivery. Internet Journal of Allied Health Sciences and Practice, 16(2) Article 2. Online. Available at: nsuworks.nova.edu/ijahsp/vol16/iss2/2/

Hines, M., Bulkeley, K., Lincoln, M., et al., 2017. Telepractice for children with complex disability: Guidelines for quality allied health services. Wobbly Hub Research Team, The University of Sydney, Sydney. Online. Available at: ses.library.usyd.edu.au/handle/2123/17369.

Hüzmeli, E.D., Duman, T., Yıldırım, H., 2017. Efficacy of telerehabilitation in patients with stroke in Turkey: A pilot study. Turkish Journal of Neurology, 23(1), 21–25.

Jaffe, T.A., Hayden, E., UScher-Pines, L., et al., 2021. Telehealth use in emergency care during coronavirus disease 2019: A systematic review. JACEP Open 2, e12443.

James, H.S.E., Smith, A.C., Thomas, E.E., et al., 2021. Exploring paramedics' intention to use a specialist palliative care telehealth service. Progress in Palliative Care, 29(2), 106–113.

Kamei, T., Kanamori, T., Porter, S.E., 2018. Detention of early-stage changes in people with chronic diseases: A telehome monitoring-based telenursing feasibility study. Nursing in Health Science, 20, 313–322.

Kruse, C.S., Atkins, J.M., Baker, T.D., et al., 2018. Factor influencing the adoption of telemedicine for treatment of military veterans with post-traumatic stress disorder. Journal of Rehabilitation Medicine, 50, 385–392.

Li, X., Wu, F., Khan, M.K., et al., 2018. A secure chaotic map-based remote authentication scheme for telecare medicine information systems. Future Generation Computer Systems, 84(2018), 149–159.

Lin, K.H., Chen, C.H., Chen, Y.Y., et al., 2014. Bidirectional and multi-user telerehabilitation system: Clinical effect on balance, functional activity and satisfaction in patients with chronic stroke living in long-term care facilities. Sensor, 14(7), 12451–12466.

Liu, F., Cai, H., Tang, Q., et al., 2013. Effects of an animated diagram and video-based online breathing program for dyspnea in patients with stable COPD. Patient Preference and Adherence, 7(2013), 905–913.

McDuffie, A., Oakes, A., Machalicek, W., et al., 2016. Early language intervention using distance videoteleconferencing: A pilot study of young boys with Fragile X Syndrome and their mothers. American Journal of Speech-Language Pathology, 25, 46–66.

Moss, B., 2020. Communication skills in health and social care, 5th ed. Sage, London.

New Zealand Ministry of Health, 2017. Post-implementation review report of the National Telehealth Service. Ministry of Health, Wellington.

NSW Agency for Clinical Innovation, 2015. Guidelines for the use of telehealth for clinical and nonclinical settings in NSW. NSW Agency for Clinical Innovation, Sydney.

O'Brien Cherry, C., Chumbler, N.R., Richards, K., et al., 2017. Expanding stroke telerehabilitation services to rural veterans: A qualitative study on patient experiences using the robotic stroke therapy delivery and monitoring system program. Disability and Rehabilitation Assistive Technology, 12(1), 21–27.

Parsons, D., Cordier, R., Vaz, S., & Lee, H., 2017. Parent-mediated intervention training delivered remotely for children with autism spectrum disorder living outside of urban areas: Systematic Review. Journal of Medical Internet Research, 19, 1–18.

Pickard, K.E., Wainer, A.L., Bailey, K.M., Ingersoll, B.R., 2016. A mixed-method evaluation of the feasibility and acceptability of a telehealth-based parent-mediated intervention for children with autism spectrum disorder. Autism, 20(7), 845–855.

Reese, R.M., Braun, M.J., Hoffmeier, S., et al., 2015. Preliminary evidence for the integrated systems using telemedicine. Telemedicine and eHealth, 21(7), 581–587.

Rogante, M., Grigioni, M., Cordella, D., & Giacomozzi, C., 2010. Ten years of telerehabilitation: A literature overview of technologies and clinical applications. NeuroRehabilitation, 27(2010), 287–304.

Rush, K.L., Hatt, L., Janke, R., et al., 2018. The efficacy of telehealth delivered educational approaches for patients with chronic diseases: A systematic review. Patient Education and Counseling, 101(2018), 1310–1321.

Sibson, L., 2021. Sometimes it's good to talk. Journal of Paramedic Practice, 13(2), 54.

Sitton-Kent, L., Humphreys, C., Miller, P., 2018. Supporting the spread of health technology in community services. British Journal of Community Nursing, 23(3), 118–122.

Speyer, R., Denman, D., Wilkes-Gillan, S., et al., 2018. Effects of telehealth by allied health professionals and nurses in rural and remote areas: A systematic review and meta-analysis. Journal of Rehabilitation Medicine, 50, 225–235.

Stavas, N., Shea, J., Kedden, S., et al., 2018. Perceptions of caregivers and adolescents of the use of telemedicine for the child sexual abuse examination, Child Abuse and Neglect, 85, 47–57.

Surantha, N., Atmaja, P., Wicaksono, M., 2021. A review of wearable Internet of Things device for healthcare. Procedia Computer Science, 179, 936–943.

The Royal Australian College of General Practitioners, 2014. Implementation guidelines for video consultations in general practice, 3rd ed. RACGP, Melbourne.

van der Meer, V., Bakker, M.J., van den Hout, W.B., et al., 2009. SMASHING (Self-Management in Asthma Supported by Hospitals, ICT, Nurses and General Practitioners) Study Group. Internet-based self-management plus education compared with usual care in asthma: A randomized trial. Annals of Internal Medicine, 151(2009), 110–120.

van Houwelingen, C.T.M., Barakat, A., Best, R., et al., 2015. Dutch nurses' willingness to use home telehealth: Implications for practice and education. Journal of Gerontological Nursing, 41(4), 47–56.

van Houwelingen, T., Ettema, R.G.A., Bleijenberg, N., et al., 2020. Educational intervention to increase nurses' knowledge self-efficacy and usage of telehealth: A multi-setting pretest–post-test study. Nurse Education in Practice, 51, 102924.

van Houwelingen, C.T.M., Moerman, A.H., Ettema, R.G.A., et al., 2016. Competencies required for nursing telehealth activities: A Delphi study. Nurse Education Today, 39(4), 50–62.

Victorson, D., Banas, J., Smith, J., et al., 2014. eSalud: Designing and implementing culturally competent eHealth research with Latino patient populations. American Journal of Public Health, 104(12), 2259–2265.

Vismara, L.A., Young, G.S., Rogers, S.J., 2012. Telehealth for expanding the reach of early autism training to parents. Autism Research and Treatment, 2012, 1–12.

Voerman, S.A., Nickel, P.J., 2017. Sound trust and the ethics of telecare. Journal of Medicine and Philosophy, 42, 33–49.

Wilkes-Gillan, S., & Lincoln, M., 2018. Parent-mediated intervention training delivered remotely for children with autism spectrum disorder (ASD) has preliminary evidence for parent intervention fidelity and improving parent knowledge and children's social behaviour and communication skills. Australian Occupational Therapy Journal, 65, 245–246.

Websites for guidelines and/or policies

Australian National Privacy Principles: www.oaic.gov.au/privacy/australian-privacy-principles

Australian state and territory privacy laws: www.oaic.gov.au/privacy/privacy-legislation/state-and-territory-privacy-legislation/state-and-territory-privacy-legislation

Australian Psychology Society, Principles for choosing videoconferencing technology: www.psychology.org.au

Canadian Association of Occupational Therapists (CAOT). 2011 CAOT position statement: tele-Occupational Therapy and e-Occupational Therapy. caot.in1touch.org/document/3717/Telehealth/eOccupationalTherapy.pdf

Guidelines for Telepractice for children with complex disabilities: ses.library.usyd.edu.au/handle/2123/17369, or for the project brief for these guidelines: ses.library.usyd.edu.au/handle/2123/17243

The Australasian Telehealth Society: www.aths.org.au

Royal Australian College of General Practitioners: www.racgp.org.au

Speech Pathology Australia (SPA), 2014. Telepractice in Speech Pathology Position Statement: www.rcslt.org/wp-content/uploads/media/docs/Telehealth/0520150113PositionStatementTelepracticeinSpeech.pdf

Telehealth: www.racgp.org.au/telehealth

Computer and information security standards: www.racgp.org.au/ehealth/ciss

Standards for General Practice: www.racgp.org.au/running-a-practice/technology/clinical-technology/telehealth

Telehealth Medical Board Guidelines released by Ahpra 2012 (NSW Outback Division of General Practice LTD) Ph: (02) 6872 4777) Outbackdivision.org.au

World Health Organization. Consolidated telemedicine implementation guide: www.who.int/publications/i/item/9789240059184

For a list of useful guidelines for telehealth services, including various healthcare professions in Australia and New Zealand: www.aths.org.au/online-resources

CHAPTER 22

Documentation: "one-way" professional healthcare communication

Chapter objectives

Upon completing this chapter, readers should be able to:

- reflect upon the importance of producing respectful documentation
- list documentation typical of healthcare
- list the results of quality, understandable documentation in healthcare
- reflect upon the effect of documentation on themselves and their health profession
- demonstrate understanding of the types and requirements of electronic documentation
- state elements of documentation to facilitate mutual understanding, including features of professional writing
- discuss the importance of considering the purpose, audience, ethical requirements, content and organisation of documentation in healthcare
- explain the importance of using a professional style in all professional documents.

Effective "one-way" or "audience-absent" communication is a reality for every healthcare professional. Such communication in healthcare should reflect the first components of the model of Person/Family-centred Care: respect (Martinez & Candilis 2011). This is required regardless of the presence or absence of the audience or recipient. In order to demonstrate respect, the healthcare professional refers to the Person/s, by name rather than their condition (McDonald et al 2015). This requires use of Person-centred expressions to avoid devaluing or marginalising the Person/s (American Psychological Association (APA) 2020). Such expressions focus upon the Person/s rather than the disability; for example, *the child (John) who has Down Syndrome* **not** *the Down child*, or *the Person (Mr Johns) with a left (L) lower limb (LL) amputation* **not** *the amputee in room 11*. The healthcare professional can also demonstrate respect by using the preferred name chosen by the Person/s; for example, *Mr Johns* **not** *Tom*, or *Jess* **not** *Jessica* (or, conversely, *Jessica* **not** *Jess*).

In healthcare, non-interactive or "one-way", audience-absent, visual forms of communication are a fundamental reality. In healthcare, these forms of communication or documentation commonly occur in computer-mediated or electronic forms (Gagnon & Sabus 2015), with electronic or digital forms gaining popularity (Antheunis et al 2013; Bardach et al 2017; Shaw et al 2018; Veale et al 2015). The accessibility of electronic forms of communication encourages their use for both personal and professional communication (Moss 2020; Sitton-Kent et al 2018). Such forms of information provision or documentation include reports (including discharge summaries), referrals, case-notes, funding applications, occasional messages and other forms of communication such as emails, SMS (many health services send appointment confirmations using SMS (Fedoruk 2014b), along with providing relevant information) and social media, including blogs, YouTube, podcasts, X (Twitter), Facebook, MySpace, LinkedIn, Google+, Research Gate and so on (see Chapter 23). In this world, texting and use of social media is an accepted manner of communicating information of many kinds (Beesley et al 2023). Despite its use, there are limitations with electronic records, including reduction of person-to-person communication with colleagues, reduced confidence the entry is available for all relevant healthcare professionals, differences in style of completing such records, availability of computers at required times and for the required length of time to complete the document, the complexity of documenting, along with often slow sign-in processes (Bardach et al 2017; Li et al 2018). Some healthcare professionals, for example, ask whether texting healthcare-related information suits everyone, especially the aged or those without adequate internet coverage (Shaw et al 2018). There are also the issues of security, including confidentiality and privacy of all documents.

The need for secure ways of providing and storing Person-related documents is essential. This requirement is becoming more problematic with increases in electronic documentation and skills in breeching security or "hacking". Regardless of these limitations, there is a global reality of the use of electronic records in healthcare. These particular limitations require consideration by system managers, with many healthcare services including particular security requirements along with using standardised forms for particular types of documents.

One-way forms of communication do not have the receiver or audience present to moderate or clarify the message. However, in common with spoken or auditory messages, the purpose of the communication is to achieve mutual understanding between the sender and the receiver of the message (Resnick & Soliman 2011). This places the responsibility on healthcare professionals to produce quality, accurate and clearly understandable documentation for all audiences (Bonk 2022; Fedoruk 2014a; Resnick & Soliman 2011). This chapter explores how to acquire and use skills in professional documentation.

Documentation: information recording and provision

Documentation is a significant responsibility for any healthcare professional. Healthcare documentation guides decision-making in the healthcare of the Person/s (Fedoruk 2014b; Wills 2011). Healthcare professionals are therefore required to record observations, results of assessments, details of interventions and interactions, improvement over time and any other information relevant to the experiences, issues and needs of the Person/s (Gateley 2023). They may also provide educational information for the Person/s relating to their condition, with relevant interventions/programs and clinical guidelines, thereby increasing health literacy (Briglia et al 2015; Lambert & Keogh 2014a; Lambert & Keogh 2014b). Health literacy is the ability of the Person/s to access, comprehend and use relevant health information to inform their health decisions (Rudd 2015). Attempts to enhance health literacy demonstrate respect for the dignity of the Person/s, reflecting the integrity of the healthcare service (Nairn 2014). In addition, it contributes to achieving mutual understanding, effective communication and improved outcomes (Duman 2015).

Quality, understandable documentation

All healthcare documentation must be accurate, understandable, well written and professional (Bonk 2022). This documentation not only justifies services (Childers 2005), it records appropriate professional reasoning (Crosthwaite et al 2017), thereby advocating for and representing the particular profession, potentially affecting the reputation of that profession (Lang 2015). Documentation provides a record of services (Kearney & Laverdure 2018; Levett-Jones & Reid-Searl 2022; Moss 2020, Rosen 2014), potentially contributing to consistent care while avoiding negative consequences for the Person/s (Shaw et al 2018, Wills 2011). It also records details of interventions, ensuring continuity of services (McDonald et al 2015, Sames 2023). In addition, understandable documentation provides an evaluation and comparison of past and present changes in the condition and function of the Person/s. It records different interventions and the related outcomes of any interventions, as well as recording appropriate measurement of the outcomes (Florin 2012). It is the best evidence of interactions between the Person/s and the healthcare professional (Gateley 2023). Thus, all relevant interactions with the Person/s should be recorded in the appropriate form and place. If not recorded, the reader cannot assume the details of any interaction. In fact, failing to document details of interactions or results of assessments suggests that interactions did not occur and/or the omission of an assessment. This can adversely affect the care of the Person/s, along with the reputation of the healthcare professional. In reality, clear and concise documentation or record-keeping relating to the Person, is as important as all other aspects of the healthcare process (Florin 2012). These reasons highlight the importance of quality documentation in healthcare (Kearney & Laverdure 2018; Lieberman & Thomas 2012).

Furthermore, every sent message, whether spoken or written, communicates something about the sender. Thus, healthcare professional documentation is a reflection upon the healthcare professional and healthcare processes relevant to their profession (Gateley 2023; Lang 2015). Therefore, such documents communicate information about the individual healthcare professional and their particular profession, thereby increasing understanding of that profession. Well-written, clear, easily understood documentation also potentially engenders respect for, and trust in, the healthcare professional creating the document, along with trust in their skills and the integrity of the content of the document. In the busyness of practice it is easy to forget the power of the written word (Rosen 2014): potentially to engender confidence in the content and the writer or to raise doubts about the reliability of the content and the writer (Resnick & Soliman 2011).

Documentation requirements in healthcare

Documentation in healthcare should facilitate understanding of the healthcare process unique for that particular Person/s (Martinez & Candilis 2011). This is the fundamental requirement of all healthcare professional documentation. However, documenting in a professional manner requires consideration of particular elements of written communication (Nelson & Weatherald 2014). Remember, the healthcare professional must produce professional, objective, clear, understandable, succinct and accurate documentation (Lindsay 2020), thereby ensuring effective communication and consistent care (Crowson 2013; Wills 2011).

Before exploring these elements of professional writing, it is important to note that learning to write quality documentation requires commitment, time and practice (Moor et al 2012; Zak 2014). However, there are basic steps to assist in the production of accurate and appropriate quality documentation.

Step 1: Consider the purpose

When preparing to produce a document in healthcare it is important to consider the purpose of the document and the audience reading the document (Allan & Grisso 2014; Eslava-Schmalbach & Gómez-Duarte 2013). When *preparing* to write the document, the purpose informs the information-gathering process and choice of content. When *producing* the document, the purpose informs the focus, the details, the content and the length.

Step 2: Consider the audience

When writing in healthcare it is essential to consider who will read the document (Resnick & Soliman 2012). Remember, different healthcare professions have their own dialects or terms not always known by others (Crowson 2013). This reality therefore requires clear explanation of such terms. If a document is for several "audiences" it is appropriate to use language and constructions suited to the individual who is least familiar with healthcare terminology. Thus, if the information is recorded in a portal where both a specialist and the Person/s will receive copies of a document, it is important either to use commonly understood terms or explain all jargon and technical terms (Shaw et al 2018). If the document will be read only by other healthcare professionals, it is beneficial to explain only those terms that are not commonly known or are specific to the particular health profession.

Research highlights a connection between health literacy and positive outcomes (Berkman et al 2011). Therefore it is essential to ensure audience understanding (Briglia et al 2015; Lambert & Keogh 2014a; Resnick & Soliman 2011; Rudd 2015). This reinforces the need for explanations of all professional jargon as a means of contributing to increasing health literacy, thereby improving health outcomes. It is also important to remember that medical records, whether electronic or hard copy, may be requested as evidence in court. This indicates the need for professionally written documentation outlining all aspects of the relevant healthcare process.

Step 3: Consider ethical requirements

When preparing particular types of documentation, healthcare professionals must also consider the ethical requirements of their particular profession (Martinez & Candilis 2011; Zonana 2011, See the particular requirements specific to your profession). Conforming to these requirements should result in clear, accurate and secure recording of all relevant information appropriate for the purpose of the document (Allan & Grisso 2014; Gateley 2023). Remember, ethical requirements include consideration of confidentiality and privacy in order to protect the rights of the Person/s (Allan & Davidson 2013; Resnick & Soliman 2012; Scott 2013; Zonana 2011). This involves more than divulging names, it is also about protecting the identity of the Person/s by not disclosing diagnoses or any other information (such as gender, age, address or locality) that might inappropriately identify the Person/s (Yap & Tiang 2014) if discussing them at a conference or in publications.

In small groups, explore the implications of electronic records.

- How are entries protected?
- What is important to remember if you are interrupted while making an entry?
- How might accessibility be controlled?
- How can you ensure the Person/s has access to their records? (It is considered a right that the Person/s can access their records.) ***Note:*** The use of portals may remove the need to consider how the Person might access their healthcare records.

Ethical considerations are essential in healthcare documentation. These considerations include specific actions when documentation is electronic, such as minimising uncompleted documents on-screen if interrupted before submitting or filing them, and ensuring all records are password-protected and always entered into the appropriate folders. Some services ask the healthcare professionals to PDF and "lock" all documents before submitting them or sending them to another service, or the Person/s.

In groups, consider the following scenario.

A student purchases a notebook specifically for use during their placement. It fits conveniently in their pocket. In it they record relevant details of the Person/s they see each day. These details include name, patient/client number, date of birth (DoB), address, diagnosis or reason for referral and relevant observations, assessments or interventions performed during their interactions with each Person. The student takes care to keep the notebook with them at all times. Thus they take it in their backpack, to and from home, on the bus each day.

- Discuss the ethical implications of this notebook for confidentiality.
- Decide if having the notebook password protected is enough to ensure privacy and confidentiality of the information about all Person/s in the notebook.
- Decide how best to assist the student to maximise their learning and protect the confidentiality of the Person/s.
- How might the student protect confidentiality at the completion of the placement and still keep a record of the learning achieved during the placement?

Step 4: Consider content and document organisation

The content and organisation of healthcare documentation often depends upon the requirement of particular healthcare professions and/or healthcare services (Moss 2020). It is important to become familiar with relevant requirements when commencing practice within a particular service. Changes in policy or guidelines may produce changes in expectations (Zonana 2011). The healthcare professional has the responsibility to be familiar with current guidelines and documentation expectations. Individual services may have slightly different guidelines. However, they typically have relevant templates for completion of particular types of documents or records (Moss 2020). In some services, particular types of documents may be auto completed from the records of the Person. This requires accurate entry of all relevant information into those records (Shaw et al 2018).

Step 5: Consider professional style

Individuals often write using words, expressions and sentence construction reflecting colloquial or everyday-spoken language. Increasingly, written documents prepared by healthcare professionals also reflect an informal spoken style. There is an unspoken expectation that a written document employ "plain English" or everyday language. This style of writing seems appropriate when writing to a friend. However, when creating documents for professional healthcare records, such as a report or case notes about a Person/s, using an informal style is inappropriate and often unacceptable. Thus healthcare professional documentation requires a level of formality and a **professional writing style**. Nelson and Weatherald (2014) highlight an increasing demand for clear and well-written documentation within the healthcare professions.

A professional document should use correct grammar, spelling and a logical progression of ideas (Resnick & Soliman 2011). A poorly written document lacking clarity, brevity and accuracy may not only have negative legal ramifications, it can potentially mean the Person/s may not experience optimal care and thus outcomes (Florin 2012; Wills 2011).

Every written form of communication in healthcare is a legal document, with legal implications (Buchanan & Norko 2011; Fedoruk 2014a). They can be used to legally support particular opinions. These realities mandate a specific standard and style of writing.

In groups, discuss these questions:

- Why explore the skills involved in professional writing? (We can just write sentences, and use spell and grammar check!)
- Why relearn how to write with a professional style when many textbooks, articles and written resources fail to use this style?
- Why continue to learn and write with a professional style even when other people may not use this style in practice?
- List the implications of unprofessional documentation for the healthcare professional.
- List the implications of unprofessional documentation for the Person/s.

Characteristics of a professional writing style

When preparing documentation, healthcare professionals should employ the characteristics of professional writing. These include use of a formal style of expression and formal word choice (see points 1, 1a, 1b, 1c); production of a cohesive, coherent document (see point 2) and use of a particular sentence structure by either skilfully using or avoiding particular grammatical features (see points 3, 3a–f, 4, 4a, 5).

Point 1: The use of formal expression and word choice

The use of informal or colloquial language, the type typical of everyday conversation, is generally inappropriate in professional documentation (American Psychological Association (APS) 2020). See these examples of colloquial expressions, with a more formal replacement:

look at	becomes: *explore, examine* or *consider*
Johnson (2013) says it's OK	becomes: *Johnson (2013) states it is appropriate*
gets in the way of	becomes: *restricts* or *limits*
the way to do ...	becomes: *the appropriate method of ...*

Colloquial expressions can produce misunderstandings. Therefore, it is best to avoid them when documenting in healthcare.

In groups, consider the following colloquial English expressions:

1. ... whatever she can **come up with**
2. ... whatever timeframe **works for him**
3. ... depends when he can **get back to it**
4. **... by the way**
5. ... **open to** ...
6. contact me to advise where **you are up to**.
   - Explain their *literal* meaning.
   - Consider how each expression might cause confusion for native English speakers and for people who have English as an additional language to their first language.
   - Suggest a more formal alternative for each colloquial expression.

Point 1a. A more *formal word choice* includes use of particular *types of nouns* (naming words for ideas or concepts and objects) not specific to particular professions. Examples are: "activity", "appearance", "area", "category", "characteristic", "consideration", "creation", "demonstration", "development", "factor", "implication", "intention", "purpose", "production", "requirement", "variation", and so forth. These types of nouns reflect a more formal style of expression.

Point 1b. Formal expression also involves the use of particular *types of adjectives and/or adverbs* (words providing additional information). Adjectives provide additional information, adding meaning about a noun. Adverbs, as their name suggests, provide additional information about a verb, typically recognised by "-ly" at the end of the word. (Please Note, not all words ending with "-ly" are adverbs!)

Examples of adjectives: "appropriate", "effective", "intentional", "necessary", "numerous", "repetitive", "variable", "various".

Examples of adverbs: "appropriately", "effectively", "intentionally", "necessarily", "repeatedly".

Certain adjectives and adverbs can be interpreted differently by different individuals, and should be avoided in healthcare documentation. Examples are: "bad", "beautiful", "extremely", "good", "great", "happily", "large", "long", "quickly", "short", "shortly", "slowly", "small", "tall", "very".

As different people typically assign different meaning to such words, it is appropriate to avoid their use in professional documentation (APA 2020).

Developing a database of formal words (nouns, adjectives, adverbs and relational verbs: see point 3a) for use when producing documents could assist healthcare professionals learning to create professional documentation.

Point 1c. Formal expression should maintain *an objective perspective* by using appropriate pronouns (Gateley 2023). Despite the tendency towards increased use of some pronouns in scientific journals, an objective perspective requires avoiding particular personal pronouns including "I", "my", "mine", "we", "our", and "you". The use of "they", "theirs, "them" to replace "she" or "he" is acceptable in Australian professional writing. Regardless of country, it is important to differentiate between opinion and factual information in all professional documents (Resnick & Soliman 2012). Thus, instead of using "I", it is beneficial to name the particular health profession (Gateley 2023). For example, instead of using "I", use phrasing such as:

- *The attending healthcare professional observed ...*
- *The dental hygienist/exercise physiologist/nurse/occupational therapist/osteopath/physician/physiotherapist/podiatrist/speech pathologist/social worker observed ...*
- *Range of Movement (ROM) was within normal range (rather than I found ROM was normal).*

Point 2: Creating a cohesive document

Professional writing uses *signals* (called *cohesive* or *linking devices*). These signals assist the reader to predict and link the content of the entire document within sentences and/or paragraph/s.

These "signals" **connect** the ideas in the document. They create a coherent, complete whole by connecting the ideas, words, sentences and paragraphs in the entire document. These devices also **communicate intentions** to the reader. They provide the reader with expectations about the contents of the following sentences and paragraphs. This cohesion allows the reader to easily and accurately understand the document. Such devices can also provide the reader with information concerning the organisation of the document. Words signalling this organisation include "firstly", "in addition", "lastly", "similarly" and "furthermore".

Such signalling devices may also include particular pronouns or words referring to concepts or points made elsewhere in the document and sometimes a concept outside the text. Examples of such pronouns are "it", "this", "these", "those".

Linking devices or signals can also *introduce* ideas, points and arguments; for example, "Initially" and "The *purpose* of *this* report /entry ..."

In addition, such devices can indicate the importance of a point; for example, ***This** is significant, **It** is essential, **Also** relevant is, **It** is worth noting,* and so on. Notice the use of "this" and "it" in these sentences; they are referring to an idea in another part of the document, perhaps something before or after the signalling word. There are many types of linking or signalling devices. When used appropriately they assist the reader to achieve understanding, as well as reflecting the professional nature of the document.

In pairs, underline the *cohesive devices* used in the above passage (point 2). Circle each one and draw an arrow to the related idea. Decide whether they reflect the organisation of the passage, refer to another point in the passage or suggest the importance of a point.

Point 3: Sentence structure

There is a particular **sentence structure** typically used in professional writing. This simple sentence structure is an important feature of professional writing (Crowson 2013). It promotes succinct and clear expression. This structure consists of two linked *noun phrases.* A relational verb (see point 3a) links or relates these noun phrases, thereby connecting the ideas. Therefore, in a well-constructed professional sentence it is possible to imagine an equals sign replacing the verb. Sometimes to maintain the structure, one of the noun phrases is short, while the other long.

Point 3a. Professional writing uses particular verbs and types of verbs. These include: the verb "*to be*" and the verb "*to have*", as well as *relational verbs* (relating ideas and concepts) and *modal verbs.*

The verb "**to be**" is commonly used in professional writing. It can be expressed using the words "is" and "was" when discussing only one (singular) and "are" or "were" when discussing more than one (plural). For example:

This issue is ...	*These issues are ...*
This issue was ...	These issues were ...

The verb "**to have**" can be expressed by the words "has", "have" or "had". For example:

It has	*It had*
They have	*They had*

Relational verbs connect or relate the ideas at the beginning and the end of a simple sentence. Examples of relational verbs are: "affect", "appear", "attempt", "classify", "complete", "create", "decrease", "develop", "emerge", "envelope", "examine", "explore", "include", "increase", "identify", "indicate", "intend", "occur", "produce", "reflect".

Modal verbs are often used in professional writing. They reflect either a *tentative* ("may", "can", "could", "shall", "should") or *definite* ("must", "will", "would") expression of ideas. In healthcare professions there are various factors potentially changing information, especially information based on opinion. Therefore, modal verbs are typically used when the message is not verified by factual information. The definite modal verb ("will", "would") is used only when there is assurance of the truth of the statement.

Point 3b. The simple sentence structure *avoids phrases and sentences finishing with prepositions or verbs*; for example, *these must be prepared **for**, she feels comfortable **with**, group sessions were **facilitated***. While such sentences reflect everyday spoken structures, it is inappropriate in professional documentation. *Prepositions* relate a noun or pronoun to another word, often introducing an idea or point or indicating the position of that point. They include "at", "above", "between", "by", "for", "from", "in", "into", "of", "on", "onto", "to", "under", "with".

Point 3c. The use of *simple present tense* also maintains a professional sentence structure. This tense typically uses the **active voice**, where the beginning of the sentence or the subject is completing the "action". The verb indicates the action. Active voice assists to ensure the sentence has a beginning and an end with a verb connecting them. This maintains an appropriate professional sentence structure. For example:

- *The report examines the health of the refugees.*
- *This chapter considers the features of professional writing.*

Sentences can be rewritten in the active voice. See the following:

PASSIVE	ACTIVE
Self-esteem is affected by body image.	becomes: *Body image affects self-esteem.*
Wellbeing is impacted by poor health and living conditions.	becomes: *Poor health and living conditions impact wellbeing.*
Some suggest obesity is produced by overeating and limited exercise.	becomes: *Some suggest, overeating and limited exercise produce obesity.*
The health and wellbeing of the population is improved by healthcare professionals.	becomes: *Healthcare professionals improve the health and wellbeing of the population.*

The original form of the above four sentences uses the **passive voice**. The passive voice is typically recognised through the presence of the word "by". In such sentences the idea at the **end** of the sentence affects the idea at the **beginning** of the sentence. Passive voice is sometimes used in health documentation. It can, however, cause misunderstandings. It is also interesting to note that use of the active voice reduces word usage, producing more succinct expression. The reader may also find the document written in active voice easier to read.

In pairs, consider each of the following phrases. Rewrite them to reflect an appropriate structure and voice. Consider word choice to assist in producing the structure.

For example:

In this paper, first principles of sentence structure and basic punctuation were introduced.

To produce appropriate sentence structure, this becomes:

This paper introduces first principles of sentence structure and basic punctuation.

- *This highlights the importance of examining the environment they are in.*
- *... to ensure local ethical, cultural and legal obligations are covered.*
- *... ensure all relevant categories are identified.*
- *... the ideas they were struggling with.*
- *... were used to explore the themes identified.*
- *... finally ethical issues were addressed.*

Point 3d. The use of *gerunds* also assists in maintaining this structure. A gerund is a verb appearing to function as a noun, typically recognised by an "-ing" ending; for example, "avoiding", "developing", "including" when used without another verb (e.g. *is developing, has been developing*). However, words with "-ing" positioning or adding meaning to a noun are not gerunds (e.g. *the **following** sentences*).

Point 3e. A professional writing style also uses the *infinitives* of verbs in order to maintain this sentence structure; for example, "to appear", "to imply", "to create", "to indicate", "to require".

Point 3f. In order to maintain the sentence structure professional writing often changes the *verb into a noun phrase,* for example:

exercising	becomes: *the use of exercise*
considered	becomes: *the consideration of*

In pairs, using the passage from point 2 above, complete the following tasks:

- Identify the relational verbs and suggest alternative relational verbs to maintain the meaning.
- Identify the modal verbs. Suggest reasons why they have been used with this point.
- Identify the gerunds. Suggest alternative forms to express the related ideas, while maintaining a professional writing style. Check the word usage and decide which version is most succinct.
- Identify the infinitive forms of the verbs – state how they contribute to maintaining a professional sentence structure.

Point 4: Abbreviations

Abbreviations (*short form*) or symbols are commonly used in documents in healthcare. Abbreviations reduce the time required to complete a report or entry. Abbreviations specific to the healthcare are common in medical records (e.g. Ax = assessment, Rx = treatment). It is important to use only commonly known abbreviations. Different healthcare services may use variations of abbreviations. Some have prepared lists to be used by employees. Therefore, it is important to become familiar with the abbreviations specific to a particular health service. Not all abbreviations used will be specific to particular healthcare professions.

Point 4a. A common form of abbreviation is an *acronym*. When using an acronym for the first time it is essential to write the full meaning (e.g. Computer-Mediated Communication = CMC or World Health Organization = WHO). In some cases, healthcare professionals can invent previously unknown abbreviations (e.g. Therapeutic use of Self = TuoS) and thus it is important to clearly document the intended meaning of any acronym before using the acronym.

Point 4b. *Apostrophes* can create another form of abbreviation. There is consistent **misuse** of apostrophes in personal and professional writing. It is common to see apostrophes used incorrectly in everyday life. However, for a healthcare professional, it is embarrassing, reflecting poorly upon the individual and their profession, especially where such misuse occurs regularly.

> *No matter that you have a PhD and have read all of Henry James twice, if you persist in writing, "Good food at it's best", you deserve to be struck by lightning, hacked up on the spot and buried in an unmarked grave (Truss 2006, p. 43–44).*

While this humorous quote appears extreme, it highlights the importance of accurate use of apostrophes, punctuation and grammar, regardless of the opinion of the writer about the need for such details.

Misuse of apostrophes conveys limited understanding of grammar and punctuation. Correctly used, the apostrophe indicates either shortening or possession. Shortening occurs consistently every day in spoken language, in phrases such as *I don't want coffee, I'm hungry not thirsty, let's sit for a min, "n" you drink "n" I'll eat!* In each case, the apostrophe indicates removal of a letter or letters, to shorten the message. Such shortening is **not** appropriate in a professional document with communicative and legal implications. The other use of an apostrophe is to indicate possession (ownership). Typically, a noun (name of an individual, idea or thing) owns something; for example: *The healthcare professional's reputation is affected by poor writing, The Person's emotions dominated all communication.* The use of apostrophes of possession, unless in the name of a condition, should also be avoided in professional healthcare documentation.

In pairs, choose which sentences and phrases should, and which should not, have an apostrophe.

- *Healthcare professional's reports should be clear, succinct and accurate.*
- *Healthcare professional's assist Person/s to achieve relevant goals.*
- *Some healthcare professional's encourage improved ability when moving.*
- *... for a Person's functioning in society.*
- *How might the carer's opinion assist the healthcare professional?*
- *OT's often enable Person/s in everyday activities.*

Together, consider the sentences grammatically requiring an apostrophe and decide how to express the idea without an apostrophe.

Point 5: Punctuation

Punctuation assists in clarifying meaning. Commonly used punctuation marks include commas, full stops, semicolons and colons. They provide signals for the reader, producing coherence, flow and understanding. In this way, punctuation contributes to achieving mutual understanding and effective communication.

Consider how the use of punctuation changes the meaning of this sentence:

A woman, without her man is nothing.

A woman: without her, man is nothing.

- Discuss the implications of the misuse of punctuation in healthcare documentation.
- Suggest possible negative results.

Report or letter writing: formatting and content

It is important to comply with the requirements of the particular health service when formatting any written document. Whether or not electronic, a report or letter should be created on the letterhead of the health service to ensure inclusion of the correct contact details of the service.

There are differing opinions about the preferred length of reports (Buchanan & Norko 2011). The purpose of the report should guide choices about points to include and thus the ultimate length of the report. Remember, the reader may lose concentration after the first one and a half pages. This highlights the importance of succinct expression of all relevant points (Resnick & Soliman 2011). Regardless of these requirements, it is always essential to remember that documenting healthcare requires respect and in some situations collaboration or shared decision-making (Martinez & Candilis 2011).

Reports and letters require gathering of information; considering or examining the gathered information; evaluating the information according to the focus of the particular healthcare profession; prioritising points within the information and effectively communicating these synthesised points (Wills 2011).

Reports and letters typically outline results of assessments, intervention outcomes or changes in status. However, letters may contain specific items not generally necessary in a report (such as a salutation to the reader: "*Dear ...*"). Reports may have particular formats with headings clearly outlining positioning of relevant information (often specifically formatted for particular health services). Despite differences, letters and reports generally include a statement of the **reason** for the document. The position of the reason varies, depending on the format of the letter or report. Reports may provide their reason in a heading at the top of a page, for example, *Initial Assessment, Home Visit Report, Progress Report, Discharge Summary*, or *Worksite Assessment*. Letters may have the name of the Person or the reason centred and before the first paragraph – something to draw the attention and focus of the reader. Reports and letters are best written to ensure mutual understanding between the writer and all possible recipients. As mentioned above, this suggests considered use of professional jargon.

While the length of some points included in reports will vary when compared to letters, reports and letters should generally include:

- the date
- identifying details of the Person/s, which may include name, identification number and/or address, age, gender, diagnosis and often reason for referral
- well-organised points, either with each point beginning a new paragraph or using bullet points or numbers to make it easy to access particular information within the report/letter. Some reporting formats use headings in bold. This can also assist the reader to readily access particular information
- where appropriate, use examples of needs to validate and verify the stated points
- some healthcare professions require a clear statement for each Person/s of the identified issues and the related action plans. Numbering each issue and related action plan with the same number is essential. This not only informs the reader about the reasoning of the particular profession, it also avoids confusion
- a signature with the name of the healthcare professional signing, their particular health profession and, if appropriate, their specific contact details. Electronic systems typically record the details of the particular healthcare professional as a result of their log in.

Letters should generally also include:

- a salutation (e.g. "*Dear ...*"); use the family name of the person to avoid offence
- a clear statement of the reason for the letter in the first paragraph
- a concluding paragraph indicating required future action or details of future requirements or events
- an appropriate salutation related to the tone of the letter before your signature (e.g. "*Yours sincerely*", "*Thank you*").

Points to remember

- It is important to distinguish between fact and opinion in all written records (Allan & Grisso 2014). The results of standardised assessment tools do not require qualification (*Results of the ROM assessment indicate*...OR *results of a pressure assessment indicate* ...); however, it is important to use appropriate words to indicate the recording of opinion or interpretation based upon observation (e.g. *It appears .... It seems*...).
- Do not forget to read, correct and edit *content, grammar* and *spelling* (remember this document reflects upon you and your profession); sign, date, ensure it is a locked PDF and file all reports and letters before sending them.

Chapter summary

There are many elements of the documentation process in healthcare. Different types of documents in health require particular consideration. When preparing documentation, it is essential to use respectful wording when referring to the Person/s, thereby avoiding alienation and preserving their dignity. In addition, it is important to remember that every document has the potential to improve the health literacy of the Person/s and their understanding of particular health professions. The possible effects of any document include advocating for the particular Person/s and health profession, providing results of assessments and or details of intervention outcomes (improvement or otherwise), changes in the condition or status, therefore guiding decision-making about the need for and type of future services.

All documents are legal records and can be used to support particular opinions in court. Preparing appropriate and relevant documents in healthcare requires commitment, time and practice. Quality documents must be easily understood, accurate and succinct. It is important to consider: the purpose of the document; the reader/recipient; ethical implications (electronic records require consideration specific to that platform); the appropriate content (often related to the purpose of the document), and organisation of that content (may be defined by the particular health service), along with the characteristics of professional writing. While there are different types of documentation in healthcare, reports and letters are common. There are particular required details that should accompany all relevant documents in healthcare. It is essential to ensure every entry or document is signed and "locked" before sending or submitting. Documentation is a requirement of every healthcare professional.

How do I act on this? It's not easy to understand.
15.00
REFERRAL
REPORT

16.20
ASSESSMENT RESULTS
CARE PLAN

I need to ensure I record this more clearly and professionally than the last healthcare professional.
17.05
INTERVENTION DETAILS
PROGRESS

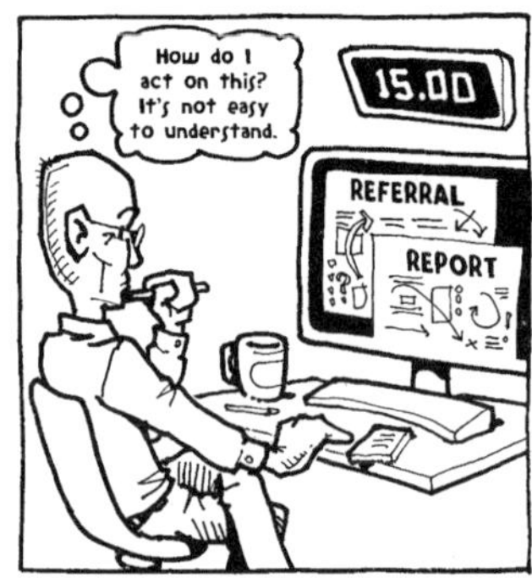

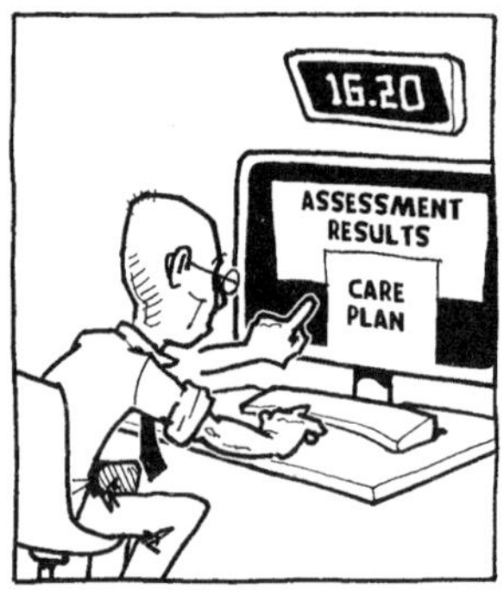

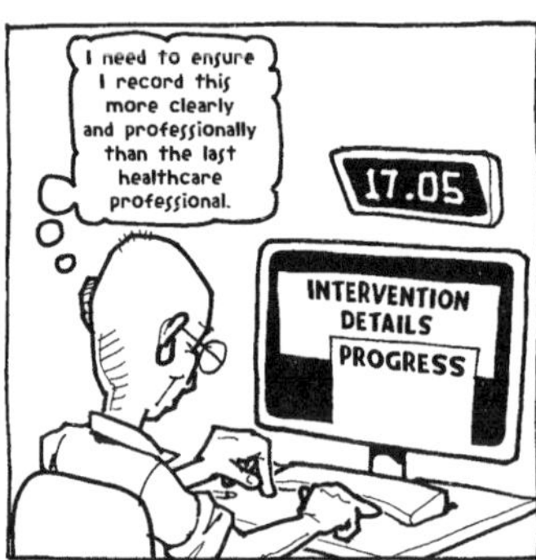

FIGURE 22.1
It is important to have clear documentation.
Courtesy Roger Harvey © Elsevier Australia.

REVIEW QUESTIONS

1. Outline how a healthcare professional can demonstrate respect when creating health documentation.

2. List three characteristics of a quality document.

   i. ______________________________

   ii. ______________________________

   iii. ______________________________

3. What are six potential reasons for preparation of quality documents in healthcare?

   i. ______________________________

   ii. ______________________________

   iii. ______________________________

   iv. ______________________________

   v. ______________________________

   vi. ______________________________

4. What is health literacy?

____

____

____

____

5. State why it is important to encourage health literacy.

____

____

____

____

6. Explain why it is important to consider the recipient of written/digital documents, whether they be the Person/s, a colleague healthcare professionals or other professionals.

7. Suggest reasons for considering the privacy and confidentiality (ethical considerations) requirements of documentation.

8. List what should always be recorded in a report or letter, whether or not electronic.

9. State the details a healthcare professional should include that are specific to a letter.

10. List the things to remember before sending a report or submitting an entry into a database.

____

____

____

____

References

Allan, A., Davidson, G.R., 2013. Respect for the dignity of people: What does this principle mean in practice? Australian Psychologist, 48(5), 345–352.

Allan, A., Grisso, T., 2014. Ethical principles and the communication of forensic Mental Health assessments. Ethics and Behaviour, 24(6), 467–477.

American Psychological Association (APA), 2020. Publication manual of the American Psychological Association, 7th ed. APA, Washington, DC.

Antheunis, M.L., Tates, K., Nieboer, T.E., 2013. Patients' and health professionals' use of social media in health care: Motives, barriers and expectations. Patient Education and Counseling, 92, 426–431.

Bardach, S.H., Real, K., Bardach, D.R., 2017. Perspectives of healthcare practitioners: An exploration of interprofessional communication using electronic medical records. Journal of Interprofessional Care, 31(3), 300–306.

Beesley, P., Watts, M., Harrison, M., 2023. Developing your communication skills in social work, 2nd ed. Sage, London, UK.

Berkman, N.D., Sheridan, S.L., Donahue, K.E., et al., 2011. Low health literacy and health outcomes: An updated systematic review. Annals of Internal Medicine, 155, 97–107.

Bonk, R.J., 2022. Writing for today's health care audiences, 2nd ed. Broadview Press, Ontario.

Briglia, E., Perlman, M., Weissman, M.A., 2015. Integrating health literacy into organizational structure. Physician Leadership Journal, 2(2), 66–69.

Buchanan, A., Norko, M.A., 2011. Report Structure. In: Buchanan, A., Norko, M.A. (eds), The psychiatric report: Principles and practice in forensic writing. Cambridge University Press, Great Britain.

Childers, K., 2005. Paying the price for poor documentation. Nursing, 35, 32–34.

Crosthwaite, P., Cheung, L., Jiang, F., 2017. Writing with attitude: stance expression in learner and professional dentistry research reports. English for Specific Purposes, 46, 107–123.

Crowson, M.G., 2013. A crash course in medical writing for health profession students. Journal of Cancer Education, 28(3), 554–557.

Duman, M., 2015. Better measures needed on the impact of health communication. Journal of Communication in Healthcare, 8(1), 3–4.

Eslava-Schmalbach, J., Gómez-Duarte, O.G., 2013. Scientific writing, a neglected aspect of professional training. Colombian Journal of Anesthesiology, 41(2), 79–81.

Fedoruk, M., 2014a. Essential competencies for the registered nurse. In: Fedoruk, M., Hofmeyer, A. (eds), Becoming a nurse: An evidence-based approach, 2nd ed. Oxford University Press, Melbourne.

Fedoruk, M., 2014b. Health Information systems and technologies. In: Fedoruk, M., Hofmeyer, A. (eds), Becoming a nurse: An evidence-based approach, 2nd ed. Oxford University Press, Melbourne.

Florin, J., 2012. An overlooked skill for counsellors: Writing. Addiction Professional, 11(3), 40.

Gagnon, K., Sabus, C., 2015. Professionalism in a Digital Age: Opportunities and considerations for using social media in health care. Physical Therapy, 95(3), 406–414.

Gateley, C.A., 2023. Documentation manual for occupational therapy, 5th ed. Slack, Thorofare, NJ.

Kearney, K., Laverdure, P., 2018. American Occupational Therapy Association. Guidelines for documentation of occupational therapy. American Journal of Occupational Therapy, 72(Supplement 2), 1–7.

Lambert, V., Keogh, D., 2014a. Health literacy and its importance for effective communication. Part 1. Nursing Children and Young People, 26(3), 31–37.

Lambert, V., Keogh, D., 2014b. Health literacy and its importance for effective communication. Part 2. Nursing Children and Young People, 26(4), 32–36.

Lang, T., 2015. Medical writing up close and professional: Establishing our identity. American Medical Writers Association (AMWA) Journal, 30(1), 10–17.

Levett-Jones, T., Reid-Searl, K., 2022. The clinical placement: An essential guide for nursing students, 5th ed. Elsevier, Sydney.

Li, X., Wu, F., Khan, M.K., et al., 2018. A secure chaotic map-based remote authentication scheme for telecare medicine information systems, Future Generation Computer Systems, 84(2018), 149–159.

Lieberman, D., Thomas, J., 2012. Guidelines for documentation. OT Practice 17(22), 7.

Lindsay, D., 2020. Scientific writing = thinking in words, 2nd ed. CSIRO Publishing, Collingwood.

Martinez, R., Candilis, P.J., 2011. Ethics. In: Buchanan, A., Norko, M.A. (eds), The psychiatric report: Principles and practice in forensic writing. Cambridge University Press, Cambridge.

McDonald, K.E., Hartwig Moorhead, H.J., Neuer Colburn, A.A., 2015. Teaching writing skills to counseling students for clinical competence and professional advocacy. Journal of Counselor Leadership and Advocacy, 2(1), 80–91.

Moor, K.S., Jensen-Hart, S., Hooper, R.I., 2012. Small change, big difference: Heightening BSW faculty awareness to elicit more effective student writing. Journal of Teaching in Social Work, 32, 62–77.

Moss, B., 2020. Communication skills in health and social care, 5th ed. Sage, London.

Nairn, T.A., 2014. What we have here is a failure to communicate: The ethical dimension of health literacy. Health Progress, 95(4), 61–63.

Nelson, P., Weatherald, C., 2014. Cracking the code: An approach to developing Professional writing skills. Social Work Education: The International Journal, 33(1), 105–120.

Resnick, P.J., Soliman, S., 2011. Draftsmanship. In: Buchanan, A., Norko, M.A. (eds), The psychiatric report: Principles and practice in forensic writing. Cambridge University Press, Cambridge.

Resnick, P.J., Soliman, S., 2012. Planning, writing, and editing forensic psychiatric reports. International Journal of Law and Psychiatry, 35, 412–417.

Rosen, D., 2014. Vital conversations: Improving communication between doctors and patients. Columbia University Press, New York.

Rudd, R.E., 2015. The evolving concept of health literacy: New directions for health literacy studies. Journal of Communication in Health Care, 8(1), 7–9.

Sames, K.M., 2023. Documentation in Practice. In: Gillen, G., Brown, C., Willard and Spackman's occupational therapy, 14th ed. Wolters Kluwer, Philadelphia PA.

Scott, R.W., 2013. Legal aspects of documenting patient care for rehabilitation professionals, 4th ed. Jones & Bartlett Publishers, Burlington, MA.

Shaw, T., Hines, M., Kielly-Carroll, C., 2018. Impact of digital health on the safety and quality of health care. Australian Commission of Safety and Quality in Health Care, Sydney.

Sitton-Kent, L., Humphreys, C., Miller, P., 2018. Supporting the spread of health technology in community services. British Journal of Community Nursing, 23(3) 118–122.

Truss, L., 2006. Eats, shoots and leaves: The zero tolerance approach to punctuation. Profile Books, London.

Veale, H.J., Sacks-Davis, R., Weaver, E., et al., 2015. The use of social networking platforms for sexual health promotion: Identifying key strategies for successful user engagement. BMC Public Health, 15, 85.

Wills, C., 2011. Preparation. In: Buchanan, A., Norko, M.A. (eds), The psychiatric report: Principles and practice in forensic writing. Cambridge University Press, Cambridge.

Yap, K.Y.-L., Tiang, Y.-L., 2014. Recommendations for health care educators on e-professionalism and student behaviour on social networking sites. Medicolegal and Bioethics, 4, 25–36.

Zak, L., 2014. Exploring valued patterns of stance in upper-level student writing in the disciplines. Written Communication, 31(1), 27–57.

Zonana, H., 2011. Confidentiality and record keeping. In: Buchanan, A., Norko, M.A. (eds), The psychiatric report: Principles and practice in forensic writing. Cambridge University Press, UK.

CHAPTER 23

Social media or "not present in person" communication and the healthcare professional

Chapter objectives

Upon completing this chapter, readers should be able to:

- demonstrate understanding of various electronic forms of communication
- list the advantages and disadvantages of social media communication
- discuss the often-forgotten realities of personal electronic communication, specifically social media, relevant to healthcare professionals
- discuss characteristics and implications of cyberbullying
- reflect upon the potential implications of healthcare professionals using personal social media
- demonstrate understanding of the use of social media for professional communication
- develop strategies for appropriate use of electronic communication, including social media.

The twenty-first century has produced remarkable changes in methods of communicating, and of quickly providing and accessing information about many different topics (Conti et al 2023; Gagnon & Sabus 2015; Irwin et al 2021; Teles da Mota et al 2022; Verner Venegas-Vera 2020). These changes have produced the electronic forms of communication using commercial wireless signals and related networking services. There is evidence that during disasters and/or challenging situations (e.g. the global pandemic COVID-19) there is an increase in the use of social media (Gottlieb & Dyer 2020). These forms of communication, some mentioned in the previous chapter, can include such media as emails, short message services (SMS), Viber, Telegram, YouTube, Flickr, Snapchat, chat rooms, discussion forums including Reddit and Whirlpool, webinars and social media or social networking sites, including Facebook, Facebook Messenger, TikTok, Instagram, Google+, WeChat, Weibo, WhatsApp, MySpace, blogs and microblogs (X [Twitter]), "patient" portals and so on. They have increased the ease of communicating across distances (Pentescu et al 2015; She et al 2023; Verner Venegas-Vera 2020). These internet-based forms of communication are becoming a common method of quickly communicating and providing healthcare, worldwide (Verner Venegas-Vera 2020).

In 2011 the World Health Organization (WHO) estimated that 85 per cent of the population of the world had the potential to use these forms of communication. The increased popularity of social media as a form of information exchange in recent years (Antheunis et al 2013; Shahbaznezhad et al 2021) has more than achieved this prediction. Individuals using social media typically use it for personal communication (Benetoli et al 2017). There is also evidence of individuals using social media being empowered to manage their health. Benetoli and colleagues (2017) also indicate improvement in Person–healthcare professional relationships because of the use of social media for health information. In fact, in 2011 over 90% of healthcare professionals were using social media for both personal and professional communication (Long 2018). The use of blogs and webcasts for professional development and information dissemination has continued to increase throughout this century. In healthcare, the use of such technology to communicate appears to both improve care while also reducing costs (Sitton-Kent et al 2018). It is interesting to note the use of social media by companies to engage customers, with the result of growing participation of these consumers (Shahbaznezhad et al 2021).

Electronic communication typically allows simultaneous access of multiple people to messages in an easy, cost-effective manner. It promotes expectation of instantaneous communication (Jandt 2020) and constant (although not in person) connection with others, thereby potentially reducing feelings of social isolation (Martin & Nakayama 2018). It is a social, public form of communication that has ethical and potentially legal implications (Boggs 2023; Henderson & Dahnke 2015). While providing opportunities for connection, social media has the potential to provide both reliable information and incorrect information (Gupta et al 2020). Access to electronic forms of communication requires particular devices (mobile phones, iPads or tablets, laptops) and relevant software applications (Apps). Such mobile devices and Apps provide opportunity for communicating without the need for face-to-face or personal contact. Readily available access to electronic forms of communication is changing both the effects of and content of communication (Fedoruk 2015; Griffiths et al 2012; Han 2020; Hjorth & Hinton 2019).

In groups, consider and discuss the following:

- Consider the amount of time group members spend using electronic communication. How many hours a day does each individual spend communicating via text messages (SMS), the internet (email, apps such as Viber, WeChat and Telegram, along with social networking sites such as Facebook, Instagram, X [Twitter]) and Skype, Zoom or Teams, or other forms of instantaneous electronic communication?
- Why do individuals use these particular forms of electronic communication?
- Decide which of these forms of electronic communication experience the most out-of-your-control disruption.
- With which form of electronic communication do individuals feel most comfortable? Why? Does everyone you know feel the same?

Share these ideas with the entire group.

The global changes in forms of communication, whether used for professional or personal communication, highlight the need to consider content and the effect of the message upon a diverse audience. It also mandates consideration of privacy and security (Brewster et al 2014; Harvey & Harvey 2014; Henderson & Dahnke 2015). Another relevant consideration is that all healthcare professionals have socially constructed identities (Monrouxe 2010). In reality, individuals have both a personal and a professional identity. These identities interrelate, impacting and informing each other, and thereby affecting communication. In addition, others interpret the quality of these identities, assigning characteristics to the identities according to interactive events – these events include posts on social networking sites.

Social networking sites

Social networking is currently a significant pastime for many people (Kaplan & Haenlein 2010; Knight et al 2015; Kuss & Griffiths 2017; She et al 2023). However, overuse of social media can reduce the ability to concentrate, while producing mood changes, limited in-person social activities, low self-esteem and often sleep disorders (Maji & Abhiram 2023). In addition, individuals using social networking sites often access and use social media while completing other tasks. Thus, social networking does not always have the full attention of the participants. Despite this, social networking can facilitate creativity as well as social engagement and support (Stehr 2023). In addition, such sites are useful for both personal learning and teaching purposes (Archee et al 2023; DiVerniero & Hosek 2011). Many people in the busy modern world use such sites as a social outlet, often their only connection point with particular people. Some use social media to ask friends with particular qualifications for professional advice and assistance. Others use them to communicate news about their life, often sharing images. Research indicates that people using social networking sites can have an extensive number of social interactions beyond their immediate locality (Archee et al 2023). However, there is also an indication that the relationships within social media are often superficial (McCallion & McCallion 2021). In addition, there is evidence that the presence of a positive comment encourages and increases the number of positive comments, with the presence of negative comments increasing the incidence of such negative responses (Waddell & Sundar 2017).

In groups, consider the following:

- Do social networking sites help you to know people well? The way you would know them if you related in person?

Remember, in person you can see their non-verbal messages and hear any changes in their voice. You can also touch them to encourage them or if they need a hug and so forth.

Share these ideas with the entire/large group.

The nature of social networking often means that individuals from particular sites invite other people to join those sites. It is often therefore difficult to know who has access to each site. In fact, your employer or a future employer might be on a site. This means they can observe and evaluate you, perhaps making judgements about your credibility and employability (Yap & Tiang 2014).

Social media sites appear to be a permanent feature of communicative life (Gagnon & Sabus 2015). They provide an easy interface to share information about personal and/or professional life and social events. They can also be helpful for people experiencing social anxiety and loneliness, or those who have limited verbalising skills or reduced mobility. As healthcare professionals must spend a considerable amount of time actively within the reality of the Person/s, it is important they have time in their own reality. This seems reasonable and appropriate; however, if the healthcare professional fails to continue to be critically self-aware and other-aware, their messages and interactions may NOT have positive effects. They may in fact, suggest a self-focused individual or indeed suggest a different image of the healthcare professional to their actual self.

In groups, consider the questions relating to these comments on a social networking site.

NOTE: All identifying features have been removed to protect the identity of the relevant individuals.

The following Facebook interactions occurred between student healthcare professionals who failed to remember who else might be connected with this Facebook site. This site included all students enrolled in and staff teaching in this particular healthcare professional degree (over 400 students).

Male Student 1, Thursday at 11.10 am

I was studying with fellow Male Student 1a the other day and he was wondering if our practical assessment would involve assisting a lady to remove her bra. Can anyone clarify this, as he is bugging me about it and I don't know the answer?

Male Student 2, Thursday at 11.20 am

Unsure, but just in case – I am sure I can help the ladies out with a one-on-one session.

Female Student 1, Thursday at 11.25 am

Are you guys actually wing manning [one male attempts to find a female for another male friend] using an assessment? That is a whole new level.

Male Student 1, Thursday at 11.26 am

This depends. Male Student 1a says it depends if you are available or not for practice!

Female Student 1, Thursday at 11.39 am

Grow up, I have a boyfriend. I meant this is a whole new level of sad and disgusting.

Male Student 1, Thursday at 11.41 am

Don't take it personally, it was a joke. Just like the whole post was.

Male Student 2, Thursday at 11.42 am

Male Student 1a is a handsome, caring and sensitive guy who cares about his education and therefore I am sure will help, so no wing manning present or needed.

Male Student 3, Thursday at 12.12 pm

The education of Male Student 1a is of the utmost importance and thus if this is in the assessment, he should be allowed to practise this skill.

Discuss the following points:

- Consider what each entry might communicate about each individual.
- How might Male Student 1a feel about this? Might he consider this defaming?
- Discuss the possible impact of these entries upon the other Facebook users.

- Do you think the people making these comments on Facebook considered the possible consequences before entering these comments?
- Why do you think Female Student 1 had to clarify her meaning?
- Is it appropriate to "make a joke" at the expense of others on Facebook?
- Might the time between each entry suggest anything about the individuals responding to the comments?
- How would you feel if people with such attitudes (whether making a joke or serious) were your healthcare professionals? Explore and discuss the reasons for your responses.
- What are the implications of healthcare professionals using social networking sites?

In non-face-to-face or one-way social networking interactions, there is the illusion of control (Hjorth & Hinton 2019). However, the sender communicating with an absent receiver does not have instantaneous feedback about the effect of the message; they experience no personal verbal responses or non-verbal cues (Li et al 2012). This distances separates the sender from the consequences of the message. This also increases the self-focus while also alleviating the sender of the responsibility of considering the receiver and their responses. This distancing has the potential to change the content and quality of the message. This can mean the sender fails to consider the receiver when composing the message. As this could be the situation, the sender may compose self-focused, inappropriate and potentially upsetting messages. Such messages not only communicate the intended message, they also suggest not-always-flattering ideas about the sender, creating a negative impression of the sender (Yap & Tiang 2014). This reality indicates the possibility of comments on social media having negative effects on people experiencing anxiety. This may therefore result in addictive use of and dependence on support through social media (O'Day & Heimberg 2021).

It is important when using electronic communication, whether for professional or personal reasons, to understand that the quality and potential meaning of the message can change without face-to-face interaction. The absence of the receiver highlights the disconnection between the offline world (reality) and the online world (Han 2020; Park et al 2014). This can cause a disconnection between the sender and reality, producing sometimes untrue and insensitive comments. It can result in the sender disengaging from usual moral behaviour because of apparent control and limited immediate consequences (Han 2020; Park et al 2014).

Research has identified a perception among social media users that online behaviour is separate from, therefore does not affect, offline professional life (Prescott et al 2012). In addition, users of social media often perceive entries on such sites as personal and targeted for their friends or group members. Therefore, they post whatever they like without fear of scrutiny (Yap & Tiang 2014). These factors have implications for usage of personal networking sites by healthcare professionals, suggesting the need for care and thought when communicating on these sites (Griffiths et al 2012; Yap & Tiang 2014). The following example indicates the possible unintended results of posts on social networking sites. This highlights the need for healthcare professionals to consider how others might misunderstand and therefore misuse their information and comments on these sites.

After the earthquake in Nepal (April 2015) many distressed and caring people sought ways to assist the many victims of the disaster. As a result, in less than a week, a photograph of two young children huddled together became the focus of social media worldwide. The caption for the heart-wrenching photograph was "Two-year-old sister protected by four-year-old brother in Nepal". As a result there were attempts to locate the children among the victims and there was a call for donations to assist the children. However, the Vietnamese photographer who took the photograph told the BBC he had taken the photograph in a Vietnamese village in 2007. The children were playing in front of their house and the girl, afraid of the stranger, began crying. Her older brother hugged his sister to comfort her. He took the photograph because it was both moving and cute! At the time the photographer published the photograph on his personal blog. He, however, failed to indicate copyright details on the photograph. A few years later he was surprised to discover the Vietnamese Facebook users had shared the photograph with the caption "abandoned orphans"! Some of the users had created intricate stories to explain the picture, stating their mother had died and their father had left them! In another country the same picture was entitled "two Burmese orphans", and [in] still another country, "victims of the civil war in Syria". So while this photograph has been shared repeatedly, it consistently did not receive the correct interpretation of the events surrounding the children.

(Nga Pham, BBC News 4 May 2015, Haunting "Nepal quake victims" photo from Vietnam.)

In groups:

- Consider why individuals using social media seek opportunities to express ideas that do not always reflect the truth.
- How might you explain the different captions for the picture?
- Are there any negative implications for the children because of these erroneous tales? Any for the photographer?
- Why is it important to make comments based upon reality and truth on social networking sites?
- What does this event imply for healthcare professionals?

The use of social media can reinforce a particular perspective of the perceived "reality", which may be based on opinion, rather than actually reflecting reality. The use of algorithms to connect and contact the user, results in the user being connected with people who share similar opinions or biases, regardless of the truth or connection of these opinions with reality (Carter & Perriam 2021; Hjorth & Hinton, 2019; McCallion & McCallion 2021; Verner Venegas-Vera et al 2020).

Cyberbullying

The expansion of available electronic communication, both in devices and internet coverage, in combination with the apparent disconnection from the offline world (reality), has seen an increase in the incidence of bullying (Francisco et al 2014). Bullying is considered to be an intentional, deliberately aggressive act, intending to harm, repeatedly performed by an individual or group towards an individual who is typically unable to defend himself or herself (Archee et al 2023; Bannink et al 2014; Francisco et al 2014; Modecki et al 2014). **Cyberbullying** is deliberate and repeated expressions of aggression intending to harm, using an electronic form of communication (Yi & Zubiaga 2023). It can take the form of sexual innuendo, labelling, ridiculing, threatening or lying (Archee et al 2023). On both personal and professional sites, it can also include personal attacks designed to obstruct or question professional abilities (Forssell 2020). The potential to remain anonymous by adopting pseudonyms may contribute to continuing acts of cyberbullying.

There are potentially three roles involved in bullying: the perpetrator, the victim and the observer (Alipan et al 2020; Levy et al 2012). Regardless of the role, research indicates there are particular effects from cyberbullying that have the potential for enduring negative consequences (Archee et al 2023; Bannink 2014; Francisco et al 2014; John et al 2018; Kwan et al 2018; Modecki et al 2014; Park et al 2014).

Individually, consider the following questions.

- If you were the victim of cyberbullying, explain how you might respond. Why?
- If you were an observer, what are the possible actions you might take? Explain why.
- If observing, what is your responsibility relating to the perpetrator?
- What is your responsibility to the victim?

In groups:

- consider the consequences of cyberbullying and discuss how to manage it if you experience or observe it
- decide when you should report breaches of rights or bullying to a "higher" authority. Discuss how you might do this.

Share group thoughts with the entire group.

The consequences of cyberbullying may lead to serious mental health conditions and even suicidal ideation or actual suicide (Bannink et al 2014; Doumas & Midgett 2022; John et al 2018; Kwan et al 2018; Langos 2014). While it is possible to terminate access for the bully, it is difficult to manage or remove the psychological damage for the victim (Price & Dalgleish 2010; Yi & Zubiaga 2023), and in some cases, the observer. In many cases, cyberbullying is not reported to other individuals due to feelings of shame, helplessness, concern about the reaction of others and a desire to be self-sufficient (DeLara 2012; Watts et al 2017). As the impact of all entries into social networking sites has implications both for the sender and the receiver/s, it is important that senders always consider the effects and potential implications of their messages.

Other factors relating to the use of social media

Social media usage has further implications for every healthcare professional. Comments on any social networking site, in common with emails, are not only permanent, but also may have legal implications (Boggs 2023). Such comments exist in a public domain and are widely available; in fact, they are potentially there for everyone to see (DiVerniero & Hosek 2011). This reality can have long-term consequences for every healthcare professional using this media.

In groups, explore the following questions:

- How might we develop a social conscience related to the use of social media?
- Together, identify the barriers affecting the development of such a conscience.
- Suggest strategies to overcome these barriers.
- Suggest guidelines for ethical and considerate use of social media.

Share the group ideas with the entire group.

Another factor affecting the use of social media is different personal interpretations of comments on such sites. Insufficient care when composing a comment may result in an easily misunderstood message. Misunderstandings may also result from the particular emotional wellbeing of the individual interpreting the comment, regardless of the intention of the individual making the comment. This personal interpretation may then be discussed elsewhere, leading to further misunderstandings and potentially negative emotions. This can produce potential confusion and negative emotions in other people and ultimately potentially harmful consequences for the individual making the original comment. It is important to remember that everything you post communicates something either negative or positive about you and possibly about the focus of the post.

In groups, consider this scenario and the related questions.

A final-year healthcare professional student was completing a professional placement as part of their degree. At around week two of this 12-week placement, the student mentioned on a social networking site that they were ***not enjoying the particular context*** of this placement. What was meant, but not stated, was that they were not enjoying the time pressures: limited time for developing a therapeutic relationship or providing actual interventions in the acute setting. After the completion of this placement, a healthcare professional working at the site of this placement was talking to a second-year student from the same profession and training institution, at a social event. This student mentioned that from a comment on a social networking site it was obvious that the final-year student had not enjoyed this placement, and that other students had decided that, if possible, they would avoid ever completing a placement at that site. The healthcare professionals at the site were both surprised and concerned, as the final-year student seemed to have had an honest relationship with the immediate supervisor and the rest of the team and had not mentioned anything to indicate lack of learning or enjoyment during the placement. When this information was communicated to the final-year student, they were amazed that their comment could be interpreted in that manner. The student had really enjoyed the placement, had learnt a great deal about being a healthcare professional and would definitely recommend it to any other student. They admitted the comment had indicated their personal struggle with an unfamiliar fast-paced acute context, but had never intended to mean the site produced a difficult, unenjoyable placement, one to be avoided by other students. The comment had been interpreted as an indication of a "bad" placement site rather than a personal reaction to an unfamiliar setting and pace of practice.

- What could the final-year student have done to avoid this situation? Remember, they were time pressured.
- Suggest guidelines for the use of social media relating to professional practice.

In this case, the final-year student decided the best course of action for future contributions to any social networking site was to implement the advice of the media. This advice states that everyone should *avoid* making any comments on any social networking site relating to anything about their workplace, but especially feelings about or interactions within their workplace.

Many people using social media do not remember that their comments are permanent, whether or not they are removed from view, and can have professional and potentially legal implications. In addition, it seems that people commenting on such sites do not remember that the interpretation of others using the site can adversely affect the meaning and thus the focus of any comment. Even though any interpretation is the responsibility of the reader or message interpreter, it may not be linked to the individual interpreting, but rather to the individual making the original comment. It is this individual who will hold the legal responsibility of the comment and any resultant discussion of the comment. This incident highlights the need for all healthcare professionals to reflect upon the realities and implications of electronic communication. It is essential that healthcare professionals promote trust within their local community. This therefore requires particular healthcare professional behaviour to develop this trust.

Another important aspect of using social media is the evidence suggesting a tendency to addiction, both visually and psychologically (Kuss & Griffiths 2017; McCallion & McCallion 2021). This is something requiring careful, regular and efficient consideration of how to control this tendency for both the healthcare professionals and also the Person/s they assist in practice.

Netiquette: a mnemonic to guide personal electronic communication

Social networking sites communicate particular messages about the sender. Therefore, it is important to consider the content and effect of any comment made on a social networking site. There are several questions that social network users can ask themselves to guide their online posts – *Would I say this to someone face-to-face? If not, why say it electronically? How would I feel if someone else posted this about me? Do I really want the world to know this about me?* There are also characteristics essential for future healthcare professionals to consider when communicating online, whether on personal or professional sites.

The components of the following mnemonic ("NETIQUETTE") reflect appropriate characteristics of positive social networking comments. It is important to ask yourself these questions before posting anything on a social networking site.

N ECESSARY: Is this comment necessary, and if so, what makes it necessary?
E STIMABLE: Is this comment admirable and worthy of esteem? Why?
T RUE: Is this comment true with evidence to support it? Are you sure? Consider the perspective of all site users.
I NSPIRING: Is this comment inspiring, encouraging and positive? How?
Q UOTABLE: Is this something other people will be proud to repeat? Why?
U SEFUL: What makes this comment useful for the diverse audience? How?
E FFICACY: What are the consequences of this comment for you and others?
T RUSTWORTHY: Does this comment indicate you are worthy of trust? How?
T IMELY: Is this comment appropriate considering the other comments? Why?
E MPATHIC: Does this comment demonstrate empathy for others? How?

NETIQUETTE is essential for healthcare professionals because of the complex interaction between and often blurring of professional and personal identity (Long 2018). It is also essential because of the potential risk associated with using social media (Koteyko et al 2015). The ability of potential employers to assess the social networking profiles of individuals seeking employment with their service also highlights the importance of NETIQUETTE (Levett-Jones & Bourgeois 2022; Yap & Tiang 2014).

Communication using electronic interfaces for social networking appears to have advantages and disadvantages. In order for healthcare professionals to benefit from the advantages, they must develop strategies to overcome the disadvantages. This is important, as there is increasing use of social media among healthcare services and healthcare professionals to implement healthcare and health promotion. Therefore, it is essential for all healthcare professionals to consider the related laws and guidelines of their registration organisations to ensure achievement of those guidelines when using social networking sites.

Professional communication using social media

Health information is more often available online. In the past few years, there has been an increase in the popularity of such sites (Veale et al 2015). Lober and Flowers (2011) consider the social milieu (e.g. podcasts, YouTube, webinars, blogs, Facebook, X [Twitter]) to be an enabler for connecting and empowering Person/s to engage in positive health behaviours. There is evidence indicating that the use of social media to access health-related information is empowering for Person/s (Benetoli et al 2017; O'Kane 2020). Antheunis and colleagues (2013) highlight the use of Facebook and X when Person/s explore or discuss health needs, while healthcare professionals use LinkedIn or X. Use of these sites indicates a change from the early e-health practices of individuals merely searching for condition-related information to possibilities of enabling Person/s to engage in supportive communication and potentially health-producing behaviours.

The use of social media within healthcare practice for empowering health and relationships with healthcare professionals is expected to continue increasing (Benetoli et al 2017). Technical advancement has produced continual high-speed internet access in many locations, with associated changes in ways of exchanging information. This also indicates a need for healthcare professionals to adjust their practice to fulfil the needs of the Person/s using social media (Gagnon & Sabus 2015; Knight et al 2015). It also indicates the need for healthcare professionals to adjust their style of communicating to accommodate the audience (Li & Mao 2015). Why? Social media presents healthcare professionals with an extensive interface for providing continued meaningful professional and personal relationships and accurate healthcare information (Henderson & Dahnke 2015; Long 2018). Establishing a personal social networking account for all personal communication and a different one for professional communication is becoming a common method of ensuring appropriate use of this form of communication, along with maintaining the reputation of the healthcare professional.

In small groups:

- suggest possible advantages of using social media in healthcare.
- suggest possible challenges of such use and how to overcome these challenges.

Research highlights the associated advantages and challenges of using social media for provision of healthcare. Person/s use social media to increase knowledge of conditions, ensure current understanding of the latest developments relevant to their conditions and to either provide or receive support and/or advice from people with experience of their condition (Bartlett & Coulson 2011). Healthcare professionals use social media to provide and receive current information and immediate advice relating to individual needs for Person/s and colleagues (Jaffe 2021). This may include receiving advice and recent research outcomes from their colleagues through specifically established online webinars, social groups or social networking groups. These platforms are usually designed to provide information, support and encouragement, while also potentially increasing the profile and understanding of healthcare professions (Health and Care Professions Council 2017). In addition, they promote increased health literacy (O'Kane 2020), mutual sharing or networking (Williams et al 2021), and empowerment for both the Person/s and the healthcare professional (Health and Care Professions Council 2017). This sharing reduces feelings of isolation encouraging increased Person-participation in the healthcare process (Bartlett & Coulson 2011; Benetoli et al 2017). However, a requirement of such use of these forms of communication is maintaining Person/s confidentiality (Doherty 2021; Health and Care Professions Council 2017). This requires consideration and removal of all identifying details of the Person/s, when sharing information, images and comments relating to that (or any other) particular Person/s.

Maintaining professional boundaries is one challenge associated with use of social media in healthcare (Basevi et al 2014; Doherty 2021; Health and Care Professions Council 2017). Relating with the Person/s on a social networking site has the potential to blur the professional boundaries of the therapeutic relationship. Depending upon the interactions (remember the possibilities for misinterpretation), it also has the potential to negatively affect the reputation of the healthcare professional and possibly their profession. This may explain the opposition from some healthcare professionals to using social media. Ginory and colleagues (2012) found that some healthcare professionals avoided social media in order to protect the healthcare professional/Person relationship and the privacy of the healthcare professional. However, these healthcare professionals also expressed concern that declining a "friend" request from a patient may negatively affect the therapeutic relationship, also possibly resulting in cyber-stalking. Alternatively, some Person/s avoid social networking sites, as they do not wish to be known as a patient (Antheunis et al 2013). Some Person/s are concerned about privacy, not wanting to discuss personal information on the internet. Others, along with many healthcare professionals, doubt the reliability of information from the internet, while others lack skills in using social media (Antheunis et al 2013).

Ongoing use of social media in healthcare mandates robust guidelines for such use, to protect the privacy of the Person/s and the healthcare professional, while also promoting ethical boundaries in the relationship between the healthcare professional and the Person/s (Basevi et al 2014; Doherty 2021; Frankish et al 2012; Yap & Tiang 2014). While further research is required about the impact of social media upon health behaviour and health outcomes (Antheunis et al 2013), there is some evidence of positive health outcomes. However, these guidelines are developing and being tested, healthcare professionals have an ethical responsibility to use social networking sites with respect and care, according to their professional board and organisations, employers, national law and or relevant legislations (Australian Health Practitioner Regulation Authority (Ahpra) 2019).

Chapter summary

Healthcare professionals around the world commonly use electronic communication due to changes in forms of communication and accessibility of services. Despite the advantages and disadvantages of electronic forms of communication, it appears that one such form – social networking – is a permanent feature of the twenty-first century. This form of communication provides opportunities for connecting and interacting with individuals, regardless of their location or verbalising abilities. However, realities about social media require consideration. These often-forgotten realities include issues relating to privacy, security and legality. They affect all individuals interacting through these sites. Therefore, healthcare professionals using social media must consider these realities and the legal implications of any of their comments on these sites. They must also avoid commenting about anything, whether feelings, opinions or events, relating to their workplace. The elements of the mnemonic NETIQUETTE may assist healthcare professionals using social media for personal communication to avoid negative consequences. They may also assist when using social media for professional communication, either with colleagues or the Person/s. The popularity of social media highlights the importance of healthcare professionals using this medium of communication, both responsibly and carefully in order to empower the Person/s and achieve effective communication and Person/Family-centred healthcare.

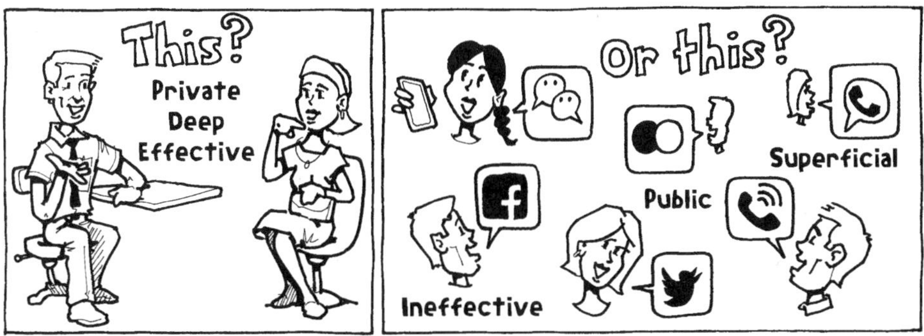

FIGURE 23.1
Social media does not always achieve effective communication.
Courtesy Roger Harvey © Elsevier Australia.

REVIEW QUESTIONS

1. i. Using your own words, define personal electronic communication.

   ii. List devices and Apps used for personal electronic communication

   iii. Suggest five different types of personal electronic communication.

2. Suggest two consequences of an absent audience/receiver of messages.

3. i. Define "social networking site".

   ii. Suggest two reasons for communicating using social media.

4. Make a table with two columns, one listing at least seven advantages and the other listing at least seven disadvantages or challenges of social networking sites.

5. List things to consider when commenting on any social networking site.

6. i. Define cyberbullying.

   ii. Suggest two explanations for cyberbullying.

   iii. State two researched consequences of cyberbullying.

7. Using the characteristics of NETIQUETTE and your relevant law or healthcare profession guidelines for use of social media, develop your own guidelines for positive and appropriate interactions through personal and professional electronic communication sites.

References

Alipan, A., Skues, J.L., Theiler, S., et al., 2020. Defining cyberbullying: A multifaceted definition based on the perspectives of emerging adults. International Journal of Bullying Prevention, 2, 79–92.

Antheunis, M.L., Tates, K., Nieboer, T.E., 2013. Patients' and health professionals' use of social media in health care: Motives, barriers and expectations. Patient Education and Counseling, 92, 426–431.

Archee, R., Gurney, M., Mohan, T., 2023. Communicating as professionals, 4th ed. Cengage Learning, Melbourne.

Australian Health Practitioner Regulation Authority, 2019. Social Media Policy. Ahpra, Sydney.

Bannink, R., Broeren, S., van de Looij-Jansen, P.M., et al., 2014. Cyber and traditional bullying victimization as a risk factor for mental health problems and suicidal ideation in adolescents. PLoS ONE 9(4), 1–8.

Bartlett, Y.K., Coulson, N.S., 2011. An investigation into the empowerment effects of using online support groups and how this affects health professional/patient communication. Patient Education and Counseling, 83, 113–119.

Basevi, R., Reid, D., Godbold, R., 2014. Ethical guidelines and the use of social media and text messaging in health care: A review of literature. New Zealand Journal of Physiotherapy, 42(2), 68–80.

Benetoli, a., Chen, T.F., Aslani, P., 2017 How patients' use of social media impacts their interactions with healthcare professionals. Patient Education and Counselling, 10(3), 439–444.

Boggs, K., 2023. Interpersonal relationships: Professional communication skills for nurses, 9th ed. Elsevier, St Louis, MO.

Brewster, L., Mountain, G., Wessels, B., et al., 2014. Factors affecting front line staff acceptance of telehealth technologies: A mixed method systematic review. Journal of Advanced Nursing, 70(1), 21–33.

Carter, S., Perriam, J., 2021. Algorithms. In: Perriam, J., Carter S. (eds). Understanding digital societies. Sage & Open University, London.

Conti, M., Pajola, L., Triconi, P.P., 2023. Turning captchas against humanity: Captcha-based attacks in online social media. Online Social Networks and Media, 36(2023), 100252.

DeLara, E.W., 2012. Why adolescents don't disclose incidents of bullying and harassment. Journal of School Violence, 11(4), 288–305.

DiVerniero, R.A., Hosek, A.M., 2011. Students' perceptions and communicative management of instructors' online self-disclosure. Communication Quarterly, 59(4), 428–449.

Doherty, R.F., 2021. Ethical dimensions in health professions, 7th ed. Elsevier, St Louis, MO.

Doumas, D.M., Midgett, A., 2022. Witnessing cyberbullying and suicidal ideation among middle school students. Psychology in the Schools, 60(4), 1149–1163.

Fedoruk, M., 2015. Health Information systems and Technologies. In: Fedoruk, M., Hofmeyer, A. (eds), Becoming a nurse: An evidence-based approach, 2nd ed. Oxford University Press, Melbourne.

Forssell, R.C. 2020. Cyberbullying in a boundary blurred working life: Distortion of the private and professional face on social media. Qualitative Research in Organizations and Management, 15(2), 89–107.

Francisco, S.M., Veiga Simão, A.M., Ferreira, P.C., et al., 2014. Cyberbullying: The hidden side of college students. Computers in Human Behavior, 43(1), 167–182.

Frankish, K., Ryan, C., Harris, A., 2012. Psychiatry and online social media: Potential, pitfalls and ethical guidelines for psychiatrists and trainees. Australasian Psychiatry, 20(3), 181–187.

Gagnon, K., Sabus, C., 2015. Professionalism in a Digital Age: Opportunities and considerations for using social media in health care. Physical Therapy, 95(3), 406–414.

Ginory, A., Sabatier, L.M., Eth, S., 2012. Addressing therapeutic boundaries in social networking. Psychiatry, 75(1), 40–48.

Gottlieb, M., Dyer, S., 2020. Information and disinformation: Social media in the COVID-19 crisis. Academic Emergency Medicine, 27, 640–641.

Griffiths, F., Cave, J., Boardman, F., et al., 2012. Social networks: The future of health care delivery. Social Science and Medicine, 75(12), 2233–2241.

Gupta, L., Gasparyan, A.Y., Misra, D.P., et al., 2020. Information and misinformation on COVID- 19: A cross-sectional survey study. Journal of Korean Medical Science, 35, e256.

Han, B-C., 2020. The disappearance of rituals. Polity Press, Oxford, UK.

Harvey, M.J., Harvey, M.G., 2014. Privacy and security issues for mobile health platforms. Journal of the Association for Information Science and Technology, 65(7), 1305–1318.

Health and Care Professions Council (UK), Guidance on the use of social media. Online. Available at: www.hcpc-uk.org/globalassets/resources/guidance/guidance-on-social-media.pdf

Henderson, M., Dahnke, M.D., 2015. The ethical use of social media in nursing practice. Medical–Surgical Nursing, 24(1), 62–64.

Hjorth, L., Hinton, S., 2019. Understanding social media, 2nd ed. Sage, London.

Irwin, T.J., Prtiz, R., Barone, A.A.L., 2021. Are all posts created equal? A review of academic plastic surgery residency programs' social media engagement statistics. Plastic and Reconstructive Surgery, 148(4), 700e–702e.

Jaffe, T.A., Hayden, E., UScher-Pines, L., et al., 2021. Telehealth use in emergency care during coronavirus disease 2019: A systematic review. JACEP Open, 2 e12443.

Jandt, F.E., 2020. An introduction to intercultural communication. Identities in a global community, 10th ed. Sage, Thousand Oaks, California.

John, A., Glendenning, A.C., Marchant, A., et al., 2018. Self-harm, suicidal behaviours and cyberbullying in children and young people: A systematic review. Journal of Medical Internet Research, 20(4), e129.

Kaplan, A.M., Haenlein, M., 2010. Users of the world, unite! The challenges and opportunities of social media. Business Horizons, 53, 59–68.

Knight, E., Werstine, R.J., Rasmussen-Pennington, D.M., et al., 2015. Physical therapy 2.0: Leveraging social media to engage patients in rehabilitation and health promotion. Physical Therapy, 95(3), 389–396.

Koteyko, N., Hunt, D., Gunter, B., 2015. Expectations in the field of the Internet and health: An analysis of claims about social networking sites in clinical literature. Sociology of Health and Illness, 37(3), 468–484.

Kuss, D.J., Griffiths, M.D., 2017. Social networking sites and addiction: Ten lessons learnt. International Journal of Environmental Research and Public Health, 14, 311.

Kwan, I., Dickson, K., Richardson, M., et al., 2018. Cyberbullying and children and young people's mental health: A systematic map of systematic reviews. Cyberbullying, Behaviour and Social Networking, 23(2), 72–82.

Langos, C., 2014. Cyberbullying: The shades of harm. Psychiatry, Psychology and Law, 22(1), 106–123.

Levett-Jones, T., Bourgeois, S., 2022. The clinical placement: An essential guide for nursing students, 5th ed. Elsevier, Sydney.

Levy, N., Cortesi, S., Gasser, U., Crowley, E., et al., 2012. Bullying in a networked era: A literature review. Harvard University, Berkman Centre Research Publication, Harvard.

Li, M., Mao, J., 2015. Hedonic or utilitarian? Exploring the impact of communication style alignment on user's perception of virtual health advisory services. International Journal of Information Management, 35(2), 229–243.

Li, Q., Smith, P.K., Cross, D., 2012. Research into cyberbullying: Context. In: Li, Q., Cross, D., Smith, P.K. (eds), Cyberbullying in the global playground: Research from international perspectives. Wiley-Blackwell, Oxford.

Lober, W.B., Flowers, J.L., 2011. Consumer empowerment in health care amid the Internet and social media. Seminars in Oncology Nursing, 27(3), 169–182.

Long, N.D., 2018. The good, the bad and the ugly of social media: How to navigate through the noise. Emergency Medicine Australasia, 30(3), 412–413.

Maji, S., Abhiram, A.H., 2023. "Mental health cost of the internet": A mixed-method study of cyberbullying among Indian sexual minorities. Telematics and Informatics Reports, 10(2023), 100064.

Martin, J.N., Nakayama, T.K., 2018. Intercultural communication in context, 7th ed. McGraw-Hill, New York.

McCallion, M., McCallion, K., 2021. Reflections on social media. Academia Letters, article 329. doi.org/10.20935/AL329.

Modecki, K.L., Minchin, J., Harbaugh, A.G., et al., 2014. Bullying prevalence across contexts: A meta-analysis measuring cyber and traditional Bullying. Journal of Adolescent Health, 55(5), 602–611.

Monrouxe, L.V., 2010. Identity, identification and medical education: Why should we care? Medical Education, 44, 40–49.

O'Day, E.B., Heimberg, R.G., 2021. Social media use, social anxiety and loneliness: A systematic review, Computers in Human Behaviours Reports, 3(2021), 100070.

O'Kane, D., 2020. Communication in healthcare practice. In: Barkway, P., O'Kane, D., 2020. Psychology: An introduction for health professionals. Elsevier, Sydney.

Park, S., Na, E.-Y., Kim, E.-M., 2014. The relationship between online activities, netiquette and cyberbullying. Children and Youth Services Review, 42(1), 74–81.

Pentescu, A., Cetina, I., Orzan, G., 2015. Social Media's impact on healthcare services. Procedia Economics and Finance, 27(2015), 646–651.

Prescott, J., Wilson, S., Becket, G., 2012. Students want more guidelines on Facebook and online professionalism. Pharmaceutical Journal, 289, 163.

Price, M., Dalgleish, J., 2010. Cyberbullying: Experiences, impact and coping strategies as described by Australian young people. Youth Studies Australia, 29(2), 51–59.

Shahbaznezhad, H., Dolan, F., Rashidirad, M., 2021. The role of social media content format and platform in users' engagement behaviour. Journal of Interactive Marketing, 53(1), 47–65.

She, R., Mo, P.K.H., Li, J., et al., 2023. The double-edged sword effect of social networking use intensity on problematic social networking use among college students: The role of social skills and social anxiety, Computers in Human Behavior, 140(2023), 207555.

Sitton-Kent, L., Humphreys, C., Miller, P., 2018. Supporting the spread of health technology in community services. British Journal of Community Nursing, 23(3), 118–122.

Stehr, P., 2023, The benefits of supporting others online – How online communication shapes the provision of support and its relationship with wellbeing. Computers in Human Behavior, 140(2023), 07568.

Teles da Mota, V., Pickering, C., Chauvenet, A., 2022. Popularity of Australian beaches: Insights from social media images for coastal management. Ocean and Coastal Management, 217(2022), 106018.

Veale, H.J., Sacks-Davis, R., Weaver, E., et al., 2015. The use of social networking platforms for sexual health promotion: Identifying key strategies for successful user engagement. BMC Public Health 15, 85.

Verner Venegas-Vera, A., Colbert, G.B., Lerma, V.E., 2020. Positive and negative impact of social media in the COVID-19 era. Reviews in Cardiovascular Medicine, 21(4), 561–564.

Waddell, T.F., Sundar, S.S., 2017. #thisshowsucks! The overpowering influence of negative social media comments on television viewers. Journal of Broadcasting and Electronic Media, 61(2), 393–409.

Watts, L.K., Wagner, J., Velasquez, B., et al., 2017. Cyberbullying in higher education: A literature review. Computers in Human Behavior, 69, 268–274.

Williams, A., Martin, S., Coates, V., 2021. Being person-centred when working with people living with long-term conditions. In: McCormack, B., McCance, T., Bulley, C., et al., Fundamentals in person-centred healthcare practice. Wiley Blackwell, Oxford.

World Health Organization (WHO), 2011. mHealth: New horizons for health through mobile technologies: Second global survey on eHealth. Global observatory for ehealth series, vol 3. WHO, Geneva.

Yap, K.Y.-L., Tiang, Y.L., 2014. Recommendations for health care educators on e-professionalism and student behavior on social networking sites. Medicolegal and Bioethics, 10.2147/MB.S60563.

Yi, P., Zubiaga, A., 2023. Session-based cyberbullying detection in social media: A survey. Online Social Networks and Media, 36(2023), 100250.

Useful websites relating to policies for use of social media

Australian Association of Social Workers: www.aasw.asn.au
Ethics and Practice Guidelines – Social media, information and communication technologies: Parts 1 and 2: www.aasw.asn.au/about-aasw/ethics-standards/ethics-and-practice-guidelines/

Australian Health Professional Regulation Agency (AHPRA) Social Media Policy: www.ahpra.gov.au/Publications/Social-media-guidance.aspx

Health and Care Professions Council (UK), Guidance on the use of Social Media: hcpc-uk.org

Medical Board of Australia: www.medicalboard.gov.au/Codes-Guidelines-Policies/Social-media-policy.aspx

Nursing and Midwifery Board of Australia: www.nursingmidwiferyboard.gov.au/Codes-Guidelines-Statements.aspx

New Zealand Government Guidance: www.publicservice.govt.nz/guidance/guidance-use-of-social-media-for-public-servants/guidance-for-public-servants-official-use-of-social-media

Nursing Council of New Zealand Guidelines: www.nursingcouncil.org.nz/Public/NCNZ/nursing-section/Standards_and_guidelines_for_nurses.aspx?hkey=9fc06ae7-a853-4d10-b5fe-992cd44ba3de

Nursing Council of New Zealand Guidelines Social Media: www.nursingcouncil.org.nz/Public/Nursing/Standards_and_guidelines/NCNZ/nursing-section/Standards_and_guidelines_for_nurses.aspx?hkey=9fc06ae7-a853-4d10-b5fe-992cd44ba3de

SECTION 4

Scenarios to guide communication: Opportunities for healthcare professionals to practise communicating effectively with "the Person/s"

Introduction

Section 4 (Chapters 24–28) was designed to promote awareness of the effects of the different styles and types of communication outlined in Sections 1 to 3 of this book. The section was also created to develop, through guided interactions or observation of these interactions, awareness of personal attitudes and skills in communication. The scenarios in this section provide the opportunity to develop skills in communicating with the Person/s typically seen and assisted by healthcare professionals within the potentially "safe" context of learning. They are not necessarily definitive, meaning individuals using them may be able to add relevant points from their personal experience. The scenarios facilitate exploration of the possible needs of the Person/s, encouraging use of the communication skills discussed in the first three sections of the book. These communication skills include introductions; providing and gathering information; questioning; validating and comforting; noting and responding to non-verbal cues; effective listening; considering the needs of the Person/s and environmental factors; avoiding misunderstandings and strategies for communicating with culturally diverse Person/s.

The scenarios in Chapters 24 to 28 are outlined to promote role-play opportunities as a learning milieu. Each scenario describes the context of an interaction between either a female or a male Person (Person 1) and a healthcare professional or an appropriately trained professional (Person 2). The information outlined in each scenario provides the details of the particular Person and typical reasons and reactions associated with the outlined issues. This is designed to assist the individuals assuming the particular role to "act" as though they actually are that Person or healthcare professional. It is important to carefully read the details of your role before commencing the role-play. In pairs, each individual has the opportunity to assume one of the roles and "act out" an interaction using the description of the context. In some circumstances it may be appropriate to assign an observer to record the use of particular communication skills, to encourage greater awareness of personal skills and associated responses.

It is also possible to use the scenarios with actors (or drama students) who assume the role of the Person, while the budding healthcare professional attempts to effectively communicate with them.

It is important for healthcare professionals to realise they must remain controlled and calm in order to achieve effective communication, *regardless* of the Person or the circumstances.

There are suggestions throughout Sections 1, 2 and 3 relating to the content of the particular chapter for use of these scenarios. The following provides suggestions for how to use them during training sessions, as paired or group activities.

One possible session outline – role-plays

NOTE: You may wish to focus on development of particular aspects of communication. This would mean the individual taking the role of the healthcare professional, for example, would focus on questioning and validating OR perhaps listening and non-verbal expression, while seeking to achieve communication focusing upon the needs of the Person/s.

1 Begin by *choosing the focus of the session* from one of the five scenario themes:
   - Person/s experiencing strong negative emotions (Chapter 24)
   - Person/s in particular stages of life (Chapter 25)
   - Person/s fulfilling particular life roles (Chapter 26)
   - Person/s experiencing particular conditions (Chapter 27)
   - Person/s in particular contexts (Chapter 28).

2 With the entire class group, discuss the following points:
   - Consider the definitions provided for each need or life reality within the scenario theme (see the relevant chapter). If the group does not agree, decide upon an alternative appropriate definition.
   - Discuss how it might feel if experiencing each need or life reality.
   - Suggest how each one might affect your daily routine and expectations of others.

3 Divide the group into pairs. If using observers, assign one or two observers to each pair. If focusing upon particular aspects of communication, the observers would need to concentrate on how the "healthcare professional" uses these aspects of communication.

4 Each pair then chooses a particular scenario within the particular theme.

5 Allocate roles to each member of the pair OR have them choose their role.

6 Allow no more than 10 minutes for everyone to read the information relevant to his or her role. Both should read:
   - the description of the need or life reality AND the description of the individuals most susceptible to that need or life reality, adding any other points as necessary.

   The "Person" should also read:
   - expected behaviours of someone experiencing that need or life reality AND possible reasons for that need or life reality, again as required, adding additional points.

   The "healthcare professional" Person 2 should also read:
   - principles for effective communication with a Person/s experiencing that need or life reality AND strategies for communicating with someone experiencing that need or life reality. Remember you may have additional ideas to add to these lists.

   Observers should read all relevant information and prepare a list of communication styles they wish to "critique" during the role-play.

7 The pairs enact the scenario.

8 Discussion and evaluation of the interaction with the pairs and observers.
   - Discuss the responses of both communicators. If there is a focus upon one aspect of communication, discuss the demonstrated skills of the healthcare professional in that aspect.
   - Explore any emotional responses and the possible reasons for these responses.
   - Identify the most effective communication strategies and explain why they were effective.

9 If possible, repeat the process until everyone wanting to assume the role of the Person in the scenario has had the opportunity to play that role and discuss the interaction.

It is important to identify what has been learnt about effective communication through the role-play with the entire group, not just the pairs. During large group discussions, emphasise use of particular aspects of communication to demonstrate respect and empathy to develop trust.

This process can be adapted and repeated using any of the 33 sets of scenarios included in this section (Chapters 24 to 28).

Alternative session outline – small-group discussions

1 Choose the focus of the discussion from among the five scenario themes:
   - Person/s experiencing strong negative emotions (Chapter 24)
   - Person/s in particular stages of life (Chapter 25)
   - Person/s fulfilling particular life roles (Chapter 26)
   - Person/s experiencing particular conditions (Chapter 27)
   - Person/s in particular contexts (Chapter 28).

2 In groups of no more than eight, discuss the impact or reality of the chosen theme on communication and everyday life.
3 Consider the implications of two or three scenarios within each theme.
4 Discuss the relevance of the listed communication strategies for each of the chosen scenarios to the need or life reality. Explain why they might or might not be appropriate to the particular scenarios.
5 Consider each chosen scenario and suggest what about the Person/s is most relevant and requires discussion from the perspective of their particular healthcare profession/s.

NOTE*:* The scenarios are fictitious, so if any of the scenarios cause discomfort or negative emotions of identification, it is essential the individual seeks assistance to achieve resolution. Resolution of discomfort will ensure a consistent ability to provide the best care for both self and the Person/s while providing healthcare.

Chapter 24

Person/s experiencing strong negative emotions

Chapter objective

Upon completing this chapter, readers should be able to apply knowledge and have emerging skills in communicating effectively with Person/s experiencing strong negative emotions.

Healthcare professionals assist vulnerable people who experience a range of emotions. This chapter considers six strong negative emotions that may be a barrier to effective communication: aggression, extreme distress, neurogenic shock, depression, severe, overwhelming and consistent anxiety and reluctance to engage or be involved in communication or intervention.

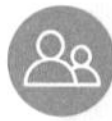

Strong negative emotions

1. Aggression
2. Extreme distress
3. Neurogenic shock
4. Depression
5. Severe, overwhelming and consistent anxiety
6. Reluctance to engage or be involved in communication or intervention.
    - Decide what it means to be experiencing the strong emotions listed above.
    - List the specific behaviours that might indicate the presence of these strong emotions.
    - List the individuals who are most susceptible to feeling these strong emotions.
    - Decide the possible events or environments that might produce the strong emotions and explain why.
    - List principles for effective communication to remember when communicating with a person experiencing these strong emotions. Give reasons for the need to remember these principles.

- Suggest strategies for communicating with a person who is experiencing these strong emotions. Decide why you might see such a person in your particular health profession.
- Check your answers against the information below, noting any additional thoughts or ideas.

NOTE: Small group discussion may prove more appropriate than role-plays when considering scenarios that incorporate Person/s experiencing strong negative emotions.

1. Person/s behaving aggressively

(Key words: angry, aggressive, insistent, forceful, violent)

Definition of aggression

Consider anger at one end of a continuum and violence at the other end, with aggressive behaviour in between. A person who behaves aggressively may demonstrate anger initially and violence ultimately.

A Person who behaves aggressively is someone who:

- exhibits apparently unprovoked behaviours that threaten those around them
- feels vulnerable and out of control
- wants their "own way" and will intimidate or threaten to fulfil their desires
- may confuse aggression with assertion
- may believe aggressive behaviour is the only way they can "win" or achieve their desired results
- ... and so on (this list is not exhaustive).

Individuals most susceptible to behaving aggressively

A common belief suggests that individuals who behave aggressively are found mostly in mental healthcare settings. This is not always true: aggressive behaviour can occur anywhere.

Individuals may be susceptible to behaving aggressively because of:

- eroded self-esteem
- emotional trauma (e.g. disappointment, loss, frustration, bewilderment)
- unresolved anger or frustration
- stress
- unfulfilled desires
- inability to understand a situation or event.

People who behave aggressively may have an emotional reason (e.g. unfulfilled desires) to which they respond with aggressive behaviour. However, such people do not always behave aggressively in the environment that provides the trigger for their emotions.

Possible reasons for aggression

Individuals may become aggressive because of:

- loss of something important (e.g. family, employment, health)
- unexpected events
- excessive use of addictive substances or withdrawal from addictive substances
- reaction to medication
- chronic pain
- forgetting to take or deciding not to take medication.

Possible behaviours related to aggression

An aggressive Person might:

- be verbally abusive and loud when interacting
- threaten (verbally or in writing) to physically harm someone or something
- use non-verbal gestures to indicate feelings of aggression.

Principles for effective communication with a Person/s behaving aggressively

When communicating with a Person who behaves aggressively, it is important to:

- respond with patience and understanding
- empathise with the Person, not necessarily with their feelings
- use active listening and careful observation
- if appropriate, focus on the problem and possible solutions
- avoid responding to the aggressive statements or threats with aggression – do not retaliate
- demonstrate interest, attention and concern through non-verbal behaviours
- remember the principles of assertive communication (see Chapter 13); however, some people may become more aggressive if you attempt to discuss what they are expressing at that time
- validate if appropriate
- avoid confronting if they are violent
- always remember safety of self and others
- position yourself closest to the door
- use emergency call buttons or duress alarms if necessary and available.

If there is a risk of violent behaviour, it is important to:

- inform the immediate supervisor of the possible risk
- wherever possible, have another healthcare professional present
- ensure the health service knows the exact whereabouts of the health professionals who work with the Person, whether on- or offsite
- plan the interaction carefully, considering the safety of all involved individuals
- be alert for the safety of everyone involved and if necessary remove self and others from the scene
- stay close to the door or exit
- avoid attempting to physically connect with the Person
- call the police if necessary.

Strategies for communicating with a Person/s behaving aggressively

- Remain calm to maximise observation and problem-solving skills.
- Ask the Person to "tell you their story" to explain their strong emotions. This may allow them to become calm.
- If the Person is still in control, state they are being inappropriately aggressive. This may stop the behaviour, potentially providing an opportunity to become calm.
- Be aware of non-verbal behaviours and remove yourself if the Person is expressing extreme agitation. Among group members, brainstorm ways to respond verbally so you can remove yourself safely.
- Engage the Person in consideration of their plans for the future and how they might fulfil these plans.

See the Introduction to Section 4 for instructions about how to use these scenarios for role-play or group discussion. Remember the principles of effective communication and Person/Family-centred Care.

Scenario one: The male and the healthcare professional

Person 1: Your name is John. You are a 35-year-old man who had an accident at work 5 years ago. You have been experiencing chronic lower back pain since that time. You were on modified duties for 2 years and have not been employed full-time during the past 3 years. You have seen four doctors and several physiotherapists, chiropractors, podiatrists, massage therapists and rehabilitation providers. You are very frustrated and fail to see how this recent referral will achieve anything different. You feel your divorce a year ago was a result of your pain over the past 5 years. You want to see more of your two children, but your pain makes this difficult.

Person 2: You are the healthcare professional. The referral indicates this man is prone to aggressive behaviour. You want to avoid aggressive behaviour in order to develop a therapeutic relationship and some appropriate goals.

Scenario two: The female and the healthcare professional

Person 1: Your name is Jessi. You are a 16-year-old girl who always passively allows other people to have what they want, regardless of what you may want. You do this because you desperately want to have a "place" in a particular group at school. However, now you cannot control the emotions resulting from repeated hurt, frustration and bewilderment because of your non-assertive responses to those around you. You now respond aggressively to everyone, even your closest friends and family.

Person 2: You are the healthcare professional doing a routine assessment and check-up with Jessi. Her responses are aggressive and rude.

- How should you complete the check-up?
- As a large group, discuss the observations, emotions and outcomes of the role-plays. Suggest possible alternative strategies that may increase the effectiveness of the communication in a similar situation.

2. Person/s experiencing extreme distress

(Key words: overwhelming emotion, fear, anxiety, grief, frustration)

Definition of extreme distress

An extremely distressed Person is someone who is experiencing overwhelming negative emotions, including sadness, anxiety, fear and loss.

Individuals most susceptible to extreme distress

Individuals may be susceptible to extreme distress because of:

- strong emotions, including fear, anxiety and grief
- enduring chronic situations such as war or displacement from safety
- conditions causing chronic pain
- loss, including loss of control over their circumstances.

Possible reasons for extreme distress

Individuals may become extremely distressed because of:

- the impending death of a child, sibling, spouse or parent
- an accident
- an attack
- lack of understanding of events or the environment.

Remember there are cultural variations in the expression of emotion. A particular culture might consider extreme emotional expression to be an appropriate response to something that another culture might consider to be a minor event.

Possible behaviours related to extreme distress

An extremely distressed Person might:

- express the depth of their emotions silently through non-verbal behaviours
- express emotion uncontrollably through paralinguistic means (e.g. crying or sobbing)
- depending on their personality, withdraw from contact with others.

Principles for effective communication with a Person/s experiencing extreme distress

When communicating with a Person who is extremely distressed, it is important to:

- empathise and validate
- listen actively – encourage them to say whatever they need to say
- be silent, if appropriate
- comfort in an affirming and encouraging way that does not fulfil the needs of the healthcare professional.

Strategies for communicating with a Person/s experiencing extreme distress

- Be willing to sit in empathic silence.
- Avoid mind reading.
- Be aware of the appropriate use of touch.
- Consider whether gender-specific care might be important (i.e. male to male and female to female).
- If a young Person, remember environmental factors (see Chapter 11) when communicating. Young people are often more susceptible to situations that cause distress, and if distressed can have less ability to control their emotions.
- If an Indigenous Person, involve an appropriate Indigenous health worker.
- Remember to debrief confidentially, if required, to maintain "self".

Remember the principles of effective communication and Person/Family-centred Care.

Scenario one: The male and the healthcare professional

Person 1: Your name is David and you are a 40-year-old father of three children. Your eldest son is in the final stages of leukaemia. No-one really knows when he will die. The emotions you feel make it difficult to continue working and supporting your wife, who is also overwhelmed by the situation. You are extremely distressed, but desperately trying to appear OK whenever you are with your son or with members of your immediate family. The energy involved in maintaining this appearance is exhausting, but you feel it is necessary. You are now sitting in a waiting area, waiting to see a healthcare professional for an unrelated reason. Although it is only 8.30 a.m. you can only sit with your head in your hands. You would really like to cry, but are not accustomed to crying in public places.

Person 2: You are the healthcare professional. You have a busy day ahead and the first person for the day is someone who is new to your service. When you enter the waiting area and see a man sitting with his head in his hands, you wonder what is wrong and why he looks like that at 8.30 a.m. You wonder whether this person works night shifts or is unwell. You discover this man is the next person you are scheduled to see.

- How will you respond?

Scenario two: The female and the healthcare professional

Person 1: Your name is Alice. You are a 16-year-old girl who was born with a deformity of your spine, which produces high levels of pain. You have limited success managing your pain with medication, but use medication episodically under careful supervision. You find the level of pain you experience limits your ability to join your peers in various age-related activities, which at the moment is causing you extreme frustration.

Person 2: You are the healthcare professional who has been attempting to assist Alice to increase her involvement in age-related activities. She is demonstrating extreme levels of distress today and has been crying uncontrollably whenever you speak to her.

- What will you do?

Some health services offer services for distressed people and thus the healthcare professionals working in such services will often encounter extremely distressed people. However, it is possible for all healthcare professionals to encounter distressed people in the course of their working life, regardless of the particular context of the healthcare professional. When relating to such people, it is challenging but essential to communicate in a manner that fulfils the needs of the individual(s) and considers the communicating people.

3. Person/s experiencing neurogenic or psychological shock

Definition of neurogenic or psychological shock

Psychological shock occurs whenever an individual experiences or observes an unexpected traumatic /stressful experience. In some cases such experiences may result in developing post-traumatic stress disorder (see Chapter 27).

Possible behaviours related to experiencing psychological shock

- Avoidance of activities or places that trigger memories of the event
- Sometimes hostile actions
- Social isolation and withdrawal
- Lack of interest in previously enjoyable activities
- Unable to follow instructions
- Arguments with family members
- Difficulty in maintaining relationships
- Obsessive and compulsive behaviours

- Substance abuse to "dull" the pain
- Constant tension and vigilance: expecting danger
- Acting to protect self and others
- Self-destructive behaviours.

Possible causes of psychological shock

- Car accident or narrow escape
- Relationship breakdown
- Your child having an accident
- Financial stress
- Being stopped by the police
- For some, even going to the dentist!
- Experiencing fear – for example, being told you have a life-threatening illness, or a chronic condition
- Witnessing something traumatic
- Hearing that someone you know has had a traumatic experience – for example, a child drowning, child experiencing a head injury from falling off a horse
- Sometimes news stories – for example, caught in a building during a fire, children and parents being separated during severe weather conditions.

Possible emotions a Person who experiences psychological shock might exhibit

- Confusion
- Disbelief
- Numbness – blocking all feelings
- Overwhelming fear
- Nervous and easily startled
- Inadequacy
- Grief
- Anxiety
- Agitation
- Anger
- Shame
- Irritability
- Possibly feelings of loss, depending on the cause of the shock.

Possible reasons for the emotions relating to psychological shock

- Unexpected intrusive thoughts about the event
- Nightmares
- Visual images of the event
- Insomnia
- Loss of memory and concentration
- Disorientation
- Mood swings
- Detachment from other people and from emotions

- Depression
- Panic attacks and restless
- Fatigue and exhaustion – tachycardia
- Changes in sleeping and eating patterns
- Chronic muscle aches and pain – stiffness throughout the body
- Sexual dysfunction
- Guilt – they should have been able to prevent the event, so now feel ineffective or inadequate
- Loss of previously important personal belief systems.

Principles for effective communication with a Person/s experiencing psychological shock

When communicating with a Person experiencing psychological shock, it is important to:

- ensure the environment is as predictable as possible – avoid unexpected events
- demonstrate interest and concern verbally and non-verbally
- develop trust, rapport and a trusting therapeutic relationship
- use active listening and observation of all non-verbal messages
- respond patiently and with understanding.

Strategies for communicating with a Person/s experiencing psychological shock

- Clearly explain everything that will occur during the interaction.
- Ask relevant questions to achieve mutual understanding of their current status.
- Consider all non-verbal messages, verifying and validating them.
- If appropriate, after discussing the idea with the Person, refer them to another relevant healthcare professional and, where possible, introduce them to this healthcare professional yourself.

Remember the principles of effective communication and Person/Family-centred Care.

Scenario one: The male and the healthcare professional

Person 1: Your name is Justin, you are 34 years old and married to Janice. You have two children, an active and healthy son aged 7 and a clever, gorgeous daughter aged 4 years. You typically enjoy taking them to the park and to games during cricket and soccer seasons. You recently experienced a car accident while driving home from work. A car you did not see ran at speed into your car. As a result, you were trapped in the car for several hours. During that time, you experienced various emotions while they removed you from the car – ranging from anger to overwhelming fear that you would never see your family again. After being removed from the car, you were taken to the hospital to assess for internal damage. Several hours passed, during that time, your very worried wife arrived (the children were with the neighbour); you saw several different healthcare professionals and had various scans. They then treated you for minor cuts and bruises, but nothing major. Since that time, you do not enjoy driving and certainly avoid taking the children to the park or to sporting events. You have regular disagreements with your wife, with whom you have previously always been in agreement. You are attending a healthcare appointment today because of aches and pains you now experience in different parts of your body. You do NOT want to talk about the car accident – you want to forget it!

Person 2: You are an experienced healthcare professional named Joshua. You are seeing Justin today for the first time –the notes/referral indicate he is experiencing aches and pains throughout his body. It should be a simple matter of identifying the cause of his symptoms.

Scenario two: The female and the healthcare professional
Person 1: You are Abigail, mother of 2-year-old Emily, who you are currently sitting alongside at the hospital, looking at her lying in a cot in a coma, with tubes and masks and monitors to keep her alive. You find yourself replaying the events leading to Emily being in hospital. You left her in the care of your husband while you did the household shopping. You were surprised to return to the house to find an ambulance and paramedics rushing out the door carrying a motionless Emily, on a stretcher. Your husband rushes over to you, saying he's glad you are home and that he needs to follow the ambulance to the hospital. You say you want to come too and rush inside with the bags of shopping. In the car you ask your husband what happened. He tells you Emily was in the backyard with him after swimming together in the backyard pool. Emily was cold so he ran inside to grab a towel, believing Emily would not go into the pool without someone being there with her. When he returned Emily was on the bottom of the pool – he dived in and placing her on the side of the pool began resuscitation. It did not seem to be making any difference, so he called for an ambulance indicating the need for haste. He cannot explain how it happened – but what they needed now was go to the hospital and hope something could be done.

Two weeks later as you sit watching Emily, holding her lifeless hand – you think about the regular arguments with your husband since then and what the future holds possibly without Emily. Nothing seems important except little Emily.

Person 2: You are the healthcare professional who met Abigail the day Emily drowned in the family pool. You try to see her regularly as you have established rapport with Abigail. Today you visit knowing the doctors are considering turning off the life supports for Emily.

4. Person/s experiencing depression

(Key words: depression, depressed, common)

Interesting facts

Different types of depression require different management. Depression can take different forms and have different affects depending on the time of life. Rates of depression in women are twice as high as they are in men.

Definition of depression

Depression is a mood disorder recognised by a lack of interest in previously enjoyable activities and/or limited feelings of pleasure in life. It may include feelings of helplessness and hopelessness.

Individuals most susceptible to feelings of depression

- People feeling worthless
- People with limited social contact
- People who have lost a significant other
- People constantly feeling they make mistakes
- People feeling guilty

- People overcommitted financially
- People experiencing loss of employment
- Women who have recently given birth
- People experiencing constant pain
- Individuals feeling high levels of fatigue.

Possible reasons for feelings of depression

- Loneliness
- Lack of social support
- Recent stressful life experiences
- Family history of depression
- Marital or relationship problems
- Financial strain
- Early childhood trauma or abuse
- Alcohol or drug abuse
- Unemployment or underemployment
- Health problems or chronic pain.

Possible behaviours related to feelings of depression

Men who are depressed may experience fatigue, irritability, sleep problems, and loss of interest in work and hobbies. They may exhibit anger, aggression, violence, reckless behaviour and substance abuse. Men experiencing depression are at a higher suicide risk, especially older men.
Women are more prone to experience feelings of guilt, sleep excessively, overeat and gain weight.
Adolescents will often be irritable when experiencing depression. They may be hostile, grumpy or easily lose their temper. Unexplained aches and pains are also common in young people with depression. They may experience difficulties at home and school, indulging in drug abuse and self-loathing.

People experiencing depression may:

- sleep a lot *or* very little
- lack interest in eating *or* eat too much and gain weight
- have difficulty concentrating, making decisions and remembering things
- engage in escapist behaviour, including substance abuse, reckless driving, dangerous sports
- be angry, short-tempered and irritable, sometimes aggressive
- demonstrate self-loathing attitudes and language.

Principles for effective communication with a Person/s experiencing depression

When communicating with a Person experiencing depression, it is important to:

- demonstrate unconditional positive regard
- validate their feelings
- employ active listening
- clarify their understanding of any discussed procedures or information
- use positive non-verbal messages
- confront false beliefs and attitudes (if appropriate) to emphasise reality
- where appropriate, provide information about depression
- if they are not receiving specific assistance, explain where they can receive assistance.

Strategies for communicating with a Person/s experiencing depression

- Relate consistently.
- Do not ignore any attempts they make to discuss their depression.
- Remain willing to discuss their feelings if they initiate the conversation.
- Reinforce the truth about their abilities and their life.
- Provide regular encouragement and positive affirmation.
- Sensitively challenge negative self-talk.

Avoid saying things like:

- *It's all in your head.*
- *We all go through times like this.*
- *Look on the bright side.*
- *You have so much to live for. Why do you want to die?*
- *What's your problem? Just snap out of it.*
- *What's wrong with you?*
- *Shouldn't you be better by now?*
- *I can't do anything about your situation.*

Remember the principles of effective communication and Person/Family-centred Care.

Scenario one: The male and the healthcare professional

Person 1: You are a 17-year-old young man named James, who lives in a rural setting. You are preparing for your final school exams, which will decide your future. You are friendly and helpful and this year you are school captain. The staff and the students at the school affirm you, even those in the primary or junior school. You usually perform well in all your subjects at school and enjoy playing for the school soccer team. You have recently been feeling overwhelmed by all the responsibilities you have at school, find it difficult to motivate yourself to attend school and have been consistently avoiding soccer training. You do not seem to enjoy it anymore, even though the coach wants you to try out for the state team in a few weeks. You are really not interested anymore and have begun to think that life is not worth living. You have not told anyone this and find it hard to talk about how you are currently feeling. However, recently you have been experiencing pain in your right knee and your mother has insisted you see a healthcare professional for assistance with your knee.

Person 2: You are the healthcare professional seeing a young man called James for the first time. You have heard of James and know he is the captain of the local regional high school. You know he is an excellent soccer player and a state coach is visiting town in a few weeks to assess the local outstanding soccer players, so you are eager to help him with the pain in his knee, so he can continue playing soccer and maybe even join the state team.

Scenario two: The female and the healthcare professional

Person 1: You are 29-year-old Rachel, who has recently given birth to your first son, Jackson. He is a bonny, cute baby who is developing well – but he keeps you awake at night, produces an amazing amount of extra work and seems to eat constantly and need his nappy changed and then washed "every time you turn around". You are finding it very difficult to understand why he cries all the time, and you need more sleep. You usually pride yourself on keeping a clean and tidy house and are currently unable to find basic things like bills to pay, because the house is so messy. There is a constant pile of washing and the kitchen is always full of dirty dishes as your husband works long hours and travels an hour to work every day. Some days you wish you could just crawl away and ignore everything, but that makes you feel guilty and a failure because you are unable to manage all the demands on your time. This little baby, that constantly demands your attention and needs so much, is making you wish you could "run away". You have a community nurse coming today to monitor the development of the baby and how you are managing breastfeeding – you feel hopeless because the house is so dirty and messy.

Person 2: You are the healthcare professional who must visit Rachel and her baby today. You notice the mess in the house and wonder how Rachel is managing. You also wonder if she has any postpartum depression.

5. Person/s experiencing severe, overwhelming and consistent anxiety

(Key words: anxious, nervous, worried, apprehensive, restless, tense, fearful, dread)

Interesting facts

Most people experience anxiety in their life, relating to potentially stressful circumstances or events. However, uncontrollable, sustained and excessive worry has severe, overwhelming and consistent effects on life, usually producing anxiety disorders. Such disorders are common mental illnesses.

Definition of severe, overwhelming and consistent anxiety

Sustained, extreme and ongoing feelings of worry, ongoing emotional distress, feelings of helplessness, severe feelings of apprehension, restlessness, can result in panic attacks and/or fear that interrupts daily activities, making it difficult to complete daily tasks. Chronic anxiety typically results in difficulty controlling unnecessary worry, along with intrusive thoughts making concentration difficult. It may cause hot and cold flushes, palpitations, feelings of a tight chest, shortness of breath, difficulty sleeping typically resulting in fatigue, headaches, difficulty concentrating on something except the causes of the worry. Such anxiety may cause depression.

Individuals most susceptible to feelings of severe, overwhelming and consistent anxiety

Those experiencing:

- stress in their daily life for an extended period of time
- ongoing fear of events
- consistent fear of people
- constant fear of the expectations of others
- fear of being unable to effectively complete particular tasks
- feelings that there is danger everywhere
- continuing change and uncertainty.

Possible reasons for feelings of severe, overwhelming and consistent anxiety

- Stress relating to particular events, people or expectations.
- Fear of pending events
- Fear of possible danger
- Fear of disappointing significant others
- Fear of "not being good enough"
- Change which they cannot control
- Fatigue
- Particular physical condition affecting their everyday functioning.

Possible effects related to feelings of severe, overwhelming and consistent anxiety

People experiencing continuing anxiety may:

- avoid anything causing their anxiety
- isolate themselves typically due to fear of the results of interacting
- reduce effective communication with others
- be unable to concentrate or to think clearly and thus problem-solve
- have difficulty concentrating on anything except the issues causing the worry
- have difficulty sleeping
- make excessive use of alcohol, cigarettes, caffeine, recreational drugs.

Principles for effective communication with a Person/s experiencing severe, overwhelming and consistent anxiety

When communicating with a Person experiencing severe, overwhelming and consistent anxiety, it is important to:

- ensure the use of all components of Person-centred Care
- encourage the Person to express their feelings and anxieties
- use clear and simple validating statements, repeating them as often as may be necessary
- demonstrate interest and concern verbally and non-verbally
- develop trust, rapport and a trusting therapeutic relationship
- use active listening and observation of all non-verbal messages
- respond patiently and with understanding
- encourage stress management and relaxation techniques (refer to relevant healthcare professional as necessary).

Strategies for communicating with a Person/s experiencing severe, overwhelming and consistent anxiety

- Ensure the environment is calm and well controlled, avoiding unexpected occurrences.
- Consider whether gender-specific care might be important (i.e. male to male and female to female).
- Relate in a calm and caring manner.
- Be respectful and accepting in order to build a trusting, therapeutic relationship.
- Identify and state their skills and areas of competence to develop their confidence.
- Encourage them, validating their abilities.

- It may not be appropriate to assist in identifying the causes of the anxiety; however, referral to a relevant healthcare professional to identify and manage the anxiety could be helpful.
- After identification of the causes of the anxiety, encourage the use of a journal to identify how to effectively manage the causes.

Remember the principles of effective communication and Person/Family-centred Care.

Scenario one: The male and the healthcare professional

Person 1: You are Dave and have just had spinal surgery from a recent work injury. You are being discharged tomorrow. The surgery has resulted in restrictions in bending and lifting and an inability to stand or sit for long periods of time. You have always been strong, independent and focused on assisting others, whether at work, in shopping centres or at home. Now these restrictions in movement produce worries about how you will manage at work (you have recently been promoted to a managerial position, requiring sitting for extended periods of time); worries about not being able to assist family members as you always do; worries about how to dress yourself (putting on socks will be difficult without help); worries about showering without help (you enjoy your shower time and the privacy of that time); worries about how you will manage maintaining the lawn and garden, something you love doing; worries about carrying the shopping into the house for your wife (something you routinely do for her and feel it is part of who you are; your identity); worries about the 30 minute drive to and from work, the list is long – everything you think of, that is typically part of your daily life creates consistent and enduring anxiety – it feels overwhelming. You feel unable to do anything and this is creating a desire to stay in hospital for a few more days.

Person 2: You are the healthcare professional who must ensure that Dave is ready for discharge. You feel confident that he will continue to improve and will fully recover from the surgery, with some limitations in his movements. However, you are sure that Dave will be able to continue his life as he did previously, after he makes the appropriate adjustments.

Scenario two: The female and the healthcare professional

Person 1: Your name is Sally. You are currently pregnant and are expecting to have the baby in a week. You are feeling quite anxious about the process. It is a well-known process to you, as you are a midwife. However, you have had two previous pregnancies. The first ended at 20 weeks in a miscarriage. The second was full term, but the baby was stillborn – or born dead. You have been finding it difficult to sleep because of constant worry, apprehension and fear about the birth of this child. All scans indicate everything is progressing well, as they did for the previous stillborn child. You find yourself thinking about all the things that could go wrong (you have seen quite a few births and are fully aware of the possible complications). This simply increases your overwhelming anxiety. Your husband is aware of your struggles and decides to ask a mutual friend, who is also a healthcare professional, to spend some time with you. While you know this friend well, you are unsure how this could possibly help, especially as you are unable to think clearly and you do NOT want to talk about your feelings as it makes you more anxious. However, you agree to see the friend – but ask them to come to your house, as you have become anxious about leaving the house, except to go to work. Despite really enjoying your midwife role, you have recently found it quite anxiety-provoking and now do not always enjoy going to work.

Person 2: You are a healthcare professional who has been asked to spend time with a good friend as she is close to giving birth and is not managing the stress related to this event. You are aware of her previous stillborn experience, but of no other reasons for her level of stress.

6. Person/s reluctant to engage or be involved in communication or intervention

(Key words: uncertain, avoidant, reluctant, resistant)

Definition of reluctance to engage

A Person who is reluctant to engage or be involved is someone who may be:

- unwilling to be or do in a particular situation, environment or context
- unsure about the situation, environment or context
- unsure about something particular in the situation, environment or context
- unsure about someone in the situation, environment or context.

Individuals most susceptible to feeling reluctant to engage

Individuals who may be susceptible to feeling reluctant to engage or be involved include:

- children
- older adults
- individuals scheduled for complicated procedures
- individuals attending a health service for the first time
- individuals who are unfamiliar with something or someone in the health service
- individuals with a previously negative experience of a health service
- individuals with inability in some area(s).

Possible reasons for reluctance to engage

Individuals may be reluctant to engage or be involved because of:

- apprehension from the unfamiliarity of the situation, environment or context
- fear about possible events in the situation, environment or context
- a previous experience of negative emotions in that particular situation, environment or context, or in a similar one
- reluctance to move because of pain or discomfort
- not being in the situation, environment or context by choice, but because (i) of an emergency, (ii) of a forced admission (Community Treatment Order) into a mental health institution, or (iii) their family might be "pushy"
- not accepting, or denying their need
- feeling unsure about the expectations of the situation, environment or context
- not understanding what they are being asked to do or say
- not understanding the particular role or expectations of the healthcare professional
- feeling they are unable to perform the required tasks or requested actions
- being physically unable to perform the required tasks or requested actions.

In common with all Person/s the healthcare professional meets, reluctant people are feeling vulnerable for many different reasons.

Possible behaviours related to feeling reluctant to engage

A Person who is reluctant to engage or be involved might:

- verbally or non-verbally refuse to engage, be involved or collaborate
- deny there is a problem
- take action that appears cooperative, but resist non-verbally
- express themself through aggression and sometimes violence

- avoid looking at the healthcare professional by turning their head away
- withdraw as far from the healthcare professional as possible.

Principles for effective communication with a Person/s reluctant to engage

When communicating with a Person/s who is reluctant to engage or be involved, it is important to:

- make introductions
- listen actively
- validate their feelings
- question them sensitively
- provide clear information in various forms
- take care to ensure all non-verbal messages of the healthcare professional are positive
- confront false beliefs and attitudes (if appropriate) to emphasise reality.

Strategies for communicating with a Person/s reluctant to engage

- Remain calm.
- Check they understand the language you are speaking.
- Consider your non-verbal behaviours – avoid overbearing or intimidating body language.
- Validate their responses.
- Clearly explain the reasons for each occurrence.
- Clearly explain the expectations or expected events.
- Clarify wherever there is uncertainty.
- Ask if they do or do not want anything, and, if possible, do that to reassure them.
- If violent, indicate their behaviour is inappropriate and call for assistance.

Remember the principles of effective communication and Person/Family-centred Care.

Scenario one: The male and the healthcare professional

NOTE: When working with children it is important to remember that the parents and siblings are part of their environment, and thus must be considered when gathering information. The parent is usually the expert in terms of knowledge about the skills and behaviour of their child.

Person 1: You are a 10-year-old boy called Carl and you need assistance from a healthcare professional. As you arrive with your mother for the first appointment you are reminded of the last time you went to see a healthcare professional. That person was not friendly – they kept talking to your mother, not to you, and they physically hurt you. You do not want to relate to the healthcare professional because they look just the same as the last one. You stand behind your mother and cling to her, hiding your face in her back. You refuse to look at the healthcare professional or respond to any of their attempts to talk with you.

Person 2: You are Carl's mother. You are very surprised at Carl's behaviour because he does not usually behave like this and you have no idea why he is clinging to you. You have no idea how to respond to promote a relationship between Carl and the healthcare professional.

Person 3: You are the healthcare professional. You know 10-year-old boys do not usually relate in this manner and you would like to tell him to "get over it" and act his age! However, you remember the three steps in effective communication and wish to apply these to this boy and his mother who are seeking your assistance.

Scenario two: The female and the healthcare professional

Person 1: You are a 79-year-old woman who prefers to be called Mrs Jones. You love attending for treatment and try to be very cooperative despite the discomfort you sometimes feel because of the treatment. You often require assistance to find the toilet and are easily disoriented when trying to find the exit after treatment. One day you could not actually find your car in the parking lot. You are anxious to hide the fact that you have been experiencing more confusion lately because you do not want to be made to leave your home, where you have lived for 30 years. You manage well when at home in your familiar environment. You always say you are fine when you are at home – that there really is not a problem – whenever the healthcare professionals suggest they contact the home-care organisation. You do not want anyone in your house; you just want to be able to stay there and be independent.

Person 2: You are the healthcare professional. You have noted the regular disorientation Mrs Jones exhibits when attending for treatment. You note that Mrs Jones appears to take pride in her appearance because she is always well dressed and clean. But you are wondering whether her appearance is an attempt to pretend that things are OK. You are concerned about her safety and think Mrs Jones might require some assistance at home. You ask her if she would like you to contact the appropriate organisation to arrange some assistance with cleaning and preparing meals at home.

As a large group, discuss the observations, emotions and outcomes of the role-plays. Suggest possible alternative strategies that may increase the effectiveness of the communication in a similar situation.

There are many reasons for reluctance to engage on the part of the Person/s. A healthcare professional may require more than a warm, friendly persona to achieve positive outcomes. The healthcare professional may require specific communication skills and strategies to encourage the Person/s who is reluctant to engage in order to achieve Person/Family-centred Care.

Chapter 25

Person/s in particular stages of life

Chapter objective

Upon completing this chapter, readers should be able to apply knowledge and have emerging skills in communicating effectively with Person/s in particular stages of life.

An individual in any of the five different stages of life – child, adolescent, young adults, older adults and a Person who is older and ageing – may present with particular attitudes and associated needs. When assisting such Person/s, it is important to remember the abilities and events typical of these stages.

Stages of life

1. Children
2. Adolescents
3. Young adults
4. Older adults
5. People who are older and ageing

- Define the above stages of life
- List some of the specific behaviours that might occur during these stages of life.
- List the individuals most susceptible to experiencing difficulty when seeking assistance from a health service during these stages of life.
- List possible negative emotions someone in these stages of life might experience when seeing a healthcare professional and explain why.
- List principles for effective communication to remember when communicating with a Person in these stages of life. Give reasons for the need to remember these principles.
- Suggest strategies for communicating with a Person who is in these stages of life and experiencing issues related to that stage. Decide why you might see such a Person in your particular healthcare profession.
- Check your answers against the information below, noting any additional thoughts or ideas.

A child

(Key words: child, children, childhood, dependent, underage)
When assisting children it is essential to remember the parent is the expert about the child. They are familiar with the skills and abilities of the child and if they indicate the child can do something you do not witness, they will probably be correct. It is important to avoid talking about children when they are present. Whether the child can understand the words or not, they are able to understand non-verbal cues and therefore will respond with a particular emotion or behaviour.

Definition of a child

For the purpose of this section, a child is a Person aged 0–16 years.

Children most susceptible to experiencing difficulties when attending a health service

Such children include those who:

- have a history of negative experiences in life
- are very young and are not accustomed to separating from a parent
- are from a different cultural background
- are unfamiliar with healthcare settings
- are experiencing physical or emotional pain
- are very ill
- have had a previous negative experience with a healthcare professional
- are a victim of an accident, attack or natural disaster
- have communication difficulties
- have a visual or auditory impairment.

Possible emotions a child might experience when attending a health service

A child might experience emotions related to:

- fear and anxiety
- physical or emotional "pain" from any source, causing frustration and despondency
- boredom
- isolation and displacement.

Possible reasons for these emotions

Children may experience these emotions due to:

- awareness that they are different to other children
- physical pain
- uncertainty and discomfort because of lack of familiarity with the environment, people and procedures
- difficulties at home, school or in the neighbourhood.

Possible behaviours related to being a child

The behaviour of a child will depend on their age, their personality, their culture, the experiences of their upbringing, the stability at home, their sense of security, the reason for the referral and the presence of a significant adult.

A child might be:

- quiet and non-engaging
- shy and hiding
- crying and clinging
- happy, but initially untrusting
- looking to their parent for assurance
- angry and aggressive
- curious and wanting to explore.
- distractible and avoidant.

Principles for effective communication with a child

When communicating with a child, it is important to:

- make introductions at a different language level for the parent compared to the child
- demonstrate empathy
- carefully observe the responses of the child
- validate their perceptions (it may be necessary to validate the perceptions of the parent if the child is unable to communicate)
- make appropriate use of non-verbal behaviour – if there is no common language, non-verbal or visual communication is essential to develop rapport and a therapeutic relationship
- allow time for the child to trust you; to feel comfortable and safe
- monitor the language level – use simple explanations and provide warnings about upcoming events and termination of the session
- touch only if appropriate
- establish boundaries and expectations for behaviour
- relate consistently with consistent expectations
- practise holistic communication
- disengage with, if appropriate, with indication of a future meeting
- ensure **Family**-centred Care.

Strategies for communicating with a child

- Talk directly to the child.
- Where possible, either position yourself down at their level or raise them up (if safe) to your level.
- Avoid talking about the child with the child present.
- Explore toys and activities that are meaningful to the child and use them to engage, comfort and relax the child.
- Provide a safe environment.
- Understand the culture of the child.
- Understand the familial, social, physical, cognitive, cultural and spiritual background, as well as the expected developmental level of the child.
- Tell the child what will happen and when it will happen. Give adequate warning about when the session will finish to facilitate smooth transition from the completion of the session to leaving the room.
- Respond to the non-verbal behaviours of the child with verbal questions or reflective comments about the observations.
- Avoid touching the child wherever possible, or ask permission to touch the child from the child and the parent.
- Avoid distractions and use silence if appropriate to encourage concentration and focus.

See the Introduction to Section 4 for instructions about how to use these scenarios for role-play or group discussion. Remember the principles of effective communication and Person/Family-centred Care.

Scenario one: The male and the trained volunteer

Person 1: You are Mohammad, a 12-year-old Sudanese boy whose family has taken refuge from Sudan. You have learnt some English, but still do not understand many of the behaviours of those around you, and you cannot read or write English yet. Your older brother was killed just before your family left Sudan. Your father does not have a job yet and your mother works until late at night for little pay, washing dishes in a Chinese take-away shop. You do not feel accepted at school, even by the other Sudanese who have been there longer than you and often tease you in Arabic. Your little sister seems happy and has several friends. You have been feeling angry and you have begun to verbally abuse teachers and the other boys from Sudan at school. You do not enjoy relating to anyone other than your family.

Person 2: You are a trained volunteer for the local multicultural centre and you run a group for "at-risk" boys with refugee status. This afternoon is the first time you will meet Mohammad. You know he is sometimes violent, but that is all you know. Many of the at-risk Sudanese boys are violent. You want to assist Mohammad to settle and integrate.

Scenario two: The female and the healthcare professional

Person 1: Your name is Elise and your 2-year-old daughter, Jenny, has just been diagnosed with an intellectual disability. She is your only child and has been a joy to your immediate family. You are confused and unsure. You are afraid of the future and while you wait to see the healthcare professional you become sad and teary. You watch Jenny play on the floor at your feet. What does this mean for her future? She is so beautiful and you had such wonderful plans for her.

Person 2: You are the healthcare professional who must assess Jenny's abilities. When you enter the waiting area you call Jenny's name and notice a woman flinch and look up. She smiles at you and lifts Jenny from the floor. How will you relate to Jenny and Elise in this initial session? What are your communication priorities?

- Elise does not want Jenny to leave her lap, and nor does Jenny want to leave it. How will you encourage them both?

Children are often the focus of a specialty health service. However, healthcare professionals from many contexts may need to relate to children. It is both challenging and rewarding to work with children, for whom particular skills are required to ensure effective communication and Family-centred Care.

NOTE: There are many groups and associations that provide information and support for parents of children with particular conditions (e.g. Autism Associations, NextSense Royal Institute for Deaf and Blind Children).

An adolescent

(Key words: adolescence, adolescent, teenager)

Definition of an adolescent

An adolescent is someone who is:

- a youth
- between childhood and maturity
- growing up or maturing
- experiencing physical changes in their body that indicate development to maturity
- experiencing emotional insecurity, social and cognitive challenges, and often spiritual independence.

The age of maturing varies depending on gender and ethnicity. In some cultures there are expectations of particular genders at a certain age. Once these expectations are met, regardless of age, the individual assumes the role and responsibilities of an adult and is considered an adult in all aspects of their existence.

In most Western cultures, age determines the arrival of adulthood. Individuals, regardless of gender, assume some of the responsibilities of adulthood from 14 years onwards (e.g. paid employment at 15 years, driving a car at 17–18 years), but are not considered adults until they reach 18–21 years (when they can vote and purchase cigarettes and alcohol). It is not the emotional, intellectual and social maturity of the individual that officially indicates the arrival of adulthood, but rather age.

Adolescents most susceptible to experiencing difficulties when attending a health service

Adolescents susceptible to experiencing difficulties when attending a health service include those who:

- are different to their peer group
- do not want to receive assistance from a healthcare professional
- are from a different cultural background
- are unfamiliar with healthcare settings
- have difficulties adjusting to the changes occurring in their body
- experience physical or emotional pain
- have had a previous negative experience with a healthcare professional
- are a victim of an accident, attack or natural disaster
- have a visual or auditory impairment
- have an intellectual disability.

Possible emotions an adolescent might experience

Emotional responses in adolescents are complex and often unpredictable for both the individual and those around them. An adolescent may experience extremes of emotion, including:

- anger
- loneliness
- confusion
- isolation
- restlessness
- conflict and stress
- feelings of rejection
- dissatisfaction
- feelings of inadequacy

- feeling like they "do not fit"
- hatred of their appearance
- insecurity
- anxiety
- feelings of unimportance
- boredom
- high energy.

Possible reasons for these emotions

An adolescent undergoes complex changes in their physical, emotional, cognitive, social and spiritual self during adolescence. An adolescent may experience extremes of emotion because of:

- hormones
- social pressures
- school pressures
- home pressures
- cultural differences
- a dominating need for social interaction
- focusing on their own needs
- their friends.

Possible behaviours related to being an adolescent

An adolescent may:

- engage in high-risk behaviours
- exaggerate their actions (act out) to gain attention
- withdraw and keep to themselves
- behave in ways that create direct conflict with their values in order to maintain a position in a social group
- be verbally abusive and argumentative
- experiment with various substances
- behave in a happy and carefree manner.

Principles for effective communication with an adolescent

The principles of effective communication apply to all individuals seeking assistance. However, it may be more difficult to communicate using these principles when relating to an adolescent unless the healthcare professional is aware of the needs of the adolescent, and is self-aware about the effects of their own experience of adolescence.

When communicating with an adolescent, it is important to:

- be self-aware – of own experiences, values and beliefs
- practise holistic communication
- understand and be sensitive
- demonstrate unconditional positive regard
- demonstrate respect
- adhere to ethical boundaries
- accommodate cultural differences
- effectively confront inappropriate self-talk, values and beliefs
- observe their non-verbal behaviours.

Strategies for communicating with an adolescent

- Aim at Person/Family-centred Care.
- Establish a safe environment, both emotionally and physically.
- It is vital to use a holistic approach because the physical symptoms may be covering underlying needs.
- Be aware of personal limitations – the healthcare professional does not need to meet all the needs of every adolescent seeking their assistance.
- Relate consistently with consistent reactions and explanations.
- Be committed to and compassionate for the Person, not necessarily their behaviour.
- Demonstrate understanding and interest through the use of activities they find meaningful.
- Be aware of the non-verbal behaviours of all communicating individuals.
- Explicitly state the expectations of behaviour.
- Establish clear boundaries.

Remember the principles of effective communication and Person/Family-centred Care.

Scenario one: The male and the healthcare professional

Person 1: Your name is Jake. You are nearly 17 years old and in your final year at school. You have found adolescence difficult. It has been difficult to concentrate and therefore learn at school. You are not sure why your parents insisted you stay at school because you rarely pass your exams. The teachers do not really understand you and only one or two seem to care. You have some great friends and do outlandish things together – not life-threatening things, just "out-there" fun things. Recent assessments indicate you have attention deficit hyperactivity disorder (ADHD) and you have begun to take medication for this. You do not like the medication because, although it makes you calm and gives you greater control, you no longer feel you are yourself. You love working outside in gardens and have begun working in the grounds of a local health service, mostly during your school holidays.

Person 2: You are a healthcare professional who often has lunch in the grounds of the health service. You have begun chatting with one of the new grounds people, Jake, and find he lacks confidence and a sense of self-worth. While this is typical of many adolescents, you feel there is more involved with Jake than typical adolescence. You have decided to befriend, encourage and affirm him, so you often have lunch with Jake.

- Do you need to be able to encourage and affirm Jake? Why?
- How can you encourage and affirm him?

Scenario two: The female and the healthcare professional

Person 1: Your name is Ruth and you are a well-known local 15-year-old with a promising career in surfing. You are the leading junior female surfer in the country. You were excited when you signed a contract with an international surfing label for sponsorship and promotions. You are popular with teachers and students, and your parents often tell you how proud they are of you. You have applied yourself at school and at the local surf club. You love surfing and at every opportunity you are at the beach on patrol or on your board.

In a recent and unusual shark attack, you lost your right arm below the elbow. The experience was very traumatic, but you have other things to concern you. What about the contract you have with the surf label? And your surfing career – what happens now? You are devastated because surfing is your life and you cannot imagine surfing without your lower arm and hand. You were hoping to be school captain in a few years, but think no-one would nominate someone without an arm. You are right-handed and you cannot imagine how you will ever write without your right hand. You are sure that boy you like in the surf club will not even look at you now. You were looking forward to driving; you often imagined driving up the coast with your board on top of the car and not a care in the world. How will you ever drive a car without your right hand? You have so many questions and fears. All your parents can say is ***You're alive – that's all that matters!***

You wish you could find someone who understands your fears and could answer your questions. However, you do not enjoy talking about or feeling negative emotions, so you need convincing to openly discuss your feelings.

Person 2: You are a healthcare professional and also a senior member of the surf-lifesaving club of which Ruth is an active member. You have been mentoring Ruth for some years and, while you are devastated by the attack, you know Ruth has greater needs than you. You have been spending time with Ruth, but feel helpless. You know of another young woman who surfs without an arm because of a car accident, and you have contacted her to organise a time to meet with Ruth. You go to see Ruth to tell her about the other woman and arrange a time to meet, but first you want to be sure that Ruth is willing to talk about her experience and associated feelings.

Adolescence can be an uncomfortable time for most people: the adolescent and those around them. Adolescents feel vulnerable because of their stage of development. If an adolescent requires the assistance of a healthcare professional, their feelings of vulnerability may multiply exponentially and thus the healthcare professional must communicate using all of the principles of effective communication.

An adolescent values their peer group and thus, wherever possible, it can be beneficial to include individuals of the same or similar age in the assistive process. Adolescents with similar experiences can be very therapeutic for an adolescent who requires assistance from a healthcare professional.

A young adult

(Key words: early adulthood, semi-independent, limited responsibilities, enjoy excitement)

Definition of a young adult

A young adult may have reached physical maturity. They seldom have others dependent on them and thus rarely have responsibility for others. They may only meet some of their everyday needs. They may drive, have some employment, often make their own decisions and live at home or in shared accommodation. They appreciate making their own choices and doing what they enjoy, rarely considering the possible effects for themselves or others. They may also act without consideration of the legal requirements in particular situations; for example, speeding when driving.

Young adults most likely to experience difficulties when requiring healthcare

- Those requiring care because of an unexpected event.
- Those who have not had previous contact with a healthcare service.

- Those who may have had negative experiences with healthcare services.
- Those from a different cultural background.
- Those who find unknown places difficult.
- Those who may have pre-existing conditions or needs.
- Those who do not enjoy having little control over things around them.

Possible emotions a young adult might experience when requiring healthcare

- Confusion
- Anger
- Frustration
- Impatience
- Guilt
- Grief (depending on the event and the consequences of the event)
- Insecurity.

Possible reasons for these emotions

- Often wonder how and why they require healthcare.
- The event causing the need for healthcare was totally unexpected and was NOT supposed to happen.
- They should have control over everything in their life.
- They want the cause of this need to be solved quickly.
- Feel responsible for the result of the event causing the need for healthcare.
- The unknown and unpredictable environment.
- Unknown people in the environment.
- Have had previous negative experience with a healthcare professional.

Principles of effective communication with a young adult

The principles of effective communication apply to all individuals seeking assistance. However, it may be more difficult to communicate using these principles when relating to a young adult. Therefore, the healthcare professional must be aware of the typical expectations and needs of a young adult, along with being self-aware about the effects of their own experiences and behaviours as a young adult.

When communicating with a young adult, it is important to:

- demonstrate unconditional positive regard
- demonstrate respect
- be self-aware – of own experiences, values and beliefs
- practise holistic communication
- understand and be sensitive
- adhere to ethical boundaries
- accommodate cultural differences
- where appropriate, confront inappropriate self-talk, values and beliefs.

Strategies for communicating with a young adult

- Remember and use all components of Person/Family-centred Care.
- Relate to the whole Person, using holistic communication.

- Communicate acceptance.
- Observe and respond to all non-verbal behaviours.
- Consider and answer all of their questions.
- Respond appropriately to all their concerns, clarifying expectations.
- Explain and outline any procedures or actions.
- Outline any expectations or future events.
- Maintain professional boundaries, while acting to communicate equality.

Remember the principles of effective communication and Person/Family-centred Care.

Scenario one: The male and the healthcare professional

Person 1: Your name is Matt. You have recently passed the test for your licence. You live in the country. You been having fun at a party with some friends. You were the individual in the group who had had very little alcohol, so everyone decided you should drive home, especially as the three other male friends were staying at your house that night. You had not driven that car before, nor on that road very often, but felt confident to drive home. However, the other friends in the car were telling you to drive faster and you lost control of the car on a bend in the road. The car rolled several times and finally stopped when it hit a large tree. You became unconscious, the friend in the front passenger seat was killed on impact with the tree, and the two friends in the back were able to contact an ambulance. It took some time for the ambulance to arrive because of the distance from the ambulance station.

You have just woken from a coma, lying in a hospital bed. You really do not remember what happened, or why you are in hospital. Your head is painful and you try to move it. You suddenly realise you do not seem to be able to feel your legs.

Person 2: You are the healthcare professional in the room when Matt wakes from a coma. He has been in a coma for just over 2 weeks and looks confused. You know that he was driving a car in the country and that the friend in the front seat was killed, while the two friends in the back were able to return home after attending emergency. You are unsure of what Matt remembers about the accident.

Scenario two: The female and the healthcare professional

Person 1: Your name is Clare. You are a well-known local soccer player, recently chosen for the national soccer team. Soccer has been the most important thing in your life for many years. You are excited to be chosen for the national team. Today, you were playing in a local game when you fell due to some uneven ground. You were experiencing pain in your back and your right knee, so the coach had you taken to hospital, to ensure immediate diagnosis and care. You are afraid this may affect your ability to play in the national team and want immediate care to ensure a complete and quick recovery. However, you have been waiting for over an hour to be seen by someone. This is making you feel both angry and frustrated, especially as you are in pain as you lie on the rather hard bed. The people who bought you to the hospital have left. You were hoping one of your parents would come soon after your arrival at the hospital. However, no-one has come and for the moment you are not enjoying being alone.

Person 2: You are the healthcare professional who has to assess the immediate needs of Clare. There are some standard questions requiring answers to ensure appropriate assessment and thus intervention. The resultant assessments will determine whether Clare will be admitted or sent home. You are aware of her recent acceptance to the national soccer team.

An older adult

(Key words: Adulthood, independence, responsible, decision-maker, adult, financially independent)

Definition of an older adult

An older adult has completed their growth and development, assumes responsibility for their own needs and often the needs of those who are dependent upon them. In some cultures adulthood is defined according to age, in other cultures according to achieving particular skills and assuming specific responsibilities.

Older adults most susceptible to experiencing difficulties when attending a health service

Older adults with:

- an unexpected illness or emergency
- pain of unknown origin
- previous negative interactions with a healthcare professional or health service
- an ill significant other
- a partner in labour
- limited knowledge of the health service environment
- limited knowledge of the roles of particular healthcare professionals.

Possible emotions an older adult might experience when relating to a healthcare professional

The emotions an older adult might experience include:

- confusion
- fear
- frustration
- despondency leading to depression
- anger
- disappointment.

Possible reasons for these emotions

Reasons for experiencing these emotions include:

- change in life situation
- illness of a family member
- desire to protect significant others
- overwhelming financial commitments
- retrenchment
- inability to achieve goals.

Principles for effective communication with an older adult

When communicating with an older adult, it is important to:

- use friendly but professional introductions
- be honest
- demonstrate empathy

- respond to non-verbal messages and questions
- acknowledge strengths and difficulties
- use active listening
- clarify understanding
- validate and encourage
- use calm and clear explanations
- affirm
- use appropriate assertion if in conflict
- provide well-designed written information.

Strategies for communicating with an older adult

- Remember the whole Person and use holistic communication principles.
- Do not forget any significant others – use a Person/Family-centred approach.
- Use non-verbal messages to communicate acceptance.
- Allocate (invest) time to answer questions and clarify meaning or future events.
- Ensure you "follow up" their concerns and respond in a timely manner.
- Consider the need for gender-specific care if they are distressed and seeking comfort.
- Retain professional boundaries while maintaining a demeanour of equality.

Remember the principles of effective communication and Person/Family-centred Care.

Scenario one: The male and the healthcare professional

Person 1: You are Joe and your wife has just left you for another man. She and her new partner have relocated to the UK for work reasons. You have a large mortgage and two children. Sally, your 4-year-old daughter, misses her mother and cries a lot. Nathan, your 9-year-old son, has begun acting out at school and is very sullen when at home. You are struggling to work and care for the children. Your job consumes 12 to 15 hours a day and does not leave you with either energy or time to spare. However, your income allows you to hire a housekeeper, who comes every day to prepare meals and organise and clean the house. Your parents are also helpful and spend time with the children some days. Sally has caught an infection from her two days at preschool and is running a fever and coughs through the night – she cries and asks for her mother several times each night. You are exhausted and are wondering if you should resign from work and try to care for the kids. It is 11.00 p.m. and you decide to take Sally to the after-hours doctor. You wake Nathan to come with you, as you do not want to leave him in the house alone. Nathan screams and yells he is old enough to stay home alone – and says he wants to stay in bed. The three of you are finally at the surgery – there is about a one-hour wait, however, a healthcare professional comes to do a preliminary questionnaire before you see the doctor. You do not want to answer questions – besides you would not know, your wife knew all the immunisation and medical history questions – you just want to see the doctor and get the children back in bed (not to mention yourself!), which you make quite clear!

Person 2: You are the healthcare professional who does a verbal questionnaire about medical history when there are more than four people waiting to make it quicker for the doctor. You have just begun your shift, so feel fresh and relaxed, and thus are happy to chat to gain the answers. This man, however, is not very cooperative and tests your patience and skills in gathering information.

Scenario two: The female and the healthcare professional

Person 1: You are Julie and 2 weeks ago you lost your job. As the sole breadwinner for the family you would like to find other employment relatively quickly. You were not worried initially as you have substantial savings that will cover the cost of living for a few months – provided there are no unexpected expenses! You know you will find another job soon because you have a sought-after skills set. However, your husband, who has an acquired disability that means he cannot work, wants to cancel the family holiday to Europe as he is concerned about how the family will manage when the savings are gone, and the trip will consume a large portion of those savings. You received a rejection for a job application this morning, but you have two others pending, so you are trying to feel positive. On the way home from taking the children to school, your car developed a major problem with the gearbox and had to be towed to your mechanic. The mechanic looked at it and thinks it will cost several thousand dollars to make the car roadworthy. You are currently sitting in the waiting room of your local doctor because Melanie, your daughter, has a very high temperature and has been sent home from school. She has been complaining about aches and pains for a few months and while previously you thought it was not serious, you are beginning to wonder if she might have something major wrong. This will cause a problem as your health insurance was connected to your employment and lapsed when you lost your job. This is the first time you have been really worried about your lack of employment and thus you sit very quietly looking at your sleeping daughter, struggling to hold back the tears. The Person that has just entered the room sits opposite you and asks you why you are there. There is no-one else in the room and Melanie is asleep, so you decide to tell her your story.

Person 2: You are a heath professional working in the community for the doctor. You need a signature and a quick word with the doctor about someone you saw yesterday. You are not dressed in a uniform, however, as a heath professional and an employee of the doctor you can see the woman opposite you is struggling to compose herself. There is no-one else in the room, so you ask her name, and tell her you noticed she is very upset and wonder if you can assist her.

A Person who is older and ageing

(Key words: ageing, older adult, senior, over 65, frail-aged)

Definition of a Person who is older and ageing

A Person who is older and ageing may be someone who:

- experiences the constraints of "age" when moving, thinking, relating or feeling, regardless of their chronological age, joint stiffness or hair colour
- has reached the age of retirement
- is eligible to join a seniors organisation.

An older and ageing Person most susceptible to experiencing difficulties when attending a health service

Such older and ageing people include those who:

- have had negative experiences of health services
- have never experienced a health service before
- are experiencing some cognitive or hearing loss
- deny they require assistance

- have limited function and participation
- are in pain
- have recently experienced the loss of someone or something close to them.

Possible emotions an older and ageing Person might experience

An older and ageing Person might experience emotions related to:

- fear and anxiety about the future
- fear and anxiety about death and dying
- grief and sadness
- confusion and deteriorating abilities
- depression
- loneliness.

Possible reasons for these emotions

Reasons for experiencing these emotions might include:

- previous negative experiences
- chronic diseases and/or multiple conditions
- pain
- feeling that they want to die
- feeling that they do not belong anywhere and cannot offer anything of value anymore.

Possible behaviours related to being an older and ageing Person

An older and ageing Person – in common with any Person – might exhibit idiosyncratic behaviours typical of their personality, interests, culture, upbringing, generation and life experiences. Older and ageing people may not exhibit "age-related" behaviours of any kind – they may live full, independent and meaningful lives.

However, an older and ageing Person who requires the assistance of a healthcare professional might:

- insist on doing a task without assistance and without fear for their safety, regardless of their ability
- request assistance, even when they are able to complete something independently
- request information repeatedly due to difficulty hearing or remembering
- request glasses and/or written information in large print
- repeat the same information on different occasions
- attempt to monopolise the time of the healthcare professional with complex new needs at every session
- be uncooperative and sullen
- be well adjusted and enjoy attending the health service.

Principles for effective communication with an older and ageing Person

When communicating with an older and ageing Person, it is important to:

- make introductions
- demonstrate respect

- demonstrate empathy
- provide clear written information with pictures if necessary to clarify meaning
- listen actively
- provide encouraging comfort
- confront inappropriate beliefs and thoughts where appropriate.

Strategies for communicating with an older and ageing Person

- Use a holistic approach.
- Ask them what they would like to be called – they might prefer to be addressed as Mr, Mrs or Miss rather than their given name until they feel the healthcare professional is not a stranger.
- Treat an older and ageing Person as an equal, regardless of their age, gender, cultural background or abilities.
- Listen to and remember their story.

Remember the principles of effective communication and Person/Family-centred Care.

Scenario one: The male and the healthcare professional

Person 1: Your name is Ron and you are an active 78-year-old man who swims every morning. Since your wife died you have independently cared for yourself and even assisted in caring for your two granddaughters. You have recently had a fall while doing the shopping and currently you require regular treatment for a knee injury. You are not enjoying the change in your functioning and are anxious to return to swimming every day. During your treatment you are polite, but do not really enjoy requiring the assistance of anyone. You are accustomed to assisting others, not having them do things for you. This young healthcare professional is very nice, but too young to know very much about anything.

Person 2: You are the healthcare professional. You have developed a working relationship with Ron and have been attempting to establish how he feels about his recent fall, because you would like to refer him to another healthcare professional who can give him some information about avoiding falls in the future.

Scenario two: The female and the healthcare professional

Person 1: Your name is Elsie. You are an 84-year-old woman who lives alone. Despite a coccygeal fusion, osteoporosis of the upper vertebrae of your spinal column and bilateral arthritis of the hands, you have continued to spin, knit and sew. Until recently you were very active, attending line dancing and playing bowls several times a week. However, you pulled a muscle in your leg while line dancing 6 months ago and have not been the same since. You had to stop line dancing and playing bowls. Then, a month ago, just as you were recovering from your leg injury and thinking about returning to line dancing, you pulled a muscle in your shoulder while cleaning your light fittings. You are fiercely independent and despite having a gold card with the Department of Veterans' Affairs (DVA), you have never thought of using it for assistance. You see a physiotherapist at present who has asked you to consider a homecare assessment to determine whether you might benefit from assistance with your housework and washing.

Person 2: You are a healthcare professional who knows Elsie very well and have been asked to convince her to accept homecare for her safety.

People who are older and ageing bring a wealth of experience and wisdom to every interaction. Unless experiencing cognitive decline, they do not usually require variation in the style of communication. As for all individuals, effective communication with an older and ageing Person requires respect, empathy, rapport, collaborative involvement in their treatment, empowerment and, of course, Person-centred Care. These characteristics should be evident in the relationship of the healthcare professional with every older Person, regardless of any decline in the physical, social, cognitive or emotional competence of that Person.

CHAPTER 26

Person/s fulfilling particular life roles

Chapter objective

Upon completing this chapter, readers should be able to apply knowledge and have emerging skills in communicating effectively with Person/s fulfilling particular life roles.

Individuals may fulfil many roles during their lives; for example, carer, colleague, parent and single parent to a child requiring assistance, sibling, grandparent, student and group member. These roles make particular demands upon the individual, which may have a variety of effects depending on their stage of life. Healthcare professionals experience various groups in their role; therefore, the final scenario relating to roles is about the groups found in the healthcare professions. This scenario is unique and therefore contains unique steps to follow for the related small-group activity.

Particular life roles

1 Carer
2 Colleague
3 Parent to a child requiring assistance
4 Single parent to a child requiring assistance
5 Sibling
6 Grandparent
7 Student
8 Group member

- Define these particular roles.
- List some of the specific behaviours that might be typical of an individual fulfilling these particular roles.
- List the negative emotions that individuals fulfilling these roles might experience when relating to a health service.

- List possible explanations for the emotions someone fulfilling these roles might experience when relating to a healthcare professional.
- List principles for effective communication to remember when communicating with someone fulfilling these particular roles. Give reasons for the need to remember these principles.
- Suggest strategies for communicating with an individual who fulfils these particular roles. Decide why you might see such an individual in your particular health profession.
- Check your answers against the information below, noting any additional thoughts or ideas.

1. Person/s fulfilling the role of carer

(Key words: carer, legal and informal, long-term, caregiver, guardian)

Definition of a carer

A carer is someone who cares for an individual with atypical health full-time or for more than a designated number of hours each day. (The designated number of hours varies according to legislation.)

Carers might be:

- spouses, daughters, sons, siblings, close friends of the same or opposite gender, or neighbours
- an individual who is paid to provide care, by either the government or the family of the Person who requires care.

Possible emotions a carer might experience

A carer might experience emotions related to:

- fear
- anxiety
- confusion
- depression
- grief
- anger
- inadequacy
- desperation
- loneliness
- denial of the problem
- isolation: no-one can understand
- hopelessness.

Possible reasons for these emotions

A carer might experience these emotions because of:

- spending all their time caring for the Person
- social isolation
- responsibility and stress
- limited knowledge about and skill in caring
- loss of hope

- confusion about the implication of recent needs that have resulted in seeking assistance from a healthcare professional
- fear of and anxiety about the future.

Possible behaviours related to being a carer

The behaviours of a carer will vary according to the age of the carer and the condition of the Person requiring assistance. A carer might:

- act as an advocate for the Person, always indicating their needs and desires
- be constantly doing things for the Person, regardless of the abilities of the Person
- exhibit non-verbal behaviours that appear opposite to their verbal messages.

Principles for effective communication with a carer

When communicating with a carer, it is important to:

- demonstrate empathy and sensitivity
- make introductions
- listen actively
- give encouraging comfort
- validate
- clearly and honestly answer any questions
- provide clear and well-organised information about the health service and any services or organisations that will provide assistance and support.

Strategies for communicating with a carer

- Do not avoid the issues – be prepared to respond to the obvious and stated needs of the carer.
- Be prepared to respond to the non-verbal behaviours of the carer – they may send a different message to their words.
- If necessary, refer the carer to other appropriate healthcare professionals or organisations.
- If appropriate, confront the fears and feelings of the carer.

See the Introduction to Section 4 for instructions about how to use these scenarios for role-play or group discussion. Remember the principles of effective communication and Person/Family-centred Care.

Scenario one: The male and the healthcare professional

Person 1: Your name is Steve. You are 39 years old and married to Marie, who was diagnosed with multiple sclerosis (MS) seven years ago. You have recently reduced your hours of work to assist Marie with the maintenance of the house, her personal care and mobility, as well as your two children. Marie was falling at home while you were at work, so you reduced your hours to be with her when she most requires assistance. You accompany Marie to every appointment with the healthcare professionals and you know them all quite well. You sit in the waiting area, feeling tired and distressed by Marie's recent deterioration. You are not sure, but you think you need to resign from work and live on your savings and a carer pension. You find it increasingly difficult to fulfil all the roles you have, and you are not sure how you will manage when Marie finally dies. You stop, shocked at the thought – you would rather call it "passing on". Your religious beliefs have been very important to how you manage your emotions and friends from church have been supportive, often cooking meals, doing housework and mowing the lawns for you. However, you are very tired and feel like you need a rest.

Person 2: You are the healthcare professional responsible for the needs of Marie, a person with MS. Marie is being seen by a healthcare professional with different expertise today and you have decided to use the time to talk with her husband, Steve.

Scenario two: The female and the healthcare professional
Person 1: Your name is Genevieve and you are the main carer for your 6-year-old son, Damien, who has cerebral palsy (CP). Damien is a boy with a wonderful sense of humour, who is confined to a wheelchair. Although you usually anticipate what he wants, he communicates using sounds, gestures and an augmentative communication system. You are also providing meals and some house maintenance for your ageing father, who lives in the next street. You are tired and wondering how you can continue to care for both your son and your father. So much with Damien takes so long; you want to encourage him to feed himself and do some of his dressing himself, but it takes much longer when you give him time to do things for himself and you do not feel you have the time.

Person 2: You are a healthcare professional who has not met Genevieve before, but have been working with Damien on school days. Genevieve has arrived early today and you go to meet her. You are committed to Person/Family-centred Care and want to find ways to encourage Damien to feed himself at least a few teaspoons of food every day instead of being fed everything.

2. Person/s fulfilling the role of a colleague

(Key words: team, multidisciplinary team, interdisciplinary)

Definition of a colleague in the healthcare professions

A colleague in the healthcare professions is:

- any other professional, whether inside or outside the health service, who works with the healthcare professional to assist vulnerable people
- any other worker who supports the healthcare professional to assist vulnerable people.

Attitudes and/or behaviours expected of a healthcare professional

A healthcare professional should be:

- professional
- ethical
- reliable
- respectful
- punctual
- caring
- interested in people
- committed to caring
- willing to make sacrifices
- willing to assist
- self-aware
- thoughtful

- diligent
- supportive of colleagues
- reflective
- reflexive
- accepting of differences
- observant.

Attitudes and/or behaviours not expected of a healthcare professional

A healthcare professional should *not* be:

- self-serving
- self-focused
- non-reflective or non-reflexive
- personally ambitious
- lazy
- judgemental
- sexually predatory
- resistant
- uncooperative
- slovenly
- racist
- sexist.

Possible emotions a colleague might experience

A colleague might experience emotions related to:

- frustration
- guilt
- grief and loss
- disappointment
- feeling misunderstood
- betrayal
- isolation
- feeling unvalued
- feeling inadequate.

Possible reasons for these emotions

A colleague might experience these emotions because of:

- personal experiences that occur outside the work context in family or social relationships
- decisions made by the employing institution
- their own attitudes and behaviour at particular times
- the attitudes and behaviour of other colleagues
- unmet expectations
- accidents, either at work or in their personal life
- a person dying either at work or in their personal life
- attempts to fulfil the unclear expectations of others
- limited resources and pressure of work.

Principles for effective communication with a colleague

When communicating with a colleague, it is important to:

- use holistic communication
- listen actively
- validate
- clarify
- understand
- confront
- empathise
- use sensitive honesty
- provide encouraging comfort
- be assertive.

Strategies for communicating with a colleague

- Demonstrate colleague-centred communication.
- Balance acceptance of the colleague with confrontation that empowers them to change inappropriate attitudes and behaviours.
- Do not assume understanding of the behaviour of a colleague.
- Demonstrate unconditional positive regard despite the differences.
- Use "I" messages to communicate both your negative and positive emotions to a colleague.

Remember the principles of effective communication and Person/Family-centred Care.

Scenario one: The male and the healthcare professional colleague

Person 1: Your name is Ian and you are a single parent with three school-aged children. You are often called to emergencies with the children and find it difficult to balance life with work. You love your work as a healthcare professional and have excellent relationships with your colleagues and the people you assist. You work efficiently and always have positive results.

Person 2: You are new to this health service and you are Ian's immediate supervisor. You have noticed that he often arrives late and leaves early without explanation. He works efficiently when he is at work and everyone thinks very highly of him. He appears to have excellent relationships with everyone, as well as positive outcomes. You have a supervision meeting with Ian scheduled for today.

- What are your aims for this session and why?
- Role-play the session when you have established those aims.

Scenario two: The female and the healthcare professional colleague

Person 1: Your name is Paula and you have a very busy day of work scheduled in your health service. A colleague notices your schedule and offers to assist you. You are quite surprised because this colleague often appears to avoid work. Together, you agree that they will do some easy administration tasks due today that your supervisor has allocated to you. You clarify when they must be done, how to do them and where to place them upon completion. Throughout the day you notice your colleague chatting and reading a novel and you hope they have done those tasks. You have no time to do them yourself. At the end of an exhausting day, you are with this colleague and your supervisor asks for the tasks the colleague had agreed to complete. You look at the colleague, who looks away, and you say you have not had time to complete them. The supervisor is not happy that you have not completed these specific tasks and says they hold you responsible. The colleague listens and says nothing. You are angry because you had no time to complete them today. You are now in the room with the colleague, you feel angry and you ... (decide what to do).

Person 2: You are the colleague who offers to assist, then chooses to chat and read instead, thinking that you will get to those tasks later. As the day disappears you think *I can do them tomorrow.* You watch the supervisor talk to Paula, but you cannot see the problem – you said you would do them and you will try to remember to do them tomorrow. You find it difficult to understand why Paula is angry.

Healthcare professionals have a responsibility to care for themselves, their colleagues and the Person/s. Reflection is beneficial in achieving this care in a manner that considers the needs of all communicators within the health professions.

3. Person/s fulfilling the role of parent to a child requiring assistance

(Key words: parents, foster-parents, role models, family, legal guardian, uncertain)

Definition of a parent

A parent is someone who:

- has been part of creating the "child"
- is legally responsible for the "child"
- the "child" views as their parent or parent figure – their protector, provider and model. A "child" is someone who has a parent and may be of varying ages.

Parents in situations most susceptible to experiencing difficulties when attending a health service

The parents susceptible to experiencing difficulties when attending a health service may be those who:

- are young
- have an intellectual disability
- have addictions
- are unfamiliar with the healthcare system
- have unrealistic expectations
- have children with long-term difficulties
- have had negative previous experiences of health services.

Possible emotions such a parent might experience

A parent might experience emotions related to:

- fear
- anxiety
- uncertainty
- desperation

- denial
- shock
- guilt
- resignation
- being lonely
- feeling inadequate
- grief.

Possible reasons for these emotions

The possible reasons for these emotions in a parent will depend upon the age of the child and the severity of the condition for which the child requires assistance. However, the emotions, regardless of their cause, are as significant as those of the child and require management by the healthcare professional.

Family-centred Care is particularly relevant to healthcare associated with children aged 0 to 16 years. Children exist in the context of the family and should not be assisted without reference to and consideration of that context.

Parents may experience negative emotions because of:

- concern for the continued health, wellbeing, participation, functioning and safety of the child
- feeling guilt and responsibility for the condition
- loneliness and isolation
- fear of and anxiety about the future
- confusion about the meaning of their life if something happens to the child
- inadequacy and desperation
- grief for lost opportunities related to career, friendships, family and siblings, in the case of a long-term condition.

Possible behaviours related to being a parent with such a child

The behaviours related to being a parent will depend on the age of the child. Such behaviours are often related to the feelings the parent is experiencing.

When the "child" is *young*, a parent might be:

- protective and even angry on behalf of the child
- anxious to understand everything related to the child
- controlling of the child
- able to coax the child into engaging and being involved in the process
- able to reassure the child and provide safety for the child.

When the "child" is an adolescent, a parent might be some of the above and/or:

- protective and overbearing
- accusatory, depending on the cause of the need for a healthcare professional.

When the "child" is an *adult*, the behaviour of the parent might depend on the quality of the relationship with the "child" and the nature of the reason the "child" is seeking assistance from a healthcare professional.

Principles for effective communication with a parent in this situation

When communicating with a parent, it is important to:

- demonstrate empathy and sensitivity
- make introductions

- provide and explain information
- provide clear and well-organised information about any services or organisations that will provide assistance and support
- listen actively
- schedule time for discussion and answers to pertinent questions
- give encouraging comfort
- validate
- effectively disengage.

Strategies for communicating with a parent in this situation

- Invest time with the parent as well as the child to develop a therapeutic relationship.
- Clearly explain and clarify their understanding of the procedures and events regularly – avoid assuming they understand everything.
- Respond to their non-verbal messages.
- Acknowledge and use the expertise and knowledge the parent has about the child.

Remember the principles of effective communication and Person/Family-centred Care.

Scenario one: The male and the healthcare professional

Person 1: Your name is Theo. You are the 72-year-old father of 48-year-old Christopher who has recently been diagnosed with motor neurone disease (MND). You are anxious about the wellbeing of your eldest son, who has managed your concreting business for many years. Christopher has been a great son, especially since your wife, Anna, died four years ago. He has provided for his wife and your five grandchildren, managed the business expertly and, like you, loves concreting. You have no idea what MND means and you just want your son to go back to his life of participation and providing.

Person 2: You are the healthcare professional who Theo sees monthly and you have noticed recently that he is not himself. Whatever is troubling him seems to be affecting the way Theo cares for himself, so you would like to explore this and see if he requires some form of intervention.

Scenario two: The female and the healthcare professional

Person 1: Your name is Sally. You are a mother of two girls with a husband who is often away for extended periods with his job. Your eldest daughter, Suzie, is 8 years old. She seems to have difficulty learning and appears to be aggressive at school. Your younger daughter, Katie, is 6 years old. They both attend the same school and the behaviour of Suzie at school embarrasses Katie, who is becoming aggressive towards her older sister at home. You have no idea how to help either of your children and feel desperate. Suzie is gentle and loving at home, so you cannot understand her behaviour at school. You attend a health service regularly and decide to ask the healthcare professional there for assistance.

Person 2: You are the healthcare professional who has been seeing Sally for some time and feel you have a positive therapeutic relationship with her. She has always been cooperative and friendly. You have no idea about the difficulties her children are experiencing, but when she explains, you decide you would like to help, even though it may not be your area of expertise.

Parents of children who require the assistance of a healthcare professional, regardless of the age of the children, require a supportive and therapeutic relationship, along with their children. The needs of the parents may or may not be different, but the parents are a vital component of the context of the Person seeking the assistance of the healthcare professional.

Similarly, when parents are receiving assistance from a healthcare professional, the children will have similar needs and emotions to those listed in this section. In such situations, the child of the Person, whether adult or not, is an integral part of the context of the Person and will therefore require consideration and effective communication.

4. Person/s fulfilling the role of single parent to a child requiring assistance

(Key words: parenting alone, one-person parenting, sole responsibility, unsupported)

Definition of a single parent

A single parent:

- is someone who is attempting to raise the child(ren) alone
- often has no-one with whom they can share the care of the child(ren)
- is often working full-time, as well as managing the needs of the child(ren), sometimes without the support of members of an extended family.

Characteristics single parents may expect of themselves

Single parents may expect themselves to be:

- competent to meet all the needs of their child(ren)
- able to manage, regardless of life events or circumstances
- good at problem-solving
- determined
- able to persevere.

Possible emotions a single parent might experience

A single parent might experience emotions related to:

- struggle
- fear
- inadequacy
- anger
- envy
- resentment
- feeling overwhelmed
- depression
- loneliness
- isolation
- insecurity
- feeling discouraged
- frustration
- anxiety

- scepticism
- constant tiredness
- desperation
- stress
- grief
- exhaustion.

Possible reasons for these emotions

A single parent might experience these emotions because of:

- feeling rejected through divorce or separation
- any unexpected event
- responsibilities and stress related to their role
- demands of the child(ren)
- no respite or rest
- financial burdens
- friends appearing to "have it easy"
- having no sense of being valued
- considering the needs of the child(ren) above their own needs.

Principles for effective communication with a single parent in this situation

When communicating with a single parent, it is important to:

- listen actively
- encourage
- give information
- establish boundaries
- confront
- disengage.

Strategies for communicating with a single parent with a child requiring assistance

- Avoid critical comments about their parenting.
- Imagine how you would manage if you were in their situation.
- Set achievable goals.

Remember the principles of effective communication and Person/Family-centred Care.

Scenario one: The male and the healthcare professional

Paul is a single parent to his three children. His wife died three years ago and he has managed to care for the children since then. The schools the children attend have after-care facilities, but Paul finds this too expensive for three children. Each of the children is allowed one extracurricular activity. Craig (15 years old) plays soccer, Lara (14) plays the piano and

Lacey (10) settled for tap dancing because her father said horse riding was too expensive and too hard to organise.

Paul manages a department store and relies on his eldest child, Craig, to care for the younger girls until he arrives home from work each day. The younger children, Lara and Lacey, do not enjoy the time before their father returns home from work because Craig orders them to do chores around the house while he plays computer games or watches television. Their father is always tired when he arrives home and thanks Craig for the completed chores. Craig does not say he did not do them and enjoys his father's appreciation. Sometimes one of the girls makes a meal, but often Paul prepares the evening meal and then supervises their homework. They have a routine that allows everyone to fulfil their responsibilities at home, work and school. Organising extracurricular activities and sport is challenging and exhausting, but parents of friends of the children often drive them home.

Today Paul receives a call from Craig's principal requesting an interview with Paul to discuss Craig's progress. Two hours after receiving that call, a teacher from Lacey's school rings to say Lacey has fallen at school and needs medical attention. As Paul drives to the school he wishes his wife was alive, just so he could have someone with whom to talk. The teacher has assured him Lacey is all right, so he is not prepared for the swelling on her forehead or the blood on her arm. He wonders why he thought it was just a scratch and a bruise. Lacey is barely conscious, but seems to know he is there.

At the hospital Paul waits quietly by his youngest daughter, holding her hand. He misses his wife, especially at times like these because she was so good with sick people. He has no idea how he will manage if Lacey needs extra time and attention, because he only just manages now. He thinks about Craig. *That 15-year-old needs more attention than I give him,* he thinks. He remembers how hard it was to be 15 and how many temptations there were when he was growing up. He realises he has not had the time to talk with Craig about this the way his father did when he was about 12. So much of his energy goes into just getting the basic things done each day.

Someone comes to take Lacey for an x-ray; Lacey does not notice that Paul does not go with her. Another healthcare professional arrives to ask a few questions and to see what Paul needs.

- If you were that healthcare professional, what questions would you be required to ask?
- Answers to some of these questions would lead you to ask further questions – what might they be?
- How important might the story of Paul and the children be for achieving the goals associated with Lacey's care?

Scenario two: The female and the healthcare professional

Jenna is a 33-year-old woman who is a single parent to 6-year-old Jonah. Jonah is currently receiving speech pathology, occupational therapy and physiotherapy for delayed speech, attention deficits and gross motor coordination. A podiatrist has made arch supports for Jonah and this has helped his gross motor performance in some areas, but he needs assistance to develop his muscle tone and strength.

Jenna and her husband separated five years ago. Jonah always spent the weekends with his father until recently, when his father moved interstate. Jenna found that the break from caring for Jonah on the weekends helped her manage during the week. It also meant she did not have extra expenses on the weekends, because Jonah's father paid for the movies and other expensive activities Jonah liked doing on the weekends.

Since that time, Jenna and Jonah seem tense when they are together and they often yell at each other out of frustration. Jenna says she hates yelling, but she gets so frustrated when Jonah will not listen to her. Jenna says she is really struggling with being alone. She finds it difficult to be responsible for Jonah without a break because he has particular needs all of the time. She is unsure how to manage the frustration and anger she feels most of the time. She is not always frustrated with Jonah, just with their situation.

- If you were a healthcare professional involved with the care of Jonah, how would you approach this situation?
- What are the aims of communication with Jenna?

As a large group, share the main points discussed by each small group about these scenarios. Consider various strategies that may increase the effectiveness of the communication in a similar situation.

5. A Person fulfilling the role of sibling

(Key words: sibling, brother, sister, family, parents, mother, father)

Definition of a sibling

A sibling is one of two or more children with one or both parents in common, they can be a brother or a sister. A sibling may be legally adopted into the family. Siblings live in the same household with the same parents or guardians. Siblings are typically an important aspect of the lives of families.

Attitudes and/or behaviours often typical of siblings

If the sibling is older, they may:

- sometimes depending on age, care for the younger sibling/s
- be expected to be an appropriate example of behaviour
- be admired by the younger sibling/s, who want to be like their older sibling
- sometimes find the younger siblings annoying
- sometimes find their younger siblings inconvenient and embarrassing
- want to protect the younger sibling/s, keeping them safe.

If the sibling is younger, they may:

- be allowed to copy their older sibling/s when appropriate
- think of their older sibling/s as wonderful and a role-model
- really enjoy spending time with their sibling/s
- expect their older sibling/s to keep them safe.

Many of the above will depend on the differences in the ages and possibly the gender of the siblings.

Possible emotions a sibling might experience

- Pride
- Enjoyment
- Pleasure
- Acceptance

- Frustration
- Anger
- Anxiety
- Regret
- Inadequacy

Possible reasons for these emotions

- Satisfaction and delight relating to their family and their role in that family.
- Pleasure relating to and playing with their sibling/s.
- Happy with and enjoying their role as a sibling.
- Recognition of their role and of their relationship with their sibling/s.
- Irritation due to the demands of the sibling/s and sometimes their parents.
- Annoyed and sometimes resentful of the expectations of their role and their sibling/s.
- Not feeling able to fulfil the expectations of their role.
- Guilt and distress because of particular events for which they feel responsible.
- A constant feeling of not being able or good enough to fulfil the sibling role.

Principles of effective communication with a sibling

When communicating with a sibling, it is important to:

- demonstrate respect and empathy to engender trust
- use compassionate and caring non-verbal messages
- develop rapport to establish and strengthen a therapeutic relationship
- use active listening to their expressions of their sibling experience
- be willing to explore their sibling role and feelings relating to the role.

Strategies for communication with a sibling

- Do not avoid discussion of their sibling or their role as a sibling.
- If appropriate, validate their emotions relating to their sibling.
- Encourage them in their role as a sibling.
- Refer to another appropriate healthcare professional if requiring resolution of negative emotions relating to their experience in their sibling role.

Sibling relationships, the associated expectations and responsibilities may change as they grow and mature; however, the relationships remain for their lifetime, regardless of the quality of those relationships.

Remember the principles of effective communication and Person/Family-centred Care.

Scenario one: The male and the healthcare professional

Person 1: You are the older brother of Emily, who has recently been diagnosed with an incurable and inoperable brain tumour. Your name is Jonathon, your family call you Jono. You have a positive sibling relationship with Emily, often playing together and reading together. You have come to the hospital today with your mother and Emily for what everyone thought was a routine check-up. You have come before and seen the healthcare professionals with Emily and your parent (sometimes your father brings Emily to the hospital). However, today there was an unexpected complication for Emily and you have been told to stay in the waiting area. You have found it very difficult to imagine life without Emily and now you sit in the waiting area alone and crying. You have told your mother you would be fine while waiting – however, you have now been overcome by grief.

Person 2: You are the healthcare professional who has been asked to see Jonathon (the older sibling of a young girl with only 6 months to live), who is sitting in the waiting room You have been told that he is managing the upcoming death of his sister well and do not expect to find him crying in the waiting area.

Scenario two: The female and the healthcare professional

Person 1: You are Kim, the older sister of Jussy (Justine a 4-year-old girl), who has just been brought to hospital due to an accident. During this accident Jussy fell and hit her head on the road surface just outside your house. This caused her to fall unconscious and although she was breathing, she was not responding to any spoken words. You feel responsible for this accident as you could have stopped Jussy from falling. It all happened so quickly. You just did not expect her to run onto the road and then fall. She rarely falls over, being quite steady on her feet. You have been experiencing overwhelming anxiety and depression since the accident. These strong emotions have been affecting your ability to live your life as you previously did, before the accident. Your parents have decided to send you to a child psychologist. You are sitting, with your mother, waiting to be seen for the first time, wondering how seeing someone to talk about your feelings could possibly help you. You have decided that if someone mentions the accident you will pretend you do not remember it.

Person 2: You are Jenny, the healthcare professional, who will be seeing Kim to assist with her overwhelming emotions. You have NOT been told about the accident involving the youngest child in the family. You are aware of various causes of overwhelming emotions for young people and assume you will be able to assist Kim to identify the possible causes of her overwhelming emotions. Initially, you intend to see Kim with her parent; however, you are intending to see her alone in future sessions. You go to the waiting area, identify Kim, introduce yourself and take Kim and her parent to your interview room. The parent is reluctant to go with you; however, you insist that for at least some of this session the parent accompanies Kim.

6. A Person fulfilling the role of a grandparent

(Key words: grandparent, family, grandmother, grandfather, grandma, grandpa)

Definition of a grandparent

A grandparent is someone who has children with children of their own. They are the parents of your parents.

Possible emotions a grandparent might experience

- Enjoyment
- Pleasure
- Acceptance
- Pride
- Satisfaction
- Gratification

- Disappointment
- Regret
- Fear
- Anxiety
- Inadequacy
- Frustration

Possible reasons for these emotions

- The role provides fun and delight.
- The grandchildren grow regularly, developing new skills.
- The grandchildren skilfully perform tasks taught by the grandparent.
- The children make decisions regarding the grandchildren different to those the grandparent feels are appropriate.
- The grandchildren expect the grandparent to be able to do anything, regardless of their actual abilities.
- Fatigue.
- The grandchildren do things that cause concern.
- The grandchildren need abilities that differ from those of the grandparent.

Possible behaviours related to the role of a grandparent

- Minding the grandchildren
- Discussing and perhaps questioning decisions with their children
- Collecting and delivering the grandchildren to different venues
- Regularly purchasing gifts of various kinds for the grandchildren.

Principles of effective communication with a grandparent

When communicating with a grandparent, it is important to:

- demonstrate respect and empathy to engender trust
- develop rapport to strengthen the therapeutic relationship
- be willing to explore their grandparenting role and their feelings relating to the role
- use active listening to their expressions of pride in their grandchildren

Strategies for communication with a grandparent

- Do not avoid discussion of the grandchildren or their role as grandparent.
- If appropriate, validate their positive emotions relating to grandparenting.
- Refer to another appropriate healthcare professional if requiring resolution of negative emotions relating to their grandparenting role.

Remember the principles of effective communication and Person/Family-centred Care.

Scenario one: The male and the healthcare professional

Person 1: Your name is James or Granddaddy Jim to your four grandchildren. You are 58 years old and live with your wife, Jody. You have been happily married for 36 years. You have previously played competitive soccer and have taught three of your four grandchildren to play soccer. Your grandchildren are Jack (10 years old); Jeremy (8 years old); Jaime (6 years old) and Jamima (3 years old). You currently coach a local soccer team, in which two of your grandchildren play. You often play soccer with your three eldest grandchildren at the local soccer fields, after school. Jeremy has just been chosen to play in a state soccer competition. While playing with three of your grandchildren you tripped, fell and fractured your ankle, also tearing a tendon in your knee. You have just begun attending a healthcare service for intervention. Despite your mobility restrictions, you still manage to watch the soccer games each week, to see your grandchildren play. You are very proud of Jeremy and eager to tell everyone his news.

Person 2: You are a recent healthcare graduate called Justine. You are seeing James for the first time today. You are very focused on appropriately performing your role as a healthcare professional. You follow the guidelines for initial interviews and know you will need to remain focused on those guidelines to complete the interview and any relevant assessment in the allocated time.

Scenario two: The female and the healthcare professional

Before using this scenario, the individual playing Lizzy will need to choose a health condition relevant to her health profession and that of their partner, and tell the individual playing the healthcare professional her chosen health condition.

Person 1: You are Lizzy, a 72-year-old widow, who is a proud grandparent of two beautiful grandchildren, Noah (6 years old) and Ava (4 years old). Ever since their birth you have been an integral part of their lives. They call you "Mum Mum". You regularly have them stay at your house, minding them three days a week while their parents work. You enjoy playing with them and cooking for them. They love staying with you and they love your cooking. You also have a weekly evening meal with them at their house. It has been wonderful, as you have not missed your husband as much since they were born. Their parents have recently told you they are moving to another location, 1000 kilometres away. While you tried not to communicate it, you feel devastated. You wonder how you will manage without them – what will you do with your days. How will you manage being alone? You have your regular appointment today with a health service to monitor your health because of your healthcare needs. You are sitting quietly in the waiting area, with your head down not relating to anyone.

Person 2: You are Linda, who has worked at this health service for several years. You see Lizzy regularly for her 6-monthly appointments to monitor her health status. Today you notice while Lizzy is in the waiting room, she is not her usual happy self. She would typically smile and acknowledge you when you walk through the room, but today she sat with her head down not relating to anyone. You wonder if her health is deteriorating and despite having a busy day, you decide to explore the cause of her mood when you see her for her appointment in 20 minutes.

7. Person/s fulfilling the role of a student

(Key words: studying, learning, professional practice, clinical experience, applying theory)

Definition of a student in the healthcare professions

A healthcare professional student is someone who is not fully qualified in their chosen healthcare profession. Students usually visit clinical settings to consolidate theory and learn skills, and may become excellent healthcare professionals in their particular profession. They might be observing, practising or consolidating, but ultimately they are connecting theory with practice.

Being a student, means individuals might:

- feel underpaid and overworked!
- feel isolated if away from family
- find balancing work and study hard
- feel pressure to party and abuse alcohol
- feel inadequate
- feel pressure to achieve high grades.

Possible emotions a student might experience

A student might experience emotions related to:

- insecurity
- loneliness
- fear
- lack of confidence
- disappointment
- frustration
- anxiety
- pressure
- feeling overwhelmed.

Possible reasons for these emotions

A student might experience these emotions because of:

- lack of knowledge or skills
- pressure to perform and achieve
- feelings of inequality
- social isolation – away from family
- financial pressure and struggles
- different learning styles
- relationship issues
- peer pressure
- poor self-management skills
- imbalance in the activities of life
- different personality types.

Possible behaviours related to being a student

A student might:

- observe enthusiastically
- attempt to compensate for inadequacy
- engage in risk-taking behaviours
- not ask questions
- chatter about irrelevant things.

Principles for effective communication with a student

When communicating with a student, it is important to:

- make introductions – to everything!
- consider their non-verbal behaviours

- demonstrate respect and empathy
- understand
- be consistent in communication
- confront when necessary
- provide information
- listen actively
- give encouraging comfort
- disengage appropriately.

Strategies for communicating with a student

- Provide clear and detailed information about the expectations of the student while they are on placement.
- Avoid making assumptions about what they know and their life experience.
- Become familiar with their learning style and manner of managing information.
- Provide immediate and specific feedback in a format that reflects their learning style.
- Communicate positive and negative feedback clearly with suggestions of definite behaviours to improve. Be specific.
- Address the causes of their issues not the symptoms.
- Adjust your communication style to be approachable – being friends with students is acceptable.
- Avoid intimidating facial expressions and behaviour.
- Allow them time to process information.

Remember the principles of effective communication and Person/Family-centred Care.

Scenario one: The male and the healthcare professional

Person 1: Your name is Ryan and you are a third-year student completing a 5-week clinical placement. You were punctual and relaxed on the first day, but each day since then you have been late and you appear anxious. On the Friday of the first week you lose a medical record required by another healthcare professional. This becomes a major issue because the record for this person is required in court on Monday.

Person 2: You are the supervisor responsible for Ryan, and, as such, you are responsible for the lost record. Respond to Ryan to achieve the best outcome for all involved individuals.

Scenario two: The female and the healthcare professional

Person 1: Your name is Sharon and you are a 19-year-old student healthcare professional. You are currently on placement at a health service with five other students from different health-care professions. This health service provides activities and education for people who are high functioning, but who have a history of mental illness. You have been enjoying the placement. You relate well to the various people who attend the service for assistance. You are young, attractive and naturally friendly to everyone. The other students are from other cities and you invite them to the pub after work. A particular male who attends the centre for assistance, Tom, is present when you make the arrangements and assumes he is included in the arrangements. When you arrive at the pub Tom is there waiting for you. You think he is there with his mates. You say *Hi* and then ignore him, not realising he is there to join you. Some of the other students notice that he leaves in a distressed state. You do not worry, saying, *It's a free world – he can do what he likes and so can I. I meant no harm; he should have known the arrangements were only for the students.*

Person 2: It is Monday morning and you are the student supervisor for this health service. Several qualified staff have heard that Tom was admitted to hospital on Friday night. One of the students feels guilty because she knew Tom was in the room when Sharon arranged to go to the pub, and she knew it was not appropriate to make the arrangements in the presence of a Person seeking the assistance of the centre. This student has told you everything that happened at the centre and the pub. You ask to speak with Sharon privately to hear her side of the story and to ensure she does not behave in this way again.

Student healthcare professionals are the future of their profession. They deserve and require effective communication and opportunities to develop their skills in communication, as well as specialised assistance to successfully complete their program.

8. Groups in the healthcare professions

(Key words: group work, group dynamics, group growth)
The healthcare professional might encounter two major kinds of groups during their practising life. The first type of group is one in which they are a member of a team or group of people. Such multidisciplinary or interdisciplinary teams may be found in public or private health services. Such teams aim to help those seeking their assistance. These teams may consist of people with different roles and different skills. The people may work for the same health service or for different services. As a member of a multidisciplinary team, it is important to understand the workings of a group and the possible experiences groups may provide. The second type of group often has therapeutic or educational goals, and is one in which the healthcare professional may be the leader or facilitator of the group.

Each of these groups require trust, commitment to group goals and participation in group activities from all participants, whether group members or group leader. Groups have a life of their own and, while beneficial, require particular knowledge and skills to maximise the benefits.

Groups in the healthcare professions

- Decide what types of groups occur in the healthcare professions.
- List the stages of growth in a group.
- List the emotions typically experienced in a group.
- List the expectations of group behaviour (group norms) for a multidisciplinary healthcare professional team, considering the possible needs of group members and the health service.
- List the expectations of group behaviour (group norms) for a therapeutic group, considering the possible needs of group members.
- List principles for effective communication to remember when communicating within a group. Give reasons for the need to remember these principles.
- Suggest strategies for communicating effectively within a group. Relate the strategies to the goals of your particular healthcare profession.
- Check your answers against the information below, noting any additional thoughts or ideas (of the group or from the information below).

Types of groups offered in health services

Health services may offer:

- educational groups
- therapeutic activity groups
- life skills groups
- healthy lifestyle groups
- condition-specific groups (e.g. stroke groups, autism groups)
- therapeutic play groups
- craft groups
- staff development groups
- professional development groups
- support groups
- seniors' groups
- leisure groups (e.g. non-professional sporting, music, dancing and drama groups).

Stages of group growth

Groups experience growth and change as group members become familiar with each other. Initially, group members experience uncertainty and possibly limited trust; they then experience differing levels of conflict as the members adjust to ways of relating within the group, and finally most groups achieve working relationships that facilitate group cohesion and productivity. Group members establish their roles and patterns of interrelating as they develop an understanding of self and of other group members. The development of trust and "working" group relationships facilitates fulfilment of group goals. Various theorists describe the stages of group growth (see Table 26.1). Some describe groups with psychosocial goals and others describe groups with task-oriented goals.

Each of the theorists in the table describe group stages using words that indicate groups will experience tension followed by ease of relating that facilitates positive outcomes. It is important to remember these stages whether you are a member of a group or the leader of a group.

Johnson & Johnson (2021) describe a group as having a leader who guides the group into productivity. The stages they describe often occur when the group is task-oriented. However, being a task-oriented group does not mean the group will be free of tension, because time is

TABLE 26.1
Stages of group growth

Tuckman & Jensen (1977)	Schutz (1973)	Mosey (1996)
Forming	Inclusion	Orientation
Storming	Control	Dissatisfaction
Norming	Affection	Resolution
Performing		Production
Mourning		

required to establish mutual understanding and commitment to the goals of the group. The stages take place as follows:

- defining and structuring procedures
- conforming to procedures and getting acquainted
- recognising mutuality and building trust
- committing to and taking ownership of the goals, procedures and other members
- functioning maturely and productively
- terminating.

Emotions typically experienced in a group

Yalom & Leszcz (2005) describe the therapeutic factors of groups that create particular emotions for all group members. While the dynamic of interdependent relationships within groups is challenging, they indicate that therapeutic factors occur because of the existence of the group and because of the complex interplay of the experiences typical of group membership. They highlight 11 primary factors that create particular emotions and demonstrate the therapeutic nature of groups. These therapeutic factors include the instillation of hope and the feeling of universality, both of which develop from the fact that other group members have similar experiences. Another therapeutic factor occurs because of feelings that arise from regular expression of experiences and feelings (catharsis) and the sharing of various types of information. Groups allow members to relate with selflessness (altruism), as they develop understanding of the feelings and needs of others through interpersonal learning. This provides opportunity to develop socialising techniques by observing and imitating the positive behaviour of other group members. Groups provide opportunity for positive group experiences that contribute to group cohesiveness and override possible negative experiences of family groups. They provide opportunity to understand existential factors relating to responsibility, because group membership requires particular behaviour to avoid unpleasant consequences.

Overall group aims

There are always overall goals for the existence of a group, whether the group is a healthcare professional team or a therapeutic group. It is important that each group member understands and is committed to these goals. Healthcare professional teams may have mission statements, and therapeutic groups will always have an overall aim. Clear explanation of the overall aim(s) is important to ensure appropriate expectations and behaviour from all group members. Both types of groups assemble for meetings, which have particular goals that contribute to the overall aim of the group. A therapeutic group may have a specific number of meetings and thus a limited group life.

Events of specific group sessions and associated emotions

Each group session contributes to the growth of the group and thus the movement through the stages of group development. The events within each session will elicit particular emotions for group members. The structure and preparation of each session will assist in management of any negative emotions associated with the session.

The events typical of a group session are as follows:

- **Welcome and aims:** Discussing the aims of the particular session allows group members to leave the events of everyday life and focus on group members and the forthcoming group events. This stage is important because it relaxes group members and allows them to remember their "place" in the group and the "place" of the other group members.

- **Warm-up:** A warm-up allows group members to reconnect with the group norms and goals, and with other group members.
- **Main activities:** The main activities usually fulfil the aims of the overall purpose of the group and the aims of the particular session.
- **Warm-down/wrap-up:** A wrap-up allows group members to reflect upon the events of the group and their relative success in achieving the aims of the session. It allows group members to reflect on the effect of the group session upon themselves and other group members. It also allows disengagement from the group members until the next group session.

Group norms: expectations of group behaviour

Group norms are the values that govern behaviour within a group. They are essential in any group because they promote cooperation and cohesion between individuals with different personalities, skills, knowledge and opinions. A group norm is the shared agreement and acceptance of rules that govern behaviour within a group. Norms include expectations regarding acceptable appearance when attending the group, punctuality, expression of emotions, acceptance of group members and confidentiality. A norm can also govern the rate, quality and method of producing outcomes if the group has a task focus. Explicit discussion of group norms in the initial stages of the group process facilitates openness concerning the expectations of particular behaviour within the group.

Principles for effective communication within groups

When communicating within groups, it is important to:

- remember that non-verbal behaviour is very powerful and can be easily misinterpreted in a group
- give non-judgemental encouragement to all members
- respect, accept, encourage and use all other elements of effective communication.

Strategies for communicating as a group leader

- Be well prepared with the required equipment and material to facilitate the group effectively and efficiently.
- Clarify and clearly state the group goals. The goals must be relevant and easily implemented, create positive interdependence, and encourage commitment from group members.
- Establish and state group norms and revisit them whenever necessary.
- Encourage open and accurate expression of ideas and feelings without judgement.
- Encourage participation, inclusion, acceptance, support and trust of each group member.
- If appropriate, share the leadership among all group members.

Remember the principles of effective communication and Person/Family-centred Care.

Scenario one: A two-day team/group development program

A health service has about 24 staff members who work full-time and part-time within the service. The person in charge has noticed there are difficulties in the relationships among many of the staff. They have organised a two-day team-building experience to attempt to develop trust and cohesion among the staff. They expect everyone to attend, including the administration staff, the cleaners, the people who work in the grounds and all healthcare professionals.

There is a mixed reaction on the first day because some people feel the cleaners should not be there and others feel the administration staff should not be there.

- Decide who should be there and explain why.
- How do you think the person in charge should manage these responses, which are contrary to the purpose of the two days?

Scenario two: An education group

A group educates its members about their condition and how to manage the condition. It runs for 6 weeks for 1½ hours each week. You facilitate the group and have other healthcare professionals attend at different times to provide a holistic consideration of the particular condition.

- Choose a condition relevant to your healthcare profession that could require an educational group.
- Using the specifications listed above (i.e. 6 weeks for 1½ hours per week) decide upon the overall goals of such a group, the possible aims of each session and the content.
- Indicate whether you will include any other healthcare professionals in the overall program. If so, devise the information and instructions you might give them as a guide for their involvement in the group.

References

Johnson, D.W., Johnson, F.P., 2021. Joining together: Group theory and group skills, 12th ed. Pearson, Boston.

Mosey, A.C., 1996. Psychosocial components of occupational therapy. Lippincott-Raven, Philadelphia.

Schutz, W.C., 1973. Elements of encounter. Joy Press, Big Sur, California.

Tuckman, B.W., Jensen, M.A.C., 1977. Stages of small group development revisited. Group and Organisation Management 2(4), 419–427.

Yalom, I.D., Leszcz, M., 2005. The theory and practice of group psychotherapy, 5th ed. Basic Books, New York.

CHAPTER 27

Person/s experiencing particular conditions

Chapter objective

Upon completing this chapter, readers should be able to apply knowledge and have emerging skills in communicating effectively with Person/s experiencing long-term conditions.

Particular conditions

1 Post-traumatic stress disorder (PTSD)/complex post-traumatic stress disorder (C-PTSD)
2 Spinal injury
3 Decreased cognitive function
4 Life-limiting illness
5 Mental illness
6 Chronic (long-term condition), with comorbidities (multiple physical conditions)
7 Stroke
8 Hearing impairment
9 Visual impairment

- Define these particular conditions.
- List some of the specific behaviours (and emotions if relevant) that might be typical of a person with these conditions.
- Choose one of three options:
  - list the emotions a person experiencing post-traumatic stress disorder or a life-limiting illness might experience when relating to a health service, *or*
  - consider which level of cognitive loss (mild, moderate or severe) may cause the most difficulty for an individual relating to a healthcare professional, *or*
  - consider which individuals may be most susceptible to experiencing a mental illness, hearing impairment or visual impairment.
- List possible reasons that might explain the emotions a person with these conditions might experience when seeing a healthcare professional.

- List principles for effective communication to remember when communicating with a person with one of these conditions. Give reasons for the need to remember these principles.
- Suggest strategies for communicating with a person who has these conditions. Decide why you might see such a person in your particular healthcare profession.
- Check your answers against the information below, noting any additional thoughts or ideas.

1. Person/s experiencing post-traumatic stress disorder (PTSD) and complex PTSD

(Key words: trauma, life-threatening, emotional illness, devastating life events, helplessness, fear, hopelessness)

Post-traumatic stress disorder (PTSD) is caused by exposure to traumatic events and complex PTSD (C-PTSD) by prolonged exposure to traumatic events.

Definition of PTSD

Post-traumatic stress disorder (PTSD) is an emotional illness that is classified as an anxiety disorder. It is usually associated with a horribly frightening, life-threatening or otherwise highly unsafe experience. Women are twice as likely to experience PTSD as men, while ethnic minorities are also more likely than non-minority men to develop PTSD. It is estimated that up to 40% of children have experienced at least one traumatic event in their life. Children may exhibit symptoms of PTSD in quite different ways to adults and can experience learning difficulties.

A diagnosis of PTSD requires the persistent presence of three groups of symptoms:

1. at least one symptom of experiencing recurring memories of the traumatic event, for example, nightmares, flashbacks
2. at least three symptoms demonstrating avoidance (phobia) of places, people and experiences that trigger the memories and/or a numbing of emotional responses to emotional situations
3. at least two persistent signs of hyperarousal existing for at least a month, for example, sleep disturbance, limited or poor concentration, irritability, unexplained anger, blackouts or poor memory, as well as hypervigilance (excessive watchfulness) for possible threats to their safety.

The combination of these symptoms must cause significant distress or functional impairment.

PTSD may negatively affect the social and emotional development of a child, whether they experience or observe the traumatic event.

Susceptibility to PTSD

Different people consider different things to be traumatic. As individuals define traumatic experiences differently, different people will respond differently to the same traumatic experience.

People who might develop PTSD include:

- people who live in war zones or locations that regularly experience traumatic events
- people with an emotional condition prior to experiencing a life-threatening or horrifying event
- people with limited social support who experience a traumatic event
- children and adolescents with learning difficulties, after a traumatic experience
- people who experience violence in the home

- people who experience, even by observing, a horrific event or emergency
- people who experience a similar event (although less traumatic) that trigger memories of the traumatic event.

Possible emotions a Person/s with PTSD might experience

A Person with PTSD might experience:

- anxiety
- fear
- uncertainty
- guilt
- difficulty regulating emotions
- persistent depressive emotions
- persistent overwhelming negative emotions.

Possible reasons for these emotions

Reasons for experiencing these emotions might include:

- re-experiencing or reliving the traumatic event
- repeated and consistent nightmares or visual representation of the event
- difficulty sleeping, creating extreme fatigue
- isolation and limited social support
- blaming themselves for the event
- receiving extremely disturbing news; for example, a diagnosis of a severe condition.

Possible behaviours typical of a Person/s with PTSD

People experiencing PTSD may:

- avoid places or people that remind them of the traumatic experience
- detach or distance themselves from people, even avoiding social interaction with significant others
- overuse addictive substances, for example, cigarettes, alcohol, marijuana
- have difficulty remembering particular appointments
- have difficulty sleeping
- experience lack of interest in previously enjoyed activities
- have difficulty regulating emotional responses, but may avoid expressing emotions
- have suicidal ideation that affects their ability to interact
- express feelings of hopelessness and/or helplessness
- avoid making plans for the future
- seek assistance for a seemingly unrelated condition, such as depression, substance abuse, manic depression or an eating disorder.

Principles for effective communication with a Person/s experiencing PTSD

When communicating with someone with PTSD it is essential to consistently demonstrate all aspects of Person/Family-centred Care:

- Be self-aware of your personal experience in resolving or not resolving your own emotions relating to any traumatic event/s in your own life.
- Demonstrate unconditional positive regard.

- Employ active listening.
- Use positive non-verbal messages.
- Clarify their understanding of any discussed procedures or information.
- Confront false beliefs and attitudes (if appropriate) to emphasise reality.

Strategies for communicating with a Person/s experiencing PTSD

Person/s with PTSD require specialised psychological intervention and often medication to reduce the severity of the symptoms.

- Provide education about the illness and include the significant others.
- Include significant others in discussions and, where appropriate, interventions.
- Listen and discuss the particular traumatic event if they initiate this conversation.
- Reinforce reality and discuss any negative thought patterns.
- Seek advice from their treating psychologist if unsure of how to proceed.
- Ensure consistency by maintaining regular contact with other healthcare professionals assisting the Person/s with PTSD.
- Reinforce appropriate strategies to manage the symptoms, including management of sleeping difficulties.
- Encourage positive thoughts about self and positive lifestyle habits.
- Encourage talking with others they trust for support.
- Reinforce their chosen relaxation techniques when discussing their life challenges.
- Reinforce principles of conflict resolution for their significant others.
- If they are not receiving specific assistance, explain where they can receive assistance.
- Educate all relevant parties about PTSD and strategies to manage the symptoms.

See the Introduction to Section 4 for instructions about how to use these scenarios for role-play or group discussion. Remember the principles of effective communication and Person/Family-centred Care.

Scenario one: The male and the healthcare professional

Person 1: You are 37-year-old Tom, who was previously a member of a national sports team. You are currently sitting in the waiting room waiting for an appointment with a healthcare professional. You are wondering what you will tell the healthcare professional today as last week they indicated that during the next appointment they wanted to talk with you about other ways to manage your symptoms. While waiting, your mind goes over a traumatic event that occurred some years ago. During this event you witnessed a severe car accident that caused the death of your beautiful wife, Beth, and your adorable 3-year-old son, Jordan. While you found this very traumatic at the time and experienced extreme amounts of guilt, you no longer relive the experience of trying but failing to remove Jordan, who was screaming uncontrollably from the car. You have resumed your life and are now happily married to Mel. You are expecting your first child together in a few weeks. Since you were told that this baby might have Down Syndrome you have begun experiencing nightmares again, in which you relive trying but failing to save Jordan. You have not told Mel about the nightmares, but she has begun asking you if everything is all right, saying you seem more withdrawn. She has also commented on the fact that you no longer take your morning jog, something you did every day regardless of your location or the weather, or watch the cricket, something you previously loved doing with her. You have begun experiencing aches and pains, so you have been seeing a healthcare professional, who has been assisting to resolve the symptoms. However, when one symptom resolves, another seems to begin. As the healthcare professional acknowledges they are ready for you, you remember that today they want to talk about other ways of resolving your symptoms. You are doubtful there is another way and do not really want to talk about your current emotional state. You believe your symptoms have a physical origin and do not relate to your current emotional distress.

Person 2: You are the healthcare professional who has seen Tom several times for a simple and treatable condition, which seems to resolve with the appropriate intervention. However, Tom keeps returning, indicating he has developed new symptoms or similar ones that require your assistance. You are wondering if there is something else troubling Tom, and last week mentioned to Tom that you want to explore other options, rather than provide the usual intervention at his next appointment.

Scenario two: The female and the respite volunteer

Person 1: Your name is Cindy and you are an only child. You are a 14-year-old girl who watched your father try to murder your mother a few months ago. Your father is now in prison, your mother is in hospital with fractured C3 and C4 vertebrae, and your grandparents live in the UK. The foster family you currently live with are caring, but you miss your mother. You visit her in hospital daily and she always appears pleased to see you, but she is not able to relate to you because of immobility, pain and emotional shock. Whenever you try to sleep at night you see the attempted murder scene all over again, and if you do sleep you usually cry yourself to sleep. At school you keep to yourself, you tell yourself it is because you do not want anyone except the principal and two teachers to know about the event. However, at the moment anything makes you cry and you find this embarrassing. In addition, you simply feel like you do not want to relate to people, so you say no when your friends ask you to go to the local shopping mall with them (something you previously loved doing with them). The shopping mall has bad associations for you since this traumatic event, as it was a family trip to that mall that triggered the event. You keep reliving it and it reminds you of how much you miss your mother.

Person 2: You are a trained volunteer assigned to provide respite for foster families. You usually enjoy this role and develop very good relationships with the adolescents for whom you provide respite. However, Cindy is very difficult to relate to – she is either emotionally withdrawn or cries with little provocation whenever you are with her. The foster family suggest this experience is not the first distressing experience for Cindy, but she will not talk to them about her previous life. You have a day scheduled with Cindy before she goes to the hospital and are thinking it might be good to go to the local shopping mall together.

2. Person/s with a spinal injury

Key words: spinal cord, paralysis, sensory loss, paraplegia, tetraplegia (quadriplegia), incontinence

Definition of spinal injury

A spinal injury occurs when there is damage to the spinal cord, affecting both the motor and sensory function. Damage above the first thoracic vertebra may cause tetraplegia and damage below may cause paraplegia. These two conditions relate to the inability to move or feel particular parts of the body.

Person/s most susceptible to spinal injury

Individuals involved in car accidents, plane crashes, diving accidents and particular types of sporting accidents

Possible emotions a Person/s with a spinal injury might experience

(These emotions typically change over time as the Person/s adjusts and develops life skills)

- Depression (want to die)
- Frustration
- Anger
- Fear
- Devastation
- Anxiety
- Despair
- Moodiness
- Isolation
- Feeling overwhelmed
- Shock
- Sentimental
- Grief
- Loss

Possible reasons for the emotions relating to having a spinal injury (to name a few!)

- Sudden unexpected injury
- Asking themselves, *"Why me?"*
- Lack of certainty about the future
- Inability to live life as they have previously
- Inability to care for self
- Fatigue
- Incontinence
- Change in sexual functioning
- Loss of their previous activities
- Inability to easily join friends
- Sometimes pain.

Possible behaviours typical of a Person/s with a spinal injury

These behaviours will vary depending on personality, social support and severity of damage.

- If unsure, they may not ask for clarification
- Avoid social interaction
- Avoid anything related to the cause of the injury
- Be reluctant to engage in their healthcare

- Be totally motivated to engage in healthcare
- Persevere to improve.

Principles of effective communication with a Person/s with a spinal injury

As with any person, whenever interacting with the Person/s or their significant others, it is essential to consistently demonstrate the characteristics of effective communication to achieve Person/Family-centred Care.

- Positive and engaged introduction to develop rapport
- Active listening and interest
- Validation of their emotions
- Empathy: verbal acknowledgement of their condition, exploration of associated symptoms
- Mutual understanding gained about their symptoms and perceived abilities
- Clarification and confirmation of their understanding of all procedures and future events
- Encouragement and affirmation of all their efforts and achievements.

Strategies of communication with a Person/s with a spinal injury

- Clear explanation of your role, allowing time for discussion and processing of all information
- Refer to other appropriate healthcare professionals as necessary
- Consider discussing what has happened since seeing you – the positive events and accomplishments
- Outline the plan for interventions, discuss any questions or concerns
- Remember to find reasons to laugh with the Person/s and their family.

It can sometimes be helpful to have another Person/s with a similar spinal injury but a few years after their injury, to regularly connect in-person with this individual.

In groups discuss: Why in-person interactions, not through social media?

Remember the principles of effective communication and Person/Family-centred Care.

Scenario one: The male and the healthcare professional

Person 1: Your name is Tran, and you are a 12-year-old adolescent from Vietnam. Your family has lived in Australia since you were 18 months old. You sustained an incomplete L2/3 spinal injury causing paraplegia, while playing ice hockey 7 weeks ago. You have not been able to feel or move your legs since then. You also have very little control of you bladder or bowel, which you find very embarrassing. You remember lying on your back for most of the last 7 weeks staring at the very boring ceiling – and although you are still not able to roll over in bed, two days ago you were allowed to sit up and now you can see your surroundings. Currently you need help to do this, because of the three fractured ribs, which hurt when you move you upper body. Your family visit every day – you wonder how your father is managing his business as you helped him after school the days you were not playing ice hockey. Whenever you think of ice-hockey you nearly cry (crying is something you do not do when other people are present) – you know you will never play it again, and playing on the national team like your older brother was your dream. Also, while you did not always enjoy school (the kids did not like you because you look different), you love maths and were about to represent your school in a state maths competition. You see several healthcare professionals every day and some weekly, but you cannot always understand the words they use. You grew up speaking Vietnamese, but speak English everywhere outside your home, so not understanding everything the staff say is confusing you. One, who has just begun seeing you, rarely speaks; however, this staff member has just come into your room.

Person 2: Before beginning the role-play choose an assessment relevant to your health profession requiring verbal interaction to use with Person 1/Tran.

You are a healthcare professional, who has been seeing Tran regularly for the last few days. He seems like a nice young man. You assume he has limited English, so while you are smiling and friendly, you rarely speak to him. However, today you must complete an assessment requiring Tran to talk. How will you manage the interaction today?

Scenario two: The female and the healthcare professional

Person 1: Your name is Joanna. You are a 16-year-old school student who sustained a complete C4/5 spinal injury causing tetraplegia (quadriplegia) following a fall during an international gymnastics competition. It is nearly 4 months post-injury. You have no control over your bowels or bladder, which is a little tiring! You do, however, have a little shoulder and elbow movement, but currently need assistance to do everything, except breathing, talking and thinking! You felt pleased with yourself when you were able to drink using a straw, if it is positioned appropriately for you. You have just begun rehabilitation at a new centre, everything is new, including the people! They all seem friendly enough, but you miss some of the people from the previous centre; they understood you, your feelings and your needs, and they had something planned every day. You miss playing computer games with your brother, Matt, who is two years younger than you. You also miss school and love your friends visiting. At first you thought you would not be able to think or talk about gymnastics again – but one of your friends is also on the national team and she visits regularly. She talks about some of her movement challenges in particular routines and you have been able to make appropriate suggestions to assist her. Every time she visits she is able to tell you that your suggestion has helped her to improve. You begin to think maybe you could be a gymnastics coach.

While you are adjusting to the move to the new centre, you want to go home and back to school as quickly as possible – you do not understand why you had to move. You have been here two days and not done anything!

Person 2: You are Ireni, a healthcare professional who is seeing Joanna for the first time. When you enter the room Joanna is lying down. You have been told Joanna appears to be a quiet and shy person, reluctant to engage with anyone at this centre. The notes from the previous service indicate Joanna is a happy girl with a sense of humour and committed to her healthcare goals. You need to establish rapport with Joanna and discuss plans relating to your healthcare profession.

3. Person/s with decreased cognitive function

(Key words: dementia, Alzheimer's disease, intellectual disability, addictive behaviours)
It is important to note that children with decreased cognitive function due to Down Syndrome or an intellectual disability do not fall into the same category as someone who has lost cognitive function because of ageing, head injury or addictive behaviours. Such children have specific needs, but are able to learn and are very able in many areas. Alternatively, in most cases, people experiencing a loss of cognitive function find it difficult to compensate for that loss after a particular level of deterioration.

Definition of decreased cognitive function

A Person with decreased cognitive function may be experiencing a mild, moderate or severe decrease in cognitive function.

A person with a *mild* decrease in cognitive function is someone who may:

- function independently
- choose to participate in the activities they perform well and enjoy
- perform their self-care activities
- assist others in basic tasks they enjoy performing
- understand others and express themselves to facilitate understanding
- develop and use compensatory strategies to participate and function
- learn and thus remember with repetition and perseverance
- "work" in a structured environment with varying levels of support
- enjoy social interaction.

A Person with a *moderate* decrease in cognitive function is someone who may:

- function with some level of assistance
- know what they enjoy performing, but may have difficulty making choices
- perform some self-care activities independently (e.g. dressing and toileting; may require a reminder to bathe)
- not always use words to communicate, but may understand others
- learn simple tasks with repetition and visual cues
- be able to "work" in a supported workplace with repetitive activities
- enjoy social interaction with particular familiar people.

A Person with a *severe* decrease in cognitive function is someone who may:

- require assistance with all personal care needs and with all other activities, except activities relating to mobility
- require constant supervision if they tend to wander and become lost
- be incoherent and unable to consistently communicate; however, may respond randomly to particular people, pictures or objects
- recognise familiar people they see constantly, but not consistently recognise others
- be repetitive in the sounds they make and in their behaviours
- be violent at particular times and sweet and passive at other times.

Individuals with decreased cognitive function most susceptible to experiencing difficulty when relating to a healthcare professional

A Person with a moderate decrease in cognitive function is most likely to experience difficulty when relating to a healthcare professional.

In groups, discuss and explain why.

Possible emotions a Person/s with decreased cognitive function might experience

A Person with decreased cognitive function might experience emotions related to:

- confusion and fear because of a change in routine
- unfamiliar environments and/or people, which may cause disturbed behaviour
- a lack of connection with reality.

Possible behaviours related to being a Person/s with decreased cognitive function

The behaviours of a Person with decreased cognitive function will vary according to the severity of the decrease in function. A Person with decreased cognitive function might:

- be illogical, irrational and unpredictable
- be perfectly happy sometimes
- repeat particular behaviours
- ask the same irrelevant questions repeatedly
- become easily distressed without provocation
- wander for no reason
- be violent – although not all individuals with a decrease in cognitive function will be violent
- behave in socially unacceptable ways.

Principles for effective communication with a Person/s with decreased cognitive function

When communicating with a Person with decreased cognitive function it is important to:

- demonstrate respect
- demonstrate empathy and understanding
- be consistent
- have a sense of humour
- give clear instructions with visual cues if necessary
- practise holistic communication.

Strategies for communicating with a Person/s with decreased cognitive function

- Invest time to develop a therapeutic relationship.
- Do not take anything personally that the person might say to you or about you.
- Consider the whole Person.
- Communicate gently and consistently.
- Avoid expressions of anger and frustration.
- Communicate with patience and a "go-with-the-flow" attitude.
- Aim to maintain a feeling of safety, happiness and comfort for the Person wherever possible.
- Remember they are generally unable to change the way they relate, how they behave and what they say.

Remember the principles of effective communication and Person/Family-centred Care.

Scenario one: The male and the healthcare professional

Person 1: Your name is Fred. You are 75 years old and you live alone in a large house. The major outing you have each week occurs when a bus collects you to attend a group for older persons. You are worried about where your wife has gone and what happened to the custard tarts you were going to eat with your cup of tea.

Person 2: You are the healthcare professional who has Fred in a weekly group. Fred is a friendly man; however, recently he has begun repeatedly asking you where his wife has gone (she died 10 years ago), and if you have eaten his custard tarts. Because Fred lives alone, you are very concerned about his safety and his ability to care for himself. You know his daughter visits daily, cleans his house and provides him with a hot meal. However, you are still concerned about his safety. Have a conversation with Fred and decide if he may be safer in the familiarity of his own home than elsewhere.

Scenario two: The female and the healthcare professional

Person 1: Your name is Sarah. Your mother, Irene, is 82 years old and is currently in a rehabilitation unit because she recently had a right cerebrovascular accident (CVA) or stroke. Prior to the stroke your mother and father, Harry, lived together in their house for 35 years. While your father is frail, he is mentally able and has been successfully caring for your mother with your support. You realise your mother has decreased cognitive function that was present before the stroke and has been worsened by the stroke, and that it might be suitable for her to be placed somewhere for people with her stage of dementia. However, you are worried about how your father will manage emotionally if they are separated in this permanent manner.

Person 2: You are Irene and you have little control over your behaviour. You often wander and disappear, only to be found undressing and trying to get into bed with any man you can find on a bed. Some of the males in the ward think it is amusing, while others find it disturbing.

Person 3: You are 86-year-old Harry. As Irene's husband of 53 years, you really want to continue caring for her. You do find her exhausting and are aware that you are not as strong as you once were. You feel you can continue caring for her with the support and assistance of your daughter.

Person 4: You are the healthcare professional who needs to speak with the family, including Irene, to determine whether she will return home or go to a high-dependency ward of a nursing home.

Working with individuals with decreased cognitive function can be both challenging and rewarding. However, such work – even on an occasional basis – does not suit all healthcare professionals.

4. Person/s experiencing a life-limiting illness and their family

(Key words: life-limiting illness, critical care, terminal illness, death, grief, loss, palliative care)

Facts about people who know they are dying and their families

A person who knows they are dying and the members of their family or circle of friends will experience emotions according to the "cycle of grief". Kubler-Ross (1969) and Kubler-Ross and Kessler (2005) suggested that there are stages of grief. However, it is now recognised that people who know they are dying can experience the emotions typical of a particular "stage" at various times throughout the process of the disease. They do not experience them in order, nor do they move through the emotions as though they are stages. They may experience them repeatedly before they reach acceptance. The emotions include denial, rage, resentment, envy, bargaining, depression and finally acceptance.

It is important to note that an individual experiencing loss of any kind may experience these emotions while attempting to grieve and adjust to the loss. Family members or friends of a Person who is dying usually experience the cycle of grief and the related emotions.

People who have a life-limiting illness often receive services from palliative care units. These units generally follow national policies, standards and guidelines specifically developed for palliative care situations (see Palliative Care Australia [www.palliativecare.org.au] or New Zealand Palliative Care Strategy [www.health.govt.nz/publication/new-zealand-palliative-care-strategy]).

The World Health Organization (WHO 2023) states that palliative care is an approach that improves the quality of life of people and their families facing the problems associated with a life-threatening illness. This is achieved through the prevention and relief of suffering by means of early identification and impeccable assessment, as well as treatment of pain and other problems (physical, psychosocial and spiritual).

WHO (2023) states that palliative care aims to assist people with life-limiting illnesses to experience quality of life until the moment of their death. Palliative care should provide relief from pain and other distressing symptoms. It should affirm life, but regard death as a normal part of life. Palliative care should neither hasten nor postpone death. Palliative care considers the whole Person, integrating psychological and spiritual care for the benefit of the Person and their family members. Palliative care is committed to supporting the family during the course of the illness and after death.

Core values of Palliative Care Australia

- Dignity of the Person, caregivers and each member of the family
- Respect and empowerment of all of these individuals
- Compassion for all involved individuals, regardless of age
- Equity in access to services
- Excellence of provision of care
- Family-centred Care.

Definition of a life-limiting illness

A Person with a life-limiting illness is someone who has 0–6 months to live. This may be due to:

- cancer
- a progressive neurological disorder
- end-stage cardiac, renal or respiratory disease
- AIDS
- other degenerative diseases
- experiencing a serious accident, attack or natural disaster
- experiencing an unexpected and serious life-threatening medical occurrence (e.g. stroke [CVA] or cardiac arrest [CA]).

Possible emotions a Person/s experiencing a life-limiting illness, their family members and friends might experience

A Person might experience emotions related to:

- bargaining (*If I do this it will cure me*)
- denial
- rage
- resentment
- envy

- depression
- anxiety
- confusion
- fear
- despair
- hopelessness
- desperation
- acceptance
- peace or agitation.

A Person experiencing a life-limiting illness may experience physical, emotional, social, cognitive and spiritual distress.
Physical distress may include:

- pain
- fatigue
- anorexia
- restlessness
- breathlessness
- oedema
- disfigurement
- loss of strength and range of movement
- bladder and bowel disturbances
- neurological dysfunction.

Psychological or emotional distress may include or be caused by:

- sadness
- shock
- uncertainty
- fear
- anxiety
- depression
- despondency
- loss of emotional control
- role changes
- loss and grief
- change in self-esteem
- change in body image.

Social distress may include:

- isolation
- lack of support
- financial issues
- family conflict
- inability to manage social situations
- inability to perform community-based or home-based tasks
- carer stress.

Cognitive distress may include:

- negative self-talk
- decreased cognitive function.

Spiritual distress may include:

- search for meaning
- crisis in faith
- asking:
  - *What is death?*
  - *What will death be like?*
  - *What about my life?*
  - *Is there life after death?*
- religion
- paranormal experiences
- review of priorities
- review of values.

Family members and friends may experience a range of emotions for many reasons also related to the components of the whole Person/s.

Possible behaviours a Person/s experiencing a life-limiting illness might exhibit

A Person experiencing a life-limiting illness will exhibit a range of behaviours that might include:

- acting as though nothing is wrong one day and being totally withdrawn the next
- being quiet and thoughtful one day and chatty the next
- forcing themself to do something, regardless of their pain or fatigue
- sleeping excessively because of pain medication, fatigue and depression
- being unable to sleep and thus being awake all night
- being short-tempered and dismissive towards carers and healthcare professionals
- being teary sometimes
- wanting to discuss spiritual issues or beliefs about life after death.

Principles for effective communication with a Person/s experiencing a life-limiting illness, their family members and friends

When communicating with a Person experiencing a life-limiting illness, or with their family and friends, it is important to:

- be self-aware – of your own values, beliefs and needs relating to experience of or thoughts about life-limiting illnesses
- demonstrate respect
- show empathy and compassion
- be silent when necessary
- listen actively
- be sensitive to non-verbal behaviours and voice
- touch if appropriate – hugs can be good
- demonstrate ethical behaviour
- provide company for the dying Person or for a family member or friend
- use an interdisciplinary approach – you cannot do it alone
- always behave with integrity and honesty.

Strategies for communicating with a Person experiencing a life-limiting illness or with their family and friends

- A family-centred approach is essential when someone is dying.
- A holistic approach is also vital when a Person is dying.
- Be committed to and aware of the quality of life of the Person.
- Be willing to discuss the practical aspects of dying.
- Be aware of personal limitations – the healthcare professional does not need to meet the needs of every Person seeking their assistance.
- Consider the need for debriefing at various times with other team members.

Remember the principles of effective communication and Person/Family-centred Care.

Scenario one: The male and the healthcare professional

Person 1: Your name is James and you are a 47-year-old pastry chef. You love working in your local bakery and have lots of friends who come into the shop. You contracted a virus eight months ago, which you thought was from walking for half an hour to work at 2.00 a.m. every day. However, the cough did not improve and you began to lose weight rapidly. After four months of having the terrible cough, the local doctor sent you for tests. You knew deep down there was something seriously wrong, but you did not want to think about it because it was less than a year since your mother had died unexpectedly.

Then, 2 months ago the doctors told you that you have final-stage cancer, an aggressive form of cancer that is in the major organs of your body and your lymphatic system. You know you have a limited time to live, but you do not know how long. You are home from hospital and you are struggling to get through each day. You try to do something every day – you go for a walk or talk to the neighbours, but you need to sleep a lot. Although you want to remain positive for the sake of your brothers and sister, it is very difficult to remain positive and you just want it all to end. You are confused, and while you want to think about dying, you are not sure what it means, what it will feel like and what will happen to you when you die. You have questions but no-one who you feel you can ask about them.

Person 2: You are a healthcare professional who lives next door to James. You see him over the back fence most days and try to encourage him to talk about what he is feeling and the things he wants to discuss. You are willing to talk about whatever he wants, even the spiritual issues he is facing.

Scenario two: The female and the healthcare professional

Person 1: Your name is Janice. Your mother died of breast cancer when she was 42 years old, a few years ago now. She was diagnosed, had treatment, lived for 5 years, then had a relapse and died 4 months after the recurrence of the cancer. The doctor has just told you that you have breast cancer. You are sure there was a mix-up with the pathology sampling and ask for more tests. It just cannot be true.

Person 2: You are the healthcare professional who has to tell Janice the result of the extra tests is positive – she does have breast cancer.

Many individuals who seek the assistance of a healthcare professional experience a sense of grief and loss – not always about their life, but about their identify and their ability to function or participate in life. Healthcare professionals who understand this reality can communicate more effectively with people experiencing a life-limiting illness, as well as people experiencing a loss of any kind. Please refer to p. 458 for references relating to life-limiting illness.

5. Person/s experiencing a mental illness

(Key words: mental illness, psychiatric, DSM-5, mental health)

Definition of a mental illness

A Person experiencing a mental illness is someone who for various psychosocial reasons is unable to manage the demands of life. People with particular conditions require assistance from a mental health service from time to time. Some of these conditions include anxiety, personality disorders, psychosis, paranoid schizophrenia, bipolar disorder, post-traumatic stress disorder, depression, alcoholism, drug addiction, obsessive compulsive disorder, phobias and combinations of the above.

Individuals most susceptible to experiencing a mental illness

The individuals susceptible to experiencing a mental illness include people who:

- have addictions
- have experienced previous episodes of any mental illness
- have a reduced sense of worth or self-esteem
- self-harm
- are suicidal
- believe someone is attempting to hurt them
- say they hear voices that tell them what they should do.

Individuals with a mental illness most susceptible to experiencing difficulty when relating to a healthcare professional

These individuals include:

- those who are acutely unwell
- those who have ceased taking their medication
- those who have been admitted against their will.

Possible emotions a Person/s with a mental illness might experience

A Person with a mental illness might experience emotions related to:

- rejection
- hopelessness
- changing cultures
- having no place to belong
- feeling undervalued
- loss of any kind
- never being "able" or competent

- paranoia
- cognitive dysfunction
- having always been told they were not good enough
- feelings of failure
- negative self-talk
- addiction
- loss and grief
- hallucinations
- failure to take medication
- reactions to medication.

Possible behaviours related to a Person/s experiencing a mental illness

A Person attending a mental health service may behave in a variety of ways depending on their condition, compliance with medication, current stability, the predictability of events in their life and their consistency of participation in health-sustaining behaviours.

A Person experiencing a mental illness might be:

- withdrawn with no desire or ability to relate
- aggressive and sometimes violent
- repetitive in actions or words
- behaving in a manner that does not indicate connection with reality
- perfectly coherent and conversant.

Principles for effective communication with a Person/s experiencing a mental illness

When communicating with a Person experiencing a mental illness it is important to:

- make introductions
- demonstrate respect
- show appropriate honesty
- give clear explanations
- confront if appropriate
- listen actively
- demonstrate unconditional acceptance.

Strategies for communicating with a Person/s experiencing a mental illness

- Explore and resolve your own personal biases relating to mental illness.
- Understand that the Person is vulnerable.
- Remember the Person is not always aware of the consequences of their behaviour.
- Do not take comments the Person makes personally.
- Do not believe the accusations of the Person about anyone else.
- Therapeutic groups can be effective.
- Outline clear and consistent expectations.
- Set clear and consistent boundaries.

Remember the principles of effective communication and Person/Family-centred Care.

Scenario one: The male and the healthcare professional

Matthew is a 28-year-old man who is addicted to alcohol and currently in hospital for detoxification. He has developed a good relationship with a male student healthcare professional. They have very different backgrounds, but are the same age and share common interests. The student visits Matthew one morning to find him writhing in pain, sweat pouring off his brow and looking terrible. Matthew seems desperate and surprises the student by grabbing his wrist. Matthew is trembling and he says that the doctor caring for him has not been assisting him. He pleads for a "drink", saying all he needs is one – just one would get him through this and he would never touch another drop.

The student feels sorry for Matthew; he knows Matthew has had a very tough life and feels he has suffered enough. He wants to help Matthew to stop him from suffering.

A nurse sees the student leaving Matthew's room and says, *You have to be careful of alcoholics when they are at this stage – they will do anything for a drink.* This comment seems unfeeling and callous to the student, who simply thinks that Matthew has suffered enough.

- What would you do?
- How would you feel if you were the student healthcare professional?
- What would you think if you learnt the student gave Matthew a drink?
- What would you think if you learnt the student was so disturbed by this situation he overused alcohol himself that night?

Scenario two: The male and the healthcare professional

Rod is a 56-year-old secondary school teacher who loves teaching mathematics. However, he has recently found the behaviour of some of the 15-year-olds upsets him and makes him angry. He is usually patient and understanding, able to relate well to the needs of young people. He is finding his impatience disturbing and has begun to think it means he is not a good teacher. He begins to feel discouraged about his ability to teach and to relate appropriately to the students. He believes he no longer has the ability to teach successfully and begins to feel he must find another profession. He feels he is too old to re-train, so he applies for a curriculum development position, but is unsuccessful. Several weeks after this, his mother and twin brother suddenly die in a car accident. He now often feels hopeless and alone. These emotions continue for over a year. He is constantly tired and finds it difficult to sleep. When asked if he is feeling unwell, he simply states he is tired. His wife, colleagues and friends notice he is withdrawn with limited affect. His wife notes that he seems depressed and suggests he seeks assistance. He says he is fine; however, several weeks later he unsuccessfully attempts suicide.

- What do you think? What would you do if you were Rod?
- How would you communicate with Rod?
- What do you feel is important when communicating with people similar to Rod?

Scenario three: The female and the healthcare professional

Mia is a 20-year-old woman with a history of treatment for anorexia. She is no longer haunted by the thoughts that caused the anorexia and is enjoying studying to be a healthcare professional. She has recently begun to experience what she describes as panic attacks. She says she knows she can successfully complete the courses in the program, but finds herself having these attacks whenever she thinks about the amount of work she has to complete. She says she has trouble breathing and her heart races, her palms become sweaty and she wants to vomit. The symptoms usually pass after a few hours, but they are occurring more frequently and lasting longer. She decides to ask a close friend for advice about this.

- What would you say to Mia?
- How would you relate to Mia?
- What elements of communication do you feel are important when relating to Mia?

There is a particular stigma associated with people who experience mental illness. Both the media and social misconceptions support and sustain this stigma. However, it is not the symptoms and behaviours associated with mental illness that are the focus of the healthcare professions, but rather human beings with particular needs and desires.

NOTE: It may be necessary to consider any stigma you personally feel about people experiencing a mental illness. It is essential you change that response to a positive one when interacting with people experiencing a mental illness.

6. Person/s experiencing long-term (chronic) and/or multiple physical conditions

(Key words: amputations, arthritis [e.g. psoriatic, rheumatoid or osteoarthritis], particular cardiac and/or respiratory conditions [e.g. cardiomyopathy or chronic obstructive pulmonary disease], cirrhosis of the liver, diabetes, some neurological conditions, strokes, traumatic or acquired brain injuries, persistent renal disease, surgery-induced conditions.)

The above key words are a few examples of the long-term or chronic conditions a Person/s may have when relating to healthcare professionals.

Definition of long-term or multiple physical conditions/comorbidity

A long-term or chronic condition is one that is of long duration with little change in symptoms or function, or it may be a condition with slow progression. Individuals with a long-term condition often develop other conditions related to their chronic condition, that is, a comorbid condition.

Susceptibility to acquiring long-term or multiple physical conditions

- Susceptibility varies depending on the hereditary status of previous generations and current family members, predisposing factors, age and in some instances gender.
- Arthritis may result from particular infections.
- Individuals who engage in extreme sports or extreme behaviours may acquire a long-term physical condition.

Individuals with long-term or multiple physical conditions most susceptible to experiencing difficulty when relating to a healthcare professional

Such individuals include those who:

- are experiencing constant pain with limited relief
- have a long history of relating to healthcare professionals

- are new to a service and have been referred because of evidence of a new condition or because of geographical relocation.

Possible emotions a Person/s with long-term or multiple physical conditions might experience

Emotions such individuals might experience include:

- frustration
- distress
- depression and despondency
- resignation
- anxiety about the future
- positive acceptance.

Possible reasons for these emotions

Reasons for these emotions might include:

- chronic pain
- repeated medication trials
- feeling like "a guinea pig!"
- acceptance of little improvement
- lack of certainty about their future
- lack of positive things to anticipate.

Possible behaviours typical of a Person/s with long-term conditions or comorbidities

Personality, age and culture can affect responses to having a long-term or chronic condition.

Person/s with a long-term or chronic condition may:

- seek opportunities to pursue particular activities
- withdraw from social interaction and demonstrate depressive symptoms
- enjoy spending time with particular friends or members of their family
- complain repeatedly, often about their pain or limitations
- be reluctant to relate to or engage with healthcare professionals
- avoid the activities or movements that might exacerbate their symptoms
- if diagnosed with such a condition at a young age, show resilience and adaptation to their limitations, demonstrating minimal limitations in daily life
- demonstrate behaviours similar to those experiencing loss.

Principles for effective communication with a Person/s experiencing long-term or multiple conditions

When communicating with a Person/s experiencing long-term or multiple conditions, it is important to use:

- clear and warm introductions to engender trust
- active listening and validation
- empathy through verbal acknowledgment of their condition and associated symptoms
- honesty without removing hope

- affirmation of their achievements
- encouragement
- clarification and to confirm their understanding of all procedures and future events.

Avoid saying: *You'll be OK.* or *Don't worry, I'm sure things will get better soon.*

Strategies for communicating with a Person/s experiencing long-term or multiple physical conditions

As with any person, it is essential the healthcare professional consistently demonstrates the characteristics of effective communication alongside Person/Family-centred Care whenever interacting with the Person/s or the significant people in their lives.

- Suggest strategies to them and their significant others to manage the many symptoms associated with their condition/s.
- After actively listening and validating their emotions, if appropriate, reinforce relevant strategies when the Person/s appears distressed about a particular symptom.
- Engage them in conversation about positive experiences they have had since you saw them last.
- If appropriate, involve any significant children in their interventions.

Remember the principles of effective communication and Person/Family-centred Care.

Scenario one: The male and the healthcare professional

Person 1: You are Hilton, a 76-year-old Aboriginal man married for 35 years to Deidre, a non-Indigenous person. You have a daughter who is a successful sociologist and academic, a son-in-law who is a mechanic and three grandchildren aged 5, 7 and 11. In your youth you were an Olympic-class athlete and very active, swimming and jogging every day, along with playing competition squash. You have worked all your life as a mechanic and really love this work. Many years ago you were diagnosed with diabetes and are now insulin-dependent; however, this has not previously affected your daily life. Ten years ago you suddenly developed multiple physical disorders that limited your physical activities and reduced your level of fitness. These conditions include psoriatic, rheumatoid and osteoarthritis, high blood pressure, a left-sided stroke and a large hernia. These have resulted in many surgical procedures and admissions to hospital. Some of the procedures included bilateral knee replacements and removal of around 30 cm of your bowel. You live for your three grandchildren: the eldest is school captain this year, and you love attending things at the school whenever possible because you are so proud of your granddaughter. However, your pain levels have made this difficult in the last few months. You are currently recovering from a shoulder replacement after eight months of pain from a fall and an unsuccessful shoulder reconstruction. You have *not* been told what to expect and your arm is *not* recovering at the rate you had expected from comments made by the surgeon: *You will not know yourself; you will have a perfect shoulder after this.* You are feeling sore, uncertain and depressed, and you find the pain difficult to tolerate at night. You are expecting a visit from a healthcare professional today, but you are becoming impatient with healthcare professionals (even though you are usually very patient) who relate to you from their stereotypes of Aboriginal people and who also indicate they think you should be back to "normal" when you are not – despite taking the precautions and doing all the exercises.

Person 2: You are a healthcare professional going to visit Hilton, an Aboriginal man who you have never met before. You are sure his shoulder will be almost back to normal as that is the expected recovery rate for shoulder replacements. When you arrive, a woman answers the door and takes you in to see a man who has skin you believe is too pale for him to be an Aboriginal man, and even though this man has a wrapped shoulder indicating he could be Hilton, you ask to see Hilton. They look shocked and indicate the person in front of you is Hilton. You feel embarrassed and wonder how you can overcome the possible offence you may have caused them and develop some rapport.

Scenario two: The female and the healthcare professional

Person 1: You are Caroline and you have epilepsy, which you developed as a child. You are a shy, modest person who does not usually like meeting new people. You have been married to Mick, a bioscientist, for 25 years. He married you knowing you had epilepsy and always said that did not worry him. In the last 25 years your cognitive functioning has deteriorated because of the severity and uncontrollable nature of your seizures (you have endured many tests and regimens to try to control them – to limited effect). You are currently able to manage the necessary household tasks and you make a wonderful lasagne, considered by your in-laws to be very authentic Italian lasagne. Mick always assists you with the shopping, and you sometimes become disoriented if you leave the house alone. You have become more childlike in some of your responses and you often find your mother-in-law, Maria, very frustrating and unreasonable in her demands of Mick. Mick is the eldest son of an Italian family. When you married him you did not realise that meant his mother would live with you if something happened to his father and Maria was not able to manage in her own home. Maria also has decreased cognitive functioning that makes her quite demanding and often appear rude. Maria found it very difficult that Mick married you as you were not Italian, and when she realised you had epilepsy she tried to persuade Mick not to marry you. She finally accepted you into the family and speaks fondly about you to everyone. You are currently in hospital because there have been some recent changes in treatment of your type of epilepsy, but that means more tests and you are experiencing fear and confusion. You have been through many tests before and there has been little change, and you feel this admission is also hopeless and a waste of time. You are also very agitated because you have been placed in a ward with two men and you find that very difficult. You wish Mick could be with you all day and count the minutes until he arrives every afternoon. You sometimes find yourself thinking that even a visit from Maria would be better than being in this room with these noisy men, who do not always close the door when they go to the toilet and each have the television on different channels. You are scheduled for the longest and most tiring test today and thus are feeling more vulnerable than usual. You do not want to talk to anyone except Mick, and are determined you will not relate to the unfamiliar healthcare professional who has just come to talk with you.

Person 2: You have not previously met Caroline, but have to gather some information about her history before she has the test. You realise she may be frustrated with all the healthcare professionals asking her questions, but you have not had time to check her records and want to build rapport and understand Caroline, as you will be relating to her after her discharge.

7. Person/s experiencing a stroke

(Key words: stroke, paralysis, numbness)

Definition of a stroke

A stroke occurs when there is either reduced flow of blood to the brain (ischaemic stroke) or sudden bleeding within the brain (haemorrhagic stroke).

Possible symptoms a Person/s with a stroke might experience:

- Muscular: paralysis and/or weak muscles on one side of the body, difficulty walking, problems with coordination, stiff muscles, overactive reflexes
- Visual: blurred vision, double vision, sudden visual loss, or temporary loss of vision in one eye
- Whole body: fatigue, light-headedness, or vertigo
- Speech: some have difficulty speaking with slurred speech, or speech loss
- Sensory: pins and needles or reduced sensation of touch in the affected side of the body
- Facial: muscle weakness or numbness particularly on one side of the body
- Limbs: numbness or weakness on the affected side of the body
- Comprehension: difficulty understanding words and sometimes actions
- Incontinence
- Also possible: balance disorder, difficulty swallowing, headache, inability to understand, mental confusion, or rapid involuntary eye movement

Possible emotions a Person/s with a stroke might experience

- Confusion
- Depression and despondency
- Distress
- Despair
- Hopelessness
- Frustration
- Loneliness
- Anxiety
- Some may experience resignation (*This is my life now!*)
- Some might try to find ways to "make the best" of their situation.

Possible reasons for these emotions

- Lack of certainty about what will happen in the future (*Will I ever be able to live life again?*)
- Inability to understand or be understood
- Inability to move one side of the body
- Difficulty eating (problems chewing food and swallowing)
- Wonder if the feeling in their body will ever return
- Inability to complete everyday tasks: for example, walking, showering, dressing, eating

- Unsure of what people are doing
- No familiar people while in hospital
- Unsure how the family will manage if there is no improvement
- Not wanting to be a burden on the family
- Fatigue after doing anything.

Principles for effective communication with a Person/s who has had a stroke

When communicating with a Person/s who has experienced a stroke, it is important to:

- consider the importance of the non-verbal messages of all healthcare professionals
- demonstrate compassion and respect
- indicate when you will touch the Person, before touching them
- when speaking – use only a few simple words, stating them slowly and clearly
- validate their emotions wherever possible
- always affirm any achievement – often by clapping if words are not understood
- actively listen to any attempts to speak – trying to understand and repeating the word/s
- encourage them to keep trying to develop particular function.

Strategies for communicating with a Person/s who has had a stroke

As with any Person, it is essential the healthcare professional consistently demonstrates the characteristics of effective communication alongside Person/Family-centred Care whenever interacting with the Person/s or the significant people in their lives.

- When appropriate, as encouragement, introduce them to someone who has had a stroke some time ago and is recovering some function, including walking.
- Suggest strategies to them and their significant others to manage the many symptoms and related difficulties associated with their condition/s.
- Carefully observe their non-verbal messages and validate their emotions.
- If appropriate, reinforce relevant strategies (way to manage or overcome) when the Person appears distressed about a particular symptom.
- Where possible and appropriate, involve any significant family members in their interventions.

Remember the principles of effective communication and Person/Family-centred Care.

Scenario one: The male and the healthcare professional

Person 1: You are Kim, a 78-year-old Vietnamese man who is recovering from a recent stroke. You were discharged home a few days ago. You have limited movement in your right arm, but are now able to walk with a walking stick. You have limited English, but have been able to understand most of what is said by the Vietnamese interpreter, who assists when relating to English speakers. You are finding it difficult to shower and dress yourself. This means you only shower once a week and your wife helps you. You do not always change your pyjamas, only when someone is visiting. This has also meant you do not attend the appointments made for you with allied health staff at the health service. You are able to swallow, but you have difficulty chewing. You wife makes you liquid food every mealtime. You have difficulty sleeping due to the spirits of your previous wives keeping you awake. This makes it difficult to keep doing your exercises due to fatigue. You are expecting a healthcare professional to visit today. This has meant you have made sure your wife has helped you with showering and dressing. You are sitting waiting in a comfortable chair.

Person 2: You are the healthcare professional visiting Kim today. You can speak Vietnamese, so there is no need for an interpreter. You are hoping Kim will have improved since his discharge. However, he has not attended any of the appointments at the health service since his discharge.

PLEASE NOTE: for this role play – use English when acting the roles, as you may not speak Vietnamese!!

Scenario two: The female and the healthcare professional

Person 1: You are Rosemary, a 68-year-old, previously fit lady who had a stroke affecting her non-dominant side, a week ago. You are still dazed and confused, often crying. You understand that you had a stroke, but are very withdrawn and reticent to relate to any staff from the health service. You are not completely paralysed, having some movement in both your affected arm and your leg. However, you have lost strength in both limbs, with reduced control of your movements. You are able to verbalise and understand what people say to you.

You cannot stop thinking about a dear friend of yours who died a few weeks after having a stroke. You are afraid you will die in the next few weeks. You also think about your grandchildren, who you enjoy minding after school 3 days a week. You cry whenever you think about not being able to do that. You are sure that if you do not die, you may not be able to care for them again. You wonder if you will be able to walk, drive, prepare meals, even eat, as at the moment you find chewing and swallowing difficult. You cry whenever you think of all these things. You currently live alone in your own house, since your husband died, and you do NOT want to move or be a burden on your family.

You have no idea what will happen or how you will manage your everyday life.

Person 2: You are a healthcare professional who has been seeing Rosemary every day since her admission. She seems to be relatively happy when you come into her room and does not cry or disengage when you talk to her. Today you have to talk to her about moving her to a rehabilitation centre as she has potential to regain some functioning in her arms and legs. You know from experience that this may take a few months.

8. Person/s experiencing a hearing impairment

(Key words: hearing loss, deafness, hard of hearing, deaf, industrial deafness, Auslan, New Zealand Sign Language, American Sign Language)

Definition of a hearing impairment

A Person with a hearing impairment is someone who:

- finds verbal or aural communication difficult because of an inability to hear
- finds comprehension of cultural cues difficult to understand because of a hearing impairment.

Individuals most susceptible to a hearing impairment

The individuals susceptible to experiencing a hearing impairment are:

- unborn babies with family members who are deaf – hereditary
- babies who do not develop appropriately in utero – congenital
- babies who have undetected meningitis

- premature infants who receive antibiotics with ototoxic side effects
- individuals who experience trauma to the head or neck
- individuals who experience an industrial accident
- children with recurring undetected or untreated ear infections
- individuals who do not wear earmuffs in areas of high noise
- older people who experience age-related hearing loss
- individuals from countries that do not have work, health and safety standards to protect their hearing
- individuals from countries or regions that have limited health services.

Possible emotions a Person/s with a hearing impairment might experience

Emotions such individuals might experience include:

- anger
- frustration
- rejection
- fear
- confusion
- vehemence and stubbornness
- isolation
- anxiety.

Possible reasons for these emotions

A Person with a hearing impairment might experience these emotions because of:

- seeing what is happening, but not being able to hear or understand everything
- having people shout at them because they think speaking loudly will assist their ability to hear
- people talking too quickly and/or with unclear articulation when they are trying to lip-read
- people talking to the hearing people in a situation, but not including the Person with a hearing impairment
- people speaking or signing to an interpreter rather than to the individual with the hearing impairment.

Principles for effective communication with a Person/s experiencing a hearing impairment

When communicating with a Person experiencing a hearing impairment, it is important to:

- show patience and perseverance – keep trying to achieve understanding
- avoid responding with frustration
- clarify understanding – avoid making assumptions about the meaning
- validate
- disengage effectively – this is very important
- avoid using humour, as subtle nuances of language associated with humour are difficult to perceive, understand or explain
- use predictable and well-articulated speech if the Person is lip-reading.

Possible behaviours typical of a Person/s experiencing a hearing impairment

A Person with a hearing impairment will exhibit different behaviour according to the age at which they developed their impairment, whether they grew up in the deaf community or a hearing population, whether they have learnt to lip-read, and whether they can read and write. Sources of information on hearing impairment are listed in Table 27.1 overleaf.

A Person with a hearing impairment might:

- often communicate with strong non-verbal gestures and facial expressions
- make intense efforts to be understood, sometimes appearing aggressive
- appear rude or inappropriate if they do not hear many auditory cues (the social or cultural cues of hearing people may have different meaning or no meaning to an individual with a hearing impairment)
- demonstrate behaviour typical of mistrust
- behave in a stubborn manner.

Strategies for communicating with a Person/s experiencing a hearing impairment

- Use alternative methods of communication if you do not share a common language.
- If working with individuals who have a hearing impairment on a regular basis, consider learning the appropriate sign language for your country (e.g. Auslan [Australian Sign Language] for Australia and some of the Pacific).
- Try to communicate, even if you do not understand.
- Use written words or pictures wherever possible.
- If communicating with someone who lip-reads, stand directly in front of them, articulate clearly and speak at a steady pace.
- Do not assume they want to have good hearing, because lack of hearing may be part of their identity.

Remember the principles of Person/Family-centred Care.

Scenario one: The male and the healthcare professional

Simon is a 10-year-old boy who was diagnosed with a severe hearing impairment at the age of six. The hearing impairment was discovered during a routine medical check-up at school. By that time Simon had been labelled as having a behaviour problem, because he would never sit still to listen in class and was always the last to finish any work. His written work was good when he could copy, but he was never able to write a story or read words.

Simon has always been a child who loves to move and thus he rarely played games that required hearing. He rarely spoke before attending school, but seemed to understand spoken words and instructions. He is a loving boy and has a supportive mother who trained as a teacher's aide to assist him with his schoolwork. He has recently had cochlear implants, which have restored 70 per cent of his hearing in both ears. However, Simon is still behind other children his age with his schoolwork and requires constant assistance with his work.

- How will you relate to Simon?
- What will be your goals in communicating with him?

Scenario two: The female and the healthcare professional

Rhonda is a 24-year-old beautician. She was born without hearing to parents who could hear. They did not consider that Rhonda should learn sign language and insisted she learn to lip-read and verbalise. They sent her to a non-specialist local school with her siblings. Rhonda learnt to read and write, as well as lip-read. She is intelligent and thus is able to compensate for her hearing impairment by guessing the meaning of situations if she cannot actually understand. She is determined and has studied hard to become a beautician. She is very difficult to understand when she speaks, and, in an attempt to be understood, she often repeats words. She is confident, but very moody when others are talking without including her. According to the culture of the hearing population, her non-verbal behaviours are exaggerated and often appear rude.

- How will you relate to Rhonda?
- What will be your goals when communicating with her?

There are many different sign languages worldwide. Within Australia there are two main dialects of Auslan. The northern dialect is based on French Sign Language and the southern dialect on British Sign Language. New Zealand Sign Language was adopted as the official sign language of New Zealand in 2006. Sign languages are languages in their own right, unrelated to the spoken language of the people who live in the same country. (Auslan, for example, is not the same as Signed English, which uses a sign to represent each English word.)

Users of sign languages use signs to indicate particular meanings and may express a whole concept with one sign, where it might take many words to express the same concept in a

TABLE 27.1
Sources of information on hearing impairment

Australia	
Australian Hearing	www.hearing.com.au
Auslan Sign Bank (Royal Institute for Deaf and Blind Children)	www.auslan.org.au
New Zealand	
Deaf Association of New Zealand	www.deaf.org.nz
National Foundation for the Deaf and Hard of Hearing	www.nfd.org.nz
United States	
National Association of the Deaf	www.nad.org
United Kingdom	
Royal Society for Deaf People	www.royaldeaf.org.uk

spoken language. Each sign language also has alphabet signs for fingerspelling. Many use a two-handed method of spelling letter by letter. However, American Sign uses a one-handed fingerspelling system. Alphabet signing/fingerspelling is a small component of signing for sign language users, only used if needing to communicate an English name or word, or with people who are not fully competent in the sign language.

Individuals who are born with a hearing impairment into a hearing population have a very different identity to individuals born deaf into a community of deaf individuals ("the Deaf community"). The Deaf community believe that being deaf is part of their identity and are sometimes vehement about maintaining that identity. Thus, they may choose not to have cochlear implants, despite the possibility of being able to hear.

9. Person/s experiencing a visual impairment

(Key words: visual loss, blindness, blind, visual impairment)

Definition of a visual impairment

A Person/s with a visual impairment is someone who:

- is unable to experience the world visually because of a loss of visual acuity – the ability to see clearly
- has less than 6/60 corrected visual acuity in both eyes
- has a field of vision constricted to less than 10 degrees of arc around the central fixation in either eye.

Individuals most susceptible to a visual impairment

The individuals most susceptible to a visual impairment are those who:

- have a family disposition to blindness
- have degenerative eye conditions
- have congenital causes
- experience trauma to the head or face
- experience an industrial accident
- have repeated and untreated eye infections
- are children with poor nutrition
- are children who live in environmentally deprived situations
- do not wear goggles in designated work areas
- are from countries that do not have work, health and safety standards to protect their sight
- have diabetes
- are children with juvenile diabetes
- are from countries or regions that have limited health services.

Possible emotions a Person/s experiencing a visual impairment might experience

A Person/s with a visual impairment might experience emotions related to:

- interest or curiosity
- insecurity
- confusion
- frustration

- fear
- sadness
- envy
- resentment
- helplessness
- determination.

Possible reasons for these emotions

A Person with a visual impairment might experience these emotions because of:

- other people assuming they know their needs
- other people assuming they must require assistance because they are blind
- strangers feeling sorry for them
- hearing things, but being unable to see them
- hearing threatening sounds to which they cannot respond because they cannot see the cause
- having limited control when in unfamiliar situations.

Possible behaviours related to a Person/s experiencing a visual impairment

A Person with a visual impairment will exhibit different behaviour according to the age at which they developed the visual impairment – whether they were born with no sight or lost their sight at a later age, whether they experienced special education specifically designed for people with visual loss, and whether they can read and write.

A Person with a visual impairment might:

- move confidently with particular self-controlled assistance
- move timidly when in an unfamiliar environment
- have limited facial and non-verbal behaviours, depending on the situation
- show well-adjusted behaviour and ease of mobility.

A Person who is losing their vision slowly might:

- walk close to a wall
- have poor posture
- move hesitantly or with short steps
- squint or tilt their head
- spill or knock over food and other items
- bump into objects
- look closely at items such as printed material
- request changes in lighting
- be sensitive to light
- easily become lost
- be unable to find items
- no longer recognise people by sight
- demonstrate altered emotional states, such as anxiety, tearfulness, frustration and embarrassment
- stop taking care of their appearance
- stop socialising in a group
- stop reading or sewing
- stop participating in activities.

Principles for effective communication with a Person/s experiencing a visual impairment

When communicating with a Person experiencing a visual impairment, it is important to:

- touch – remember to ask permission first
- validate
- clarify
- ensure use of physical contact to demonstrate your presence if using silence
- provide information – use Braille or computer technology if appropriate
- verbally disengage.

Strategies for communicating with a Person/s experiencing a visual impairment

- Identify yourself – do not assume the Person will recognise you by your voice.
- Speak naturally and clearly. Loss of eyesight does not mean loss of hearing.
- Continue to use body language. This will affect the tone of your voice and give a lot of extra information to the person.
- Use everyday language. Do not avoid words like "see" or "look" or talking about everyday activities, such as watching television or DVDs or streaming services.
- Name the Person when introducing yourself or when directing conversation to them in a group situation.
- In a group situation, introduce the other people present.
- Never channel conversation through a third person.
- Never leave a conversation with a Person without saying you are doing so.
- Use accurate and specific language when giving directions, for example, *The door is on your left* rather than *The door is over there.*
- Avoid situations where there is competing noise.
- Always ask if they require assistance – do not assume they do.
- In dangerous situations say *Stop* rather than *Look out.*
- Relax and be yourself.
- Do not assume you know what they want or what will help them. Ask them.

Remember the principles of effective communication and Person/Family-centred Care.

Scenario one: The male and the healthcare professional

Person 1: Ronny lives in a rural area. He is 64 years old and last week received the diagnosis of trachoma after experiencing conjunctivitis for some time. He lives with his extended family. There is only one income to support seven people. He is happy, but finds his fading vision disturbing because he is not as mobile these days and loves watching the local children play in the schoolyard next to his house. He finds it difficult to watch television, but has it turned on for company when the others are away.

Person 2: You are the healthcare professional who needs to have a conversation with Ronny and collaborate to set achievable goals. You know that his visual loss may be permanent.

- What is important for Ronny?
- What might you need to know in order to assist him to maintain meaning in his life?

Scenario two: The female and the healthcare professional

Person 1: Your name is Tania and you are a 24-year-old woman with an Indigenous background. You are a well-respected early intervention teacher who manages a local preschool. You love everything about your job – the paperwork, the children, the parents, seeing the children develop skills and grow taller, as well as having them proudly display their work before they leave each day. The parents, staff and children say you have excellent skills in observing and interpreting the non-verbal cues of children, parents and staff. However, you have recently lost your vision after an accident and have not been able to work. Your boyfriend of four years – now your fiancé – is supportive, but you sense he is afraid and unsure of your future together.

Person 2: You are meeting Tania for the first time and you want to assist her to establish some appropriate short-term and long-term goals.

Sources of information on visual impairment are listed in Table 27.2.

TABLE 27.2
Sources of information on visual impairment

Australia	
Vision Australia	www.visionaustralia.org
See Differently (Royal Society for the Blind)	www.seedifferently.org.au
New Zealand	
Blind Low Vision NZ (Royal New Zealand Foundation of the Blind)	blindlowvision.org.nz

References

Life-limiting illness

Kubler-Ross, E., 1969. On death and dying. Routledge, London.

Kubler-Ross, E., Kessler, D., 2005. On grief and grieving: Finding the meaning of grief through the five stages of loss. Simon & Schuster, London.

New Zealand Palliative Care Strategy. Online. Available at: www.health.govt.nz/publication/new-zealand-palliative-care-strategy

Palliative Care Australia. Online. Available at: www.palliativecare.org.au

World Health Organization (WHO), 2023. Palliative care essential facts. Online. Available at: www.who.int/health-topics/palliative-care

CHAPTER 28

Person/s in particular contexts

Chapter objective

Upon completing this chapter, readers should be able to apply knowledge and have emerging skills in communicating effectively with Person/s in particular contexts.

Healthcare professionals assist vulnerable people in a range of contexts. This chapter considers people in five contexts that may be a barrier to effective communication: an emergency, people living in an aged-care facility, domestic abuse, people who are homeless, and those with a different language to the healthcare professional.

Particular contexts

1 People experiencing an emergency
2 People living in an aged care residential facility
3 People experiencing domestic abuse
4 People who are homeless
5 People with a different language to the healthcare professional.

- Decide what it means to be a Person in these contexts.
- Choose one of five options:
  - List the specific behaviours that might relate to being a Person who experiences an emergency, *or*
  - Suggest the emotions a Person recently relocated to a residential aged care facility might experience, *or*
  - List the emotions a Person experiencing domestic abuse might experience when relating to a health service, *or*
  - Suggest the emotions a Person who is homeless might experience when relating to a health service, *or*
  - Discuss which individuals may be most susceptible to the emotions associated with not being able to speak the language of the healthcare professional.

- List possible reasons that might explain the emotions a Person in these contexts might experience when seeing a healthcare professional.
- List principles for effective communication to remember when communicating with a Person in these contexts. Give reasons for the need to remember these principles.
- Suggest strategies for communicating with a Person in these contexts. Decide why you might see such a Person in your particular health profession.
- Check your answers against the information below, noting any additional thoughts or ideas.

1. A Person/s who experiences an emergency

Definition of a Person/s who experiences an emergency

(Key words: emergency, near-death experience, accident, disaster, attack, trauma)

A Person who experiences an emergency is someone who experiences suddenly adverse bodily harm because of an accident, attack or natural disaster. This may occur because of a myocardial infarction (heart attack), sudden onset of a stroke (cerebral vascular accident) or a sudden onset of or deterioration in any medical condition.

Behaviours related to being a Person/s who experiences an emergency

A Person who experiences an emergency might be:

- impatient and angry, even aggressive
- irrational and incoherent due to shock
- chatty and apparently unconcerned
- quiet and unresponsive
- frustrated – expressed verbally or non-verbally
- completely passive.

Individuals most susceptible to emergencies

The individuals most susceptible to emergencies are anyone who lives, breathes and moves, regardless of age, racial group and gender! However, people may be especially susceptible to emergencies if they:

- play sport or do extreme sports (e.g. mountain climbing, abseiling)
- drive
- work with machinery, whether in cities or rural areas
- are involved in violent encounters.

Possible emotions a Person/s who experiences an emergency might experience

A Person who experiences physical or emotional harm because of an emergency may feel:

- fear
- anger

- shock
- guilt
- despondency
- impatience
- disbelief
- anxiety
- frustration from being asked to answer the same questions by different healthcare professionals
- a lack of control over the things being done to them.

Principles for effective communication with a Person/s who experiences an emergency

When communicating with a Person who experiences an emergency, it is important to:

- make introductions
- demonstrate empathy to build a therapeutic relationship
- validate the Person and their experience
- provide and explain information
- remember that such people are often in pain and may be impatient and angry if asked the same questions repeatedly; instead, make statements to verify the gathered information
- recognise that shock can affect the cognitive functioning of an individual
- recognise that the Person may respond differently to their actual feelings if medicated for pain
- verify or clarify the interpretations of perceptions
- comfort and reassure through encouragement – they may be afraid of the implications of the emergency for their future
- remember that the Person may experience social isolation in hospital if they were airlifted from a rural area
- remember the Person did not intend to have or cause the accident.

Strategies for communicating with a Person/s who experiences an emergency

- Consider the whole Person – they will have more than physical needs.
- Observe the non-verbal behaviours of the Person closely and ask for verification or clarification of the interpretations of those perceptions.
- Gather information from notes and other healthcare professionals rather than asking the same questions repeatedly. If unsure about the accuracy of the information, make statements and ask for verification; this allows the Person to simply nod or affirm in some manner.
- Give non-verbal cues or visual indication of what is happening or what the Person needs to do.
- Express sensitivity and compassion, regardless of the cause of the emergency.
- Remember the family members of people seriously hurt because of an emergency – they are often terrified and have feelings of helplessness.

See the Introduction to Section 4 for instructions about how to use these scenarios for role-play or group discussion. Remember the principles of effective communication and Person/Family-centred Care. Before acting the roles, you may wish to decide what type of assistance Person 1 requires. If it is not possible to role-play these scenarios, consider and explore the possible responses and communication strategies that will achieve effective communication and Person/Family-centred Care.

Scenario one: The male and the healthcare professional

Person 1: Your name is Malcolm. You are a 28-year-old man who shattered your right tibia and fibula playing football. You are no longer in the acute ward, but you vividly remember your experience in the emergency department (ED).

You arrived in an ambulance, were hurriedly transferred to a cubicle in ED, with the curtains drawn and left alone in pain for what seemed like hours. Thirsty and exhausted, you realised you wanted to go to the toilet. You were not comfortable calling for help. Finally, a nurse came in with a tray. Without introducing himself, he asked particular questions and filled in a form. Then, without explaining what he was doing, he rolled up your sleeve. You pulled your arm away, not sure what was coming next. He grabbed the tray and left. As he disappeared through the curtains you quickly said you needed to go to the toilet. You heard the nurse *say The one with the broken leg is uncooperative and wants a bottle.* Sometime later a different nurse arrived with a bottle. Every person who came in after that asked you the same questions. There were several hours of waiting and your lower back was hurting. A doctor finally arrived. She examined you and asked the same old questions. She explained you would need surgery, which would take place in about an hour. There were no explanations of anything and no time to ask questions or find out what happened to your expensive football boots. Your parents were an hour away and you had just terminated your relationship with your girlfriend of 5 years. You thought about how you were studying full-time and working part-time doing deliveries. You lay in emergency worrying about how you would pay your rent, drive your car and continue your studies. You felt lonely and unloved.

You are now attending a rehabilitation service and find it difficult to trust most healthcare professionals because of the treatment you received on that first day, the day you broke your leg during that tackle. You are meeting a new healthcare professional today. You are not interested in another change – it will mean more of the same questions.

Person 2: You are the healthcare professional assigned to assess Malcolm. You have heard he is not trusting and, although motivated to improve, he is often sullen and reluctant to develop a relationship.

Scenario two: The female and the healthcare professional

Person 1: Your name is Rachel and you are a solicitor in a big law firm. You are 40 years old and divorced, with two children aged 12 and 14 who live with you every alternate week. Your parents are ageing and quite frail. While you were driving to work a young driver drove through a red light, hitting the driver's door next to you. You fractured four ribs and your right femur and lost some teeth in the accident. You are now in an emergency department. You are very worried about your children and the future, including paying the mortgage for your recently purchased, beautiful new apartment. You cannot think clearly or remember what has happened since the accident. Fear, anxiety and pain limit your ability to concentrate and understand what is happening around you.

Person 2: You are the healthcare professional who must explain a procedure or future event to Rachel.

Group discussion

As a large group, discuss the observations, emotions and outcomes of the role-plays. Suggest possible alternative strategies that may increase the effectiveness of the communication in a similar situation.

Not all healthcare professionals relate to people who experience emergencies immediately after the emergency. However, many will communicate with people who remember the experience of an emergency, either as a victim or an observer. Such individuals require communication that considers the various aspects of their lives influencing their everyday roles, participation and functioning.

2. A Person/s living in a residential aged care facility

Definition of a Person/s living in a residential aged care facility

A Person living in a residential aged care facility is typically, but not always, over 80 years of age, who cannot live with their family or is unable to afford a live-in carer.

Individuals most susceptible to living in a residential aged care facility

- Person/s living alone requiring regular monitoring to maintain safe daily functioning
- Person/s with chronic health conditions limiting their safe functioning at home
- Frail Person/s who are ageing and losing their functional capacity.

Possible behaviours related to being a Person/s living in a residential aged care facility

- Sitting quietly in a public area
- Watching television in their room all day
- Wandering around going into any room with the door open
- Talking to anyone who looks at you whether or not you know them
- Sitting in a public place talking to everyone.

Possible emotions a Person/s living in a residential aged care facility might experience

(These emotions may depend on the circumstances surrounding the move to the facility.)

- Happiness and contentment
- Comfortable
- Peaceful
- Neglected
- Angry
- Despair
- Fear

- Isolation and loneliness
- Rejection
- Conflict and ambivalence

Possible reasons for these emotions

- Grieving the loss of their "home"
- Financial drain
- Inability to see significant members of their family or social group regularly
- The food is not their preferred choice!

Principles for effective communication with a Person/s living in a residential aged care facility

When communicating with a Person living in a residential aged care facility, it is important to:

- clearly demonstrate empathy
- validate their feelings about residing in an aged care facility
- develop rapport and a therapeutic relationship
- consistently use active listening.

Strategies for communicating with a Person/s living in a residential aged care facility

- Encourage them to find reasons to enjoy their days
- Discuss the positive aspects of their life
- Avoid disagreeing with the Person
- Avoid saying they should be in this facility
- If possible, refer them for regular attendance at a program for older adults.

Remember the principles of effective communication and Person/Family-centred Care.

Scenario one: The male and the healthcare professional

Person 1: You are an 80-year-old man called Michael. Until recently you were living at home in a single-storey house with your 78-year-old wife, Elaine. You are quite a heavy man and your wife, while active and involved in many community activities, is not very strong. You have also been forgetting things lately and often going outside and forgetting why you are outside. You recently had a fall in your backyard; although unhurt you were unable to stand up to go into the house and had to wait for Elaine to return from shopping. When she did return, you called loudly to Elaine, asking for assistance. She eventually found you; however, was unable to help you onto your feet. After this event, Elaine worried about you every time she left you alone at home, which was a regular occurrence. As a result, she suggested you move into the local residential care facility, which she volunteered at once a week. You were not happy with that idea; however, felt it would help Elaine, who repeatedly reminded you that it was only a few streets away, therefore she could see you every day. So you moved to the facility – the people are helpful and the meals are acceptable (but not as good as those meals Elaine cooked). Since that time, Elaine and your children visit you regularly, but you often think you need something from home or want to see if Elaine is OK and thus walk home.

Person 2: You are Olivia, a healthcare professional, who regularly sees Michael at the residential aged care facility. You have a relaxed and trusting relationship with Michael. You have been asked to talk to him about his walks to his previous place of residence, to encourage him to stop walking "home". During your discussion, you feel Michael has mild dementia. What do you need to do in response to this observation?

Before using the following scenario, the individual playing the healthcare professional will need to decide on the care they provide for Kerry. It should be relevant to their particular health profession.

Scenario two: The female and the healthcare professional

Person 1: You are 92 years old and your name is Kerry. Despite decreased mobility, you have been living independently in your two-storey home with a cleaner, who does your washing as well as cleaning the house; meals on wheels and nurses to shower you every second day. You used a walker on the second level of your home to access the kitchen, your bedroom, living area, bathroom and toilet. You had a stair lifter to help you manage the stairs in your house and could easily manage the controls for this. You used a wheelchair when taken out of the house. You had a myocardial infarction a few years ago and recently had a fall at home. The geriatrician has told you it is time to move to a facility with permanent staff to monitor your functioning, safety and health. A vacancy at a residential aged care facility close to your eldest son has meant you now live there. While you understand this move, you do not necessarily enjoy it. Your eldest son and often his wife have been taking you out in your wheelchair for lunch on Saturdays and for a weekly evening meal for several years and they continued to do this after your move to the aged care facility. You look forward to these excursions (even in a wheelchair) as they give you something to look forward to and it gives you time away from the facility. You recently had a fall and fractured your neck of femur. After more than a month you have returned to your room in the residential aged care facility. Even though your personal possessions are in the room, you are sure you do not belong in this room and repeatedly mention this. You regularly say you want to go home. You are currently unable to stand, transfer or walk, even with a walker and thus cannot have your regular outings with your son. You have to be moved in your wheelchair to the dining room for your meals. You are unhappy and frequently express the desire to die.

Person 2: You are Raelene, a healthcare professional scheduled to see Kerry to provide relevant care. You are aware of her decreased mobility and her confusion since fracturing her neck of femur and try to accommodate these in your care for her.

3. A Person/s who experiences domestic abuse

(Key words: domestic violence, domestic abuse)

Definition of domestic abuse

Domestic abuse occurs when individuals in a family experience physical or emotional abuse in direct or indirect forms from a member of the same family.

Domestic abuse can take the form of:

- physical aggression, that is, an attack causing physical harm
- emotional manipulation or accusatory blaming

- deprivation of needs by controlling money
- isolation from friends and family
- constant expectation of explanations of behaviours and whereabouts.

Both men and women experience domestic abuse; however, the majority of people experiencing domestic abuse are women. Domestic abuse can occur in heterosexual and homosexual relationships. Another form of abuse is elder abuse. This abuse may occur in families or aged care facilities. Elder abuse can be as undetected and destructive as domestic abuse.

Individuals who experience domestic abuse have many needs. They need first to understand that women or men generally and them specifically do not have to submit to abusive relationships. They will not benefit from discussion about suspected domestic abuse until they establish this understanding. Once individuals accept that they do not have to remain in an abusive relationship, they will require particular assistance from an appropriate service. They will require a safe place to live, appropriate care for any children, financial assistance and child support, a means of becoming financially self-supporting and, possibly, legal protection.

Many people who experience domestic abuse find it difficult to leave because they believe the person will change. The abusive relationship usually includes patterns of alternating i) abuse and ii) expressions of love and promises to change and never abuse again. Fear of the abuser committing suicide, of trying to kill them or hurting the children, or fear of being alone, may stop a person from leaving an abusive relationship. If they do actually leave the relationship, they require ongoing counselling to overcome the erosion to their self-image, typically resulting from an abusive relationship.

Behaviours related to being a Person/s who experiences domestic abuse

A Person who experiences domestic abuse might:

- always act to satisfy the people around them, especially their partners
- accept any abusive or violent behaviour they experience
- avoid mentioning their experiences, regardless of the associated depth of emotion
- find it difficult to make decisions
- be passive in relationships and not mention their own needs
- show behaviour that is not assertive or acknowledging of their needs
- always take the blame when things do not go according to plan
- stay in an abusive relationship because of fear for the children or fear of being alone
- always be looking at the time – not wanting to be late or away too long
- blame themselves for having provoked the abuse.

Possible emotions a Person/s who experiences domestic abuse might experience

A Person who experiences domestic abuse might experience emotions related to:

- fear
- uncertainty
- poor self-esteem
- feeling deserving of the abuse
- anger
- guilt
- mistrust of men and/or women

- anxiety
- feeling unlovable
- insecurity
- depression
- isolation
- denial of the problem
- ambivalence.

Possible reasons for these emotions

People experiencing domestic abuse may experience these emotions because of:

- negative self-talk
- feeling that they deserve abuse
- their partner using non-verbal behaviour to control
- their partner often threatening to harm
- their partner constantly "putting them down"
- their partner not allowing access to their money
- their partner not allowing them to do paid work
- their partner stating they are not a good parent
- their partner controlling who they see and what they do
- their partner destroying their possessions
- their partner saying they deserve the abuse
- their partner threatening suicide
- their partner threatening to hurt the children.

Principles for effective communication with a Person/s who experiences domestic abuse

When communicating with a Person experiencing domestic abuse, it is important to:

- be reliable and worthy of trust
- create a safe place
- confront inappropriate beliefs
- listen actively
- observe their non-verbal communication
- validate their emotions, not their situation
- provide clear information related to all possible interventions.

Strategies for communicating with a Person/s who experiences domestic abuse

- Build rapport – this is essential.
- Be careful with touch.
- Deal with the specific issues.
- Affirm their strengths.
- Communicate to externalise the problems.
- Set achievable goals.
- Use same-gender healthcare professionals.
- Refer to appropriate services.
- Avoid criticism of their skills.

Small Group Discussion

Remember the principles of effective communication and Person/Family-centred Care. You may need to consider the requirements for mandatory communications (see Chapter 19).

Scenario one: The male

Jan loves wine and often drinks a bottle of wine over lunch and also with the evening meal. She is a friendly person, whose partner, Greg, gives her everything she wants to keep her happy and away from alcohol. She often screams and swears at Greg and even chases and hits him with whatever she can find at the time. Greg comes in for regular check-ups and has just come in for treatment. He has a broken right arm and states he broke his arm falling off a ladder more than a month ago. The next time Greg comes in he has a black eye and a hand-shaped bruise on his now-healed broken arm. He states he ran into a door, but has no answer when asked about the shape of the bruise on his arm. He quickly covers it with his sleeve.

- How should you relate?
- What should you say?
- Do your goals change?

Scenario two: The female

Alicia lives in a caravan (trailer) park with her three children and husband, who is a labourer at the local ship-building yard. He is often tired and angry when he returns from work. He expects everything exactly as he wants it when he arrives home and regularly hits Alicia if things are not as he wants. She has presented to your health service with a back injury and has bruises on her back that suggest she was hit. She maintains she hurt her back from a fall, but does not remember the details. You suspect domestic abuse.

- How should you relate?
- What are the major aims of relating?
- What do you wish to communicate?

Group discussion

As a large group, share the main points discussed by each small group about these scenarios. Consider various strategies that may increase the effectiveness of the communication in a similar situation. Decide how a healthcare professional should act in similar situations.

Healthcare professionals who suspect domestic abuse of adults or children have a duty of care to report this suspicion. It can be beneficial to discuss any suspicion with a more senior or experienced healthcare professional, in order to plan strategies for relating and the requirement to report. The realities of domestic abuse are complex and the Person experiencing the abuse may believe they deserve the abuse. They may believe that removing themselves would have far worse consequences than remaining in the relationship. Counselling to achieve skills in assertiveness may assist, although assertiveness may simply escalate the levels of violence. Communicating with people who experience domestic abuse is challenging. It requires understanding and affirmation of the Person/s to achieve Person/Family-centred Care, effective communication and appropriate outcomes.

4. A Person/s who is homeless

(Key words: homeless, homelessness, excluded, loss)

Definition of a Person/s who is homeless

A homeless Person/s is someone who, for various reasons, has no regular place to live or stay. They may live "on the street" or "lounge surf"/"lounge hop" or sometimes sleep on all-night trains, moving from one location to another, and then returning to the original location.

Individuals most susceptible to being homeless

These are some possible reasons, but there may be many other reasons for homelessness.

- Those with limited income and many financial commitments
- Those who are experiencing relationship struggles
- Those who are told to leave a family or relationship for various reasons
- Those who have to relocate for work reasons and are unable to find somewhere appropriate and permanent to live.

Possible behaviours related to being a Person/s who is experiencing homelessness

- Drug addictive behaviours
- Act with anger
- Fail to respond to anyone unknown to them
- Tendency to avoid relating to unknown people
- May lack interest in previously gratifying activities
- May act to emotionally protect themselves.

Possible emotions a Person/s who is homeless might experience

- Rejection
- Confusion and sometimes disbelief about the cause
- Feelings of loss – these will typically include loss of control of their situation
- Isolation and loneliness, despite friends attempting to provide support
- Feelings of anxiety, grief and fear (this may be overwhelming)
- Frustration
- Regret
- Feelings of desperation, resulting in either anger or hopelessness
- Denial of the problem.

Possible reasons for these emotions

- Isolation from family
- Regret for their behaviour relating to their homelessness
- Loss of hope for change and sometimes loss of previously important beliefs
- Depression
- Fear and anxiety about the future
- Insomnia and sometimes tachycardia
- Separation from previously significant people
- Changes in eating habits.

Principles for effective communication with a Person/s who is homeless

When communicating with a Person/s experiencing homelessness, it is important to:

- make introductions – consider how to develop a trusting therapeutic relationship
- demonstrate empathy and sensitivity, both verbally and non-verbally
- listen actively, while observing and clarifying all non-verbal messages
- respond patiently while providing honest and compassionate comfort
- validate their feelings
- answer any questions clearly and honestly
- provide clear and well-organised information about the health service and any services or organisations that will provide assistance and support.

Strategies for communicating with a Person/s who is experiencing homelessness

These may depend on the emotional and cognitive state of the Person/s and on the reason for their homelessness. Therefore, there may be additional, relevant strategies.

- Do not avoid the issues – be prepared to respond to their obvious and stated needs.
- Ask relevant questions to achieve mutual understanding of their current status.
- Be prepared to respond to their non-verbal behaviours– they may send a different message to their words.
- When appropriate, after clarification, validate their non-verbal messages.
- If appropriate, confront their fears and feelings.
- If agreeable to the Person, refer them to other appropriate healthcare professionals or organisations to manage their needs and/or condition.

Remember the principles of effective communication and Person/Family-centred Care.

Scenario one: The male and the healthcare professional

Person 1: You are a young man, named John. You are in the third year of an engineering degree. While you have been doing well in your studies, you have found the expectations of your parents and lecturers stressful and when someone suggested using something to make you feel better, you began using heroin. The now constant need to have some heroin and the expense of it has meant you have been stealing money to buy the drug. Your parents have been paying your university fees for you; however, you have not been regularly attending this semester and have failed three out of four of your courses. Your parents have been noticing some changes in you, especially with your results from the semester. They then learn about your drug addiction and about you stealing money to buy the drugs. They are very disappointed and angry, as they were sure you could do well and enjoy being an engineer. They tell you to leave home as they do not want to see you again. They change the locks to the home, instructing the other family members not to allow you to come onto the property or enter the house.

You do not have the money to find somewhere else to live, and most of your uni friends have stopped relating to you since you began using heroin. You meet a few other addicts who are also homeless. They show you where you can sleep and when it is cold, how to keep warm. They also show you where you can get free food.

One evening you consumed more heroin than usual, collapsing into unconsciousness as a result. The other people with you tried to wake you up as the police were nearby. When they could not wake you, they left you in the park with some cover. The police found you and called an ambulance because you were unconscious and had obviously been using drugs.

You have now been in hospital for a few days. At least it is somewhere warm to sleep and there is regular food. The difficulty is that your addiction mandates the need for heroin. You are beginning to be more aggressive than previously and increasingly irritable.

Person 2: You are the healthcare professional who has been asked to introduce John to a group for individuals who have a drug addiction and who are attempting to stop using addictive drugs. It has been noted that John had multiple needle marks on his body, evidence of heroin in his blood upon admission, and that it took some time for him to begin relating comfortably to staff. You are unsure if he has considered stopping the use of addictive drugs and will need to be careful to ensure all components of Person/Family-centred Care.

Scenario two: The female and the healthcare professional

Person 1: Your name is Melissa. You have experienced a marriage break-up because your ex has decided he prefers someone else. As your ex owns the home (it was bequeathed to him when his parents died and the Title Deed is in his name), you have nowhere to stay (your family members live in another state). You did not ever add your name to the Deed, as at the time your ex did not want to and you did not feel there was any need to do this. However, now you realise you should have insisted. You do own your car, so that means you have been able to continue working, using public transport would take over an hour to get to work. Fortunately your workplace has showers and towels, so if necessary you can shower every day. It is now 6 months since you became homeless and despite your income, you do have not the energy or clarity of mind to find somewhere to live. This is especially so as you loved your house and the location by the beach (you cannot afford anything in such a location). However, sleeping in your small car is not easy. A few of your friends have had you stay with them – usually sleeping on their lounge as they do not always have a spare room with a bed. You are experiencing what feels like depression and are having difficulty sleeping or eating. You have been losing weight. Some of your friends have noticed this and one has suggested you see someone to help you manage your “new” everyday life. You go to the local hospital to see if there is something that can be done that does not cost too much money, as your ex has removed your name from your previous healthcare fund and you are currently unable to afford to join a new fund. Your current Medicare card may not work as it has the name of your ex on it. You did not think to apply for a new one. You decide to go to the hospital. You do not feel able to manage the feelings related to seeing your GP (who you have not seen since your separation), as they previously always saw you with your ex.

Person 2: You are assessing a 27-year-old woman, who appears to have anorexia, as she is very thin. She also seems to have limited positive affect. The form she completed indicates she is having trouble sleeping at night, while finding eating difficult. You suspect there are many reasons for her current state. However, you realise it will be important to identify the reasons for her visit to the hospital today.

5. A Person/s who speaks a different language to the healthcare professional

(Key words: speaker of languages other than English [LOTE], non-native speaker [NNS], non-English-speaking background [NESB])

Definition of a Person/s who speaks a different language to the healthcare professional

A Person/s who speaks a different language to the healthcare professional is someone who is *unable* to communicate verbally or in written form in the language of the healthcare professional.

Behaviours related to being a Person/s who speaks a different language to the healthcare professional

A Person who speaks a different language to the healthcare professional might:

- show apparently aggressive non-verbal behaviours
- demonstrate apparent comprehension, even when they do not understand
- attempt to solve problems alone
- avoid asking for assistance because of embarrassment
- sit quietly and avoid indicating they do not understand
- expect the services to be the same as they are in their own culture.

Possible emotions a Person/s who speaks a different language to the healthcare professional might experience

A Person who speaks a different language to the healthcare professional might experience emotions related to:

- fear about communicating in another language
- confusion and vulnerability, even though they normally understand conversational English
- inadequacy because they understand general English, but not the English of the healthcare professional
- frustration because of trying to understand, but not being sure that they do.

Possible reasons for these emotions

A Person who speaks a different language to the healthcare professional may experience these emotions because of:

- regular breakdowns in communication
- apparently aggressive non-verbal behaviours from those around them
- regular misunderstandings
- differences in cultural and social expectations
- age and gender differences
- cultural differences.

Principles for effective communication with a Person/s who speaks a different language to the healthcare professional

When communicating with a Person who speaks a different language to the healthcare professional it is important to:

- demonstrate empathy
- respect cultural differences
- establish rapport to build a therapeutic relationship
- negotiate meaning to achieve mutual understanding
- constantly clarify the understanding of the Person
- avoid making assumptions
- consider the potential meaning of the non-verbal behaviours of the Person – do not assume the non-verbal behaviours have the same meaning in both cultures.

Strategies for communicating with a Person/s who speaks a different language to the healthcare professional

- Use an interpreter – remember to speak to the Person not the interpreter (see Chapter 16).
- Ask questions about what is appropriate in their culture. You could ask the interpreter or family members who are fluent in your language.
- Avoid using non-verbal or visual cues unless you are certain of their meaning.
- Explain how and why things are done in this health service.
- Wherever possible, avoid using family members or friends to interpret.
- Wherever possible, use a same-gender healthcare professional.
- Wherever possible, provide all information in translated written form, ensuring the translation is the correct form of the language of the Person.
- Have a known person introduce any new healthcare professionals that will assist the Person.
- Learn a few simple words and phrases of the language of the Person (e.g. *hello, thank you, please, goodbye, how are you?*)
- Avoid assuming they understand.
- Avoid assuming that the healthcare professional understands.
- Have a sense of humour.

Remember the principles of effective communication and Person/Family-centred Care. Before acting the roles, you may wish to decide what type of assistance Person 1 requires. If it is not possible to role-play these scenarios, consider and explore the possible responses and communication strategies that will achieve effective communication and Person/Family-centred Care.

Scenario one: The male and the healthcare professional

Person 1: Your name is Ahmed and you are a 45-year-old Middle-Eastern man who requires assistance from a health service. You speak very limited English and feel insecure about this unfamiliar place. Although you do not usually speak to unknown women, especially in public places, you spoke to a woman who was wearing a uniform. You hoped she might speak

Arabic and you tried to speak to her. She seemed confused when she looked at you, but obviously did not understand Arabic.

Person 2: You must assess and devise some goals for a new Person seeking assistance. He is a Muslim man, who you think appears arrogant and rude. You observed him speak to the female cleaner, who, although she does not speak fluent English, does not speak Arabic either. She appeared shocked and confused, and you assume the man was rude to her. However, you are unsure because you may be misinterpreting his non-verbal behaviours or his tone of voice.

Scenario two: The female and the healthcare professional

Person 1: Your name is Kyoko and you are a 20-year-old woman from Japan. You have been studying English and have basic conversational skills. You are planning to become a healthcare professional when you complete your English studies. You have sprained your ankle and would prefer to see the healthcare professionals in Japan, but you will not be in Japan for another 10 months, so you are sitting quietly in a health service waiting room. You remember the first time you came to this service – you were very embarrassed and distressed that a young male healthcare professional assessed you. Although he explained everything, your English skills were not proficient enough to understand all the words. You remember crying very quietly. The young man, Matt, did not notice until you were leaving, when a woman waiting asked Matt what he had done because you were crying. When he noticed, he seemed to be concerned; maybe he thought he had physically hurt you.

The next time you came he introduced a female healthcare professional and an interpreter. You were able to apologise for crying and explain that you would feel more comfortable with a female healthcare professional assisting you, if possible. During that visit, you received answers to all your questions. Matt was able to explain everything he did the last time, explaining what would happen next time. Since then, you have been seeing Rochelle and she has been helping you. You now feel comfortable going regularly to see Rochelle for healthcare.

Person 2: You are Matt. Kyoko is a lovely young lady who has been receiving assistance for several weeks. The beginning was difficult, but using an interpreter really helped for her second visit. Having Rochelle work with her also made a difference. However, today Rochelle is away and you have to see Kyoko. You are concerned and enter the waiting area with a little trepidation.

Group discussion

As a large group discuss the observations, emotions and outcomes of the role-plays. Suggest possible alternative strategies that may increase the effectiveness of the communication in a similar situation.

Glossary

Aboriginal or Torres Strait Islander peoples The original inhabitants of the country of Australia; a person of Aboriginal or Torres Strait Islander descent who identifies as an Aboriginal or Torres Strait Islander and is accepted as such by the community in which they live.

Active listening Listening that responds to the verbal and non-verbal messages to indicate interest and acceptance. It enables the healthcare professional to assist, enjoy, influence, observe and understand.

Advocacy Presenting and supporting the needs and perspectives of all relevant Person/s to relevant healthcare professionals.

Aggressive communication Communication in which perceptions, opinions and feelings are expressed in a manner that intimidates or attacks the other communicating individual/s.

Alternative communication Non-verbal forms of communication to replace the spoken word, for example, an electronic device using visual communication software.

Ambiguity A situation in which something can be understood in more than one way and initially the intended meaning is not clear.

Assertive communication Communication in which perceptions, ideas or opinions are expressed in a manner that respects the worth and rights of others to have and express perceptions, ideas or opinions, regardless of differences.

Assumption To presume or believe something that may or may not be correct about someone, something or a particular event.

Attitudes Unconscious values and beliefs.

Augmentative and alternative communication (AAC) Systems that allow non-verbal methods of communication, including visual and computer-assisted devices.

Augmentative communication Non-verbal forms of communication that highlight the spoken word through simultaneous gestures, facial expressions, signs, pictures and keyword signing.

Background The environment in which a person grows, matures, and develops their values and beliefs.

Barrier Anything that stops or restricts something from happening; can restrict function and/or participation in a particular area.

Beliefs Principles or doctrines that a person or group considers true.

Benefits Has value and advantages.

Bias An unfair preference or dislike of someone or something.

Body language Non-verbal communication that includes gesture, facial expression, posture, eye contact, gait and clothing.

Care Particular treatment and attention.

Case conference Regular meetings with all team members to discuss Person/s status and ongoing care.

Challenges Various obstacles requiring consideration.
Chronic condition Diagnosis that is long-lasting with constant or recurring symptoms.
Clan A group of families related through a common ancestor or through marriage.
Clarify To make something clear, either by asking questions to ensure understanding or by explaining any unclear information.
Cliché A phrase or statement that is overused and does not communicate care or understanding.
Closure Provides an effective and satisfying end to individual sessions, overall interventions and in particular circumstances, end of life.
Codes of conduct or behaviour Expectations and rules applied to healthcare professionals by government, registration bodies, the relevant profession and particular healthcare services. These expectations and rules define the expected conduct or behaviour of every healthcare professional.
Cognition The process of perceiving, processing, storing and retrieving information, as well as thinking and planning with intuitive thought and perception.
Collaboration Working together in a cooperative relationship.
Collaborative partnership A partnership that requires the contribution of each person to achieve a satisfactory and appropriate outcome.
Comforting The process used by the healthcare professional to ensure the Person seeking assistance feels encouraged, affirmed and empowered to continue meeting the daily challenges in their life.
Complement Working together to ensure holistic care for the Person/s.
Complementary and alternative medicine (CAM) Treatment that does not usually conform to "traditional" medicine or the medical model.
Complexity Complicated, sometimes convoluted and difficult.
Comprehensive care Care that considers all aspects of the Person/s and their needs.
Computer-mediated communication (CMC) Electronic forms of communication.
Conclusions Ending or concluding interactions and/or interventions to ensure satisfactory completion of interactions and thus effective communication.
Confidentiality Keeping information within a particular context; involves keeping information private.
Conflict A struggle or clash between two different or opposite ideas, thoughts, people or principles; can be physical, psychological, social or spiritual.
Confronting The act of challenging and sometimes disagreeing with inappropriate attitudes and beliefs in order to clarify and examine these attitudes and beliefs and ultimately change them. It is neither intimidating nor judgemental.
Consent To give permission or approval for something to happen, usually in writing.
Context Surrounding factors that affect meaning; can be situational and/or environmental.
Continuity of care To ensure enduring and connected treatment and attention.
Control The ability to manage or direct the events in life.
Critical reflective practice Involves reflection, including consideration of skills, feelings, beliefs and outcomes of relevant healthcare to identify areas of strength and those requiring improvement when providing healthcare assistance to relevant Person/s.
Cross-cultural communication Occurs when people from different cultures interact with the intention of reaching mutual understanding.
Cultural assumptions Opinions about patterns of behaving, beliefs and values that are culturally determined.

Cultural competence To understand the customs, beliefs, values and behaviours of a particular culture.
Cultural identity Characteristics that a person recognises as belonging uniquely to their own culture.
Cultural norms Standard patterns of behaviour that are considered normal in a particular culture.
Cultural safety (security) Achieved through practice that respects, supports and empowers the cultural identity and wellbeing of an individual. It allows the Person seeking assistance some control over or contribution to their health interventions and outcomes.
Cultural sensitivity Achieved through practice that accommodates the cultural identity, needs and practices of different cultures.
Culturally unsafe communication Communication that diminishes, demeans or disempowers the cultural identity and wellbeing of an individual.
Culture of disease or ill-health Individuals with illness experience adjustment to their beliefs, values and daily habits or "ways of doing".
Culture Traditions and patterns of behaviour that develop in a particular group because of the values and beliefs of that group. It influences every aspect of life.
Customs Actions that people from a particular group always perform in particular ways in particular circumstances.
Cyberbullying An intentional attempt to harm or defame an individual using social media – typically targeting an individual who is unable to defend themselves.
Data platforms Electronic databases used to record relevant Person/s information and all interactions.
Defence mechanisms (defences) Adaptive mental mechanisms that assist the individual to continue functioning, despite the presence of uncomfortable emotions, thoughts, information or wishes, by removing them from the conscious mind. A method of managing otherwise unmanageable thoughts and emotions. There are four defences that occur on a continuum: psychotic, immature, neurotic and mature.
Discharge To remove care for Person/s.
Discipline A particular healthcare profession.
Disengagement Process that leads to the disconnection of the individuals in a communicative act. It involves satisfactory completion of an interaction.
Diverse/Diversity Variety of something – cultures, opinions, beliefs, etc.
Dominant/primary personal needs Needs that dominate relationships and may negatively impact on the relationship between a healthcare professional and a Person seeking assistance.
Effective communication All people communicating have clearly understood the exact meaning of every message, regardless of the forms of the message.
Effective cross-cultural communication Involves open, receptive and responsive communication to accommodate differences because of cultural diversity; and challenges relating to variations in communication style in order to achieve mutual understanding.
Effective listening Listening that adapts to the particular individual, their non-verbal cues and the context. Requires active engagement with the Person and their message; a characteristic of a therapeutic relationship.
Effective speaking Requires interest in, enthusiasm for and knowledge about the topic and the "audience", as well as understanding of the effect of non-verbal behaviours upon the words spoken.
Efficacy The ability to produce the necessary and desired results with efficiency and accuracy.

Elder Custodians of cultural laws, ceremonies, practices, traditions and remedies. They are often the key decision-makers providing advice and leadership.
Emotions Feelings that individuals experience because of internal factors causing negative or positive agitation or disturbance.
Empathy The direct, clear and accurate understanding and expression of the emotions of an individual.
Emphasis Stress on a particular word or phrase that may change the meaning.
Empower To give the Person/s seeking assistance a sense of confidence to overcome the challenges they face.
Environment Factors external to the person, which may be physical, emotional, social, cultural or spiritual.
Equality Balance of power in a relationship through shared opportunities and mutual demonstrations of an attitude of acceptance.
Ethical communication Requires knowledge of and commitment to the requirements that result in appropriate communicative behaviour while practising as a healthcare professional.
Ethical dilemma A challenging problem or predicament with moral implications.
Ethical responsibility Protecting information about the people seeking assistance, whether read or heard, or acting in the interests of the Person seeking assistance and in accordance with the appropriate code of ethics or conduct.
Ethnocentric When an individual believes their particular method or way of approaching a situation is superior and indeed the best way.
Explaining To make the meaning of something clear by using words that are easy to understand.
Eye contact Occurs when communicating individuals look directly into the eyes of the other people interacting. Not appropriate in all cultures.
Facial expressions A type of body language in which the face is used to communicate meaning.
Function To perform any activity of choice.
Gestures A type of body language in which meaning is expressed through the use of the arms, hands or fingers.
Health A sound condition of the mind, body, emotions and spirit allowing a person to function and participate in their chosen life activities.
Health outcomes The results of any healthcare.
Healthcare discipline A particular profession dedicated to healthcare.
Healthcare professional An individual who works in a profession directly affecting the health of the people they assist while providing healthcare.
Holistic care Considers all aspects of the Person and their context; it allows the Person to have an active role in their healing.
Holistic communication Requires a willingness to communicate about contexts, experiences, thoughts, emotions, needs and desires; requires understanding of the value and uniqueness of each individual.
Honesty A characteristic that results in a sincere disposition and respectable conduct.
Humour The ability to see that something is funny. When an error has been made, the ability to laugh at oneself.
Ideal healthcare professional An excellent example of a healthcare professional because of exemplary thoughts, patterns, attitudes, values and behaviour.
Indigenous community Local Aboriginal or Torres Strait Islander peoples or Māori, or people from their place of birth.

Indigenous Peoples or **First Nations Peoples** Those who inhabited a country or region before another group came and settled the country or region as though it belonged to the newcomers.
Informed consent To give written permission or consent on the basis of real knowledge and understanding of an event or procedure.
Informing Communicating information or knowledge to the Person seeking assistance.
Instructing Teaching someone how to do something.
Integrated Different perspectives and skills of multiple healthcare professions included in the care of the Person/s.
Interdisciplinary Different health disciplines working together.
Interpersonal Interactive relationships with other people.
Interpreter Someone who translates orally or visually what is said in one language into another language to facilitate communication.
Interpreting Translating the meaning of an utterance, regardless of the word/sound spoken.
Interprofessional Activities for and interactions between individuals from different professions.
Intervention Action taken by the healthcare professional after collaboration with the Person to positively change something in the life of the Person.
Introducing oneself Presenting oneself, the role, the environment, the procedure, the people in the environment and their role with the aim of making the Person seeking assistance aware of the healthcare professional and the role of the healthcare professional in that healthcare service.
Jargon Words used in a particular context or profession which gives them specific meaning known only to those familiar with the context or profession.
Journal A helpful learning tool in which to record answers to questions and thoughts about self and reactions; can promote learning about self.
Judgement An opinion of someone based on personal values and beliefs; may not always be accurate or informed, with potential to negatively affect communication.
Kinship group People related by blood or marriage.
Large culture A culture with a large membership, or a nation.
Learning styles Styles of learning that best suit an individual.
Listening barriers Habits that limit the ability to listen, process, remember and respond appropriately to a spoken message.
Mainstream healthcare systems Services that are provided by and for the dominant cultural group, whether owned by the government or a non-government body.
Māori The people who were the first inhabitants of New Zealand.
Misunderstanding A failure to negotiate meaning; also known as miscommunication.
Model Assists in guiding healthcare.
Multidisciplinary A combination of different disciplines or healthcare professions.
Mutual respect Reciprocated or shared value and appreciation of all individuals relating in healthcare.
Mutual understanding All the people communicating understand all the factors contributing to the meaning of the message.
Nation A community of people living in a defined area and who share a common origin, culture, traditions and language.
National Boards Country-wide governing bodies of each healthcare profession.
Nationality The characteristics that an individual recognises as unique to their nation.
Non-judgemental Avoiding forming an opinion in order to ensure positive relations with acceptance regardless of differences between the people communicating.

Non-verbal communication Communication without spoken words.
Non-verbal messages Messages sent using body language or suprasegmentals of the voice.
Online Typically electronic or on-screen communication.
Open communication Accepting and accommodating differences and needs while communicating.
Over-identification Occurs when the healthcare professional introduces a similar situation or experience to the Person seeking assistance.
Palliative Relating to life limiting or end-of-life illnesses.
Paralinguistic features of the voice (paralanguage) Particular vocal effects that change meaning, including emphasis, timely pauses, tone, laughing, whining, moaning and other non-verbal sounds.
Participation Active involvement in everyday activities of choice.
Passive communication Lack of expression of perceptions, ideas or opinions because the Person feels they do not have the right or value to express themselves in that situation.
Passive-aggressive Involves fluctuating between aggressive behaviour or responses and passive (not engaged or listening) behaviour or responses depending on the context and the original event causing the response.
Pauses When the communicating individuals do not produce words or sounds, providing opportunity for thought and processing.
Perfectionism Always being as accurate as possible (right); reaching the highest standard in actions and words.
Person/Family-centred Care (P-cC) The needs and wishes of the family or Person/s and or the family are the centre of the goals and elements of their healthcare.
Person/s Any Person/s to whom the healthcare professional relates while fulfilling their role as a healthcare provider. May include colleagues, other workers in the healthcare service, the Person seeking assistance and their family and friends.
Personal space A comfortable distance between people when communicating or moving past each other; usually determined by particular cultures; can vary according to cultural perceptions.
Personality preferences Suggests particular preferred methods of communicating and of managing information. There are various theories suggesting personality types and related preferences.
Physical The aspect of the Person that relates to the external and internal parts of the body.
Pitch Frequency of sound, which makes the voice sound low or high.
Policy A strategy or plan guiding actions.
Prejudice A preformed opinion often of a negative kind, based on ignorance, irrational feelings, and uninformed or inaccurate stereotypes.
Procedural guidelines The practical and/or bureaucratic instructions, plans and/or strategies.
Procedures The actions or techniques used to provide appropriate healthcare.
Professional writing style This style of writing uses formal expression and words, particular types of verbs, accurate grammar, and simple sentence structure to produce a clear, succinct, cohesive and coherent document. It avoids using apostrophes and unexplained acronyms.
Prosodic features of the voice The vocal effects including volume, pitch, speed and rate of speech creating the unique rhythm of a language.
Psychological aspect of the individual A Person's mental and emotional processes.
Rapport A connection between two people based on trust and awareness of a common goal.

Records (medical) Documentation into the individual file of the Person/s about their current status, any provided interventions, and the results of these interventions, from the particular healthcare professional making the entry. Each entry will occur after the most recent intervention or interaction with the Person/s. These records are typically electronic.
Reflection Examination of how the reactions of the self affect interactions; using the experience and knowledge of the self, as well as theory to increase self-awareness and understand the causes of those reactions.
Reflective The revisiting of uncomfortable events in order to understand them and change behaviour in similar situations in the future.
Reflexive Considering how the self affects and is affected by particular events in order to evaluate and critique the self; facilitates internal change to benefit relationships with people seeking assistance.
Registration bodies The organisations with whom all healthcare professionals must enrol.
Remote communication Interactions that are not typically face-to-face.
Requirements The necessary actions.
Respect Unconditional positive regard for self and others regardless of weaknesses or failures, position or status, beliefs and/or values, and material possessions or socioeconomic level. It assumes all human beings have innate worth and value.
Role The expected function of an individual given their position or membership in society and the expected behaviour of that position.
Self-awareness Awareness of the beliefs, values, thoughts, inadequacies and fears affecting and driving thoughts and responses of the healthcare professional during interactions.
Self-disclosure Sharing the experiences and feelings of the healthcare professional.
Self-efficacy Valuing the worth, usefulness, abilities, effectiveness of the skills of the healthcare professional.
Sentence structure In professional writing, sentence structure is simple, requiring a verb to connect the beginning of the sentence with the end of the sentence.
Sequential interpretation The interpreter translates a small portion of the information and then waits for the next piece of information before they interpret further.
Sexual Relating to reproductive organs and the responsibilities associated with the use of those organs; may also refer to sexual preference.
Silence Absence of speaking or making any sound.
Simultaneous interpretation The interpreter interprets at the same time as the healthcare professional presents the information.
Small culture A culture with a small membership.
Social media Communicating using an electronic form of communication. It allows communication with many people simultaneously in many locations without seeing any of the receivers of the messages.
Social The aspect of a Person that relates to others as an individual or a group.
Spiritual The aspect of a Person that gives meaning to self, life and the universe. It determines the beliefs and values motivating and sustaining the Person.
Status The relative "importance" of someone in a particular group or in society.
Stereotype An oversimplified idea or image of an individual or group that may be incorrect.
Suprasegmentals Elements of the voice (not words or body language) that affect the meaning of messages. There are two types: prosodic and paralinguistic features.
Team Group of people working together to achieve similar goals.

Teamwork Cooperating and collaborating with all members of the group assisting the Person/s.
Telecommunication or **Telehealth** The use of technology to provide healthcare, while the healthcare professional is not in the room with the Person.
Therapeutic relationship A collaborative relationship between the healthcare professional and the Person/s to fulfil their needs, thereby empowering the Person/s to overcome any challenges.
Tone of the voice Indicates the feelings, attitudes or thoughts of an individual about the particular topic.
Touch A non-verbal way of physically connecting with a Person by using a part of the body, usually a hand, to connect with a part of their body.
Transliteration The exact translation of each word/sound spoken regardless of meaning; these interpretations often have limited meaning.
Trust Confidence in and reliance upon the healthcare professional to provide quality service always in the best interests of the Person seeking assistance.
Validation The healthcare professional confirms the existence of particular situations or emotions, whether or not they agree, indicating that the emotional response is understandable.
Values The measure of worth, importance or usefulness of something or someone.
Verify A healthcare professional explores their perceptions of the Person/s to establish the truthfulness of the perceptions and the appropriateness of the emotions.
Visual Anything that can be seen with the eye.
Volume of a voice Whether the voice is loud or soft. Volume can communicate particular meaning.
Vulnerable Feeling emotionally insecure and unsure about the possibility of experiencing harm.
Wellbeing A sense of feeling comfortable and safe.
Whole Person A dynamic system in which every aspect of the individual affects and interacts with the other aspects simultaneously. It consists of five fundamental aspects: the physical; the emotional, including the sexual aspect; the cognitive; the social; and the spiritual.
Workplace culture The expectations, values and principles governing the behaviour of each team member in the employing organisation.
Worth The value of someone – innate and inbuilt in all human beings.

Index

B

C

D

E

F

M

N

O

P

T